ESSENTIALS OF VETERINARY
MICROBIOLOGY

ESSENTIALS OF VETERINARY
MICROBIOLOGY

ESSENTIALS OF VETERINARY MICROBIOLOGY

G. R. Carter, D.V.M., M.S., D.V.Sc.
Department of Pathobiology
Virginia-Maryland Regional College of Veterinary Medicine
Virginia Polytechnic Institute and State University
Blacksburg, Virginia

M. M. Chengappa, B.V.Sc., M.S., Ph.D.
Department of Pathology and Microbiology
College of Veterinary Medicine
Kansas State University
Manhattan, Kansas

A. W. Roberts, B.S., M.S.
Athens Diagnostic Laboratory
College of Veterinary Medicine
University of Georgia
Athens, Georgia

With Chapters By

G. William Claus, B.S., Ph.D.
Microbiology Section
Department of Biology
College of Arts and Sciences
Virginia Polytechnic Institute and State University
Blacksburg, Virginia

Yasuko Rikihisa, M.S., Ph.D.
Department of Veterinary Pathobiology
College of Veterinary Medicine
The Ohio State University
Columbus, Ohio

FIFTH EDITION

A Lea & Febiger Book

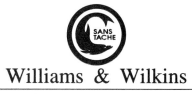

Williams & Wilkins

BALTIMORE • PHILADELPHIA • HONG KONG
LONDON • MUNICH • SYDNEY • TOKYO

A WAVERLY COMPANY
1995

Executive Editor: Carroll Cann
Developmental Editor: Susan Hunsberger
Production Manager: Laurie Forsyth
Project Editor: Rebecca Krumm

Third Edition 1986
Carter, G. R. (Gordon R.)
    Essentials of veterinary microbiology/G.R. Carter,
M.M. Chengappa, and A.W. Roberts, with chapters by G.
William Claus, Yasuko Rikihisa.—5th ed.
        p. cm.
    Rev. ed. of: Essentials of veterinary bacteriology and
mycology. 4th ed. 1991.
    Includes bibliographical references and index.
    ISBN 0-683-01473-0
    1. Veterinary bacteriology. 2. Veterinary mycology.
3. Veterinary virology. I. Chengappa, M. M. II. Roberts, A.
Wayne. III. Carter, G.R. (Gordon R.). Essentials of
veterinary bacteriology and mycology. IV. Title.
SF780.3.C37 1994
636.089′601—dc20   94-29049
                                                         CIP
                                          94 95 96 97 98
                              1 2 3 4 5 6 7 8 9 10

PREFACE

This edition has been expanded by the addition of a comprehensive section on virology. This section is the revision of an earlier book, *Essentials of Veterinary Virology.* Following the chapters dealing with introductory virology, the various virus diseases are grouped according to the host and organ system affected. This orientation, rather than the taxonomic, was thought to have practical advantages for students. The taxonomic approach is used in the sections of the book that cover bacteria and fungi, however, because these organisms are less host- and organ-system-specific than are viruses.

We have attempted to provide the latest information on all facets of the microbial pathogens of animals of veterinary interest. As in earlier editions, a special effort has been made to emphasize practical applications. The book is primarily directed to undergraduate veterinary students.

Veterinary microbiology is traditionally taught by means of lectures and laboratory exercises. This text provides the more important facts of introductory and pathogenic microbiology for the lecture portion. In the interest of economy the number of illustrations has been kept to a minimum. If laboratory exercises are adequate, students will have an opportunity to observe and study the microscopic and cultural characteristics of important microorganisms.

We have found that the teaching of the pathogenic portion of the course can be made more interesting and relevant to veterinary practice by the use of abbreviated case reports and descriptions of outbreaks of infectious disease. These can be used as the principal vehicle for conveying the lecture material or employed on occasion to stimulate interest.

A number of references are listed at the end of each chapter for students interested in additional information and greater depth in a particular topic. A glossary has been added mainly for those students who have not had courses in immunology and pathology. Only terms not explained in the text are included.

We would like to express our appreciation to the Virginia-Maryland Regional College of Veterinary Medicine, the Department of Pathology and Microbiology of the College of Veterinary Medicine, Kansas State University, and the Athens Diagnostic Laboratory of the College of Veterinary Medicine, University of Georgia for providing excellent general support. We wish to express our thanks to the following: Dr. W.L. Chapman (University of Georgia), for the use of his updated pathology lecture notes on viral diseases of laboratory animals; Ms. DeLynda Davis, for the virology illustrations; and Ms. Louri Roberts and Ms. DeLynda Davis, for typing the virology portion. With regard to the bacteriology and mycology portion of the book, we are indebted to Ms. Lori Page-Willyard and Ms. Susan Delap and staff for their excellent secretarial support. We would also like to express our appreciation to our many friends and colleagues for their support, advice, and constructive criticisms. The help of Williams & Wilkins, formerly Lea & Febiger, and their editorial staff in the preparation of the final manuscript is gratefully acknowledged.

We are also much indebted to Professors G. William Claus and Yasuko Rikihisa for their excellent chapters.

Blacksburg, Virginia   G.R. Carter
Manhattan, Kansas   M.M. Chengappa
Athens, Georgia   A.W. Roberts

CONTENTS

BACTERIOLOGY AND MYCOLOGY
G.R. Carter and M.M. Chengappa

I INTRODUCTORY BACTERIOLOGY AND MYCOLOGY

II BACTERIA

III FUNGI

VIROLOGY
A.W. Roberts

IV INTRODUCTORY VIROLOGY

V SURVEY OF VIRAL INFECTIONS

Part I

INTRODUCTORY BACTERIOLOGY AND MYCOLOGY

1

Classification and Morphology of Bacteria and Fungi

Yasuko Rikihisa

PROCARYOTES AND EUCARYOTES

In terms of intracellular organization, the cells of all living things are either *eucaryotes* or *procaryotes* (Fig. 1–1). The eucaryotic cells have a membrane-bound nucleus (i.e., a true nucleus), whereas in the procaryotic cells nuclear material is not enveloped by a membrane. Bacterial cells are procaryotes and cells of all other living organisms are eucaryotes. *Protists* are undifferentiated unicellular organisms that do not form specialized tissues and organ systems as do higher plants and animals. The protists are divided into eucaryotic (higher)

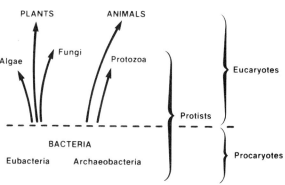

Figure 1–1. Relationships of living organisms.

and procaryotic (lower) protists. Eucaryotic protists are divided into algae, fungi, and protozoa. *Algae* have chlorophyll and cell walls. *Fungi* have cell walls but lack chlorophyll. *Protozoa* have neither chlorophyll nor cell walls.

BACTERIA

The bacteria, or procaryotes, are single-celled organisms that are distinguished from the eucaryotic organisms by the characteristics listed in Table 1–1.

In volume 1 of *Bergey's Manual of Systematic Bacteriology,* published in 1984, the kingdom *Procaryotae* is proposed to contain four divisions:

I. Gracilicutes (*gracilis.* [L.] thin) have a gram-negative type cell wall.

II. Firmicutes (*firmus.* [L.] strong) have a gram-positive type cell wall.

III. Tenericutes (*tener.* [L.] soft) lack a cell wall and are commonly called the mycoplasmas.

IV. Mendosicutes (*mendosus.* [L.] having faults) are members of *Archaeobacteria* such as methanogens, halophiles, and thermoacidophiles, which live in somewhat extreme environments. Archaeobacteria are so called because of their apparent primi-

Table 1–1. *Differences Between Procaryotic and Eucaryotic Cells*

Characteristics	Procaryotic Cells	Eucaryotic Cells
Nucleoplasm bounded by a membrane	–	+
Nucleolus	–	+
Chromosome number	1	>1
Reproduction	asexual	sexual or asexual
Mitotic nuclear division	–	+
D-amino acids, diaminopimelic acid, and muramic acid	+*	–
Cytoplasmic ribosomes	70S	80S
Endoplasmic reticulum	–	+
Mitochondria	–	+
Chloroplasts	–	+†
Golgi apparatus	–	+
Cytoplasmic streaming	–	+
Cytoplasmic membrane	sterols generally absent	sterols present
Organelles with nonunit membrane	+	–

* Except for mycoplasmas and chlamydiae.
† Plants and algae.

tiveness and dissimilarities in comparison to other bacteria.

Divisions I, II, and III are referred to as *Eubacteria.* The bacteria that are associated with or cause disease in animals belong to Eubacteria. Eubacteria are more conveniently grouped as consisting of *Cyanobacteria* and other bacteria.

Cyanobacteria (Blue-Green Algae)

This group has been treated as one of the algae; however, their typically procaryotic cell structure identifies them as bacteria. The cyanobacteria perform oxygen-elaborating photosynthesis and possess plant-type chlorophylls in thylacoid membranes. They are different from photosynthetic bacteria, which perform nonoxygenic photosynthesis and possess bacteriochlorophyll but not thylacoid membranes. On occasion livestock, pets, and wild animals may ingest toxic cyanobacteria and be fatally poisoned.

Other Bacteria

Conventional Bacteria. These include the rest of the free-living bacteria, e.g., the phototrophic, gliding, sheathed, and appendaged bacteria; rod, coccal, and spiral-shaped bacteria; both gram-positive and -negative bacteria. The phototrophic bacteria (purple bacteria and green bacteria) perform anoxygenic photosynthesis and possess a unique pigment system containing bacteriochlorophyll.

Rickettsiae and Chlamydiae. These organisms differ from conventional bacteria in that they are smaller (0.2 to 0.5 μm in diameter) and they are obligate intracellular parasites. They resemble bacteria because they contain both DNA and RNA, multiply by binary fission, have muramic acid (ex-

cept for chlamydiae), and are susceptible to some antibacterial drugs.

Mycoplasmas. Most of these organisms are parasitic on plants or animals, lack cell walls, are highly pleomorphic, are resistant to penicillin, and are the smallest of the free-living organisms.

METHODS EMPLOYED FOR OBSERVING BACTERIA

The microscope is an essential investigative tool of microbiology. The units of measurement employed in microbiology are the micron (μ) or micrometer (μm = 10^{-6}m), the nanometer (nm = 10^{-9}m) and the angstrom (Å = 10^{-10}m). The two types of microscopes available are light and electron. These types differ by the ray they use to effect magnification, i.e., light and electron beams, respectively.

MICROSCOPE

Light Microscope

Bright-Field Microscope. The conventional microscope has three objectives: low power, high power (high dry), and oil-immersion. The latter, with the usual ocular lens × 10 providing a total magnification of approximately × 1000, is used for the routine examination of stained bacterial smears and wet preparations under coverslips. The resolution of the light microscope is limited by the wavelength of visible light, which is about 0.5 μm; images less than 0.2 μm cannot be clearly resolved.

Dark-Field Microscope. This type of illumination can be used in the conventional microscope by substituting a dark-field condenser for the conventional condenser. This special condenser obliquely reflects a powerful source of light onto a wet preparation. Very small objects, including microorganisms, scatter the light and can be seen as brilliant images against a dark background. Extremely small and slender organisms such as the spirochetes, which cannot be seen with the conventional microscope, can be readily visualized using this method. Living organisms and their movement can be seen.

Fluorescence Microscope. Although various fluorescent dyes are used to stain microorganisms, the technique known as immunofluorescence (fluorescent antibody or FA procedure) is much more widely used in clinical microbiology, mainly for the identification of organisms. Fluorescent antibody reagents are prepared by coupling a fluorescent dye to a specific antibody. This conjugate will unite with its corresponding bacterial or viral antigen. The union is visually detectable by the presence of characteristic fluorescence when it is excited by the ultraviolet light of a fluorescence microscope. An indirect procedure is also used in which the conjugated (secondary) antibody is prepared against the globulin, which includes specific (primary) antibody to identify the organism. This conjugate can thus recognize whether or not the specific antibody has united with the microorganism.

Phase-Contrast Microscope. When light waves pass through transparent objects, such as cells, they emerge in different phases, depending on the properties of the materials through which they pass. In phase-contrast microscopy, a phase condenser and phase objective lens convert differences in phase into differences in intensity of light. Thus some structures appear darker than others. This method is useful in studying the fine detail of unstained living microorganisms.

Electron Microscope

The principle of this instrument is analogous to that of the light microscope. Instead of visible light, the electron microscope employs a beam of electrons that is focused by an electromagnetic field instead of by glass lenses. Because of the short wavelength, it can resolve objects as small as 0.0004 μm.

Because biologic materials are mainly composed of the elements carbon, hydrogen, nitrogen, and oxygen, which have low electron scatter-deflecting ability, special techniques are necessary to make specimens stand out against background.

Thin Sectioning. Most microorganisms are too thick for direct examination of the internal structure by the electron microscope. To make them transparent to the electron beam, thin sectioning is employed. Before sectioning, the specimen must be fixed, dehydrated, and embedded to preserve specific structures. Positive staining of the thin section with heavy metal elements is used to increase the contrast of specimens.

Negative Staining. Negative staining sets specimens against an electron-dense heavy metal element. The procedure provides a high resolution of viral and other small particles. The technique is very simple, quick, and economical, and it is often used as a quantitative device to enumerate viral particles and as a diagnostic procedure to identify the virus in stools, urine, cerebrospinal fluid, tears, blood, lavages, and blister fluids.

Freeze Fracture. In the freeze-fracture procedure, specimens are quick-frozen in freon, split or cleaved, and a carbon replica of the fractured surface is prepared at liquid nitrogen temperature. The replica surface is shadow-cast with a heavy metal to provide contrast. Chemical fixation, embedding and sectioning procedures, and accompanying artifacts are thereby avoided. This technique is especially valuable for viewing the internal structure of the biologic membrane, since fracture often occurs between the outer and inner leaflets of a unit membrane.

Localization Techniques. To determine the cellular site of enzymes and their activities, or to be able to follow the formation or incorporation of specific structures within a cell, *enzyme cytochemistry* and *autoradiography* are used. In enzyme studies, the reaction product of an enzyme is precipitated and made electron-dense, so that the position of the enzyme can be identified. Autoradiography is a method for locating radioactive substances by use of modified photographic techniques. The microorganism is incubated with a radioactive precursor and allowed to use this precursor in its normal metabolic pathways. The tissue to be examined is then fixed and routinely sectioned for electron microscopy. The section of tissue is coated with a thin film of photographic emulsion. Rays released by radioactive decay expose silver grains in the emulsion that are subsequently developed, fixed, and viewed in the microscope.

To identify the position of specific antigens, either within or on the surface of a cell, *immunolabeling* by antibody coupled with ferritin, gold particles, or peroxidase is used. Ferritin and gold particles are electron-dense and readily recognizable under the electron microscope. Peroxidase enzyme forms a complex with the substrate hydrogen peroxide. This complex reacts with an electron donor, such as diaminobenzidine tetrahydrochloride, to form an electron-dense precipitate.

High Voltage Electron Microscopy. This allows thicker specimens to be examined by obtaining a stereo image. The higher accelerating voltage of 1000 kV (1 MV) or higher results in improved resolution and penetration power. In comparison, the conventional electron microscope operates at 60 to 80 kV.

Scanning Electron Microscopy (SEM). The object is scanned with a flying spot of electrons, and the emergent secondary electrons are collected and shown on a screen of the cathode-ray tube. Three-dimensional images are obtained, but internal detail is not provided by SEM.

X-Ray Microanalysis. When an electron hits a specimen, characteristic x-rays are released from each element. In x-ray spectroscopy, an x-ray detector is used to monitor the distinct x-ray pattern produced by the interaction between the electron beam of the microscope and the chemical elements in specific areas of the specimen. This method is especially suitable for localizing specific elements in the microorganism.

STAINING PROCEDURES

Staining methods are used to determine the morphologic form of bacteria and their affinity for certain dyes. Bacteria are divided into two major groups on the basis of the Gram stain. Briefly, the procedure for the Gram stain is as follows: The cells are first fixed to a glass slide by heat, then stained with a basic dye (e.g., crystal or methyl violet) that is washed off with an iodine-potassium iodide solution (mordant), and then washed with water and cautiously decolorized with acetone or ethyl alcohol. The smear is then counterstained with safranin.

Gram-positive organisms retain the basic dye following decolorization with acetone or alcohol and appear deep violet. The gram-negative organisms, on the other hand, do not retain the violet stain but take up the counterstain (safranin) and stain red to pink. As a general rule, organisms that give a doubtful reaction are gram-positive. The gram-positive cell wall presents a permeability barrier to elution of the dye-iodine complex by the decolorizer. Aging gram-positive cells become gram-negative because autolytic enzymes attack the cell wall.

Gram-positive and gram-negative organisms differ in the structure of the cell wall:

1. Gram-negative organisms have more lipid in their cell wall.

2. Gram-positive bacteria have a thicker peptidoglycan layer, which renders them more resistant to mechanical damage. Because of these structural differences, the two groups vary in their reaction to Gram stain and their susceptibility to enzymes, disinfectants, and antimicrobial drugs.

Not all bacteria can satisfactorily be stained by the Gram method. The cell walls of mycobacteria contain lipids and waxy substances (mycolic acid) that make them difficult to stain. However, when they are stained by a special procedure called an *acid-fast stain*, they retain the carbolfuchsin even after exposure to a strong acid-alcohol (HCl and ethanol) solution.

The leptospira and treponemes are very slender and cannot be satisfactorily resolved following Gram staining, but they can be demonstrated by *silver staining. Negative staining*, employing nigrosin or India ink, is used for demonstrating capsules. The capsules appear clear and unstained, surrounded by the dark inert particles. For demonstrating flagella (around 0.02 to 0.03 μm in diameter), a *mordant* is used before staining; this precipitates on flagella and thus thickens them.

BACTERIAL STRUCTURE

SHAPE AND SIZE OF BACTERIA

The three basic morphologic forms of bacteria are the straight rod (bacillus), the sphere (coccus), and the spiral or curved rod (spirochete, spirillum, vibrio). There is considerable variation in these basic forms: coccobacillary, ovoid, and filamentous forms are frequently seen.

The cocci are found in different arrangements, depending upon their dividing planes. The staphylococci occur in bunches or clusters, the streptococci form chains, and the pneumococci are predominantly paired. Some of the micrococci occur in groups of four, or tetrads (*Aerococcus viridans*); others are grouped in packets of eight (*Sarcina*).

The various species of the Enterobacteriaceae occur as rather regular rods, but some of the smaller organisms such as *Pasteurella, Brucella,* and *Haemophilus* are both bacillary and coccobacillary. Some members of the genera *Bacillus* and *Clostridium* have rods in chain formation. The corynebacteria are remarkably pleomorphic and produce club-shaped forms. The actinomycetes (*Actinomyces* and *Nocardia*) have both bacillary and filamentous branching forms. The anaerobic *Fusobacterium* has a characteristic elongated, spindle shape. Among the spiral forms are those that are curved, comma, or S-shaped (*Vibrio* and *Campylobacter*) and those that are tightly or loosely coiled (*Treponema* and *Leptospira*).

The size of bacteria also varies considerably. Most rod forms range from 2 to 5 μm in length by 0.5 to 1 μm in width; spirochetes may be longer (up to 20 μm) and narrower (0.1 to 0.2 μm). Cocci are approximately 1 μm in diameter. The size of bacteria varies somewhat, depending upon the medium and the growth phase. They are usually smallest in the logarithmic phase of growth. An *Escherichia coli* bacterium has a volume of ~ 1 μm³ and a weight of ~ 10^{-12}g, whereas a liver cell has a volume of ~ 1,000 μm³ and a weight of ~ 10^{-9}g. For convenience, bacteria can be roughly grouped according to size as follows:

Large: Spirochetes, *Bacillus*, *Clostridium*
Medium: Enterobacteriaceae (*Escherichia coli*, *Proteus*), pseudomonads
Small: *Brucella*, *Pasteurella*, *Haemophilus*
Very small: *Rickettsia*, *Chlamydia*, *Mycoplasma*

BACTERIAL ULTRASTRUCTURE

Bacteria are enclosed by the cell envelope, which is made up of two or three layers, depending upon the organism. All, except mycoplasmas, have a *cell wall* internal to which is the cell or *cytoplasmic membrane*, and some have *capsules* external to the cell wall. Many bacteria have *flagella* and some gram-negative varieties have *pili* or *fimbriae*.

The cytoplasmic membrane surrounds the body of the organism, which consists principally of cytoplasm. Ribosomes, granular inclusions and, in some bacteria, mesosomes (infoldings of plasma membrane), are found distributed within the cytoplasm. Bacteria do not have a membrane-enveloped nucleus as do the eucaryotes, although with appropriate staining nuclear structures can be seen. The principal structural features of bacteria are shown in Figures 1–2 and 1–3.

Cell Envelope

Capsules and Slimes. These are amorphous, polymeric, often gelatinous materials lying outside the cell wall. Most are polysaccharides but several are polypeptides; some bacteria, such as *Bacillus megaterium*, have both compounds in their capsule. Special staining procedures, including negative stains, are used to demonstrate capsules. The capsules of mucoid strains of *Pasteurella multocida* and *Streptococcus equi* consist almost wholly of hyaluronic acid. Virulence may depend to some extent on the antiphagocytic properties of the capsule, e.g., *Bacillus anthracis*, *Brucella abortus*, and *Streptococcus pneumoniae*.

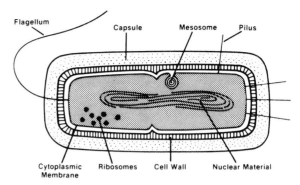

Figure 1–2. Principal structures of bacteria.

Cell Wall. There are basic differences between the cell walls of gram-positive and gram-negative bacteria. The cell wall makes up approximately 20% of the total dry weight of the bacterium. It gives the organism shape and a rigid structure that protects the cell's internal structures from severe chemical and physical actions.

The cell wall is permeable and the cytoplasmic membrane is selectively semipermeable, determining which molecules will be excreted from the cell and what concentration of the different solutes will be maintained. Movement of substances across the membrane takes place by simple diffusion and by more complex transport systems.

The supporting role of the cell wall can be demonstrated if its formation is prevented by penicillin or it is destroyed by *lysozyme*. The structures that remain are bound by the cytoplasmic membrane only and are called *protoplasts* (gram-positive) or *spheroplasts* (gram-negative). Unless placed in a hypertonic milieu, protoplasts and spheroplasts swell and burst.

Structure and Chemical Composition of Cell Walls. The cell wall's rigid structure is provided by *peptidoglycans*. These very large polymers are composed of two kinds of building blocks: (1) *N*-acetylglucosamine and *N*-acetylmuramic acid disaccharide polymers, and (2) peptides consisting of four or five amino acids, namely, L-alanine, D-alanine, D-glutamic acid, and either lysine or diaminopimelic acid (Fig. 1–4). These are unique to bacteria.

Gram-Positive Bacteria. Cell walls range from 150 to 800 Å in thickness. In addition to the peptidoglycan, some gram-positive organisms possess polysaccharides and *teichoic acids*. Table 1–2 compares some major envelope structures of gram-positive and gram-negative bacterial cells. A diagram of the cell walls of both types of organisms is shown in Figure 1–5.

Gram-Negative Bacteria. The cell wall is approximately 100 Å in thickness, high in lipid content (11

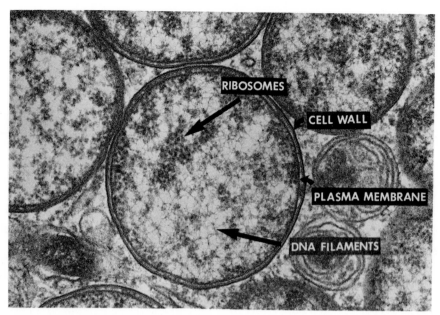

Figure 1–3.   Transmission electron micrograph of *Rickettsia.*

to 22%), and appears as a unit membrane; thus, it is called the outer membrane. A major protein of the outer membrane, called *porin,* forms transmembrane pores or diffusion channels that allow passage of small hydrophilic molecules through the outer membrane. A relatively small amount of peptidoglycan is present in the inner rigid layer, but a large amount of a lipopolysaccharide (LPS), often referred to as *endotoxin,* occurs external to the outer membrane. Endotoxin is important in the pathogenesis of some diseases. The serologic specificity of the O-antigens of gram-negative bacteria resides in the determinants of polysaccharide. The lipid moiety of the LPS, called lipid A, is the toxic component. The basic structure of *Salmonella* LPS is shown in Figure 1–6.

Periplasm. The periplasm is the space between the plasma membrane and cell wall and is visible in gram-negative but difficult to see in gram-positive bacteria. The periplasm contains various hydrolytic enzymes and binding proteins that specifi-

cally bind sugars, amino acids, and inorganic ions. These enzymes and proteins aid transport of various compounds into and out of the bacterial cytoplasm, and they are released by osmotic shock.

Appendages

Flagella. These are long whip-like structures of locomotion. They are composed of three parts: filament, hook, and basal body. The basal body is embedded in the plasma membrane and gives the flagella rotary motion, which propels the organism. The distribution of flagella on the cell is of significance in taxonomy. *Monotrichous* bacteria have a single polar flagellum; *lophotrichous* bacteria have tufts of several flagella at one pole; *amphitrichous* bacteria have flagella at both poles; and *peritrichous* organisms have a number of flagella distributed all around the cell surface. The diameter of a flagellum is 10 to 20 nm, and special staining procedures are used to demonstrate flagella. They are composed mostly of a protein monomer called

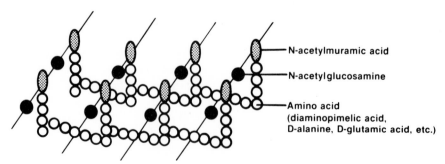

N-acetylmuramic acid

N-acetylglucosamine

Amino acid
(diaminopimelic acid,
D-alanine, D-glutamic acid, etc.)

Figure 1–4.   Schematic peptidoglycan structure.

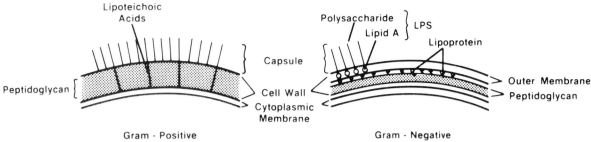

Figure 1–5. Diagram of gram-positive and gram-negative envelope structures.

flagellin. Flagella contain H-antigens and are thus useful in serologic identification of some bacterial species.

Most of the organisms that produce capsules, e.g., species of *Klebsiella, Haemophilus, Pasteurella,* and *Bacillus,* are nonmotile. None of the cocci of medical importance is motile. Motility is determined in the laboratory by the examination of wet preparations from cultures under the microscope (hanging-drop method) and by observing the kind of growth obtained when a semisolid agar medium is stabbed with an inoculum of the organism being examined. Diffuse growth into the agar indicates motility.

Axial Filament. This is a flagellum-like filament located in the periplasmic space between the inner and outer membranes of spirochetes. The spiral organisms move by a traveling helical wave along axial filaments.

Pili (Fimbriae). These are shorter, thinner, and straighter than flagella and are attached to the plasma membrane of mostly gram-negative bacteria. They are composed of a protein monomer called *pilin,* which is 4 to 20 nm in diameter and can only be seen by electron microscopy. The pili enable some bacteria to adhere to epithelial cells, thus leading to colonization of mucous membranes.

The sex pili (see Chapter 3) occur in fertility (F) factor (+) cells found among the Enterobacteriaceae and a few other bacteria. They adhere to F (–) cell surfaces and make possible the transfer of genetic material from F (+) to F (–) cells in conjugation.

Endospores

Members of the genera *Clostridium* and *Bacillus* have the capacity to produce highly resistant, thick-walled spores (Fig. 1–7). They occur when vegetative cells are deprived of some factor or nutrient necessary for growth, e.g., they may appear in the later stages of artificial cultivation. In anthrax, spores are produced when the organisms are exposed to oxygen.

Spore formation begins with realignment of DNA material into filaments and invagination of plasma membrane, forming a structure called the *forespore.* The forespore is further surrounded by the plasma membrane. The facing side of these two plasma membranes is the peptidoglycan synthesizing side, and *spore cortex,* a poorly polymerized peptidoglycan, is synthesized in the space between the two layers of plasma membranes. *Spore coat,* a keratin-like protein rich in cysteine, is formed outside the spore cortex. In some microorganisms, an *exosporium* is formed outside the spore coat. When spore formation is completed, the mature spore is released by the disintegration of the envelope of the mother cell, or *sporangium.* Each spore germinates into a single vegetative cell when conditions for growth are favorable. In gram-stained preparations, spores appear as ovoid, refractile, nonstaining objects either within the cell or free of it.

The location of the mature spore in the cell may be central, terminal, or subterminal, depending

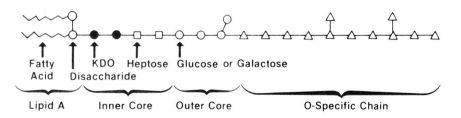

KDO: 2-keto-3-deoxyoctonic acid

Figure 1–6. Schematic diagram of lipopolysaccharide structure.

Table 1–2. *Principal Components of the Cell Walls of Gram-Positive and Gram-Negative Bacteria*

Component	Gram-Positive	Gram-Negative
Peptidoglycan	+ (thick)	+ (thin)
Teichoic acid and/or teichuronic acid	+	−
Lipopolysaccharide	−	+
Polysaccharide	+	+
Protein	Present or absent	+
Lipid	−	+
Lipoprotein	−	+

Adapted from Mandelstam, J., and McQuillen, K. (eds.): *Biochemistry of Bacterial Growth* 3rd Ed. New York, John Wiley & Sons, 1982.

upon the organism, and is useful for identification of the microorganism.

The remarkable heat resistance of spores is thought to be due to the dehydration of the spore protoplast. The irradiation resistance may be related to a high level of cystine disulfide bonds in the spore coat protein, and dehydration resistance is due to keratin-like spore coat protein.

Relatively large amounts of calcium and a compound unique to spores, *dipicolinic acid*, a derivative of diaminopimelic acid (a component of peptidoglycan), occur in the spore.

BACTERIAL TAXONOMY AND CLASSIFICATION

Taxonomy is defined as the science of classification (orderly arrangement of organisms). *Nomenclature* is the assignment of names to the taxonomic groups according to international rules.

PRACTICAL (PHENOTYPIC) CLASSIFICATION

The bacteria are placed in groups in *Bergey's Manual of Systematic Bacteriology* (volume 1, 1984) based on a few readily identifiable characteristics such as morphologic characteristics, reaction to Gram stain, and oxygen requirements. *Bergey's Manual*, the standard reference work for microbiologists, contains detailed descriptions of most known bacteria. Many different characteristics, including morphologic, cultural, biochemical, and nucleic acid (DNA base compositions, DNA ho-

mologies), are used, often in a rather inconsistent manner.

Nomenclature. The classic binomial (Linnaean) system whereby organisms are given a genus and species name is used. The taxonomic levels or ranks used in the current *Bergey's Manual* are hierarchical ones. A specific suffix is used for each category:

Class (-al): A class consists of related orders.

Order (-ales): An order contains a group of related families.

Family (-aceae): In this category are placed closely related genera or tribes.

Tribe (-ieae): A tribe contains closely related genera.

Genus: This most important category contains closely related species.

Species: Included in the same species are strains of organisms that have many characteristics in common, e.g., different strains of *Escherichia coli* will give substantially the same reactions to many biochemical tests.

Subspecies: Some species may be further subdivided into subspecies on the basis of small but consistent differences, e.g., *Campylobacter fetus* subsp. *fetus*, subsp. *intestinalis*, subsp. *jejuni*.

Strain: A strain consists of the descendants (clone) of a single isolate in pure culture. For each species there is a *type strain*, which usually is the particular culture from which the species description was originally made. Type strains are available in various culture collections.

Biovars: A strain with special biochemical or physiologic properties.

Serovars: A strain with distinctive antigenic properties.

In addition to generic (genus) and species names, well-known trivial names, such as tubercle bacillus (*Mycobacterium tuberculosis*), often appear in medical literature. When a generic name is vernacular-

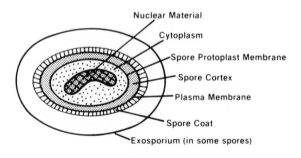

ized in English, such as bacillus and salmonella, it is neither capitalized nor italicized.

Bergey's Manual has evolved since the publication of the first edition in 1923. The manual provides a key that may be used for the identification of bacteria. It is not widely used in diagnostic laboratories except for very uncommon organisms. Microbiologists in diagnostic laboratories usually use simplified schemes to place an unknown organism into a particular genus from relatively small choices, and then reference is made to tables or flow diagrams for the identification of a species within the genus. A modified presentation of the classification of medically important bacteria according to the *Bergey's Manual of Systematic Bacteriology* (volume 1, 1984, and volume 2, 1986) is given in Table 1–3.

Since 1980, valid names of all bacterial species have been published in the *International Journal of Systematic Bacteriology*.

GENETIC BASIS FOR CLASSIFICATION

Genetic information is coded in DNA base sequence. As organisms drift apart by mutation, conjugation, transduction, and selection in different environments (i.e., evolution), their genomes change in size, nucleotide base composition, and nucleotide base sequence.

DNA Base Compositions

The proportions of the four DNA bases in the total DNA of an organism can be assayed. By convention the base composition of a DNA preparation is expressed as the mole percentage of guanine-cytosine (GC) to the total. Since GC + AT (adenine-thymine) = 100%, if the GC content is 40%, the AT = 60%. Determination of GC percentage is relatively simple and is of some value in taxonomy, e.g., all the Enterobacteriaceae from *Escherichia coli* to *Salmonella* have GC percentages ranging from 50 to 54. Similarity of base composition, however, does not necessarily signify DNA homology. The genomes of all vertebrates have a GC percentage of 44, which is the same as some microorganisms.

DNA Hybridization

DNA sequence homology between two organisms can be quantified by procedures that determine the extent of formation of molecular hybrids from two DNA strands of different origin. This approach has been useful in demonstrating relative order and degree of DNA similarity of closely related groups of bacteria. However, this technique is too specific for studying the relationships of dis-

similar bacterial groups. Hybridization between DNA molecules of two *E. coli* strains would be close to 100%, but hybridization of *E. coli* with a *Salmonella* would be about 45%. The phylogenetic definition of a species generally includes strains with approximately 70% or greater DNA-DNA relatedness.

Ribosomal RNA Hybridization or Gene Base Sequence Comparison

Ribosomal RNA (rRNA) exhibits more homology among widely dissimilar organisms than does DNA. Thus it is useful in comparing distantly related organisms. rRNA similarity values have contributed to the establishment of Division IV, Mendosicutes, in the kingdom Procaryotae.

NUMERICAL TAXONOMY

In numerical taxonomy each physiologic and biochemical characteristic is given equal weight. Bacterial strains being studied are subjected to about 50 different tests, and each strain is listed as giving a positive or negative result on each test. With a large number of strains and tests the data are analyzed by computer, making possible a comparison of each strain with all other strains to detect similarities and differences. Similarity coefficients are calculated that indicate the relatedness of each strain to another. Numerical taxonomy has little practical significance, but it is a convenient way of detecting and quantifying the finer differences among fairly closely related bacteria.

CLASSIFICATION OF FUNGI

The taxonomy of fungi is in a state of flux; it undergoes continual refinement and revision. The products of sexual reproduction such as ascospores, basidiospores, and zygospores have been used to define large, major groups of fungi. The sexual cycle, if present, can be used to confirm species identity. However, the sexual cycle of many fungi is not known and consequently classification is based on asexual and vegetative morphology. The criteria for establishing genera and families are frequently unreliable. However, comparisons of guanine and cytosine content, and DNA homologies, have helped establish some relationships. Some of the salient features of the principal fungous groups are given below.

Kingdom Mycetae

Division Mastigomycota: Aquatic fungi producing motile, flagellated cells

Table 1–3. *Classification Outline of Medically Important Bacteria*

Kingdom Procaryotae
    Division I.   Gracilicutes: Procaryotes that have a rigid or semirigid cell wall containing peptidoglycan and a negative reaction to Gram stain.
        Class I.   Scotobacteria
            Section 1.   Spirochetes
                Order   Spirochaetales
                    Family   Spirochaetaceae
                          Genus   *Spirochaeta*
                          Genus   *Treponema*
                          Genus   *Borrelia*
                          Genus   *Serpulina*
                    Family   Leptospiraceae
                          Genus   *Leptospira*
              Section 2.   Aerobic-Microaerophilic, Motile, Helical-Vibroid Gram-Negative Bacteria
                        Genus   *Spirillum*
                        Genus   *Campylobacter*
                        Genus   *Helicobacter*
              Section 3.   Nonmotile (or Rarely Motile) Gram-Negative Curved Bacteria
              Section 4.   Gram-Negative Aerobic Rods and Cocci
                  Family   Pseudomonadaceae
                        Genus   *Pseudomonas*
                  Family   Legionellaceae
                        Genus   *Legionella*
                  Family   Neisseriaceae
                        Genus   *Neisseria*
                        Genus   *Moraxella*
                        Genus   *Acinetobacter*
                  Other Genera
                        Genus   *Flavobacterium*
                        Genus   *Alcaligenes*
                        Genus   *Brucella*
                        Genus   *Bordetella*
                        Genus   *Francisella*
              Section 5.   Facultatively Anaerobic Gram-Negative Rods
                  Family   Enterobacteriaceae
                        Genus   *Escherichia*
                        Genus   *Shigella*
                        Genus   *Salmonella*
                        Genus   *Citrobacter*
                        Genus   *Klebsiella*
                        Genus   *Enterobacter*
                        Genus   *Erwinia*
                        Genus   *Serratia*
                        Genus   *Hafnia*
                        Genus   *Edwardsiella*
                        Genus   *Proteus*
                        Genus   *Providencia*
                        Genus   *Morganella*
                        Genus   *Yersinia*
                  Family   Vibrionaceae
                        Genus   *Vibrio*
                        Genus   *Aeromonas*
                        Genus   *Plesiomonas*
                  Family   Pasteurellaceae
                        Genus   *Pasteurella*
                        Genus   *Haemophilus*
                        Genus   *Taylorella*
                        Genus   *Actinobacillus*
                  Other Genera
                        Genus   *Chromobacterium*
                        Genus   *Streptobacillus*
                        Genus   *Eikennella*
                        Genus   *Gardnerella*
                        Genus   *Calymmatobacterium*
              Section 6.   Anaerobic Gram-Negative Straight, Curved, and Helical Rods
                  Family   Bacteroidaceae
                        Genus   *Bacteroides*
                        Genus   *Fusobacterium*
                        Genus   *Porphyromonas*
                        Genus   *Prevotella*
              Section 7.   Dissimilatory Sulfate- or Sulfur-Reducing Bacteria

Table 1–3. Classification Outline of Medically Important Bacteria (Continued)

Section 8.   Anaerobic Gram-Negative Cocci
  Family   Veillonellaceae
      Genus   *Veillonella*
Section 9.   The Rickettsiae and Chlamydiae
  Order   Rickettsiales
      Family   Rickettsiaceae
        Tribe   Rickettsieae
            Genus   *Rickettsia*
            Genus   *Rochalimaea*
            Genus   *Coxiella*
        Tribe   Ehrlichieae
            Genus   *Ehrlichia*
            Genus   *Cowdria*
            Genus   *Neorickettsia*
      Family   Bartonellaceae
            Genus   *Bartonella*
            Genus   *Grahamella*
      Family   Anaplasmataceae
            Genus   *Anaplasma*
            Genus   *Aegyptianella*
            Genus   *Haemobartonella*
            Genus   *Eperythrozoon*
  Order   Chlamydiales
      Family   Chlamydiaceae
            Genus   *Chlamydia*
Other Sections: Gliding Bacteria, Sheathed Bacteria, Budding and/or Appendaged Bacteria
Class III.   Oxyphotobacteria
  Order   Cyanobacteriales
  Order   Prochlorales
Class II.   Anoxyphotobacteria
  Order   Rhodospirillales
  Order   Chlorobiales
Division II.   Firmicutes: procaryotes that have a rigid or semirigid cell wall containing peptidoglycan and a positive reaction to Gram stain.
  Section 1.   Gram-Positive Cocci
    a.   Aerobic and/or facultatively anaerobic
      Family   Micrococcaceae
            Genus   *Staphylococcus*
      Other Genera
            Genus   *Streptococcus*
            Genus   *Enterococcus*
    b.   Anaerobic
            Genus   *Peptococcus*
            Genus   *Peptostreptococcus*
  Section 2.   Endospore-Forming Rods and Cocci
            Genus   *Bacillus*
            Genus   *Clostridium*
  Section 3.   Regular, Gram-Positive, Asporogenous Rod Bacteria
            Genus   *Lactobacillus*
            Genus   *Listeria*
            Genus   *Erysipelothrix*
            Genus   *Caryophanon*
  Section 4.   Irregular, Nonsporing, Gram-positive Rods
            Genus   *Corynebacterium*
            Genus   *Rothia*
  Section 5.   The Mycobacterium
      Family   Mycobacteriaceae
            Genus   *Mycobacterium*
  Section 6.   Nocardioforms
            Genus   *Nocardia*
            Genus   *Rhodococcus*
Division III.   Tenericutes: Procaryotes that do not have a rigid or semirigid cell wall.
  Class I.   Mollicutes
      Order   Mycoplasmatales
        Family   Mycoplasmataceae
            Genus   *Mycoplasma*
            Genus   *Ureaplasma*
Division IV.   Mendosicutes: Procaryotes with unusual walls, membrane lipids, ribosomes, and RNA sequences.
  Class I.   Archaeobacteria

Adapted from Krieg, N.R., and Holt, J.G. (eds.): Bergey's Manual of Systematic Bacteriology. Volume 1, 1984, Volume 2, 1986, Baltimore, Williams & Wilkins.

Division Amastigomycota: Terrestrial fungi, non-motile.

    Subdivision Zygomycotina: Nonseptate mycelium, asexual and sexual reproduction

        Order Mucorales: Asexual reproduction by sporangia, bread mold (*Rhizopus, Absidia, Mucor*)

        Order Entomophthorales: Asexual reproduction by conidia

    Subdivision Ascomycotina: Septate mycelium, sexual reproduction by a sac-like structure (ascus). *Neurospora,* morels, truffles, yeasts (*Saccharomyces cerevisiae*), *Emmonsiella capsulata.* Contains teleomorphic states of dermatophytes, *Aspergillus, Penicillium,* and some other fungi.

    Subdivision Basidiomycotina: Septate mycelium, sexual reproduction by a basidium. Puffballs, mushrooms, rusts, smuts, *Filobasidiella neoformans.*

    Subdivision Deuteromycotina (Fungi imperfecti): Septate mycelium, sexual reproduction has not been discovered.

        Class Blastomyces: Imperfect (asexual) yeasts, e.g., *Candida, Malassezia, Torulopsis, Rhodotorula, Trichosporon;* some have true hyphae and others pseudohyphae

        Class Hyphomycetes: Produce septate hyphae; reproduce asexually by conidia; most pathogenic fungi, e.g., *Aspergillus, Blastomyces, Geotrichum, Histoplasma, Microsporum, Trichophyton, Penicillium,* and many darkly pigmented (dematiaceous) fungi

SUBCELLULAR STRUCTURE OF FUNGI

Fungal growth and structure are described in the section on fungi. Fungi include unicellular yeasts and multicellular molds.

In general, fungal cells are larger than most bacteria and are eucaryotic. Thus, they possess all the cytoplasmic organelles indicated in Table 1–1, with the exception of chloroplasts (Fig. 1–8). They are not photosynthetic. The medically important structures of a fungus are the capsule, cell wall, and cytoplasmic membrane.

Capsule. Some fungi produce an external coating of slime or a more compact capsule. The capsule, or slime layer, is composed of amorphous polysaccharides that may cause the cells to adhere and clump together. The fungal capsule may be

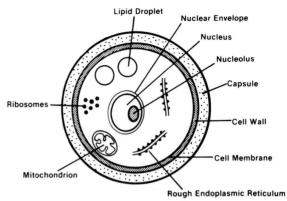

Figure 1–8. Schematic drawing of a yeast cell.

antigenic and antiphagocytic, as in *Filobasidiella* (formerly *Cryptococcus*) *neoformans.*

Cell Wall. The cell wall is the major structure of a fungus and it determines its shape and the process of fungal morphogenesis (e.g., sporulation or yeast-mold dimorphism). It lies immediately external to the cytoplasmic membrane. Unlike that found in bacteria, most of the fungal cell wall is a thatchwork of polysaccharide (chitin, glucan, mannan, cellulose) chains called *microfibrils.* The rest is protein and glycoprotein, which cross-link the polysaccharide chains. Since a wide variety of species of fungi share the same polysaccharides, many have common surface antigens. However, many unique antigenic determinants resulting from the different branching patterns of the polysaccharides are also found within a certain group. These antigens are useful for classification. Detection of species-specific surface antigens in solution provides a sensitive identification of slow-growing or poorly sporulating pathogenic fungi or both.

Cytoplasmic Membrane. Fungi possess a bilayered membrane similar in structure and composition to the cell membranes of higher eucaryotes. Unlike the bacterial membrane (except for the mycoplasmas), but similar to that of other eucaryotes, the fungal membrane contains sterols. The principal fungal sterols are *ergosterol* and *zymosterol* (mammalian cell membrane possesses *cholesterol*). This difference has been exploited in the successful use of the polyene antibiotics (e.g., amphotericin B), which have greater affinity to fungal sterol than to cholesterol.

FURTHER READING

Berbee, M.L. and Taylor, J.W.: Detecting morphological convergence in true fungi, using 18S rRNA gene sequence data. Biosystems 28:117–125, 1992.

Davis, B.D., Dulbecco, R., Eisen, H.N., and Ginsberg, H.S. (eds.): Microbiology. 4th Ed. New York, Harper & Row, 1989.

Joklik, W.K., Willett, H.P., Amos, D.B., and Wilfert, C.M. (eds.): Zinsser Microbiology: 20th Ed. Norwalk, CT, Appleton and Lange, 1992.

Krieg, N.R., and Holt, J.G. (eds.): Bergey's Manual of Systematic Bacteriology, Baltimore, Williams & Wilkins, Volume 1, 1984. Volume 2, 1986.

Moore, W.E.C., and Moore, L.V.H.: Index of the bacterial and yeast nomenclatural changes. Washington, D.C., American Society for Microbiology, 1992.

Rippon, J.W.: Medical Mycology. 3rd Ed. Philadelphia, W.B. Saunders, 1988.

2

Microbial Nutrition, Metabolism, and Growth

G. William Claus

CHEMICAL AND PHYSICAL REQUIREMENTS FOR GROWTH

An infection occurs whenever a particular microorganism carries out an active metabolism, grows, and exerts a harmful effect within the tissue of an animal's body. Whether or not this happens depends upon the environment provided by that tissue. Many microorganisms never cause an infection simply because the host tissue does not provide the physical or chemical conditions necessary to support that microbe's metabolism and subsequent growth. On the other hand, some tissues provide an excellent environment for the growth of some harmful microorganisms. An understanding of the chemical and physical requirements for growth of a microorganism will better enable you to grow it in the laboratory, and it will also help you to realize how the infected tissue provides those requirements for growth of the pathogen.

Nutritional Categories

Microorganisms may be divided into three major categories according to their ability to use various forms of energy and carbon for biosynthesis (Fig. 2–1).

Photosynthesis and Autotrophs. Photosynthetic microorganisms are those capable of using light as a sole energy source and either carbon dioxide or more reduced organic molecules as a carbon source for growth. Autotrophic (chemolithotrophic) microorganisms are those that cannot use light as an energy source but can use inorganic molecules as the sole source of energy, and they may use either carbon dioxide or more reduced organic molecules as a carbon source for synthesis and growth. There are no known strict photosynthetic or autotrophic microorganisms that are animal pathogens.

Heterotrophs. Heterotrophic microorganisms are those that cannot use light or inorganic compounds for energy and cannot use carbon dioxide as the sole source of carbon for synthesis and growth. Instead, the heterotrophs use reduced organic molecules (such as sugars, amino acids, fatty acids, and nucleic acids) both as a source of energy and of carbon for synthesis and growth. Only a few heterotrophs cannot be cultivated in artificial (synthetic) media in the laboratory, that is, outside the animal's body; these are called strict parasites. Most heterotrophs are considered saprophytes because they can be cultivated on media in the laboratory. All pathogenic microorganisms, both opportunistic and strict pathogens, are heterotrophs, and the large majority of these are saprophytes.

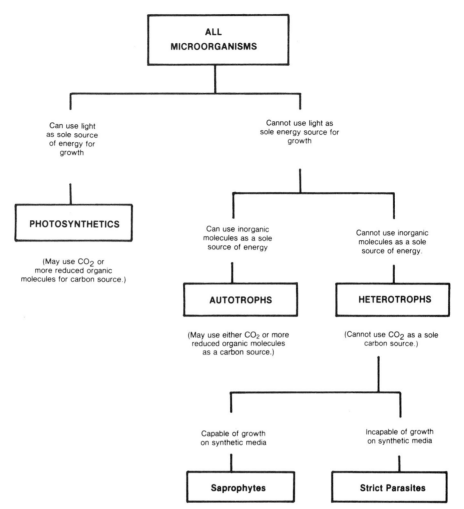

Figure 2–1. Major nutritional categories of all microorganisms. Note that the majority of microorganisms having veterinary significance are saprophytic heterotrophs.

Nutrient Requirements

Nutrients for microbial growth may be divided into two classes: (1) essential nutrients, without which a cell cannot grow; and (2) nonessential nutrients, which are used if present. All essential nutrients must be provided in an artificial medium for cultivation of a microorganism.

All cells must have a source of carbon and a source of energy to grow. In addition, all cells must have a nutritional source of nitrogen, phosphorus, sulfur, sodium, potassium, iron, magnesium, manganese, and trace quantities of many other minerals. These nutrients are essential for the growth of all microorganisms.

Some microorganisms are able to grow on media that contain only those nutrients just listed. For example, some enterobacteria will grow in a medium containing only glucose (as a carbon and energy source), ammonium ion (as the sole nitro-

gen source), phosphate ion (as a phosphorus source), sulfate ion (as a sulfur source), and trace amounts of other minerals. These cells make all the polysaccharides, fats, proteins, and nucleic acids necessary for growth solely from the carbon and energy available in the glucose molecule. These cells have a very complex metabolism with powerful biosynthetic capabilities.

Other microorganisms require complex organic compounds to grow. For example, they may need certain amino acids, fatty acids, nucleotides, or vitamins before growth is possible. These microbes are not able to make these compounds from a simple carbon and energy source (like glucose); therefore, these compounds must be supplied in the growth medium. These organic compounds are called preformed nutrients because they must be offered to the cells in a "preformed" state. If a microbe requires many preformed nutrients for growth, it is called fastidious. Fastidious microbes lack powerful synthetic capabilities.

Even though a microorganism is capable of making everything it needs from a simple sugar such as glucose, it will usually grow more rapidly in the presence of many preformed nutrients. For example, *Salmonella* species are capable of growth on a glucose plus mineral salts medium, but they will grow many times faster if provided with the preformed nutrients found in yeast and beef extracts. These extra nutrients are called nonessential because their presence is helpful but not necessary. In general, microorganisms preferentially take in preformed nutrients rather than making them on their own because this saves energy.

Microorganisms that coexist with or are pathogenic for animals seem to range all the way from those able to grow in only a glucose plus mineral salts medium to those that are extremely fastidious.

Hydrogen Ion Concentration

Some bacteria of veterinary significance are aciduduric, that is, they have the ability to survive (but not grow) for short periods of time in very acidic environments. For example, gastric fluids may have a pH value of 1.0, and gastrointestinal (GI) pathogens must first survive these stomach fluids before growing and exerting their adverse effects in the intestines. Although some microbes are aciduduric, very few are able to grow at these extremes in pH.

Each microorganism has a pH range within which growth is possible, and each usually has a well-defined optimum pH at which the cells grow at their maximum rate. Most bacteria of medical or veterinary significance grow best at a neutral or slightly alkaline pH (pH 7.0 to 7.5), the pH of most mammalian fluids and tissue.

When one prepares a medium for laboratory growth of a microbe, its initial pH (hydrogen ion concentration) is often above or below the pH that will support optimum growth of that microorganism. It is then customary to adjust the pH with an inorganic acid or base before the medium is sterilized. Autoclaving sometimes alters the medium pH; therefore, it is best to recheck the pH of one sample after the autoclaved medium has cooled.

It is desirable to maintain a relatively constant medium pH during microbial growth. However, some growing microbes excrete organic acids that increase the acidity (decrease the pH) of the growth medium, and some microbes excrete ammonium ions that increase the alkalinity (increase the pH) of the growth medium. Buffers are salts of weak acids or bases. If buffers are present in the growth medium, they respond to the microbial addition of acids or bases by taking up or giving off hydrogen ions, helping to keep the pH constant. Amino acids are good buffers, and they are naturally present in many complex laboratory media. Thus, additional buffers need not be added to complex media. Synthetic growth media often contain no chemicals having a buffering capacity, and synthetic buffers are often added to these media to maintain an optimum pH for microbial growth.

Carbon Dioxide Concentration

All microorganisms require carbon dioxide (CO_2) for both survival and growth. This is supplied either exogenously (from the environment outside the cell; the earth's atmosphere normally contains about 0.03% CO_2) or endogenously (from within the cell; produced by decarboxylation reactions during catabolism).

Some microorganisms initiate growth in the laboratory and reproduce at a more rapid rate when the CO_2 concentration is increased above that normally found in the atmosphere. This phenomenon is characteristic of many pathogens of veterinary significance. These microbes may be grown in a "CO_2 incubator" by using compressed CO_2 to replace about 10% of the atmosphere inside the incubator. Alternatively, one may seal the inoculated cultures inside a jar with a lighted candle (candle jar) and allow the candle to burn to extinction; this method decreases the amount of O_2 available and raises the CO_2 levels from 0.03% to about 3%. Often it is not clear whether it is the decreased O_2 concentration or the elevated CO_2 levels that stimulate growth (see Microaerophils further on).

Oxygen Concentration

When oxygen is dissolved in fluids, it forms a variety of ions, such as the toxic superoxide radical. As a consequence of metabolism in the presence of O_2, hydrogen peroxide is also formed, and this, too, is toxic. Therefore, cells capable of growth in the presence of O_2 must have a way to detoxify these harmful forms of oxygen. Microorganisms accomplish this by producing enzymes that break down the toxic molecules or change them into a form that is less toxic. Superoxide dismutase, catalase, and peroxidase are examples of such enzymes (Fig. 2–2).

Cells that grow in the presence of air usually use O_2 to support a respiratory type of metabolism. Other types of microbes normally live where there is only a small amount of O_2; consequently, they have only a limited ability to detoxify oxygen radi-

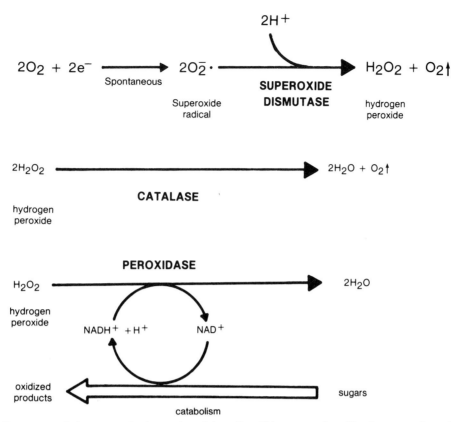

Figure 2–2. Enzymes made by some microbes and used (usually within or near the cell's plasma membrane) to destroy toxic forms of oxygen, such as the superoxide radical and hydrogen peroxide.

cals, and their cultivation in the laboratory must be under conditions in which the O_2 concentration is artificially lowered. Still other microbes live only in environments that totally lack O_2; these microbes usually lack this detoxification ability, and their laboratory cultivation must be in the complete absence of O_2.

The terms that follow reflect an organism's ability to grow in the presence of O_2, and, in some cases, even to use O_2 to their metabolic advantage.

Strict (Obligate) Aerobes. These are microorganisms that can only grow in the presence of air (O_2), and the more O_2 available, the better they grow. All filamentous fungi but only a very few bacteria are in this category. Strictly aerobic pathogens are not common but occur on the mucosa of the upper respiratory tract. They have an unusually high capacity to detoxify the toxic forms of O_2; that is, they produce large amounts of extremely active catalase and superoxide dismutase. In the laboratory, strict aerobes are usually cultivated on the surface of solid media or in well-aerated liquid media. These microbes are incapable of supporting growth from the energy supplied by fermentation. All accomplish a respiratory type of metabolism and use only O_2 as a terminal electron acceptor.

Facultatives. These microbes are able to grow in either the presence or the absence of air (O_2), but they grow better when oxygen is present. All yeasts and a large number of bacteria fit this description. Facultative pathogens are very common. They may begin to grow in well-oxygenated tissue (or laboratory media), rapidly use the dissolved oxygen, and then continue to grow in the absence of O_2 but at a slower rate. Because facultatives are able to grow in the presence of air, they must have the ability to detoxify the toxic forms of O_2. In the laboratory, facultatives are usually cultivated under aerobic conditions, but they may grow in the absence of O_2 and at all intermediate oxygen concentrations. These microbes are able to support growth from the energy supplied by either fermentation or a respiratory catabolism. While respiring, some may use inorganic ions other than O_2 for a terminal electron acceptor to support respiration. In other words, some may continue to respire, even under anaerobic conditions, if an alternate terminal electron acceptor is available.

There are many facultative bacteria associated with the animal body. For example, bacteria normally found on an animal's skin or within its intestines are often facultative. These bacteria are common opportunistic pathogens that cause tissue infections when the skin or gut wall is broken or abraded.

Microaerophiles. These microbes require oxygen, but they will not grow in air that normally contains 20% oxygen. Only a few bacteria are microaerophiles, but some of these are important animal pathogens, such as some *Actinomyces* and *Campylobacter* species. They grow in body cavities and tissues having reduced O_2 concentrations. Cultivation in the laboratory is often achieved in liquid or on solid media held in an atmosphere containing about 6% oxygen. Laboratory cultivation is also possible in semisolid media (0.1 to 0.4% agar). The agar prevents oxygen from freely mixing through the tube. Oxygen can only diffuse from the surface; thus the medium is stratified with an oxygen gradient having the most oxygen-rich layer at the surface. After inoculating the medium by stabbing deeply with a loop or needle, microaerophiles begin to grow in a discrete band located from a few millimeters to several centimeters below the surface, where the oxygen concentration is the most favorable. Microaerophiles use a strictly respiratory catabolism, with O_2 being the only terminal electron acceptor used. It is believed that microaerophiles do not tolerate normal atmospheric oxygen concentrations because they have a limited ability to detoxify the toxic forms of O_2.

Strict Anaerobes. These microbes lack the ability to grow in the presence of air, and often even small amounts of O_2 are toxic. In healthy animals, anaerobic environments are commonly found in the oral cavity (especially between the teeth and gums) and in the intestines (where the facultative microbes scavenge all available O_2). Strict anaerobes are among the normal microflora of these environments. Most infections initially contain a mixture of facultatives and anaerobes, and the facultative bacteria quickly use up the available O_2. This leaves an anaerobic environment that favors the growth of strict anaerobes. So far as is now known, only a few microbial types are strict anaerobes. The best known types of veterinary significance are in three genera: *Bacteroides*, *Clostridium*, and *Fusobacterium*. The reasons why strict anaerobes are intolerant to O_2 are not completely clear, but it may be that they lack the ability to remove toxic forms of oxygen (most lack superoxide dismutase). For this reason, anaerobes are cultivated in an artificially reduced medium in an atmosphere that contains little or no oxygen. Reducing agents such as sodium thioglycolate or dithiotreitol are commonly added to the medium to depress the oxidation-reduction (redox) potential of the medium and hold it at the correct state of reduction. A satisfactory anaerobic atmosphere is often achieved with a GasPack (BBL Microbiology Systems, Cockeysville, MD) that uses a H_2 and a CO_2 generator. The H_2 reacts with O_2 inside the sealed container to form H_2O, thereby removing the gaseous O_2. Although some strict anaerobes are capable of anaerobic respiration (using inorganic terminal electron acceptors other than oxygen), those of veterinary significance appear to support growth only from energy supplied by fermentation.

Temperature

Temperature is one of the most important environmental factors affecting the growth and survival of microorganisms. At cold temperatures, metabolic rates are very slow, and cells will survive for long periods of time (Fig. 2–3). As the temperature rises, enzymatic reactions inside the cell proceed at faster rates and growth also becomes more rapid until the optimum growth rate is achieved. Just above that optimum temperature, however, proteins, DNA, and RNA become irreversibly denatured, and the growth rate falls rapidly to zero. Continued increases in temperature will kill the microbe.

All microorganisms have an optimum growth temperature. The optimum growth temperature of most microbes associated with mammals is from 35 to 37° C, but some (such as *Yersinia* species) still grow well at room temperature (25° C). Microbiologists classify these cells as mesophiles (optimum growth from 28 to 38° C), and this category contains almost all known microorganisms.

Pathogens that have an optimum growth rate at the body temperature of one animal may not grow or may be killed when transferred to another animal that has a body temperature just a few degrees

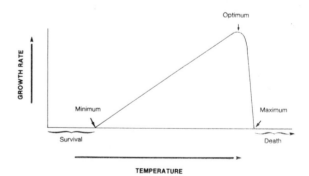

Figure 2–3. Effect of temperature on microbial survival and growth. Cell viability is preserved by temperatures below that supporting minimal growth. As temperature is increased, growth rate is also increased. As temperatures increase above that which is optimum for growth, the rate of growth decreases and then stops. Death occurs at temperatures above the maximum that will support growth.

higher. This may help to explain the species specificity of some microbial pathogens. Also, in the inflammatory response, the localized temperature increase provides an environment that is often less favorable for microbial growth, and this allows time for the body's natural defense mechanisms (e.g., phagocytosis) to capture and kill the invading microorganisms.

If the temperature is elevated above the maximum at which growth is possible, then vegetative cells (but not endospores) die. Our knowledge of these lethally elevated temperatures is used in the pasteurization of liquids to make them safe for human consumption and in the boiling or autoclaving of instruments to kill most or all of the contaminating microorganisms.

The effect of cold temperatures on microorganisms is also of considerable significance. As the incubation temperature is lowered, enzymatic reactions inside the cell proceed at slower rates, and growth rates are decreased until cells reach the minimum temperature at which growth is possible. Unlike elevated temperatures, however, temperatures below the minimum growth temperature cause no damage. On the contrary, cold temperatures preserve microorganisms. Storing cultures in a refrigerator (about 4° C), or in a freezer (about −10° C), or in a container with liquid nitrogen (about −196° C) are commonly used methods for the long-term preservation of microbial cultures.

MOVEMENT OF NUTRIENTS INTO CELLS

Movement through the Capsule and Cell Wall

The capsule surrounding many microorganisms is a loose matrix that permits the diffusion of all soluble molecules but does not allow transfer of colloid-sized particles. Thus, the capsule does not prevent entry of most available nutrients into the cell.

The gram-positive cell wall is also a permeable but rigid matrix that allows for diffusion of soluble nutrients.

The outer membrane of gram-negative cell walls, however, is thought to be a barrier to large molecules. Interspersed throughout this outer membrane are a large number of only a few types of proteins (Fig. 2–4). The concentration of each protein type in the outer membrane varies considerably, depending upon the types of nutrients in the environment. One type of proteins, almost always present in large numbers, are called porins. The porin molecules appear to form water-filled channels that span the cell-wall (outer) membrane, and these channels are of sufficient diameter to allow passage of molecules having a molecular weight up to 800 to 900 daltons. Therefore, small hydrophilic nutrients (like inorganic ions, mono- and disaccharide sugars, amino acids, and di- and tripeptides), as well as small non-nutrient molecules, can easily diffuse through these channels (pores). Thus, it is believed that the outer membrane of the gram-negative cell wall acts as a molecular sieve.

Other proteins present in the outer membrane of the gram-negative cell wall occur in smaller numbers than the porins. A number of these minor proteins seem to be receptor proteins (Fig. 2–4) that facilitate entry of molecules too large to pass through the pores (such as iron chelates, vitamin B_{12}, and degradation products of nucleic acids). These membrane-bound receptor proteins occur in larger amounts when their substrate is present in the medium. Still other minor outer membrane proteins appear to have a structural function.

Neither the outer membrane of the gram-negative cell wall nor the cytoplasmic (plasma) membrane should be thought of as static structures. There is evidence that optimal cell growth occurs only when the outer membrane of the gram-negative cell wall and the plasma membrane are in a partially fluid state.

In the region between the cell-wall (outer) membrane and the plasma membrane of the gram-negative cell, there is a rigid, girder-like polymer called peptidoglycan (Fig. 2–4). This cell wall region is referred to as the periplasm. Within the periplasm are three types of proteins. First, there are hydrolytic enzymes, such as proteases, RNA and DNA nucleases, phosphatases, phosphodiesterases, and lactamases (which destroy the β-lactam antibiotics such as penicillin). The function of the hydrolytic enzymes is to cleave intermediate-sized nutrients so that they are small enough to pass through the plasma membrane. Second, there are binding proteins that specifically bind sulfate, some sugars, and amino acids and act in concert with the plasma membrane to help translocate these nutrients into the cell. Finally, there are the chemoreceptor proteins that allow motile gram-negative cells to detect certain nutrients in the environment, so that they may direct their movement toward the nutrient source. Thus, periplasmic proteins play a predominant role in both detecting nutrients and transferring them into the cell.

Translocation Across the Plasma Membrane

Most microorganisms function best when surrounded by water containing dissolved inorganic

Outside

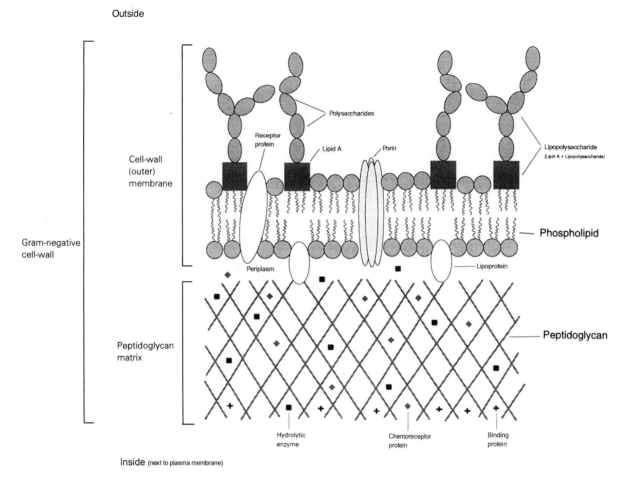

Figure 2–4.   Representation, as viewed in cross-section, of the gram-negative cell wall (not drawn to scale). The wall has two main layers: (1) an outer membrane, composed of a phospholipid bilayer containing embedded proteins and lipopolysaccharides; and (2) a rigid peptydoglycan matrix containing various types of functional proteins.

ions. Most microbes also require reduced organic molecules that are used as a carbon and energy source. In order for the cell to use these nutrients, they must first be translocated across the plasma membrane. The term translocation is used here to indicate the general movement of nutrients across the plasma membrane regardless of whether energy is required to accomplish that movement. Translocations accomplished without the expenditure of energy are called diffusion, whereas those requiring energy are called transport.

Passive and Facilitated Diffusion. Passive diffusion is probably the simplest method of translocating solutes (dissolved nutrients) into or out of the cell. It allows the free flow of solutes across the plasma membrane, it requires no carrier protein within the membrane, and it requires no energy. But passive diffusion of solutes is slow, and the concentration eventually becomes equal on both sides of the membrane. Therefore, both the intercellular concentration and the rate of uptake depend on the extracellular concentration. There are proba-

bly few, if any, nutrients that are translocated across the plasma membrane by passive diffusion.

Facilitated diffusion is similar to passive diffusion in that it requires no energy and the solute concentration inside the cell is never greater than on the outside. However, facilitated diffusion differs from passive diffusion in two important ways: (1) facilitated diffusion uses carrier proteins in the plasma membrane, often called permeases, which specifically bind the solute and facilitate its translocation. Probably because of this, (2) facilitated diffusion is more rapid than passive diffusion. Facilitated diffusion of soluble nutrients appears rare in bacteria. Glycerol is the only nutrient known to enter *Escherichia coli* by facilitated diffusion, and it appears that the same mechanism is also used for glycerol translocation in *Salmonella typhimurium* and species of *Klebsiella, Shigella, Pseudomonas, Bacillus, Nocardia,* and every other bacterium studied to date.

Both passive and facilitated diffusion probably play minor roles in nutrient translocations. This is suspected because the concentration of most nutrients is much greater inside the cell than outside. The higher intracellular concentration of nutrients allows the cell to keep its enzymes saturated with substrates, so that biochemical reactions are accomplished at the maximum possible rate. But a higher intracellular concentration of nutrients also means that they are translocated against a concentration gradient, and this requires energy. Energy-requiring translocations are only accomplished by actively metabolizing cells, and these types of translocations are usually called transport mechanisms.

Mechanisms of Transport. To date, there are two types of energy-requiring transport mechanisms known: one type is called active transport and the other is called group translocation.

Active Transport. There are three main features of active transport: (1) like facilitated diffusion, active transport requires membrane-bound carrier proteins (also called permeases) that specifically bind one type of nutrient and assist in its translocation across the membrane; (2) also like facilitated diffusion, the nutrient translocated by active transport enters the cell in an unaltered state; and (3) unlike facilitated diffusion, active transport requires energy, and this energy is provided by the protonmotive force. Before we consider how the protonmotive force drives active transport, we must first briefly consider a few key features of the metabolic process called electron transport. Note, however, that electron transport is covered in more detail later in this chapter.

The internal breakdown (oxidation) of a nutrient, which serves as the respiring cell's energy source (such as glucose), provides the cell with hydrogens (containing high-energy electrons) that are carried to a series of membrane-bound proteins collectively known as the electron transport system (Fig. 2–5). As these energy-rich electrons are passed from one electron transport protein to the next, the energy in those electrons is used to translocate protons (H$^+$) from the inside to the outside of the plasma membrane. Since the plasma membrane is relatively impermeable to both H$^+$ and OH$^-$, electron transport creates a strong positive charge (H$^+$) on the outside of the membrane and a more negative charge (OH$^-$) on the inside. This difference in charge (ΔpH) across the membrane is called the proton gradient, and the amount of energy available in a membrane having a proton gradient is called the protonmotive force. The energy in the protonmotive force can apparently be used for doing work, such as translocating ions and uncharged molecules into the cell against a concentration gradient. This process may be likened to an energy-driven pump that pushes the nutrients "upstream," that is, against a concentration gradient.

There are at least two ways that this proton-driven pump may work. The first is called symport (Fig. 2–5), where a carrier protein transports both the nutrient and one or more protons into the cell at the same time. In so doing, the proton gradient is somewhat diminished, but the cell has accomplished some useful work. It has pumped a nutrient inside the cell against a concentration gradient. At present, it appears that symport may be a primary mechanism for transporting nutrients into the cell.

The second active transport mechanism is called antiport (Fig. 2–5). With this mechanism, the carrier protein simultaneously transports two things in opposite directions. Once again, one or more protons enter the cell, along with the transport of another substance out of the cell. It is conceivable that antiport may be used by cells in the excretion of toxic waste products against a concentration gradient.

Group Translocation. There are three main features of group translocation: (1) like facilitated diffusion and active transport, group translocation requires a membrane-bound carrier protein to specifically bind one type of nutrient and assist in its translocation across the membrane; (2) like active transport, group translocation requires energy, but this energy comes from a high-energy metabolic intermediate rather than the protonmotive force; and (3) unlike active transport, the nutrient enters the cell in a chemically altered (usually phosphorylated) state (Fig. 2–5). Since the transported material is chemically different from that found outside the cell, technically speaking no concentration gradient is produced. However, the cell does accumulate a useful nutrient in much greater concentration than its precursor on the outside, so the overall effect appears similar to that accomplished by active transport.

The best studied examples of group translocations involve certain sugars, such as β-glucosides, fructose, glucose, *N*-acetylglucosamine, and mannose. Each of these appears to be phosphorylated during transport by the phosphotransferase system (PTS). The mechanism (Fig. 2–5) involves at least four separate proteins that carry the high-energy phosphate group from phosphoenolpyruvate (a common catabolic intermediate) to the incoming sugar. The first two (proteins I and HPr) contain histidine, have a low molecular weight, and reside as soluble molecules inside the cell. These two proteins are subject to genetic regulation and are formed in greater amounts when the PTS-

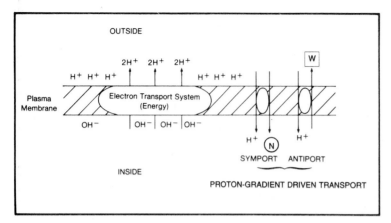

PROTONMOTIVE FORCE

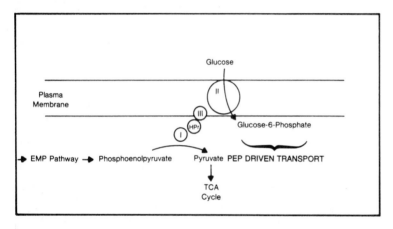

GROUP TRANSLOCATION

Figure 2–5. Two types of energy-requiring mechanisms of transport. In active transport, the cell uses the electron-transport system to translocate protons (H$^+$) outside the cell, thus creating a proton gradient. The energy established by the proton gradient (the protonmotive force) can be used to drive soluble nutrients (N) into or wastes out of the cell. With group translocation of glucose by *Escherichia coli*, the high-energy phosphate bond of phosphoenolpyruvate (PEP) serves as the initial energy source for transport, and four different proteins (I, HPr, II, and III) are also involved.

transported nutrient occurs in the environment. The next protein (III) appears to be peripheral (located on the inner surface of the plasma membrane). The last protein to carry the high-energy phosphate (II) exists tightly bound within the membrane and also serves as a carrier protein to bring the phosphorylated nutrient across the membrane.

Since group translocation does not require intermediates that are produced in great quantities only during respiration (such as ATP and high-energy electrons), this transport mechanism is thought to occur predominantly in fermenting organisms. Most strict aerobes, such as *Azotobacter, Micrococcus, Mycobacterium,* and *Nocardia,* appear to lack a phosphotransferase system. Facultatives of veterinary significance known to contain a PTS include *Escherichia, Salmonella, Staphylococcus,* and *Vibrio;* the strict anaerobes include *Clostridium* and *Fusobacterium.*

MICROBIAL METABOLISM

Metabolism refers to the integration of all chemical reactions occurring within the living cell. Metabolism starts with nutrients brought in from the environment, and the ultimate product is a new cell. For the sake of discussion here, metabolism is divided artificially into two parts: catabolism and anabolism (Fig. 2–6). Catabolism refers to those metabolic reactions that break down the nutrient serving as the cell's chemical energy source. Anabolism defines those metabolic reactions that make new cellular materials and use the energy provided by catabolism.

Catabolic pathways are exergonic, that is, they yield energy, and this energy is often trapped in the formation of new high-energy phosphate bonds, such as adding energy to ADP and inorganic phosphate (Pi) to form ATP. Catabolic pathways are oxidative, i.e., some reactions remove hydrogens (2H$^+$ + 2e$^-$) from the nutrient energy

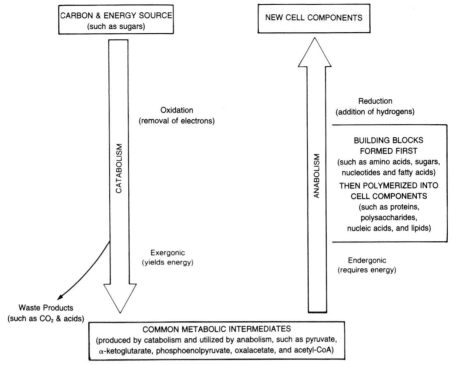

Figure 2–6. An overview of cellular metabolism. Catabolism provides the energy and electrons needed to drive anabolism. Catabolism also provides many if not all of the organic intermediates (building blocks) needed for biosynthesis of polymers during anabolism.

source and save these energy-rich hydrogens for later use by giving them to hydrogen carriers such as NAD^+ or $NADP^+$.

Catabolic pathways also produce intermediates (building blocks) for biosynthesis at many steps during the oxidation process.

Finally, when the cell can oxidize the carbon and/or energy source no further, the product of the last reaction is excreted as waste. Examples of excreted waste products are CO_2 (the most oxidized form of carbon), various organic acids or neutral compounds, and oxidized inorganic molecules.

Anabolic pathways are endergonic, that is, they require energy, and this is frequently supplied by the hydrolysis of one of the high-energy phosphate bonds on ATP. Anabolic pathways are also reductive; some reactions use hydrogens ($2H^+ + 2e^-$) supplied by reduced NAD^+ and $NADP^+$ ($NADH_2$, $NADPH_2$). Anabolic pathways begin with intermediates produced by catabolism and then use these to form building blocks such as amino acids, fatty acids, sugars, purines, and pyrimidines. These building blocks are then polymerized into new cellular materials, such as proteins, lipids, polysaccharides, and nucleic acids. All of this synthesis (anabolism) requires energy . . . *a lot of energy.*

Catabolism is integrated with anabolism in three major ways: (1) the energy (ATP) produced by catabolism is used to drive anabolic pathways; (2) the energy-rich hydrogens removed during oxidative catabolism and carried by NAD^+ or $NADP^+$ are used to support the reductive (hydrogen-requiring) anabolic pathways; and (3) some of the intermediates produced during catabolism are used to start anabolic pathways.

The three sections that follow present a brief overview of the metabolism of microorganisms having veterinary importance. They begin with a consideration of the two major types of catabolism (fermentation and respiration) and end with a succinct examination of how anabolism is integrated with microbial catabolism.

Fermentative Catabolism

Pasteur described fermentation as "life without air." Indeed, we now know that fermentative catabolism is carried out by most (but not all) bacteria and fungi growing in anaerobic environments, such as the rumen or the gut, or deep within infected tissue. Anyone who has smelled rumen fluid or the exudate from many infections has sampled a few of the many rich odors that often result from fermentations. Although not limited to fermentations, the excretion of gases and volatile organic compounds is very common to this form of catabolism.

Common Characteristics. Fermentative catabolism shows two common characteristics. First, only small amounts of ATP are formed by a process known as substrate-level phosphorylation. Oxidative phosphorylation does not occur during fermentation. Second, organic intermediates of fermentative catabolism serve as the cell's terminal electron acceptor, and a reduced organic product is excreted into the surrounding medium.

To illustrate these same characteristics of fermentation, let us use what is perhaps the simplest example: the homolactic fermentation of glucose accomplished by *Enterococcus faecalis*. Like many fermenting microbes, these bacteria are quite fastidious; that is, they will only grow in a nutritionally rich medium. Therefore, most of their biosynthetic intermediates are supplied by the growth medium, most of the glucose is oxidized only for energy, and most of the carbons from glucose end up in products excreted by the cell. Most of the excreted material is lactic acid. These bacteria use the Embden-Myerhoff-Parnas (EMP) pathway (sometimes called glycolysis) to oxidize glucose to pyruvate. This pathway is not limited to fermentation or to *E. faecalis*; it is found in both eucaryotic and procaryotic cells and is common to many fermentative and respiratory forms of catabolism.

The general scheme for the EMP pathway and for lactic acid formation by *S. faecalis* is shown in Figure 2–7. This drawing illustrates two major characteristics of fermentative catabolism. The first is that ATP is formed only by substrate-level phosphorylation. This usually occurs as a two-step process: (1) the incorporation of inorganic phosphate into a catabolic intermediate to form a high-energy phosphate bond, followed by (2) the subsequent transfer of that phosphate and the high-energy bond to ADP to form ATP. In the EMP pathway, inorganic phosphate is added to glyceraldehyde-3-phosphate to form a new high-energy phosphate bond attached to the first carbon. In the next step, this high-energy phosphate is taken from the first carbon of 1,3-DPG and used to phosphorylate ADP. Thus, one more ATP is added to the cell's ATP pool. When one molecule of glucose is oxidized to two molecules of pyruvate, the cell uses two ATPs (to form one fructose-1,6-diphosphate), but it gains four ATPs (as two glyceraldehydes are oxidized to two pyruvates); therefore, the net gain is two ATPs for each glucose oxidized to two pyruvates. To emphasize the inefficiency of fermenting glucose, compare this yield with the 36

to 38 ATPs produced in oxidizing one molecule of glucose with a respiring catabolism!

From the preceding paragraph, it is evident that fermenting microbes are not very efficient in converting their nutrients into usable forms of energy (ATP). To compensate for this inefficiency, they oxidize great quantities of their energy source. This brings us to the second characteristic of fermentative catabolism: catabolic intermediates serve as the cell's terminal electron acceptor, and the reduced organic product is excreted into the surrounding medium. The explanation focuses on the idea that all cells seem to produce only a limited quantity of hydrogen carriers (NAD^+ and $NADP^+$). During oxidative catabolism, these hydrogen carriers accept hydrogens as they are being removed from the energy source. Some but not all of these reduced carriers give up their hydrogens to support reductive anabolic reactions. Reductive anabolism reoxidizes a few hydrogen carriers, so that they can once again accept hydrogens given off during oxidative catabolism; however, most of the hydrogen carriers reduced during catabolism would remain in the reduced state in a fermenting cell if it were not for the catabolic intermediate's acceptance of electrons from the reduced carriers. For example, in *E. faecalis* (Fig. 2–7), pyruvate (the catabolic intermediate) is reduced to lactic acid when it accepts hydrogens from $NADH_2$, and the lactic acid is excreted. For every glucose molecule fermented, two glyceraldehyde-3-phosphates are oxidized to two pyruvates, and this generates two molecules of $NADH_2$. To reoxidize both hydrogen carriers, both molecules of pyruvate could be reduced to lactic acid. This accomplishes two things for the cell: (1) it reforms the NAD^+ needed for continued glucose oxidation; and (2) it gets rid of unneeded hydrogens (protons and electrons) in the form of reduced pyruvate (lactic acid).

The fermentative production of lactic acid from sugars by the EMP pathway and the excretion of large quantities of lactic acid are characteristic of the lactic acid bacteria. These bacteria are part of the natural microflora of the mouth and intestinal tract of mammals and occur on the surfaces of plants, and they are taxonomically placed in the genera *Enterococcus*, *Leuconostoc*, *Pediococcus*, and *Lactobacillus*. Depending upon the species, these bacteria may also produce varying quantities of acetic and formic acids as well as carbon dioxide, ethanol, glycerol, diacetyl, acetoin, and butanediol in addition to lactic acid. Some species are predominantly responsible for the controlled fermentation of harvested plant materials (e.g., silage production). In this process, the lactic acid (produced by

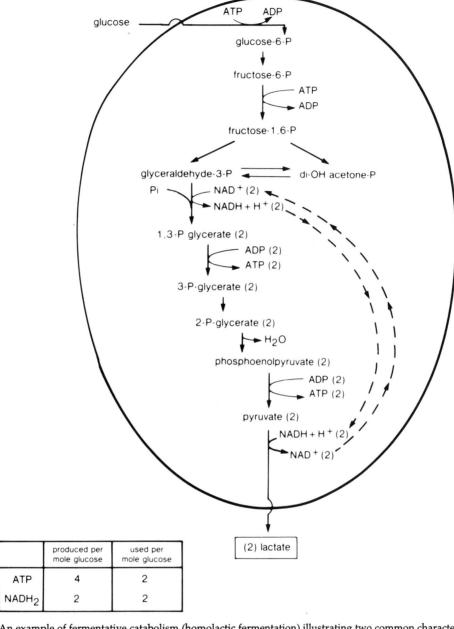

	produced per mole glucose	used per mole glucose
ATP	4	2
NADH$_2$	2	2

Figure 2–7. An example of fermentative catabolism (homolactic fermentation) illustrating two common characteristics: (1) ATP is formed only by substrate-level phosphorylation; and (2) catabolic intermediates (e.g., pyruvate) serve as the terminal electron acceptor, and the reduced organic product (e.g., lactate) is excreted into the surrounding medium.

the lactic acid bacteria) lowers the pH of the plant material, and this inhibits growth of plant-decaying microorganisms. Thus, the lactic-acid fermentation of plant materials preserves valuable vegetation so that it may be stored for later use as an animal food source. Other species of lactic acid bacteria grow between the teeth and gums, and produce acid from sugars in the animal's diet; the acid erodes the tooth enamel and causes dental caries. Still other species are opportunistically

pathogenic and may cause soft tissue infections (see Chapter 9, Streptococci).

Other Fermentations. Similar catabolic characteristics for sugars are found in most other fermentations, although the exact metabolic pathways used and the catabolic intermediate that is reduced and excreted vary widely (Table 2-1).

Although the preceding discussion centers on the microbial fermentation of sugars, it should be emphasized that amino acids, fatty acids, purines,

Table 2–1. *End Products Excreted by Microorganisms Fermenting Sugars*

Fermentation Type	Microorganisms*	Products Formed
Lactic acid	*Lactobacillus* *Streptococcus* *Leuconostoc* *Pediococcus* *Sporalactobacillus* *Bifidobacterium*	Lactic, acetic, and formic acids, ethanol, glycerol, diacetyl, acetoin, butanediol, and CO_2
Ethyl alcohol	*Saccharomyces cerevisiae* *Zymomonas* *Sarcinia ventriculi* *Erwinia amylovora*	Mostly ethyl alcohol
Butyric acid and acetone-butanol	*Clostridium butyricum* *C. kluyveri* *C. acetobutylicum* *C. pasteurianum* *C. perfringens* *Neisseria* species *Bacteroides* species *Fusobacterium* species *Eubacterium* species *Butyrivibrio* species	Varying amounts of butyric and acetic acids, butanol, acetone, ethanol, isopropanol, H_2, and CO_2
Mixed acid	*Escherichia, Salmonella, Shigella, Proteus,* and *Klebsiella*	Primarily lactic, acetic, succinic, and formic acids with little H_2, CO_2, and ethanol
Butanediol	*Enterobacter, Serratia, Erwinia, Aeromonas, Bacillus polymyxa,* and *Klebsiella*	Lots of butanediol, with some CO_2, H_2, and ethanol and only slight amounts of mixed acids
Propionic acid	*Propionibacterium* *Clostridium propionicum* *Corynebacterium diphtheriae* *Veillonella* *Neisseria* species	Primarily propionic, acetic, and succinic acids and CO_2

* If the fermentation type appears to be characteristic of the entire genus, the genus name only is given. When characteristic of several species the word "species" is used. If characteristic of only one species, the entire species named is used.

and pyrimidines are also fermented by some microorganisms living in anaerobic environments. Other metabolic pathways are involved, but the same common general characteristics appear in these other fermentations. For example, the proteolytic clostridia produce and excrete enzymes that break down proteins to a size where these short chains of amino acids can enter the cell. Once transported inside, the amino acids are fermented, and malodorous fermentation end-products are usually excreted (e.g., mercaptans, and skatole). The fermentation of dead animal and plant tissue is a necessary part of the decay process, and decay is essential for the recycling of nutrients in our environment!

Respiratory Catabolism

Characteristics. Respiratory catabolism has four common characteristics. First, large quantities of ATP are formed (much more ATP per molecule of energy source than with fermentation), and most of that ATP is formed by a process known as oxidative phosphorylation. A small proportion of ATP is also formed by substrate-level phosphorylation,

just as it is with fermentation, because some of the same catabolic pathways are used. Second, inorganic compounds (such as O_2 or NO_3^-) diffuse into the cell, are used as the terminal electron acceptor, and the reduced inorganic products (such as H_2O or NO_2^-) are excreted into the surrounding medium. Third, many more reduced electron carriers (such as $NADH_2$ and $NADPH_2$) are formed than with fermentative catabolism. Fourth, the organic energy sources used by the cell for catabolism are usually completely oxidized to CO_2 by a cyclic oxidative pathway (such as the TCA cycle).

The following sections will consider (1) the pathways common to respiratory catabolism, (2) how the hydrogens removed during this oxidation are used to make ATP, and (3) the involvement of the electron transport system and the types of terminal electron acceptors used at the end of this system. Glucose catabolism will be used as an example because it occurs in most microbes, and the oxidation of other compounds usually leads into the pathways used for glucose catabolism.

Pathways of Respiratory Catabolism. Respiring microorganisms use one or more of three pathways for the catabolism of glucose to acetyl-coenzyme A: the Embden-Meyerhoff-Parnas (EMP) pathway, the Entner-Doudoroff (ED) pathway, and the hexose-monophosphate (HMP) pathway. In many cases, microbes use either the HMP or the ED pathway along with the HMP pathway to meet the cell's needs. Only rarely is one of these pathways used exclusively. Each of these three pathways oxidizes glucose to acetyl-CoA, then acetyl-CoA is further oxidized by the tricarboxylic acid (TCA) cycle. Therefore, complete oxidation of glucose to CO_2 requires the participation of *either* of the three pathways (EMP, ED, or HMP) *and* the TCA cycle. We will consider how each mechanism serves the cell and meets the four characteristics for respiratory catabolism. For comparative purposes, one molecule of glucose will be completely oxidized to CO_2 for each catabolic sequence.

EMP Pathway Coupled With the TCA Cycle (Fig. 2–8). The EMP pathway is widely distributed among many different types of microorganisms. Perhaps the most important group of bacteria of veterinary significance is the family *Enterobacteriaceae*, which contains genera such as *Escherichia, Enterobacter, Salmonella, Shigella, Klebsiella, Proteus, Yersinia*, and *Serratia*. Note that the EMP pathway shown in Figure 2–8 is essentially identical to that shown for fermentation by the lactic acid bacteria, with one exception: pyruvate is not reduced and excreted as lactic acid. Instead, pyruvate is oxidized further to acetyl-CoA, which in turn enters the TCA cycle. When one glucose molecule is oxidized by the EMP pathway to acetyl-CoA, the following compounds are formed: (1) four molecules of ATP (but two are used in the formation of glucose-1,6-diphosphate, so the net gain is only two molecules of ATP by substrate-level phosphorylation); (2) four molecules of $NADH_2$; (3) two molecules of CO_2 (which are excreted); and (4) two molecules of acetyl-CoA (which individually enter the TCA cycle). So at this point in the catabolism, the cell has started with one six-carbon molecule (glucose), broken off and excreted two one-carbon molecules (CO_2), and two two-carbon molecules (acetyl-CoA) remain for further oxidation through the TCA cycle.

To begin the TCA cycle, the cell must have one molecule of oxalacetate, but notice that a new molecule of oxalacetate is regenerated after each turn, so this initial molecule can be considered "catalytic." Note also that one molecule of acetyl-CoA supports one "turn" of the TCA cycle. One turn of the cycle releases two molecules of CO_2, so two turns of the cycle will complete the oxidation of the glucose molecule and the release of all carbons as CO_2. Two turns of the cycle also produce two molecules

of ATP by substrate-level phosphorylation, so the cell now has a total of four ATPs produced by this method from each glucose molecule. This is twice the number formed by substrate-level phosphorylation when one glucose is oxidized during the lactate fermentation and most other fermentations. In addition, two turns of the cycle also form six molecules of $NADH_2$ and two molecules of $FADH_2$, so the cell has now produced a total of 12 molecules of reduced hydrogen carriers per glucose molecule. This large production of reduced hydrogen carriers is one of the major ways in which cells carrying out a respiratory catabolism differ from fermenting cells. But, before we consider how these hydrogen carriers are used, let's examine the two other major mechanisms of glucose oxidation found in respiring cells.

ED Pathway Coupled With the TCA Cycle. The ED pathway shown in Figure 2–9 is quite different from the EMP pathway. The enzymes supporting this pathway are widely distributed among bacteria; those having veterinary importance are species of *Pseudomonas* and *Alcaligenes*.

When one glucose molecule is oxidized by the ED pathway to acetyl-CoA, glucose is first phosphorylated to glucose-6-phosphate (using one ATP), then oxidized to gluconolactone-6-phosphate, and then it undergoes several enzyme catalyzed rearrangements to form ketodeoxyphosphoglucose (KDPG). Next, KDPG is split by an enzyme into pyruvate and glyceraldehyde-3-phosphate (G-3-P). The G-3-P molecule is then oxidized to pyruvate by the same enzymes used in the lower half of the EMP pathway. Note that this produces two molecules of pyruvate, both of which may be oxidized to acetyl-CoA.

When one glucose molecule is oxidized by the ED pathway to two molecules of acetyl-CoA, the following compounds are formed: (1) two molecules of ATP are formed during the oxidation of glyceraldehyde-3-phosphate, but one ATP is used in the formation of glucose-6-phosphate, so the net gain is only one ATP by substrate-level phosphorylation; (2) four molecules of $NADH_2$; (3) two molecules of CO_2 that are excreted; and (4) two molecules of acetyl-CoA that individually enter the TCA cycle. Therefore, the net gain up to that point is very similar to that achieved by the EMP pathway, except that the ED pathway produces two less ATPs per molecule of glucose.

Just as with oxidation of glucose by the EMP pathway and the TCA cycle, oxidation of one molecule of glucose by the ED pathway will produce two molecules of acetyl-CoA, and these will support two turns of the TCA cycle. Two turns of

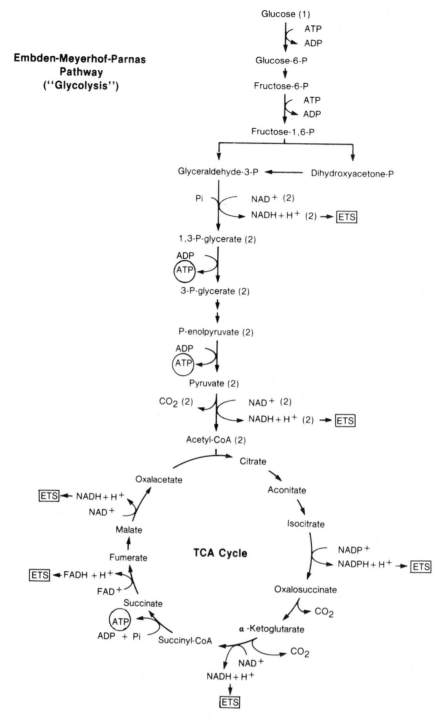

Figure 2–8. Respiratory catabolism of glucose to acetyl-CoA by the Embden-Meyerhof-Parnas (EMP) pathway and further catabolism of acetyl-CoA to CO_2 by the tricarboxylic acid (TCA) cycle. Note how oxidation of glucose through the EMP pathway and TCA cycle illustrates the four characteristics common to all respiratory catabolism (see text).

the cycle will produce four molecules of CO_2, two molecules of ATP, and eight molecules of reduced hydrogen carriers. Thus, cells using the ED pathway and TCA cycle have a net gain of three ATPs produced by substrate-level phosphorylation and 12 reduced hydrogen carriers coming from the

complete oxidation of one molecule of glucose to CO_2. In comparison with the EMP + TCA system, the ED pathway coupled with the TCA cycle produces only one fewer ATP and the same number of reduced hydrogen carriers. Remember that respiring cells may use these reduced hydrogen car-

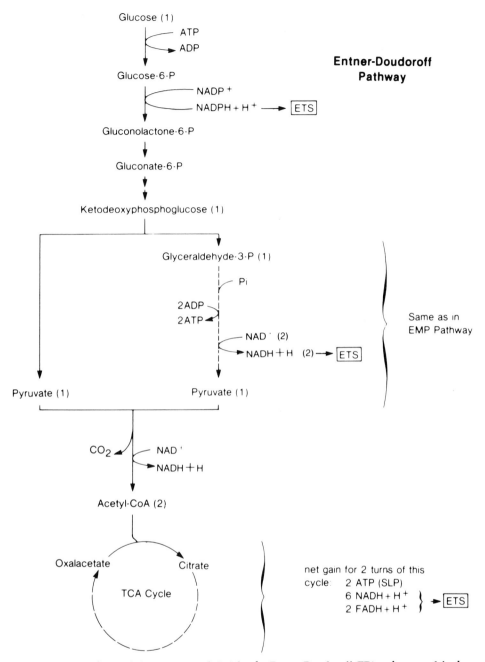

Figure 2–9. Respiratory catabolism of glucose to acetyl-CoA by the Entner-Doudoroff (ED) pathway and further catabolism of the acetyl-CoA to CO_2 by the tricarboxylic acid (TCA) cycle. Note how oxidation of glucose through the ED pathway and TCA cycle illustrates the four characteristics common to all respiratory catabolism (see text).

riers to produce many more ATP molecules by using a process known as oxidative phosphorylation. But, before we examine that process, let's comparatively examine the third major type of oxidative pathway used by cells carrying out a respiratory catabolism of glucose.

HMP Pathway Coupled With the TCA Cycle. It is well known that the HMP pathway, shown in Figure 2–10, is used to form the five-carbon sugar called ribose, which is a precursor in the formation of all nucleic acids and one amino acid. The HMP pathway also produces the four-carbon sugar

erythrose, which is a precursor for the synthesis of the aromatic family of amino acids in bacteria. Thus, the HMP pathway serves at least as a synthetic (anabolic) pathway in most bacteria. In addition, the HMP pathway appears to serve a catabolic function for many bacteria, particularly when growing in an aerobic environment. According to some research, facultative microorganisms growing on sugars shift from the EMP pathway (without the TCA cycle) to the HMP + TCA pathway when their extracellular environment goes from the absence to the presence of oxygen.

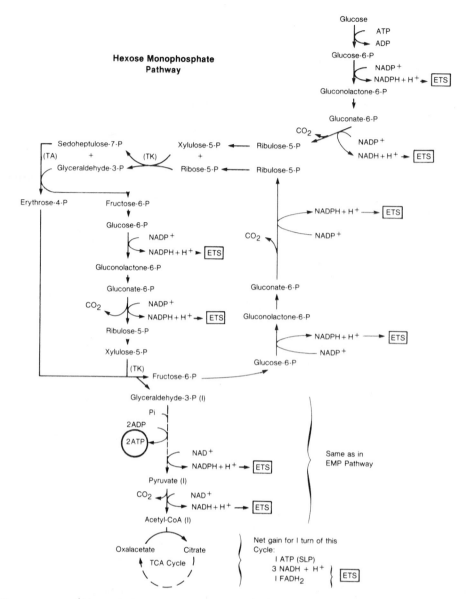

Figure 2–10. Respiratory catabolism of glucose to acetyl-CoA by the hexose monophosphate pathway (HMP) and further catabolism of the acetyl-CoA to CO_2 by the tricarboxylic acid (TCA) cycle. Note how oxidation of glucose through the HMP pathway and TCA cycle illustrates the four characteristics common to all respiratory catabolism (see text).

The oxidative HMP pathway may, for the sake of discussion, be divided into three parts: formation of ribulose-5-phosphate, the pentose-phosphate cycle, and oxidation of glyceraldehyde-3-phosphate to acetyl-CoA (Fig. 2–10).

In the first part of the HMP pathway, glucose (a six-carbon sugar or hexose) is first phosphorylated and then oxidatively decarboxylated to ribulose-5-phosphate (a five-carbon sugar or pentose). This accomplishes three things: (1) it produces two reduced hydrogen carriers ($NADPH_2$); (2) it breaks off and excretes one molecule of CO_2; and (3) it forms the pentose called ribulose-5-phosphate, which continues on into the pentose-phosphate cycle.

The pentose-phosphate cycle is the second part of the HMP pathway. To start this cycle, assume that the cell has one catalytic molecule of ribose-5-phosphate (R-5-P), just as we assumed that the TCA cycle began with one catalytic molecule of oxalacetate. An enzyme called transketolase (TK) reacts with the two pentoses (xylulose-5-phosphate [X-5-P] and R-5-P), transfers part of one to the other, and forms a seven-carbon and a three-carbon molecule. The products of this reaction are acted upon by an enzyme called transaldolase (TA) to produce a four-carbon sugar (erythrose-4-phosphate) and a six-carbon sugar (fructose-6-phosphate). Note here that the fructose-6-phosphate (F-6-P) is then oxidized to X-5-P in the same way described for the first part of the HMP, and this process accomplishes the same three things: release of one more CO_2, production of two more $NADPH_2$'s, and formation of X-5-P. The X-5-P and erythrose-4-phosphate are converted to F-6-P and glyceraldehyde-3-phosphate (G-3-P). Once again, the F-6-P is converted to glucose-6-phosphate, which is then oxidized to X-5-P in the same way described for the first part of the HMP, and, once again, the cell produces two more $NADPH_2$'s, releases one more CO_2, and forms R-5-P. Formation of R-5-P completes the cycle, and regenerates the R-5-P required to react with the X-5-P that starts the cycle over again. Thus, one turn of the pentose-phosphate cycle accomplishes four major things: (1) it releases two molecules of CO_2; (2) it yields four molecules of $NADPH_2$; (3) it produces one molecule of glyceraldehyde-3-phosphate that can be oxidized further; and (4) it regenerates the catalytic molecule of R-5-P.

Oxidation of glyceraldehyde-3-phosphate (G-3-P) to acetyl-CoA can be considered the third and final part of the HMP pathway. One G-3-P molecule is formed from one turn of the pentose-phosphate cycle, and this is oxidized to one molecule of acetyl-CoA using the same enzymes used by the EMP and ED pathways.

When one glucose molecule is oxidized by the HMP pathway to one molecule of acetyl-CoA, the following compounds are formed: (1) two molecules of ATP (during the oxidation of one glyceraldehyde-3-phosphate to pyruvate), but one ATP is used in forming glucose-6-phosphate (in the first part of the HMP pathway), so the net gain is only one ATP (by substrate-level phosphorylation); (2) eight molecules of reduced hydrogen carrier (two from part one, four from part two, and two from part three of the HMP); (3) four molecules of CO_2 that are excreted; and (4) one molecule of acetyl-CoA (which enters the TCA cycle). Therefore, the net gain in ATP production by the HMP pathway is similar to that of the EMP and identical to that produced with the ED pathway. On the other hand, there are twice as many reduced hydrogen carriers produced by the HMP and twice as many molecules of CO_2 released by the HMP compared with the EMP and ED pathways. Note, however, that there is only one acetyl-CoA formed by the HMP pathway, so that only one turn of the TCA cycle is supported per glucose oxidized by the HMP pathway.

This one turn of the TCA cycle will produce only two molecules of CO_2, one molecule of ATP, and four molecules of reduced hydrogen carrier. Thus, cells using the HMP pathway and TCA cycle to completely oxidize glucose to CO_2 have a net gain of two ATPs, produced by substrate-level phosphorylation, and 12 reduced hydrogen carriers.

One can see, therefore, that all three pathways for respiratory catabolism of glucose (EMP + TCA, ED + TCA, and HMP + TCA) have very similar gains both in ATP (from substrate-level phosphorylation) and in reduced hydrogen carriers.

One of the important features of respiratory catabolism, when compared with fermentative catabolism, is the large number of reduced hydrogen carriers produced. It is the ability to produce and efficiently use these reduced hydrogen carriers that allows respiratory catabolism to be so much more energy-efficient than fermentative catabolism. Let us now examine how respiring cells use these reduced hydrogen carriers.

Electron Transport Coupled with Oxidative Phosphorylation. Molecules such as NAD^+, $NADP^+$, and FAD^+ are called *hydrogen carriers* because they carry the hydrogens removed during oxidation of the cell's carbon and energy source such as glucose. These hydrogens are composed of a hydrogen nucleus (H^+), also called a proton, and an electron (e^-), which contains much energy. One important way in which the energy in these hydrogens (electrons) is used is the process called electron transport (Fig. 2–11). The NAD^+ and $NADP^+$ molecules are soluble and found inside the cell. Once reduced, these carriers interact with a series of catalytic proteins in the plasma membrane called the electron-transport system (ETS). The hydrogens (containing their high-energy electrons) are passed from the $NAD(P)H_2$ to the first membrane protein of the ETS, and then either the hydrogens or electrons are sequentially passed from one protein to the next in sort of a bucket-brigade process.

The type of proteins found in the electron-transport chains of respiring microorganisms vary greatly, depending upon the type of microorganism and the conditions of growth. Perhaps the most common types (listed in the approximate order that they accept hydrogens or electrons in the ETS) are flavins (flavoproteins); quinones (quinoproteins); and b-type, c-type, a-type, o-type, and d-type cytochromes. As the electrons are passed along the ETS chain, it appears that much of their energy is used to create a proton gradient across the plasma membrane (see the earlier section entitled Mechanisms of Transport). The electrons used to reduce the final electron acceptor of the ETS contain no more usable energy, so they are given to an inorganic molecule such as oxygen. This inorganic molecule is called the terminal electron ac-

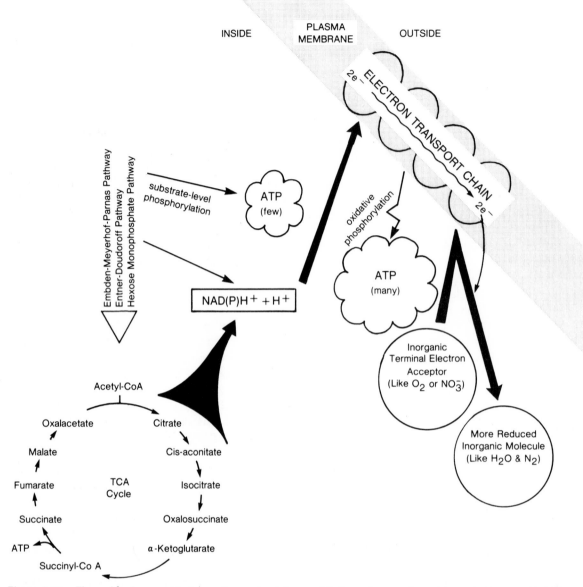

Figure 2–11. Flow of hydrogens (electrons plus protons) from catabolic pathways of respiring organisms to $NAD(P)^+$ and through the electron transport system (ETS), also called the electron transport chain. After passing through the ETS, the energy-weak electrons (e^-) combine with protons (H^+) to reduce the inorganic terminal electron acceptor. An important consequence of this electron flow during respiratory catabolism is the large amount of ATP produced by oxidative phosphorylation. The type of electron flow and ATP production is characteristic to all types of respiratory catabolism (see Fig. 2–12).

ceptor, because its function is to accept the energy-weak electron at the terminus of the ETS. The product of that final reduction (e.g., H_2O for aerobic respiration) is discarded by the cell as a waste product.

It is now believed that part of the energy in the proton gradient, which is established by cells carrying out respiratory catabolism, is used to form new molecules of ATP by a mechanism known as oxidative phosphorylation. The way in which a proton gradient is used to accomplish oxidative

phosphorylation is schematically illustrated in Figure 2–12 and described in the following way. Reduced hydrogen carriers, such as $NAD(P)H_2$, give hydrogen atoms to the first electron-transport protein, such as a flavoprotein (FP). The FP accepts two hydrogen atoms ($2H^+ + 2e^-$), but it passes along only the electrons to the next protein, which is an iron/sulfur-containing protein (Fe/S). The two protons ($2H^+$) are released on the outside surface of the cell's plasma membrane. The two electrons now on the reduced Fe/S protein have slightly less

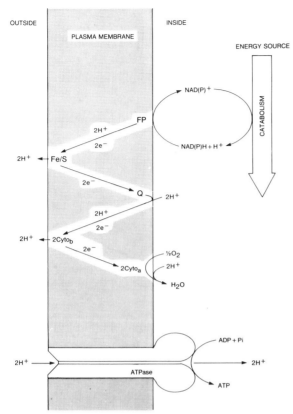

Figure 2–12. Production of a proton gradient as a consequence of electron transport resulting from respiratory catabolism, and the use of protons from that gradient to drive ATP synthesis. This mechanism of ATP formation is called oxidative phosphorylation.

energy, and these weaker electrons are next given to a quinoprotein (Q). Since the quinoprotein is able to carry hydrogen atoms, it picks up protons from the inner surface of the plasma membrane, and two complete hydrogen atoms are carried to cytochrome-*b*. However, cytochrome-*b* is able to carry only one electron, so it takes two of these cytochromes to carry these two electrons. The two protons ($2H^+$) are placed on the outside surface of the cell's plasma membrane.

The two electrons now carried by the two cytochrome-*b* molecules have slightly less energy. These two weaker electrons are next given to two terminal cytochromes (the cytochrome oxidases). These reduced cytochromes give these two energy-weak electrons to two protons and an atom of oxygen to form water. Thus, oxygen serves as the terminal electron acceptor and functions in trapping these weak electrons in a molecule (water) that can easily diffuse from the cell. In addition, electron transport has established a proton gradient (higher outside) across the plasma membrane.

An enzyme called ATPase also resides within the cell's plasma membrane. One function of this

enzyme is to catalyze the phosphorylation of ADP to form ATP (Fig. 2–12). Strong evidence now suggests that this energy-requiring reaction obtains the needed energy from the proton gradient. Because it took energy to establish the proton gradient (energy coming from high-energy electrons), use of this gradient yields energy. It now appears that two protons pass into the cell through the ATPase protein, and that this proton flow releases enough energy to phosphorylate ADP. Note in Figure 2–12 that the flow of one pair of electrons down this theoretical electron transport chain causes the translocation of two pairs of protons, so the flow of one pair of electrons through this bacterial ETS could conceivably support the generation of two molecules of ATP.

This type of ATP generation is referred to as "oxidative phosphorylation," and is a very important part of respiratory catabolism. This is the way in which the energy in the hydrogens removed from the nutrient serving as the cell's carbon and energy source are converted to a form that can be used in synthesizing new cell materials (ATP). Note, however, that oxygen is not required by all microorganisms that carry out oxidative phosphorylation as part of respiratory catabolism.

Terminal Electron Acceptors for Anaerobic Respiration. Although O_2 appears to be the most common terminal electron acceptor for the oxidation of $NAD(P)H_2$ by electron transport systems, a few microorganisms can use other types of inorganic terminal electron acceptors. This is still part of the process known as respiratory catabolism, but the use of acceptors other than O_2 is called anaerobic respiration. Some of these alternative terminal electron acceptors are part of a system that generates ATP by oxidative phosphorylation; among these are nitrate (NO^-_3), nitrite (NO^-_2), sulfate (SO^{2-}_4), and fumarate (an intermediate of the TCA cycle).

Many types of bacteria reduce nitrate if oxygen is not available, but they prefer to use O_2 as a terminal electron acceptor. These microbes are only capable of respiratory catabolism. Some reduce nitrate to nitrite and release the latter into the surrounding medium; other bacteria will continue to reduce nitrite to nitrous oxide and then reduce nitrous oxide to dinitrogen (N_2), which escapes into the atmosphere. If reduction goes all the way to N_2, this microbial process is called denitrification because it accounts for the loss of agriculturally important nitrates from the soil.

A few bacteria use sulfate as a terminal electron acceptor and reduce it to hydrogen sulfide (H_2S). Most, if not all, of these sulfate-reducing bacteria are strict anaerobes, because they are unable to alter the toxic forms of oxygen. These bacteria are often found in anaerobic muds and account for the black color and rotten-egg smell when these muds are disturbed. They play a significant part in the microbial degradation of plant tissue.

A wide variety of bacteria, under anaerobic conditions, are able to use fumarate (a TCA cycle intermediate) as a terminal electron acceptor at the end of an ETS, and they form succinate as the reduced product. This ability has been reported in *Escherichia coli* as well as in some clostridia and in *Vibrio succinogenes*, *Desulfovibrio gigas*, and *Proteus rettgeri*.

Although it is presently debated, evidence exists that CO_2 may also serve as a terminal electron acceptor for microbial electron transport chains that accomplish oxidative phosphorylation. The product of CO_2 reduction is methane (CH_4), and the microbes that accomplish this are called methanogens or methanogenic bacteria. Even though quinones and cytochromes are not found in the methanogen's plasma membrane, the membrane does contain a recently discovered type of electron carrier called F_{420}, and this may participate in an ETS that results in oxidative phosphorylation. The methanogens are widely distributed in extremely anaerobic environments such as mud, the intestinal tract, the rumen, and anaerobic digestors of sewage-treatment plants. Ruminant animals are of particular interest, because they establish a mutualistic relationship with microorganisms. Although these animals are herbivores, they cannot produce the enzyme cellulase but rather depend upon the microbes within the rumen to break down the cellulose. Various anaerobic microorganisms within the rumen convert cellulose, starch, and other polysaccharides to low-molecular-weight organic acids, CO_2, and H_2. The organic acids formed (such as acetate, propionate, and butyrate) are quickly absorbed through the wall of the rumen and enter the bloodstream, where they are oxidized aerobically by the animal to produce ATP that supports the animal's energy requirements. The methanogens appear to autotrophically use hydrogen (produced in large and otherwise toxic quantities by other microorganisms) as their primary energy (high-energy electron) source in the rumen, and they use CO_2 (produced by other microbes) as their terminal electron acceptor, resulting in CH_4 (methane) as the reduced product. The ruminant then rids itself of methane by belching.

Although not a predominant form of catabolism, anaerobic respiration does play an important role in the cycling of nutrients within our ecosystem.

Anabolism

Anabolism (biosynthesis) is the second major part of metabolism. Unlike catabolism, anabolism is the building up of reduced organic molecules, ultimately resulting in the formation of a new cell. Anabolism requires energy in the form of ATP and hydrogens (attached to reduced hydrogen carriers) that result from catabolic pathways (see Figure 2–6). In addition, anabolism requires building blocks that are provided either extracellularly as nutrients or are formed intracellularly as intermediates of catabolic pathways. The term building block refers to the starting materials from which cellular polymers are made, such as amino acids, fatty acids, purines, pyrimidines, and sugars. If their presence is not required in the medium as an essential nutrient, this means that the microbe can make that building block from intermediates resulting from catabolism of the carbon source.

Let us assume that we are working with a bacterium capable of growing in a medium containing only glucose and inorganic sources of nitrogen, phosphorus, and sulfur plus smaller quantities of other mineral salts. Since glucose is the only carbon source available to the cell, this means that all cellular polymers must be made from intermediates formed during the catabolism of glucose. It now appears that most microorganisms, whether or not they are pathogens, use similar if not identical catabolic intermediates to form these building blocks.

Many gram-negative enteric bacteria are capable of using both the EMP and the HMP pathways coupled with the TCA cycle to carry out respiratory catabolism. In the absence of a terminal electron acceptor, the TCA-cycle enzymes no longer function as a cyclic pathway, but most of these enzymes continue to produce the catabolic intermediates that are essential for biosynthetic pathways. Figure 2–13 schematically shows the EMP and HMP pathways with the TCA cycle and indicates which catabolic intermediates commonly produce building blocks for each cellular polymer.

Note that in an actively growing microorganism, a pathway like EMP + TCA cycle does not function solely for catabolism or energy production. One molecule of glucose may indeed be entirely oxidized to CO_2, but the next molecule of glucose may be oxidized only so far as pyruvate and from there it may support synthesis of the amino acid alanine and ultimately the synthesis of proteins. Therefore, the "catabolism" of glucose appears to be a dynamic process that supports both the cell's need for energy and its need to produce building blocks for biosynthesis.

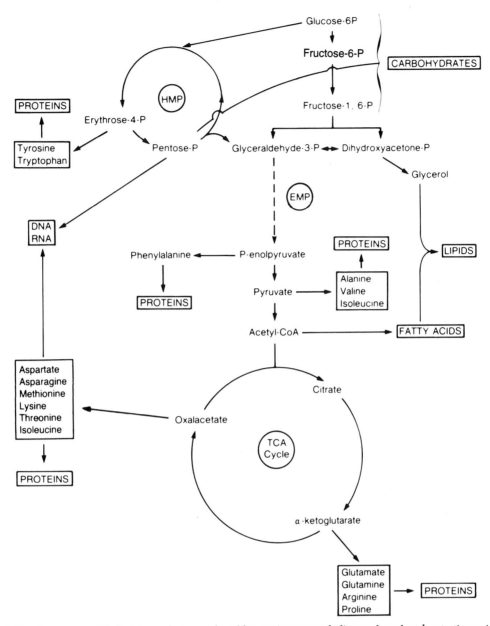

Figure 2–13. Common metabolic intermediates produced by respiratory catabolism and used as the starting point for anabolic (biosynthetic) pathways. Note that anabolism is often considered in two stages: (1) pathways for the production of building blocks (e.g., amino acids) from catabolic intermediates, and (2) mechanisms for the proper covalent bonding of these building blocks into polymers (e.g., proteins).

The ultimate function or consequence of biosynthesis is growth, or, as microbiologists define growth, the production of new cells. All cells are composed of four types of polymers: protein, lipid, RNA, and DNA. Synthesis of the building blocks to support construction of these polymers and the polymerization process itself requires the expenditure of large quantities of energy. About 70% of the dry weight of the *Escherichia coli* cell is protein, and it is estimated that about 88% of all energy obtained from glucose catabolism goes into making the cell's protein. In comparison, these same bacteria contain only about 10% RNA, 10% lipid, 5% polysaccharide, and 5% DNA, and the remaining 12% of the energy gained from glucose oxidation is used to support the synthesis of those polymers.

ESTABLISHMENT AND GROWTH OF PURE CULTURES

Pure Culture Isolation

The establishment and maintenance of pure cultures are absolute requirements of a microbiologist who wishes to study the characteristics of one type of microorganism. Indeed, Koch's postulates require the use of pure cultures in establishing the cause and effect relationship between a microorganism and an infection. In nature, however, pure cultures are rare. Therefore, a microbiologist spends considerable amounts of time and energy purifying single types of microorganisms from the environment. Sometimes this may be accomplished simply by physically separating (streaking or spreading) the culture on the surface of a general-purpose medium. Many times, however, other microbes will grow faster and outcompete the suspected pathogen on such a medium; or the suspected pathogen may be present in such small numbers that it would never appear as an isolated colony on a streak or spread plate. This common situation requires the use of either a selective medium or an enrichment culture to isolate the suspected pathogen.

Selective Media. An ideal selective medium is one that will preferentially grow only one type of microorganism. One must first determine the type of microbe that is suspected, then choose a medium that will both encourage the growth of the suspected pathogen and inhibit the growth of all other organisms common to that environment. In order to choose a satisfactory selective medium for that microbe's growth, one must make sure that all the cell's nutritional requirements are supplied by that medium. Then one can select the type of inhibitory agent that will prevent the growth of the other microbial competitors.

There are many kinds of selective media, but most employ some chemical agent that is added to the growth medium. To be selective, the organism you wish to isolate (i.e., the suspected pathogen) must be resistant to that chemical agent, and the organisms whose growth you wish to inhibit (i.e., the normal flora) must be susceptible to that chemical agent. Antibiotics, dyes, detergents, and sodium chloride are commonly used chemical agents for the selective growth inhibition of unwanted microbes. If a medium contains a substance like blood or an acid-base indicator that only certain types of microbes will respond to in a characteristic way, it is called a differential medium, because it allows one to visually differentiate between types of microorganisms.

Sometimes a medium may be both differential and selective. For example, a medium may contain blood (to differentially detect α- and β-hemolysis produced by streptococcal colonies) as well as an antibiotic (that will selectively inhibit growth of other gram-positive cocci).

Occasionally a physical agent (like high temperature) is used in combination with chemical agents to selectively allow the growth of one type and inhibit most others. For example, selective growth of enteropathogenic *Escherichia coli* is accomplished by using a temperature of 44.5° C and a medium that contains a detergent and a dye along with the required nutrients (Difco m-FC medium).

When microbiologists use the term selective medium they generally are referring to a solid medium contained in a Petri dish or test tube. These are usually inoculated with a loop or a small volume of liquid. Therefore, the microbe one is searching for must be present within that small volume. This is not always the case. Sometimes larger volumes must be examined for the suspected microorganism, and this is the purpose of enrichment culture.

Enrichment Culture. This culturing technique is used for the growth of microbes that are present in very small numbers and may represent only a very small proportion of all types of microorganisms present in a mixed culture. Usually, a relatively large volume (from 1 to 10 ml) is inoculated into a type of broth that provides a selective environment favoring the growth of one kind of microorganism. For example, one often enriches for *Shigella* species with GN-Hajna broth, *Salmonella* species with selenite broth, and fluorescent *Pseudomonas* species with asparagine broth. The types of chemicals added to these broths to make them selective, however, are often identical to those used in "selective agars." The purpose of both selective agars and enrichment broths is to enable the microbiologist to isolate a particular type of microbe so that it may be purified and studied.

Determination of Culture Purity. A pure culture is defined as one that contains cells of only one type. One can attain this by microscopic separation and subsequent cultivation of a single cell, but this method is extremely time-consuming and usually impractical. Perhaps the most practical method for obtaining a pure culture is the streak plate. Using this method, one can theoretically start with a mixed culture and physically spread this over the surface of a solid medium until each cell is physically separated from all others. Upon incubation, each cell will grow and form a colony of macroscopic size. If a colony results from the growth of a single cell, then it is a pure culture by definition.

From a practical standpoint, however, many microorganisms adhere tightly to other cells. For example, some cells produce extracellular (capsular) material. Capsular material is adhesive, and this property allows the producing cell to stick to other things such as its own progeny, solid surfaces in its environment, or cells of another type. Therefore, the appearance of a well-isolated colony is no absolute guarantee that it arose from a single cell.

On the other hand, a pure culture obtained by the streak-plate method is considered adequate in the clinical or diagnostic microbiology laboratory if it meets two criteria: (1) all cells from that culture should have the same size, shape, and Gram reaction; and (2) all subsequent streak plates should exhibit colonies of the same type. It is important, therefore, to Gram stain and streak single colonies several times to make sure they are pure.

Bacterial Growth Characteristics

Biological growth is generally defined as an increase in size or mass. However, because of the small size of the bacterial cell and the inability to determine the dry weight of a single cell, this general definition for growth of multicellular organisms is not practical for the bacteriologist. When referring to growth, the bacteriologist usually means an increase in cell numbers.

For bacterial numbers to increase, the medium must have the minimum number of essential nutrients, and the environment surrounding the medium must provide the minimum physical conditions for growth of that cell type. Both the rate of growth and the final numbers achieved at the end of growth will increase when any one of the following conditions is raised above minimum levels: the concentration of any one essential nutrient; the temperature; and the concentration of oxygen (unless the bacterium is microaerophilic or strictly anaerobic). Also, growth rate and final numbers will often increase with the addition of non-essential nutrients, because cells prefer to use environmentally supplied nutrients instead of making their own.

On the other hand, the rate of growth will either decrease or stop when nonessential or essential nutrients are depleted; when waste products accumulate to toxic levels; or when the concentration of heat, hydrogen ions, or oxygen (for some) is lowered below optimal levels. The same conditions that slow or stop microbial growth may also cause cell death.

The factors mentioned previously that increase growth rates and final population density or cell viability appear to exert these effects regardless of whether bacteria are growing on solid or liquid media.

Growth in Liquid Media. When a small number of cells from a pure culture are inoculated into a liquid medium (broth), the cells exhibit a charac-

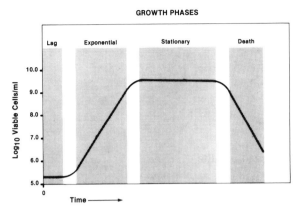

Figure 2–14. The four characteristic phases of microbial growth that occur when cells are transferred to a liquid medium in a closed container. Note that the lag phase may be eliminated if exponentially growing cells are transferred into an identical medium.

teristic growth curve that can be thought of in four phases (Fig. 2–14). Note that Figure 2–14 shows the change in the logarithm of viable cell numbers versus time.

During the lag phase, cells are shifting their metabolism so that they will be able to grow on the new medium. There are two important characteristics of the lag phase: (1) cells are rapidly making new DNA and RNA and inducing the synthesis of new enzymes needed for cell division, and thus there is a great deal of metabolic activity (including synthesis) taking place; but (2) as shown in Figure 2–14, there is no increase in cell numbers. The initiation of cell division marks the transition between the lag phase and the exponential growth phase.

During the exponential growth phase, cell division occurs at a maximum rate for the growth conditions provided by that medium and those environmental conditions. This is called the exponential phase, because cell numbers are increasing (doubling) at an exponential rate. In other words, the logarithm of the cell numbers increases linearly with time.

The rate of cell division during exponential growth is often called the doubling time. This is the time that it takes for one doubling in cell numbers. The doubling time of any culture is affected greatly by the environmental (nutritional and physical) conditions provided. The doubling time is also affected by the cell's genetic ability to carry out efficient catabolic and anabolic pathways; therefore, growth rates are often characteristic of microbial cultures. For example, *Escherichia coli* has a doubling time of about 20 minutes in nonsynthetic media under optimal conditions, whereas the doubling time of *Mycobacterium tuberculosis* may be as long as 24 hours in nonsynthetic media under optimal conditions.

This rate of cell division does not continue indefinitely, however. A test tube, flask, or plate is a closed system; that is, each contains a limited amount of medium enclosed within a vessel. Eventually, the cells may run out of nutrients, or cellular waste products may build up to toxic levels, or the population density may become so great that the rate of diffusion of nutrients between cells becomes limiting. When the rate of cell division slows below exponential levels, the cells make a transition from exponential growth to the stationary phase.

In the stationary phase, there is no net increase or decrease in cell numbers. What happens depends upon the bacterial type. Some appear to just stop growing but fully maintain their viability. Others appear to reach a state in which the rate of new cell formation is exactly equal to the rate of cell death. Regardless of the cause, the effect is always a lack of change in viable numbers. The length of this phase varies greatly among the bacteria. Eventually, there is an initiation of death or an increase in the rate of death, and this marks the transition between the stationary phase and death phase.

During the death phase, the rate of cell death in the population is exponential. On the other hand, the rate of death is not always equal to the rate of growth of the same population. It is also important to point out that cell death is defined as the loss of a cell's ability to form a colony when transferred to a plate. This does not necessarily mean that cells have lost their ability to carry out metabolism and affect their environment.

Growth on Solid Media. Growth of microorganisms on the surface of a solid medium follows the same growth characteristics shown in Figure 2–14. However, cells usually cannot become as widely dispersed as in a liquid medium, so they remain tightly packed together in a colony after many divisions. Under these conditions, nutrient diffusion rapidly becomes limiting, especially at the center of the developing colony, and those cells rapidly reach the stationary phase. However, at the colony's edge, cells continue to grow exponentially even while those at the center are in the death phase.

For reasons that are not clearly understood, bacterial colonies usually do not continue to expand indefinitely across the surface of a plate. Instead, a mature colony composed of the same type of bacteria has a well-defined edge, an elevation, a texture, and light-absorbing or light-transmitting properties that are characteristic of that bacterial type. Note, however, that these characteristics vary considerably from one type of growth medium to another; this is in part a result of differences in metabolism and changes in quantity and type of materials excreted from cells.

FURTHER READING

Brock, T.D., Madigan, M.T., Martinko, J.M., and Parker, J.: Biology of Microorganisms. 7th Ed. Englewood Cliffs, NJ, Prentice-Hall, 1994.

Gerhardt, P., et al. (eds.): Manual of Methods for General Bacteriology. Washington, D.C., American Society for Microbiology, 1981.

Neidhardt, F.C., Ingraham, J.L., and Schaechter, M.: Physiology of the Bacterial Cell: A molecular approach. Sunderland, MA, Sinauer Associates, 1990.

Pelczar, M.J., Jr., Chan, E.C.S., and Krieg, N.R.: Microbiology: Concepts and applications. New York, McGraw-Hill, Inc., 1993.

PLATE 1—BACTERIA

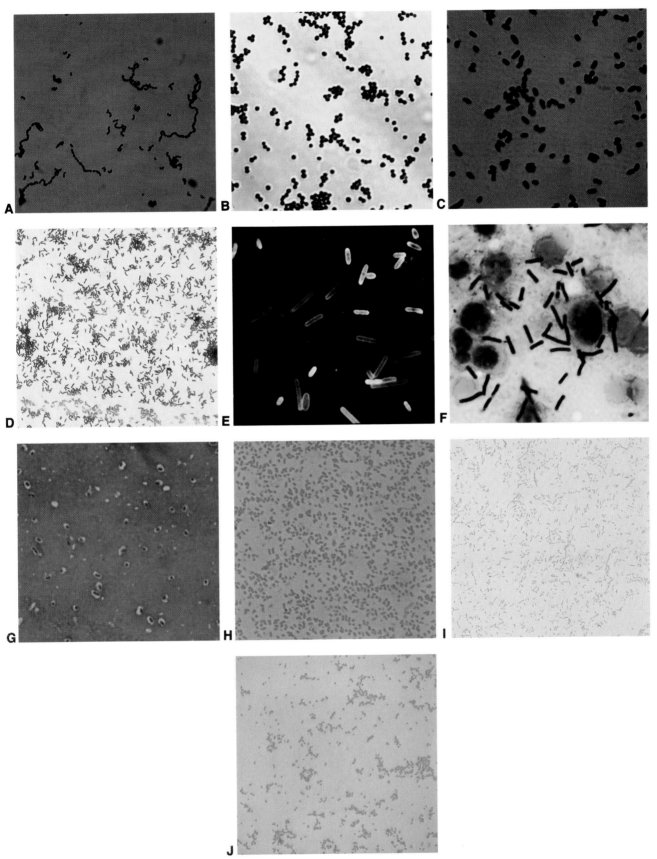

A. Gram-stained smear showing characteristic streptococcal chains of cocci. B. Gram-stained smear showing gram-positive cocci in clusters and short chains. C. Gram-stained smear of *Rhodococcus equi* showing characteristic, somewhat ovoid rods. D. Gram-stained smear of *Listeria monocytogenes* showing small gram-positive rods. E. Fluorescent antibody stain (fluorescein and rhodamine) of *Clostridium septicum* (yellow-green) and *C. chauvoei* (coral). Courtesy of Irene Batty. F. Gram-stained smear of *Bacillus anthracis* showing large, square-ended, gram-positive rods. G. Capsule stain of *Klebsiella pneumoniae*. Bacteria appear dark within a clear envelope. H. Gram-stained smear of *Pasteurella haemolytica* showing small rods and coccobacilli. I. Gram-stained smear of *Campylobacter fetus* showing weak-staining, characteristic pleomorphic forms. J. Gram-stained smear of *Moraxella bovis* showing small rods and coccobacilli.

PLATE 2—BACTERIA

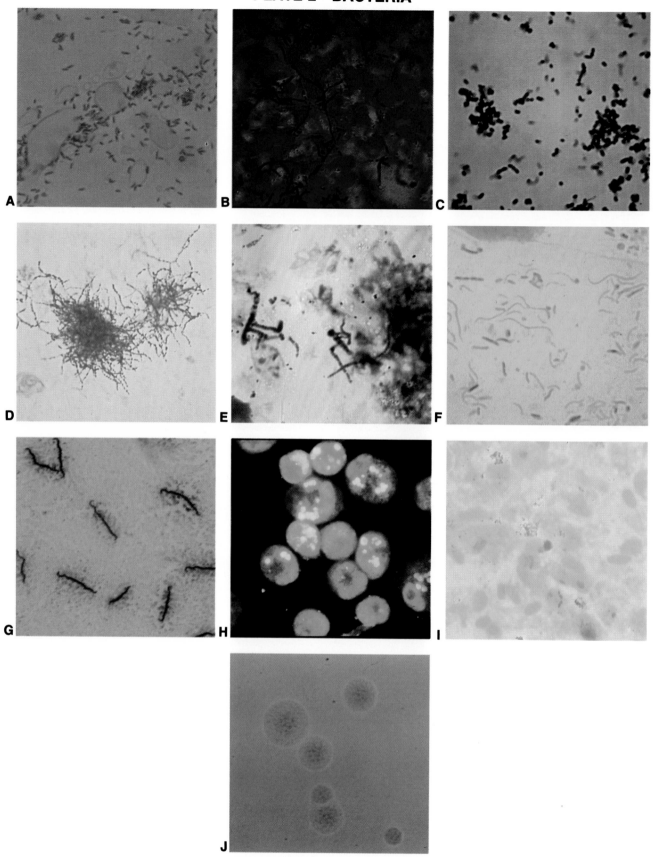

A. Small rods of *Mycobacterium paratuberculosis*. Acid-fast stain (Ziehl-Neelsen). **B.** Smear of *Actinomyces bovis* showing characteristic short and long forms. Gram stain. **C.** Gram-positive, pleomorphic forms of *Actinomyces pyogenes*. **D.** Smear showing the partially acid-fast forms of *Nocardia asteroides*. Modified Ziehl-Neelsen stain. **E.** Characteristic segmenting forms of *Dermatophilus congolensis*. Gram stain. **F.** Gram-stained fecal smear showing weak-staining, loosely coiled, short and long forms of *Serpulina hyodysenteriae*. **G.** *Leptospira pomona*. Fontana's silver stain. **H.** *Ehrlichia canis* in macrophages. Fluorescent antibody stain. **I.** Smear showing small, pink-staining forms of *Chlamydia psittaci*. Macchiavello's stain. **J.** *Mycoplasma* colonies showing characteristic fried-egg appearance. Unstained, low power.

PLATE 3—FUNGI

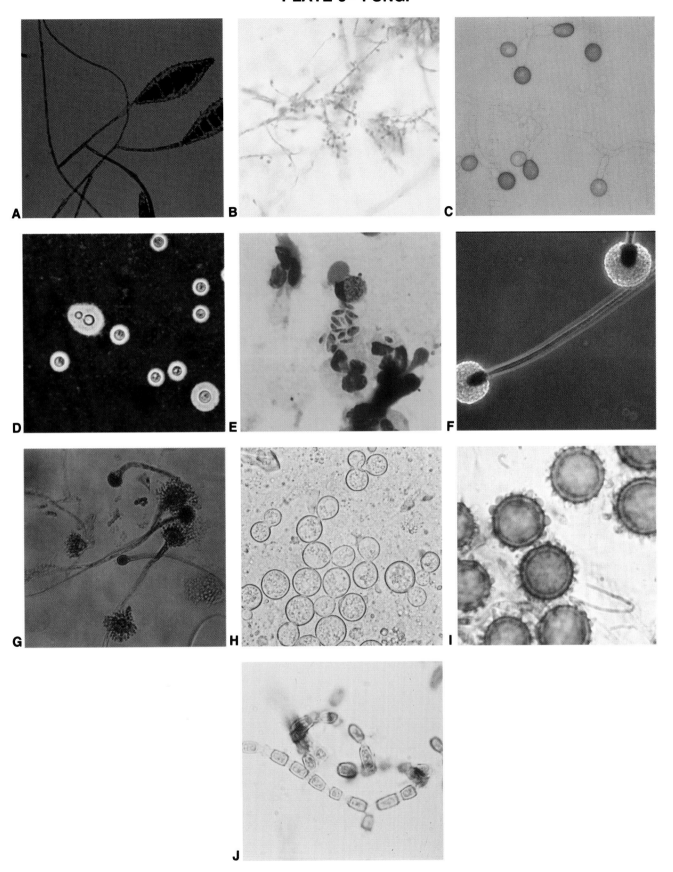

A. Macroconidia of *Microsporum canis.* Lactophenol cotton blue stain. **B.** Typical microconidia of *Trichophyton mentagrophytes.* Lactophenol cotton blue stain. **C.** Chlamydospores and pseudohyphae of *Candida albicans.* Lactophenol cotton blue stain. **D.** Large capsules of *Cryptococcus neoformans.* India ink preparation. **E.** Yeast forms ("cigar-bodies") of *Sporothrix schenkii* in a smear from a cat. Giemsa stain. **F.** Sporangia of a young *Mucor* culture borne on sporangiophores. Lactophenol cotton blue stain. **G.** Conidia of *Aspergillus fumigatus* attached to sterigmata that have arisen from a vesicle. **H.** Yeast forms of *Blastomyces dermatitidis* in lesion exudate. Unstained. **I.** Characteristic tuberculate (cockleburr) chlamydospores of *Histoplasma capsulatum.* **J.** Mycelial phase of *Coccidioides immitis* showing thick-walled, barrel-shaped arthrospores.

PLATE 4—VIRUSES

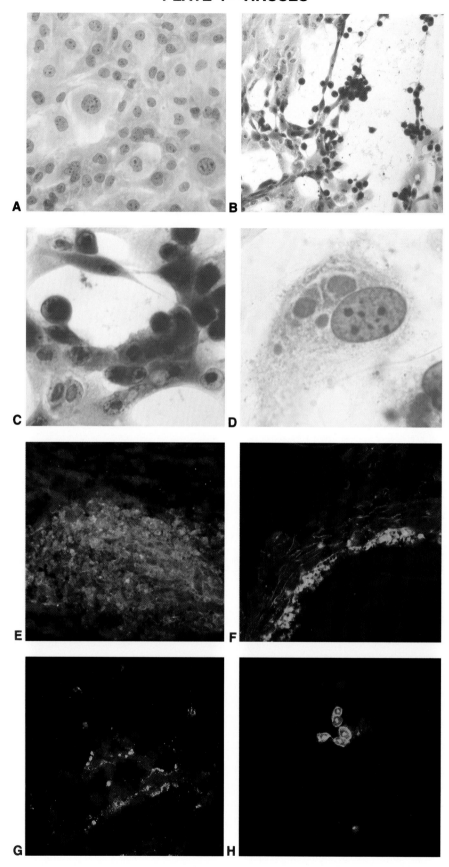

A. Normal cell culture. **B.** EHV-2 cytopathic effect. **C.** EHV-2 intranuclear inclusions. **D.** Pseudocowpox intracytoplasmic inclusions.
E. EHV-1 immunofluorescence in frozen section of equine fetal liver. **F.** CDV immunofluorescence in frozen section of canine lung.
G. CPV-2 immunofluorescence in frozen section of canine intestine. **H.** FVR immunofluorescence in feline conjunctival scraping.

3

Molecular Genetics and Genetic Variation in Bacteria and Bacterial Viruses

G. William Claus

STRUCTURE AND FUNCTION OF THE BACTERIAL GENOME

Structure and Chemistry of the Bacterial Nucleus

The term nucleus is defined as a membrane-bound organelle within a cell that contains chromosomes and nucleoli. Eucaryotic cells contain such a structure but bacteria do not. However, bacteria do contain genetic material, and its function is the same as the nucleus of eucaryotic cells. The genetic material inside a bacterium is often called a nucleoid, nuclear body, nuclear region, or bacterial nucleus.

The bacterial nucleus may be seen with the brightfield microscope after cells are stained with the DNA-specific Feulgen reagent. The bacterial nucleus may also be seen with the phase-contrast microscope when cells are suspended in a concentrated protein solution that matches the refractive index of the protoplasm, because this enhances the differences in contrast between the nuclear region and the cytosolic material that surrounds it. When observed in these ways, the appearance of the nu-

clear region varies from condensed to diffuse, often depending upon the rate of growth. The bacterial nucleus is amorphous and lacks the limiting nuclear membrane that is characteristic of eucaryotic cells.

Investigators have succeeded in isolating the nuclear region of *Escherichia coli* and other bacteria, and the chemical analyses of all appear similar. Each is composed of about 80% DNA, 10% RNA (mostly nascent), and 10% protein (mostly RNA polymerase).

In 1963, John Cairns developed a special technique that allowed him to isolate and spread out the chromosome of *E. coli* so its structure could be examined under an electron microscope. He found that the *E. coli* chromosome was circular and had the same width as one double-stranded DNA molecule and a circular length of about 1 mm. Because the chromosome's length was about 1000 times longer than the entire cell, it was immediately recognized that the molecular organization of the chromosome within the nuclear region must be very complex. More recent evidence shows that this DNA molecule (the bacterial chromosome) is supercoiled, and this accounts for its efficient packing inside the cell. In order for the double-stranded helical DNA molecule to be supercoiled, one strand must first be broken (nicked) so that the helical molecule can be twisted upon itself (supercoiled). Studies suggest that there are 18 to 20 loops of DNA in the *E. coli* chromosome and that each loop is supercoiled, so that the entire molecule is reasonably compact.

Genetic Elements of Bacteria: Chromosomes and Plasmids

Microbiologists use the term genome to mean the complete set of genetic elements occurring within a cell or virus particle. Although the chromosome is the primary genetic element in bacteria, many bacteria also contain small pieces of genetic material called plasmids that are physically separate from the chromosome. Therefore, when considering the genomic material of bacteria one should include both the chromosomes and the extrachromosomal plasmids. For the time being, however, let us concentrate on the bacterial chromosome, while remembering that much of what we say about chromosome structure and replication also applies to plasmids.

Most nongrowing eucaryotic cells are diploid, that is, they contain two copies of each chromosome per cell (pairs of matching genes). Eucaryotic chromosomes are structurally complex, and cells have a number of different types of chromosomes.

In contrast with eucaryotes, procaryotic cells (bacteria) have simple genetic systems. Bacterial chromosomes are single DNA molecules. Nongrowing cells are haploid; that is, they contain only one chromosome (DNA molecule) per cell (i.e., one set of genes). During growth, however, the bacterial cell contains at least one partial copy of its chromosome at any one time, because DNA synthesis must provide two complete copies just prior to cell division.

Overview of Molecular Genetics

Genetic processes require at least three types of polymers: deoxyribonucleic acid (DNA), ribonucleic acid (RNA), and proteins. During cell growth, all three types of macromolecules are made. Since the steps leading from DNA to RNA to newly synthesized protein require the transfer of information, DNA and RNA are often called informational macromolecules to distinguish them from other large molecules such as lipids and polysaccharides.

The cell's structural genes determine the order of placement for each amino acid during the synthesis of a protein molecule. One gene consists of a sequence of triplet purine and pyrimidine bases on the DNA molecule that codes for a sequence of amino acids as the protein molecule is being made. The base sequence in each triplet is critical, because a change in even one base may cause an inactive protein to be formed or actually stop the synthesis of that protein.

DNA does not function directly in protein synthesis, however, but through an intermediate molecule called messenger RNA (mRNA). During mRNA synthesis, one strand of the DNA serves as a template, so that the purine and pyrimidine bases on the mRNA are assembled in the proper order during synthesis. Each newly formed mRNA molecule is composed of a series of triplet bases that are complementary to those found on the DNA molecule. The triplets on the mRNA are called codons. The process of transferring information from DNA to an mRNA molecule during synthesis is called transcription. Once mRNA synthesis is complete and the new molecule binds to a ribosome, the mRNA serves as a template for protein synthesis.

Another RNA molecule made by the cell is called transfer RNA (tRNA). The tRNA molecule has two critical sites: one that will bind with only one type of amino acid, and another site (on the opposite end of the molecule) that consists of three purine or pyrimidine bases that are complementary to only one codon on the mRNA (the triplets on the tRNA are called anticodons). Each tRNA molecule binds to an amino acid and also binds to the mRNA found on the ribosome complex, so that the amino acid will be inserted in the proper order during protein biosynthesis. This process of translating the code found on the mRNA into the sequence of amino acids in a protein is called translation. Bacterial cells use complex systems to determine if protein synthesis will take place and to regulate the rates of protein synthesis once it does take place. This is probably because not all proteins are always needed by the growing cell, and some proteins are needed in greater quantities than others.

DNA Structure and Synthesis

A DNA molecule consists of two strands, each of which contains alternating units of phosphate (HPO_4^{2-}) and a sugar called deoxyribose (Fig. 3–1). Each phosphate attaches to both the 3' and the 5' position of adjacent deoxyribose molecules (ester linkages), forming what is commonly called the "sugar-phosphate backbone" of one DNA strand. At one end of each strand, the sugar phosphate has a free 3' hydroxyl, and it has a free

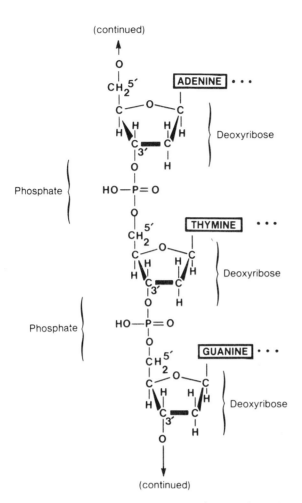

Figure 3–1. A small segment of DNA showing alternating molecules of deoxyribose and phosphate covalently bonded together to form one strand of the double-stranded DNA molecule. Each purine or pyrimidine base is covalently bonded at the 1' position of the ribose and loosely associated by hydrogen bonding ($\cdots$) to a complementary base on the adjacent strand (not shown).

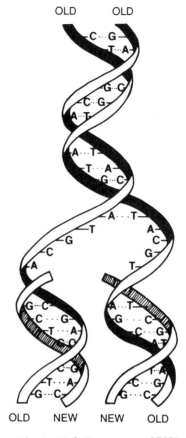

Figure 3–2. The double-helix structure of DNA during the replication process. At the top of this drawing, each sugar-phosphate strand is shown as a continuous band with the bases adenine (A), cytosine (C), guanine (G), or thymine (T) covalently bound (—) to each sugar. The two strands are held together by hydrogen bonding (. . .) between each complementary base pair. During replication, the old strands separate, and one new strand is formed that is complementary to each of the old strands.

5' hydroxyl at the other end. Attached to each deoxyribose on each strand is one of four possible purine or pyrimidine bases: adenine, thymine, guanine, or cytosine. Replication (new DNA synthesis) always begins at the 5' end and progresses toward the 3' end of each DNA strand.

The single bacterial chromosome contains two complementary (not identical) DNA strands that are wound around one another in a helical fashion, with the ends covalently bonded together to form a circular macromolecule. The purine and pyrimidine bases of each strand are arranged such that the guanine on one strand is always across from a cytosine of the adjacent strand, and a thymine is always across from an adenine (Fig. 3–2). These adjacent bases are held close to one another by hydrogen bonding. Replication occurs by unwinding the existing helix and then adding individual

sugar-phosphate-base units (called nucleotides) so that a new complementary DNA strand is built adjacent to the old existing strand (see bottom half of Fig. 3–2).

The point at which the two strands unwind is called the replication fork, the growing point, or the replicon, and it is believed that the bacterial chromosome is attached to the cell's plasma membrane at this DNA replication site. Here, during bacterial chromosome (DNA) replication, each nucleotide unit is added at the 3' hydroxyl end of the new DNA strand. Therefore, replication of these two strands runs in opposite directions (Fig. 3–3).

When the double helix opens up to begin replication, an enzyme called primase initiates the synthesis of a short DNA (primer) strand. Once the first nucleotide is in place, then another enzyme (one type of DNA polymerase) continues to covalently bond each additional nucleotide to the 3' hydroxyl end of the newly developing strand. This new

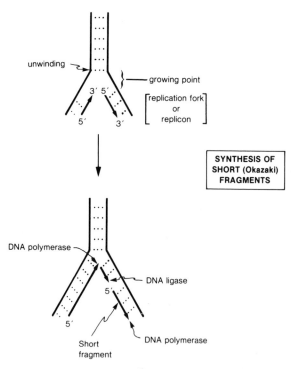

SYNTHESIS OF
SHORT (Okazaki)
FRAGMENTS

Figure 3–3. Mechanism of DNA replication. Unwinding occurs at the growing point (replication fork or replicon). The enzyme DNA polymerase connects each nucleotide only to the 3' end of each short fragment. These short (Okazaki) fragments are subsequently joined together by the enzyme DNA ligase.

DNA forms in short chains (called Okazaki fragments), and then the adjacent fragments are covalently bonded together by an enzyme called DNA ligase. With the addition of each new nucleotide, the old DNA strand acts as a template (preformed pattern) for the formation of the new strand, so that complementary base pairing occurs during this synthesis. The end result of this synthesis is two double-stranded DNA molecules (two bacterial chromosomes). Each one contains one strand from the old molecule and a new, complementary strand.

Once replicated, each chromosome is then supercoiled. Supercoiling is believed to be an important factor in both the replication of DNA and its transcription. Enzymes called topoisomerases appear to regulate the degree of DNA supercoiling and thus its ease of replication and transcription. Each time that DNA is supercoiled, it is put under strain. Because it is under strain, it unwinds more easily than if it were not supercoiled. The topoisomerase that promotes DNA supercoiling (and thus controls unwinding) at the replication fork is called DNA gyrase.

A highly schematic and oversimplified illustration of chromosome replication and the subsequent division of these two DNA macromolecules prior to cell division is shown in Figure 3–4. The exact manner in which each chromosome finds itself in a new cell is not known, but it is believed that the site of attachment of the chromosome to the plasma membrane plays an important part in this partitioning process. Evidence also suggests that rapidly dividing cells have more than one growing point (site of replication), because the time between cell divisions is shorter than the time it takes to replicate an entire chromosome. If this is true, then at any one time during rapid growth there may be at least one complete chromosome and several partial copies at various stages of completion.

RNA Structure and Synthesis

The bacterial cell's ribonucleic acids (RNAs) also play an important part in gene expression. Therefore, RNA must be understood in order to completely comprehend genetic variation in bacteria.

There are three major differences between the chemistry of RNA and that of DNA. First, molecules of RNA contain a sugar called ribose instead of deoxyribose. Second, RNA has a base called uracil instead of the base thymine. And finally, bacterial RNA is not a double-stranded molecule (some viral RNAs are double-stranded). Like all other cells, bacteria contain three major types of RNA: messenger RNA, transfer RNA, and ribosomal RNA.

Messenger RNA Synthesis. The function of messenger RNA (mRNA) is to copy (transcribe) the genetic code from the gene (chromosomal DNA) and to move that message to the site of protein synthesis (the ribosome). Transcription of the genetic code occurs during mRNA synthesis.

The site on the chromosome where mRNA synthesis begins is called the promoter region, and each gene (or set of genes) on the chromosome has its own promoter. An enzyme called RNA polymerase binds to the promoter region, and this causes the two DNA strands to uncoil, so that the code may be read (transcribed) from one DNA strand (the sense strand). The RNA polymerase then moves along the DNA sense strand while it simultaneously bonds together the ribonucleotide building blocks (adenosine triphosphate or ATP, cytosine triphosphate or CTP, guanosine triphosphate or GTP, and uridine triphosphate or UTP) to form the new mRNA molecule. The order in which the ribonucleotides are inserted into the developing mRNA is determined by the sequence of bases on the single-stranded DNA molecule. In other words, the bases on the single DNA strand act as a template for the assembly of complemen-

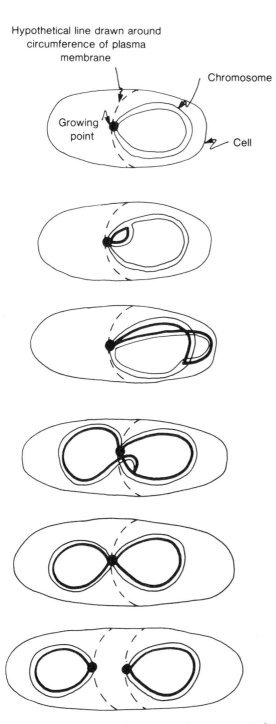

Figure 3–4. Replication of the bacterial chromosome. Each of the old strands of chromosome is represented by thin lines, and the new strands are shown with heavy lines. Sites of attachment to the plasma membrane are also sites for DNA replication (growing point). Separation of growing points may allow for partitioning of each new chromosome prior to cell division.

tary ribonucleotides, and RNA polymerase covalently bonds these ribonucleotides together and releases one pyrophosphate for each nucleotide that is bound. Therefore, the transcription process transcribes the genetic code from the DNA (gene) to the mRNA (message). As the RNA polymerase moves progressively down the DNA molecule, the double-stranded helix continues to open up; it recloses after the message has been completely transcribed.

Termination of mRNA synthesis also occurs at a specific (termination) site on the DNA molecule. This termination site determines how long the mRNA will be, and, as we will see, this in turn determines how large the protein molecule will be. Several types of termination sites on the DNA molecule have been identified, and these effectively stop the action of RNA polymerase (thus mRNA synthesis). The resulting complete, functional mRNA molecule is linear and single-stranded.

Not all mRNA molecules code for synthesis of a single protein molecule. In bacteria, some mRNAs code for synthesis of several related enzymatic proteins whose synthesis is coded on adjacent genes. For example, the genes that code for all of the enzymes needed in the synthetic pathway for formation of one amino acid may be sequentially arranged on the DNA. Instead of having one termination site at the end of the code for each enzyme, the DNA may have one termination site for the entire sequence of genes. Thus, one long mRNA molecule could be transcribed so that it would code for the simultaneous synthesis of all enzymes required for that synthetic pathway.

Several important antibiotics appear to interfere with mRNA synthesis. Actinomycin inhibits mRNA synthesis by binding to the DNA molecule in such a way that it stops mRNA formation. Two groups of antibiotics, the rifamycins and the streptovaricins, are effective against bacteria because they appear to bind to the RNA polymerase molecule and inhibit its activity. The rifamycins seem to be highly specific for bacterial RNA polymerase.

Transfer RNA Structure and Function. Transfer RNA (tRNA) is a single-stranded molecule that contains double-stranded regions as a result of the molecule folding back upon itself. These folded regions have complementary bases across from each other, and hydrogen bonding holds these adjacent strands together. The structure of tRNA is generally drawn like a cloverleaf, with three distinct loops (of unpaired bases) and a stem having two open ends.

To function properly, a molecule of tRNA (Fig. 3–5) must do four things: (1) it must bind with an enzyme that activates amino acids; (2) it must specifically bind with one type of amino acid; (3) it must recognize a specific triplet code (codon) on the mRNA, and bind with the triplet bases on that codon; and (4) it must nonspecifically bind with the ribosome to which an mRNA is bound. The structure of the tRNA molecule closely reflects how it functions in these ways during protein synthesis.

The D loop on tRNA selectively binds an enzyme called an aminoacyl-tRNA (AA-tRNA) synthetase. This enzyme does two things: (1) it specifically activates one type of amino acid; and (2) it binds that activated amino acid to the acceptor stem of the tRNA. To activate the amino acid, AA-tRNA synthetase cleaves pyrophosphate from an ATP molecule and covalently bonds the remaining AMP to the amino acid. Thus, an activated amino acid is an amino acid-AMP complex. The specificity of the tRNAs toward only one type of AA-tRNA synthetase should be emphasized here. It is extremely important that the correct AA-tRNA synthetase be attached to the tRNA molecule, because this enzyme determines which amino acid will be activated and bound to the tRNA, and this, in turn, determines which amino acid will be inserted in the developing protein during transla-

tion. Specific binding between a tRNA and an amino acid occurs in the soluble portion of the cell. Once the amino acid has been activated and the amino acid-tRNA complex leaves the enzyme, the complex migrates to a ribosome containing an mRNA molecule.

The anticodon loop on tRNA contains three bases (the anticodon) that are complementary to three bases on mRNA (the codon). The function of the anticodon on this loop is to specifically recognize and bind it to an mRNA codon. In other words, the mRNA codon specifies which activated amino acid-tRNA complex it will bind to and thereby determines which amino acid will be inserted at that point in the developing protein. Thus, the genomic message from the chromosome is transcribed by the mRNA, which then migrates to the ribosome where its message is translated by the tRNAs carrying the activated amino acids.

The TψC loop appears to bind to the 50S ribosome subunit (see next section) during the translation process to help all of these components stay in the proper configuration while the activated amino acids are being covalently bonded onto the newly developing protein molecule.

Ribosome Structure and Function. Three important types of RNA are found in all cells: messenger, transfer, and ribosomal RNA. All three types are involved in transferring information from the sequence of nucleotide bases in the DNA to the sequence of amino acids in the polypeptide chain of a protein. Almost all the proteins made by a cell are catalytically active (enzymes). One might say that the DNA carries the genetic information, the RNA translates it, and the catalytic proteins that are made express the genetic information.

In bacteria, each ribosome is composed of two subunits. Each subunit is described by the way it sediments in a high-speed centrifuge. These sedimentation properties (abbreviated "S" for Svedberg units) are determined by the size, density, and shape of the subunit. Thus, bacteria contain a ribosome that is made up of one 50S and one 30S subunit. Each subunit is made up of a number of individual proteins as well as ribosomal RNA (rRNA). The 30S and 50S subunits exist separately in the bacterial cell and come together to form a 70S particle only when they combine with a molecule of mRNA. Translation of the genetic code takes place on this ribosome-mRNA complex.

The 70S ribosome provides the structural framework that supports and aligns not only the mRNA but also the tRNAs and the many proteins required for translation. Distortion of ribosomal structure, therefore, can prevent proper functioning of this

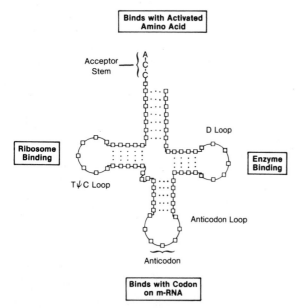

Figure 3–5. Molecular structure of a transfer RNA (tRNA) molecule showing a cloverleaf arrangement. Nucleotides (boxes or letters) are covalently bound together (—) to form a long, single-stranded molecule that is folded back upon itself. The folded tRNA is held together by hydrogen bonds (. . .) between adjacent complementary bases. Three loops are formed upon folding, and each loop has a specific function. The two ends of this single strand form the stem of the molecule that will bind one type of amino acid (see Fig. 3–6).

entire translational complex. Certain types of antibiotics appear to alter the structure of ribosomal subunits. For example, streptomycin, neomycin, tetracycline, and spectinomycin alter the structure of the 30S subunit of bacteria and therefore are specific in their action against procaryotes. Similarly, puromycin, chloramphenicol, erythromycin, and cycloheximide appear to alter the 50S procaryotic subunits. Note, however, that this is not the only mode of action of these antibiotics. Most also affect other steps in protein synthesis.

The Genetic Code

The information contained in the nucleotide sequence of the bacterial cell's chromosome (DNA) is ultimately translated into the sequence of amino acids that make up each protein. Thus, the genetic code is contained in the DNA. However, this code is transcribed from the DNA molecule to mRNA, and it is actually the mRNA that serves as a template for the assembly of amino acids during protein synthesis. Therefore, it is customary to speak of the genetic code in terms of nucleotide sequence of the mRNA molecules.

All RNAs contain four different nucleotide bases: adenine (A), guanine (G), cytosine (C), and uracil (U). Within the mRNA, three sequential nucleotide bases (triplets like CUA) are used to code for the positioning of an amino acid during translation. Each of the triplet nucleotide sequences on the mRNA strand is called a codon. Because there are four nucleotide bases and three bases in each codon, 64 different triplets (codons) are possible. However, there are only 20 different amino acids to code for. Therefore, many more codons are possible than are needed for translating genetic information from the mRNA to the developing protein. What this means is that the genetic code is redundant, with several codons capable for coding for insertion of the same amino acid into the developing protein during synthesis. For example, UCU, UCC, UCG, and UCA all code for serine insertion.

A few codons do not code for any amino acids (such as UGA, UAG, and UAA); these are called nonsense codons, and they serve as a signal to stop protein synthesis when the molecule is fully formed. Some evidence suggests that a few codons represent only starting points for new protein synthesis. These are called initiating codons. A distinct starting point is essential so that translation begins at the proper location. Without a specific starting point, the whole reading frame might be shifted and a completely different protein (or no protein at all) would be made, depending upon the extent of the reading frame shift.

Errors in translating the message on mRNA are probably rare under normal circumstances. However, those antibiotics that act on the 30S or 50S ribosome subunits are thought to increase translation errors to such an extent that the newly formed protein is abnormal, and the cell can no longer function properly. Drastic shifts from optimum pH, temperature, and cation concentration also appear to cause translation errors during protein synthesis.

Mechanism of Protein Synthesis (Expression of the Genetic Code)

Protein synthesis (translation of the genetic code from mRNA) is a continuous process that may be thought of as occurring in four steps: (1) initiation; (2) elongation; (3) termination-release; and (4) polypeptide folding.

Initiation (Fig. 3–6) requires the formation of a complex that contains mRNA, the 30S ribosome subunit, tRNA, the 50S subunit, and several proteins (called initiation factors). In bacteria, tRNA binds to the 30S subunit, and the 50S subunit binds to the 30S particle, forming the 70S ribosome. The anticodon on an activated tRNA recognizes and binds to the initiating codon on the mRNA strand, and the TψC loop of this same tRNA also binds to the 50S subunit of the ribosome. Streptomycin interferes with initiation, probably because of its effect upon the 30S subunit.

In bacteria, the first (initiating) codon on the mRNA strand is either AUG or GUG. When used as an initiating codon (only), these triplets code for an amino acid called *N*-formylmethionine, so this is the first amino acid in the sequence for each protein. This amino acid can later be enzymatically removed, so not all bacterial proteins have methionine at their amino terminal ends. Just preceding the initiation codon are three to nine nucleotides that bind the mRNA to the 30S ribosome subunit (probably by base pairing with the rRNA).

Elongation, the next step in protein synthesis, is actually a repeated series of events called recognition, transfer, and translocation (Fig. 3–6). To achieve elongation, there must be a continual supply of activated amino acid-tRNA complexes, such that the mRNA (on the ribosome) will be continually bathed in amino acid-tRNAs. However, only those with anticodons matching the next codon on the mRNA will be "recognized" and will bind to the mRNA at that position. (The antibiotics streptomycin, neomycin, and tetracycline appear to adversely affect this codon recognition.) Once the two amino acids are adjacent to one another, then the first amino acid is transferred and covalently bonded to the second amino acid. Next, the empty

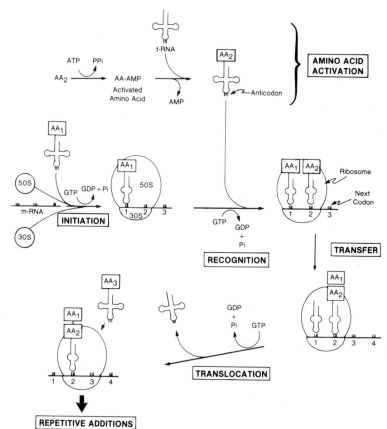

Figure 3–6. Translation of the genetic code from a messenger RNA (mRNA) molecule to the order of amino acids (AA) on a protein molecule during synthesis. Once synthesis is initiated such that the mRNA-ribosome-AA complex is formed, the addition of each additional amino acid (e.g., AA$_2$ or AA$_3$) requires four events: amino acid activation, recognition, transfer, and translocation. These four events are continuously repeated in the elongation step of protein synthesis.

tRNA on the first codon is released from the mRNA (and 50S subunit), and the tRNA molecule with its attached polypeptide chain is moved along the ribosome (translocated) to the next position. (The antibiotics cycloheximide and spectinomycin appear to interfere with ribosome translocation.) This series of events is repeated over and over again, resulting in the elongation of the polypeptide chain.

Note in Figure 3–6 that each event in the elongation process, including initiation and amino acid activation, requires molecules that have high-energy phosphate bonds (adenosine triphosphate or ATP and guanosine triphosphate or GTP). For example, formation of the initiation complex (the initiation step) requires energy, and this is provided by the hydrolysis of one GTP. High-energy compounds like GTP are supplied by catabolism of the cell's exogenous energy source. Catabolism (and anabolism too) is accomplished by enzymes (catalytically active proteins) that are made in the manner being described. Thus, catabolism of the energy source and synthesis of proteins are inseparably linked by the supply and demand for ATP and GTP, among other things.

Termination, part of the third step in protein synthesis, occurs when an mRNA codon is reached that does not code for the attachment of any AA-tRNA. (In addition to their other activities, the tetracycline antibiotics also seem to interfere with the termination of protein synthesis.) These are called termination codons or stop codons. There are three termination codons that stop polypeptide synthesis in all cell types: UGA, UAG, and UAA. Because no AA-tRNA binds with these nonsense codons, there is nothing to transfer the polypeptide chain to, so the polypeptide chain is released into the cytoplasm.

Once released from the ribosome-mRNA complex, the polypeptide chain is free to fold into an active, three-dimensional protein structure that is held in this form by weak disulfide bridges and hydrogen bonding. This is the last step in protein synthesis, known as polypeptide folding. If everything has gone correctly, the result is a functionally active enzyme that can participate in the cell's metabolism.

Regulation of Protein Synthesis

Most of the proteins contained within the bacterial cell are enzymes. Therefore, it is common to equate bacterial protein synthesis with enzyme synthesis. Some enzymes are always being made by the cell, so they are always present in relatively high concentration, and these are called constitutive enzymes. Other enzymes are only produced under certain conditions and these are called inducible enzymes.

Three mechanisms of genetic control will be briefly discussed here: (1) the induction-repression mechanism; (2) catabolite repression; and (3) attenuation. Each of these control mechanisms acts at the transcription level, that is, on the gene (DNA), as its message is being transcribed to a new mRNA molecule. And each of these mechanisms functions to turn off gene expression (ultimately enzyme synthesis) when the gene product (the enzyme) is not needed for cellular metabolism. The function of repressing enzyme synthesis seems obvious, since it would be foolish for a cell to waste energy on making unneeded enzymes.

The ability to repress enzyme synthesis is now thought to be a valuable and widespread mechanism for energy conservation by all types of microorganisms. Regulating genetic expression in bacteria (procaryotes), however, appears simpler than in eucaryotic microorganisms. The following sections will deal only with genetic control mechanisms in procaryotic cells.

Induction and Repression. Control of enzyme synthesis by induction or repression usually involves not one but a set of adjacent genes on the bacterial cell's chromosome. These structural genes are responsible for the synthesis of several enzymes that usually accomplish all or part of the catabolism of a specific energy source. This set of adjacent genes forms a functional genetic unit called an operon. The operon is located next to other parts of the DNA that regulate the expression of the structural genes, and these are called promoters, operators, and regulatory genes. The operon that has been most closely studied is the lactose (*lac*) operon from *Escherichia coli*. The *lac* operon is responsible for the initial stages of lactose catabolism in this bacterium, and it contains three structural genes (Fig. 3–7): (1) the "Z" gene that codes for production of an enzyme called β-galactosidase. This enzyme breaks apart disaccharide sugars that contain a galactoside molecule covalently joined by a β-glycosidic bond to another sugar; (2) the "Y" gene that codes for galactoside permease production, an enzyme within the plasma membrane that transports galactoside molecules inside so that they can be cleaved into separate monosaccharide sugars by β-galactosidase; and (3) the "A" gene that codes for production of galactoside acetylase, an enzyme whose function is not clearly understood.

Repression of the *lac* operon comes about in the following way. Transcription begins when RNA polymerase binds to the promoter region. The regulatory gene is the first part of the DNA sense strand transcribed. The function of the regulatory gene is to code for continuous production of repressor proteins (see Fig. 3–7).

If lactose (or another β-galactoside) is *not* present in the medium, then the repressor proteins are free to bind with the operator. In so doing, they also prevent the RNA polymerase from binding to the operator, which it must do before it can move on to transcribe the structural genes of the *lac* operon. This alteration of the operator stops further transcription and effectively inhibits synthesis of the enzymes required for lactose utilization, but note that these enzymes are not needed in the absence of lactose, so this may be thought of as an energy-conservation mechanism.

For induction, a β-galactoside (such as lactose) must be present in the medium, and the β-galactoside itself serves as the inducer (Fig. 3–8). Cells probably always have a small number of galactoside transport proteins (permeases) in the membrane, even if transcription of the *lac* operon is repressed. Therefore, if lactose is added to the medium, a small amount is initially transported into the cell. The regulatory gene continues to code for synthesis of repressor proteins; however, lactose (the inducer) binds with these repressor proteins, so that the repressor proteins will no longer bind with the operator gene. Since the repressor proteins are now inactivated, transcription of the operon genes by RNA polymerase can proceed. Thus, induction and repression both have the same underlying mechanism: control of the operator. Since induction actually interferes with the action of the repressor proteins, some microbiologists prefer to call the induction process derepression.

Catabolite Repression. Another mechanism for control of enzyme (protein) synthesis is called catabolite repression. To understand this mechanism, it is important to know that bacteria are often capable of growing on a variety of nutrient energy sources, but some of these energy sources are used preferentially. For example, *Escherichia coli* can catabolize either glucose or lactose to obtain energy for growth. If both are present, however, these bacteria will first use glucose until the supply is exhausted and then shift to lactose utilization. As previously described, the enzymes responsible for lactose utilization are inducible, but the synthesis of these enzymes (transcription of the *lac* operon) is also subject to catabolite repression. When glucose is preferentially used in the presence of lactose, glucose is the catabolite (substrate for catabolism) that acts as a repressor on the *lac* operon. Once the glucose supply in the medium is ex-

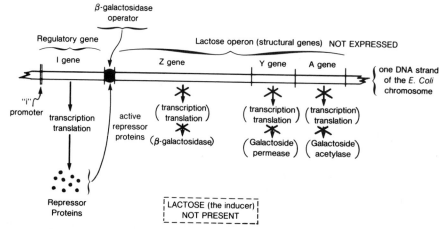

Figure 3–7.   Repression of the lactose *(lac)* operon of *Escherichia coli.* In the absence of lactose, repressor proteins remain active and bind to the operator gene, thereby preventing transcription of the structural genes that make up the *lac* operon. Because these genes are not transcribed, the unnecessary proteins are not made; thus energy is conserved.

hausted, there is no catabolite to serve as the repressor, and catabolite repression is abolished. Lactose can then induce the *lac* operon, and lactose catabolism can begin after a short lag.

The manner in which glucose acts as a catabolite repressor has only recently been determined. To understand this mechanism, it is first necessary to describe more fully how RNA polymerase binds to the sense strand of the DNA. In the previous section, it was stated that transcription (mRNA synthesis) begins when RNA polymerase binds at the promoter. However, with catabolite-repressible enzymes, binding appears to occur only if a catabolite-activator protein (CAP) has already bound to the promoter. In order for CAP to bind, it must be in the proper three-dimensional structure, and this requires a molecule called cyclic AMP (cAMP). It appears that glucose either inhibits the synthesis of cAMP or causes cAMP to be broken

down. Regardless of the reason, intracellular cAMP concentrations are low in the presence of glucose. The lack of sufficient cAMP prevents CAP binding to the promoter; thus RNA polymerase does not bind, and transcription does not occur. Therefore, catabolite repression is really the result of a glucose-stimulated cAMP deficiency.

There is some evidence that glucose-controlled cAMP concentrations regulate enzyme synthesis for a number of other catabolic pathways in *E. coli.* This suggests that enzymes responsible for catabolism of energy sources other than glucose are not made in the presence of glucose (a preferred energy source for *E. coli*). Thus, once again, the cell conserves energy by stopping synthesis of unneeded enzymes. Alternatively, when the preferred energy source (glucose) is depleted, the cell starts synthesis of other enzymes used for catabolism of other substrates. Perhaps cells capable of

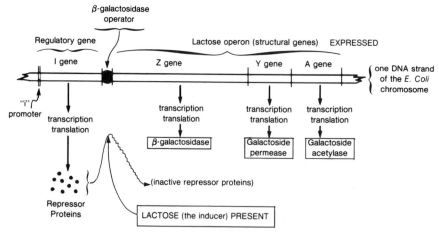

Figure 3–8.   Induction of the lactose *(lac)* operon of *Escherichia coli.* When lactose is present, it binds with the repressor proteins, thereby making them unable to bind to the operator gene. This allows transcription (and subsequent translation) of the structural genes of the *lac* operon so that all the enzymatic proteins necessary for lactose utilization are made.

such feats are more adaptable to changing environments and thus more likely to survive than those that lack such regulation mechanisms.

Attenuation. A third mechanism of regulation occurs in operons controlling synthesis of amino acids. The best studied of these seems to be the tryptophan operon. This operon contains structural genes for the five enzymes required to convert catabolic intermediates to tryptophan. The adjacent regulatory sequence includes three major regions: the promoter, the operator, and a region that seems characteristic of attenuation controlled regulatory sequences called the leader sequence. Within the leader sequence is a region called the attenuator that codes for synthesis of a peptide (small molecular weight protein) that is rich in tryptophan. This tryptophan-rich peptide is called a leader. If tryptophan is abundant in the medium and in the cell, then the leader can be assembled. On the other hand, if intracellular tryptophan concentrations are low or absent, the leader peptide cannot be made.

The critical feature of this mechanism is that synthesis of the leader peptide causes transcription of the tryptophan structural genes to stop. On the other hand, if a tryptophan deficiency stops synthesis of the leader peptide, then transcription of the structural genes will take place, and tryptophan synthesis will occur inside the cell.

Summary. Although it may appear that much is known about how protein (enzyme) synthesis is regulated, there is much more detail to learn. For example, it is not known for sure if anabolic and catabolic pathways are regulated in the same way. At the present time, however, it appears that *catabolic* (energy-yielding, degradative) pathways are controlled using either induction-repression or catabolite repression. Note that both of these mechanisms use the presence of the initial substrate (energy source) to turn *on* the synthesis of these catabolic enzymes. Alternatively, the attenuation mechanism appears to regulate *anabolic* (energy-requiring, biosynthetic) pathways, and this mechanism uses the presence of the end-product to turn *off* synthesis.

MUTATION AS A MECHANISM FOR GENETIC VARIATION IN BACTERIA

Introduction to Microbial Mutations

We previously examined the structure of the bacterial chromosome and how its genetic information is expressed and regulated under normal circumstances. Let us now shift attention to how infrequent but important changes occur in the nucleotide sequence of bacterial chromosomes. But first we need to define some terms.

A microbial strain (also called a clone) is a population of cells that are genetically identical. Pure culture techniques are extremely important for isolation and maintenance of microbial strains. The genotype of a strain refers to the genetic characteristics of the cell regardless of whether these genes are being expressed (transcribed and translated) at any given time. The phenotype of a strain is that set of genetic characteristics that can be seen or measured; in other words, phenotypic characteristics result from those genes that are expressed in that environment. If the environment is changed, genetic regulation may (by induction or repression) change genetic expression, and thereby also change the phenotype of that strain.

Microbiologists commonly refer to a strain isolated from the environment as the wild type. In the broadest sense of the term, mutation is defined as a sudden and inheritable change in the cell's chromosome (genotype). With microorganisms, however, it is often convenient to differentiate between two types of sudden and inheritable change in the DNA: (1) recombination, in which the change is caused by the introduction of new genes from outside the cell; and (2) mutation, in which changes occur that are not the result of introducing new genetic material from outside the cell. For the present, let us deal only with mutation and leave an explanation of recombination for later in this chapter.

Spontaneous Mutations

A spontaneous mutation is one that occurs without known cause. Spontaneous mutations probably result most commonly from errors made while copying the DNA during chromosome replication.

The accuracy with which DNA is copied during chromosome replication is very high (errors estimated at fewer than one in every 500,000 bases copied). Therefore, the rate of error in any one gene is very small, and the frequency of spontaneous mutation is rare. But microorganisms reproduce very quickly in the laboratory, so there are many chances for errors to occur, and, therefore microbes make excellent tools for studying mutation.

For any given gene, spontaneous mutation will occur at the frequency of only about one in every 10^5 to 10^9 cells. For example, a nutritionally deficient mutant may arise spontaneously in a bacterial population in one out of every 10^7 cells; therefore, only 10 of these mutants could be found in every

10^8 cells examined. From these numbers, it should be apparent that detection of spontaneous mutation in the laboratory is difficult unless selection techniques are used. For example, one could place a large number of cells (more than 10^7) in a medium containing growth-inhibiting concentrations of streptomycin (a selective medium), and only the streptomycin-resistant cells should grow. Such a mutation could arise due to modification of genes coding for ribosome synthesis. Since the ribosome is the target of streptomycin activity, a structurally modified ribosome would render the antibiotic ineffective.

Whether streptomycin-resistant mutants remain at the spontaneous level depends upon the presence or absence of streptomycin. Continual prophylactic or therapeutic use of any single antibiotic encourages the selection of spontaneous mutants that are resistant to that antibiotic. The predominance of these mutants in the environment drastically decreases the effectiveness of this antibiotic in combating future infections.

Spontaneous mutation frequencies vary for different genes and also for the same gene in different microbial species. It is also important to realize that the frequency of spontaneous mutation for each gene is independent of all others. Thus, if the frequency of spontaneous mutation to streptomycin resistance in a bacterial strain is one in every 10^7, and the frequency of spontaneous mutation to penicillin resistance in that same strain is one in every 10^5 cells, then the frequency of mutation of two genes in the same cell (allowing both streptomycin and penicillin resistance) is one in every 10^{12} cells. Considering this, it should be obvious why dual antibiotic therapy is often preferred.

Molecular Mechanisms of Mutagenesis

Mutations result from alteration in the nucleotide base sequences of the cell's genes (DNA). If we continue to separately consider mutation and recombination events, then there are two mechanisms that describe many (if not most) mutations: point mutations and deletion mutations.

Point Mutations. Point mutations result when one deoxyribonucleotide is substituted for another during DNA synthesis (gene replication). For example, a deoxyadenosine may be inserted instead of a deoxyguanosine, and this means that adenine would replace guanine in the sequence of bases on the new DNA strand. Therefore, point mutations are alterations of only one base in the sequence of bases that make up a single structural or regulatory gene.

Whether or not a point mutation is phenotypically expressed depends upon which base is substituted and where that substitution takes place on the gene. To explain this, let us consider a point mutation occurring in the DNA triplet that codes for the amino acid serine during translation. You may recall that the genetic code is redundant, for example, more than one triplet codes for the insertion of serine during protein synthesis. If the point mutation causes a substitution that alters the DNA triplet, such that the resulting mRNA codon will still code for serine, then there will be no alteration in the amino acid sequence of the protein made by this gene. Because the same protein is made, it will function the same, and there will be no phenotypic expression of this point mutation. This is called a silent mutation, because the protein produced by that gene is identical to that made before the mutation.

Alternatively, the DNA-base substitution resulting from point mutation can alter the triplet such that the mRNA (produced during transcription) will code for the insertion of another amino acid during protein synthesis (translation). If this different amino acid is in a critical location, such as part of an enzyme's active site, then the function of that protein could be altered or even destroyed, resulting in a phenotypic change. If that protein were critical to the cell's survival, this point mutation could be lethal. On the other hand, if the substitution altered the amino acid sequence at a point on the protein not critical for its catalytic activity, then this mutation would not be phenotypically expressed. Note that this latter mutation is not silent because the amino acid sequence of the protein produced by that gene is altered.

Deletion Mutants. A deletion mutant is one in which a portion of one strand of the DNA is removed. Anywhere from one to several hundred deoxyribonucleotides (bases) may be deleted from the DNA strand. Deletion of a single base in a structural gene will probably result in a reading frame shift, and the next three bases may be read as a nonsense codon. This would cause the cessation of transcription and hence a shorter mRNA. If this occurs at the terminal end of the gene, the alteration of the mRNA and the resulting protein may not drastically affect the protein's catalytic activity. If, however, the deletion occurs closer to the promoter end (the 5' end) of the structural gene, then the resulting (shorter) polypeptide will probably be nonfunctional and easily detected phenotypically (if this mutant strain survives). Deletion of larger segments of the DNA usually results in complete loss of the ability to produce the protein. Phenotypically detectable deletion mutations cannot be restored through further mutation.

Reversions. A revertant is a strain in which a wild-type phenotypic characteristic, originally lost due to mutation, is restored regardless of the mechanism. Reversions are often called back mutations because a second mutation is required to restore the original characteristic. Many mutations are revertable, and the reversion may occur in one of several ways. For example, a back mutation may occur at the same site (or close to the same site) of the original mutation, such that a reading frame shift, originally caused by a small deletion, is corrected. Chemical or physical agents that increase the frequency of mutation (mutagens) also stimulate the frequency of reversion.

The ability to stimulate back mutation by mutagens has a very practical application in the use of the Ames test for determining the carcinogenic potential of chemical mutagens. The Ames test (named for Dr. Bruce Ames, University of California, Berkeley) uses mutant strains of *Salmonella typhimurium* that are very sensitive to back mutation when subjected to chemical mutagens. This test is much more economical and takes far less time than using laboratory animals for initial screening of suspected carcinogens.

Mutagenesis and Carcinogenesis

It is now well known that a wide variety of chemical and physical agents induce (increase the frequency of) mutation by reacting directly with the cell's DNA. For example, some chemicals may cross-link adjacent DNA strands and cause either point mutations or deletions. Other chemicals, such as the dyes acridine orange and ethidium bromide, may insert between two base pairs during DNA replication and cause reading frame shift mutations. Physical agents (like nonionizing or ionizing radiation) may cause pyrimidine dimer formation or actually break the DNA strands. When the cell tries to repair these DNA alterations, errors may be introduced or actual deletions in the DNA strands may occur. These chemical or physical agents may increase the frequency of mutation from 10 to 100 times above the rate found with spontaneous mutation. Therefore, mutagens are frequently used in the laboratory to increase the possibility that certain mutants will be isolated.

There is good evidence that large numbers of animal cancers are caused by synthetic chemicals added to the environment. The variety of these chemicals that animals come in contact with each day is enormous. It is also important to note that good correlation exists between the mutagenic ca-

pability of a chemical and its carcinogenic ability. Therefore, laboratory procedures (like the Ames test) that assess mutagenic potential are helpful tools for screening large numbers of suspected chemical mutagens in a short period of time. It is not always true that mutagens are also carcinogens, but the correlation is quite high, and the knowledge that a chemical is mutagenic warns of a possible carcinogen. Also, if a chemical is *not* mutagenic for bacteria, this does not mean that it will not be carcinogenic for animals. Therefore, procedures like the Ames test should be used in conjunction with other tests for screening chemicals, and further confirmation of carcinogenic potential must be made with animal tests once the screening tests warn of the chemical's carcinogenic possibilities.

Veterinary Significance of Mutation

Even though spontaneous mutations are rare events, they may alter phenotypic characteristics that cause difficulties in identifying pathogenic microorganisms. The clinical microbiologist is very familiar with the isolation of strains that have all of the typical characteristics of a pathogen except one or two. Indeed, clinical isolates commonly vary in one or more phenotypic characteristics from those described for a pathogen. It is assumed that these phenotypic variations between pathogenic strains are the result of altered environments that have allowed one or more mutants to overgrow the parental strain.

A mutation may affect a wide variety of phenotypic characteristics. The general types of changes often seen are given in Table 3–1. One type of mutation commonly seen by the clinical microbiologist is the smooth-to-rough colony alteration. The smooth appearance of the colony is usually caused by the presence of an extra-cellular capsule that accumulates in the developing colony to such an extent that it makes the colony appear smooth and glistening. Smooth strains are often the more virulent strains, because the presence of a capsule helps the cell resist phagocytosis; thus it will be more evasive. Repeated cultivation on artificial media will often select for mutants that lack capsules and appear dry and granular or rough. These rough strains are usually less virulent (pathogenic) than the smooth strains. However, when rough strains are placed back into the animal, the nonencapsulated cells are engulfed by phagocytes, and only the encapsulated mutants survive if present. Hence, animal passage selects for growth of encapsulated mutants, and this may result in the apparent restoration of a smooth strain.

Table 3–1. Common Effects of Mutation on Bacterial Characteristics

Category	Nature of Change	Expressed Phenotypic Characteristic
Motility	Loss of flagella or flagellar function	Compact colonies instead of flat and spreading
Capsule	Loss or modification of capsule	Rough and somewhat small colonies instead of smooth and larger
Nutritional	Loss of enzyme in anabolic pathway	Inability to grow on medium lacking that nutrient
Energy Source	Loss of enzyme in catabolic pathway	Give no evidence of metabolic activity (e.g., acid production) on media containing that energy source (e.g., sugar)
Drug-resistant	Impermeable to drug, or drug target altered	Growth on medium having a growth-inhibiting concentration of that drug
Virus-resistant	Loss of virus receptor on cell surface	Growth in presence of large numbers of virus
Heat-sensitive†	Alters an enzyme so that it becomes more heat-labile	Inability to grow at higher temperatures that normally support growth (e.g., 37° C) but does grow at lower temperatures
Cold-sensitive	Alters an enzyme so that it becomes more cold-labile	Inability to grow at a low temperature that normally supports some growth (e.g., 20° C)

Adapted from Brock, T.D., Smith, D.W., and Madigan, M.T.: Biology of Microorganisms. 4th Ed. Englewood Cliffs, N.J., Prentice-Hall, 1984, p. 306.

† More commonly (but less descriptively) called "temperature-sensitive" in the literature.

GENETICS AND REPLICATION OF BACTERIAL VIRUSES

Structure of the Bacterial Virus Particle

All viruses are obligate intracellular parasites that lack a cellular structure and also lack the ability to carry out catabolic metabolism. The structure of bacterial viruses is very diverse, but all virus particles share two common characteristics: (1) they contain only one type of nucleic acid—*either* DNA *or* RNA (never both)—and this nucleic acid is either single- or double-stranded (never both); and (2) they surround their nucleic acid with a protein coat, called the capsid which is composed of one or several types of protein molecules (capsomeres).

The nucleic acid (whether DNA or RNA) within all virus particles functions as the viral genome, that is, it carries the genetic information for virus replication. Where evidence is available, it seems that the nucleic acid is highly folded and tightly packed inside the capsid. For example, the DNA of an *E. coli* virus called T4 contains one DNA molecule with a total length of about 50 μm, whereas the entire diameter of the virus particle is about 0.095 μm by 0.065 μm.

The protein coat (capsid) surrounding all viruses has at least two important functions: (1) it serves to protect the genome from destructive cellular enzymes (such as DNAse and RNAse); and (2) the individual protein molecules of the virus coat (capsomeres) have enzyme-like specificity that recognizes and specifically binds with surface components on the susceptible host cell. This binding occurs during the attachment step of the replicative cycle (Fig. 3–9). Binding is so specific that one type of virus usually recognizes and binds to only one bacterial species (or one type of tissue within one host).

Bacterial viruses (called phage or bacteriophage) can be divided into six categories, depending upon their structure and genomic content:

1. Icosahedral head (looks round at low magnification but is composed of 20 triangular plates) containing double-stranded DNA (dsDNA) with a contractile tail having fibrils on the distal end.
2. Icosahedral head containing dsDNA with long (often thin and flexible) noncontractile tail lacking fibrils.
3. Icosahedral head containing dsDNA with short (often apparently rigid) noncontractile tail lacking fibrils.
4. Much smaller icosahedral head (composed of large capsomeres) containing single-stranded DNA (ssDNA) with no tail.
5. Equally smaller icosahedral head (composed of small capsomeres) containing single-stranded RNA (ssRNA) with no tail.
6. Filamentous (long, hollow, flexible rod-shaped) structure (no head) containing ssDNA (forms a central spiral surrounded by the protein capsomeres).

Thus, it can be seen that the structure and genomic content of bacteriophage vary widely. It also appears that most (if not all) structural types are associated with each bacterial genus, but the significance of these structural and genomic variations is not yet clear.

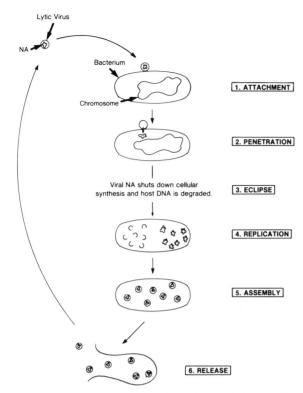

Figure 3–9. Replicative cycle of lytic bacterial viruses. Although the illustrations represent characteristics of bacterial viruses, these six steps are common for all types of lytic viruses. The virus particle is illustrated as the capsid proteins or coat surrounding the viral nucleic acid (NA).

Replication of Lytic Bacterial Viruses

Since viruses are strict intracellular parasites, they all must be capable of directing the infected host cell to make virus particles instead of more cells. The replication cycle of all lytic (cell-destroying) viruses appears similar, and this cycle is usually thought of as occurring in six separate steps (Fig. 3–9): (1) attachment (specific absorption) of the virus particle to the susceptible host's surface; (2) penetration of either the nucleic acid (all bacteriophage) or the entire virus particle (many animal and plant viruses) into the cell; (3) eclipse, in which the viral nucleic acid shuts down cellular synthesis and host-cell DNA is degraded; (4) replication, in which the altered host cell's metabolism is now directed to make each viral component; (5) assembly of the nucleic acid and protein capsomeres into fully infective virus particles; and (6) release of the new virus particles from the cell.

With bacterial cells, this process of viral (phage) replication is called the replicative cycle or the lytic cycle, because the infecting virus genome produces many new viruses and because the new viruses are released upon lysis (breaking apart) of the host cell. In contrast, many virus-infected plant or ani-

mal cells do not lyse the host cell at the end of their replicative cycle. Instead, virus particles are slowly released from these eucaryotic cells by a mechanism resembling pinocytic or phagocytic engulfment, except that the viruses move out of rather than into the cell. This "blebbing" process usually results in a virus particle that is coated with a piece of the eucaryotic cell's membrane.

A unique feature of the bacterial-virus replicative cycle appears at the penetration step. Only the nucleic acid penetrates the bacterial cell; the protein coat (capsid) remains attached to the outside surface of the bacterial cell wall. With the animal or plant viruses, however, the entire virus particle enters the cell by a pinocytosis-like process.

Lytic bacterial viruses are detected and enumerated by spreading an infected culture of a susceptible host on the surface of an appropriate growth medium, such that confluent growth will occur. Wherever lytic bacteriophage attacks a host cell, lysis will occur, and the released phage will continue to infect and lyse adjacent cells. This results in a clear area on a surface of otherwise confluent growth, and this clear area of lysis (containing many virus particles) is called a plaque. Lytic viruses may be serially diluted and spread-plated with a susceptible host to enumerate the number of lytic phage in the undiluted culture, because each virus particle will produce one plaque.

Temperate Bacterial Viruses and Lysogeny

Many bacterial viruses do not carry out a lytic replicative cycle as just described. Instead, the viral genome is inserted into the host cell's chromosome, and that insertion (called a prophage) is replicated along with host DNA between cell divisions (Fig. 3–10). Note that the prophage is replicated and transferred to new progeny along with the host's chromosome at each generation. Viruses capable of this phenomenon are called temperate, and the bacterial cell that is able to carry and replicate the prophage (temperate virus) is called a lysogenic bacterium. The entire process of infection of a lysogenic bacterium with a temperate-phage particle and the subsequent insertion of the prophage into the host's chromosome and replication along with that chromosome is called lysogeny.

In the case of lytic phage, the virus genome carries and expresses genes for the synthesis of certain enzymes and other types of proteins that are essential to virus reproduction. In contrast, temperate phage carry similar information, but the expression of these genes is temporarily blocked by a specific repressor coded for by the virus. When this repressor is inactivated, synthesis of the entire virus parti-

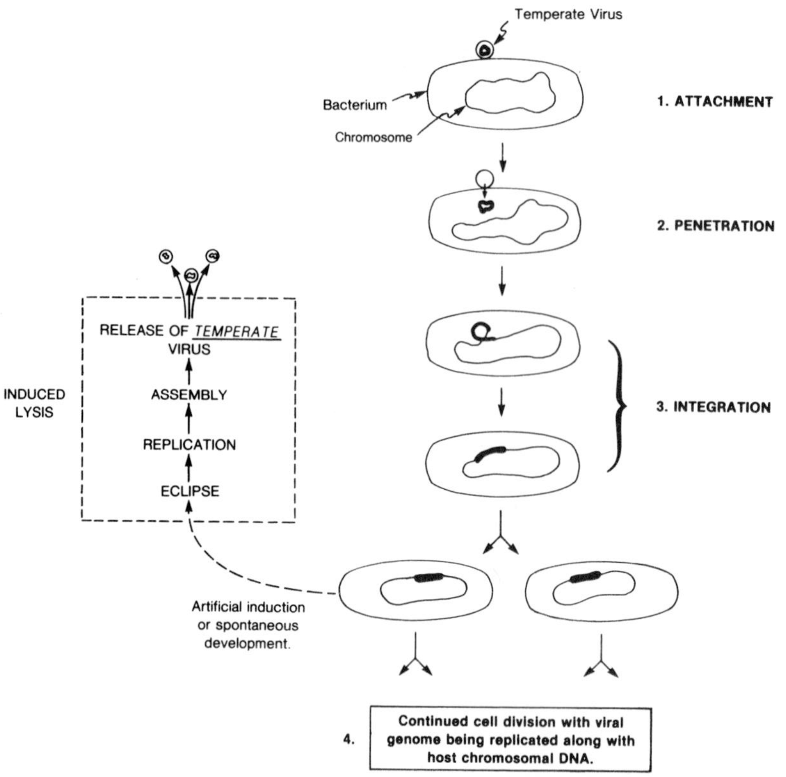

Figure 3–10. Consequences of infecting a lysogenic bacterium with a temperate virus. Attachment and penetration occur just as in the replicative cycle, but once inside the cell, the viral DNA (heavy line) becomes integrated into the host's chromosome. Expression of the integrated viral nucleic acid is normally repressed, but it is replicated along with the host's DNA. If repression is lifted (dotted arrow), the remaining steps in the replicative cycle will occur (box); however, only temperate viruses are produced.

cle occurs, but only temperate phage are produced. Once mature virus particles are assembled inside the host, the host cell will lyse and release temperate phage that can infect new cells but only establish lysogeny.

Usually, lysogenic bacteria show no sign that they are infected, but note that they carry the hereditary ability to produce complete, infective, temperate-phage particles. If a culture of infected lysogenic bacteria is treated with mutagens known to damage DNA and activate the repair process, such as ultraviolet light or nitrosoguanidine, then most if not all of the cells carrying prophage will produce mature temperate phage and lyse. This treatment is called phage induction. It is presumed that the DNA damage somehow disturbs the repression mechanism that inhibits temperate-phage replication, and this derepression allows the replicative cycle to begin and the cell to produce mature temperate phage. Note that this process produces only temperate phage, even though the host cell lyses. This is because the prophage that is induced (derepressed) to complete the replicative cycle codes only for production of temperate phage.

However, induction is not always necessary to produce mature, fully infective, temperate phage particles. In any lysogenic bacterial culture, some small fraction of the prophage-infected cells (e.g., only one in every 1000 or less) will spontaneously produce mature, infective, temperate phage and

lyse. This is why infected lysogenic cultures often produce a few cloudy (not clear) plaques on spread plates containing confluent growth.

Many strains of bacteria isolated from nature are found to carry temperate phage, and the large majority of bacterial viruses isolated from the natural environment are temperate rather than lytic. Therefore, it appears that lysogeny is a common microbiologic phenomenon. Yet, one could reasonably ask why bacteria tolerate temperate phage infections. In the following section, one may see that lysogeny is an advantage not only to the geneticist but also to the bacteria themselves, because a special type of lysogeny (called transduction) may give the host a survival advantage in a constantly changing environment.

RECOMBINATION AS A MECHANISM FOR GENETIC VARIATION IN BACTERIA

Introduction to Recombination Events

We have previously defined bacterial recombination as a "... sudden and inheritable change caused by the introduction of new genetic material (of cellular origin) from outside the cell." Recombination in bacteria involves the insertion of a genetically different piece of DNA (coming from a donor cell) into a recipient cell. Often, but not always, this foreign piece of DNA is inserted into the chromosome of the recipient cell, replicated along with the recipient's own chromosome, and the foreign genes are phenotypically expressed. Insertion of the foreign DNA by recombination may occur in one of three ways among the bacteria: (1) transformation occurs when free chromosomal or plasmid DNA (presumably released upon lysis of another bacterial cell) is inserted directly into another (competent) recipient cell; (2) transduction occurs when chromosomal DNA is also packaged inside a temperate bacterial virus, and transfer of this host DNA occurs along with the viral DNA after the virus infects an appropriate lysogenic host cell; and (3) conjugation (mating) occurs after actual cell-to-cell contact between donor and recipient cells.

Some knowledge of recombination mechanisms in bacteria is necessary to understand certain types of drug resistances and toxin formation in bacteria and for an understanding of how bacteria are genetically "engineered" with genes from animal and plant cells. The next three sections deal with the three types of bacterial recombination events, and the major section that follows shows how these principles are used in genetic engineering.

Transformation

Of the three known recombination mechanisms, transformation is the only one that appears to have evolved solely for the purpose of exchanging chromosomal DNA among bacterial cells. The other two accomplish an exchange of chromosomal DNA only as a consequence of errors in phage replication (transduction) or plasmid transfer (conjugation).

To accomplish transformation, two things are essential: an appropriate source of free DNA (from a donor strain), and competent recipient cells. A recipient cell must be capable of binding the DNA, translocating the DNA across the cell wall and plasma membrane, and then inserting the DNA into its own chromosome.

Nature of Transformable DNA. The long, continuously closed, supercoiled, helix of double-stranded DNA that serves as the chromosome within the bacterial cell does not stay in that form when the cell is lysed. Even with gentle lysis under laboratory conditions, the chromosome will break into 100 or more pieces, each piece containing about 50 genes (one average gene has a molecular weight of about 10^6 with about 1000 base pairs). A competent cell will usually incorporate only a few of these DNA fragments, so that only a small portion of genes from a donor cell can be transferred to another cell by transformation.

Natural Competence. Unaltered cells (recipients) that can take up free DNA fragments and be genetically altered (transformed) are said to be naturally competent. As will be discussed later, it is possible to force some cells to be competent by treating them with high concentrations of calcium ions and subjecting them to temperature shocks to increase the permeability of their wall and plasma membrane. This latter situation is part of a laboratory technique referred to as artificial transformation.

Natural transformation has been described with some gram-positive bacteria (e.g., *Streptococcus pneumoniae, S. sanguis, Bacillus subtilis, B. cereus,* and *B. stearothermophilus*) and with species of several gram-negative genera (e.g., *Neisseria, Acinetobacter, Moraxella, Haemophilus,* and *Pseudomonas*). The discovery of transformation involved the bacterium *Streptococcus pneumoniae.* One strain of this species was encapsulated and virulent, and the other strain of the same species lacked the genetic information needed to produce a capsule and was avirulent. When dead cells of the virulent (capsulated) strain were mixed with live avirulent (uncapsulated) cells, live virulent cells were produced. We now know that DNA containing genes for capsule production were released from the dead cells, and this DNA transformed competent cells in the live but avirulent culture.

Natural competence is affected by the physiologic state of the cells and the composition of the growth medium. For example, in the laboratory, the proportion of competent cells in a population of *S. pneumoniae* rises dramatically during the middle of exponential growth, then falls just as dramatically shortly thereafter. During this brief period when a large number of cells are competent, each competent cell produces and excretes a few molecules of a soluble protein called a competence factor, which induces cells to make about 8 to 10 new proteins. During this period, the outer surface of the competent cells seems to change, so that double-stranded DNA (dsDNA) can bind at specific sites. When this excreted protein is added to noncompetent cells (of the same strain), these cells, too, become competent. These soluble protein competence factors have only been shown in gram-positive bacteria to date.

Uptake of Donor DNA by Competent Cells. The dsDNA first binds to specific proteins on the surface of competent cells. In the case of the gram-positive bacterium *S. pneumoniae,* there are about 30 to 80 sites per cell, and only dsDNA will bind to these sites. Shortly after binding, one of the strands (of the dsDNA) is degraded by a cell-surface bound enzyme. Next, the resulting ssDNA is coated by a single, small molecular weight polypeptide, and this complex enters the cell by an unknown mechanism.

In the case of the gram-negative *Haemophilus* and *Neisseria* species studied, dsDNA is not degraded to ssDNA before it enters the cell.

Integration of Donor ssDNA into the Chromosome. Once inside the cell, the donor ssDNA from *S. pneumoniae* tries to pair with a similar region on the host cell's chromosome. When a similar region is found: (1) one strand of the host's dsDNA is opened up with an enzyme called an endonuclease; (2) the dsDNA is unwound for a short distance; (3) the opposite end of the host DNA (corresponding to the opposite end of the new donor DNA) is also cut with an endonuclease; (4) the new donor strand is inserted; and (5) enzymes called DNA ligases fuse both ends of the donor ssDNA with the adjacent host chromosomal DNA strand. As you might expect, many things can go wrong with this process, and thus the efficiency of natural transformation is usually quite low (from 0.1 to 1.0% of all cells present).

In the case of the gram-negative *Haemophilus* and *Neisseria* species studied, the dsDNA that enters the cell is closely associated with the host cell's chromosome before one strand is degraded. No free ssDNA intermediates seem to exist within the cell prior to incorporation of the donor DNA into the host chromosome. Once again, no single general mechanism appears to account for the way in which the transformed DNA is incorporated into the host chromosome in all bacteria.

Artificial Transformations. Many bacteria (including *E. coli*) appear not to have evolved natural mechanisms for transformation, and attempts to emulate true transformation of open strands of ssDNA or dsDNA into the potential recipient cell's chromosome have generally failed. There seems to be no trouble in getting the linear pieces of ssDNA or dsDNA into the cell, but once inside, these DNA strands seem to be quickly destroyed by the host cell's own nucleases before they can be integrated into the chromosome.

On the other hand, free, self-replicating forms of covalently closed strands of DNA (like plasmids and viral genomes) can be forced inside normally incompetent cells (for example, by subjecting the cells to abnormally high concentrations of calcium ions at low temperatures, or by electroporation), and the frequency of transformants in the survivors is high (about 20%). Apparently these covalently closed circular forms of DNA are not attacked by the recipient cell's intracellular nucleases. The cal-

cium and cold-shock treatment or the electroporation treatment are the most common methods for getting DNA into cells, but a freeze-thaw technique and treatment of protoplasts with polyethylene glycol also have been successfully used with some bacteria.

The process by which self-replicating forms of DNA are artificially introduced into a cell that would normally not be an appropriate host, and the expression of these new genes in the recipient cell, are essential to the field now called "genetic engineering." This topic will be more thoroughly explored near the end of this chapter.

Transduction

Transduction is defined as the transfer of host genes between bacterial strains by bacterial viruses. In terms of the transfer of genetic material, transduction accomplishes the same function as transformation. Transduction appears to result from errors that occur during the replication of the virus. Although most commonly studied in *E. coli,* transduction has been demonstrated in a wide variety of bacteria, and it probably occurs widely in nature.

During the assembly step in phage development, an occasional phage particle becomes filled with host chromosomal DNA or a mixture of both host and phage DNA rather than being filled only with phage DNA (Fig. 3–11). The resulting aberrant phage is often called a transducing particle. It is a defective phage because it never seems to cause subsequent lysis of the newly infected host. After the transducing particle is absorbed to a new host, the phage DNA or donor-host DNA (or both) penetrate the cell wall and plasma membrane. The addition of donor-host DNA to the newly infected host's chromosome and the phenotypic expression of these new genes constitute completion of the transduction event.

Two types of errors in phage development lead to two types of transduction. The difference between these two types apparently depends upon the site at which the phage genome is integrated into the chromosome of the host.

Specialized Transduction. With specialized transduction, only a few host genes are transferred, and they are the same genes each time. Specialized transduction seemingly occurs only with defective temperate phage and only with those phage whose genomes always integrate into the host cell's chromosome at one specific place (Fig. 3–11). The error occurs when something triggers (induces) the defective prophage to complete the replicative cycle. Normally when this happens, only the prophage

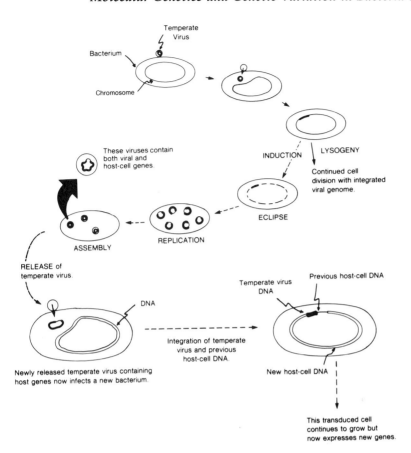

Figure 3–11. Schematic representation of specialized transduction: the transfer of genes from one type of bacterial cell to a similar type by defective temperate bacterial viruses. During virus replication, some adjacent host chromosomal DNA is also replicated. Thus, mature virus particles contain both viral and host genes, and both are integrated upon subsequent infection of a new host. Expression of viral DNA is repressed in the new host, but the newly received bacterial genes may be fully functional.

is cut from the chromosome and replicated. However, during specialized transduction, an error occurs during excision so that part of the adjacent chromosome is also removed, along with part or all of the prophage. Enough prophage DNA must be excised to allow for replication of coat proteins and other requirements for assembly and release of mature phage; otherwise, the replication process will not proceed to completion. On the other hand, the amount of adjacent host-chromosomal material cannot be too large, because there is a very limited amount of space within the capsid (phage head) for packaged DNA. It is for this reason that only a very few host genes are ever transferred during transduction. The more host DNA that is excised, the less room exists for phage DNA, and the greater the chance that assembly of mature phage will not occur. However, when mature phage are produced, most contain host gene(s); therefore, the frequency of transduction is high.

Generalized Transduction. With generalized transduction, almost any gene on the chromosome may be transferred from donor to recipient, but the frequency of transfer is often very low. For example, generalized transduction of genes from *Salmonella typhimurium* infected by phage P22 are usually about one in every 10^5 to 10^9 infected cells.

Unlike specialized transduction, generalized transduction seems to occur with either temperate or lytic phage. When a population of sensitive bacteria is infected with phage and the complete replication cycle takes place, the host DNA often breaks down into phage-genome sized pieces. If some of these chromosomal DNA pieces persist (are not fully degraded by the cell's own nucleases), then a piece of this host DNA may be incorporated inside a capsid during phage assembly. These defective particles are released, along with the normal phage during lysis of the host. When this lysate is used to infect another population of similar cells, most of this population is infected with normal phage. A few cells, however, may be infected with these defective (transducing) particles. When that happens, the donor DNA will penetrate the recipient host, and donor DNA may then be inserted into the recipient cell's chromosome. The reason for the low transduction frequencies that occur with generalized transducing phage is probably the low numbers of phage containing host DNA.

When comparing specialized and generalized transduction, the following distinctions are important. Generalized transduction requires that all host DNA is not degraded prior to assembling the virus particles, and the mistake made here is in the packaging of host DNA instead of viral DNA inside a few capsids. In contrast, the mistake made in specialized transduction is in defining the prophage boundaries for excision; some adjacent host DNA is taken out along with part or all of the prophage prior to replication. Hence the new phage will contain some host-cell genes. In addition, the defects that account for specialized transduction are only realized after inducing lysis in a lysogenic culture carrying prophage, whereas generalized transduction may also occur with lytic phage.

Veterinary Significance of Transduction. From a veterinary standpoint, perhaps the greatest significance of transduction is the ability of bacteriophage to transfer genes that allow for the bacterium to become more virulent or more invasive within the infected tissue. Examples of genes transferred from virulent to nonvirulent strains by transducing phage are: (1) those coding for botulinum toxin by *Clostridium botulinum* (types C and D); (2) those coding for botulinum toxin (type alpha) by *C. botulinum;* (3) those coding for production of alpha-hemolysin or endotoxin by *Staphylococcus aureus;* and (4) those coding for hyaluronidase in *Streptococcus equi.* It presently appears that antibiotic-resistance genes are only rarely transferred to antibiotic sensitive cells by transduction.

Plasmids and Conjugation

Before we can adequately consider conjugation as the third type of recombination event occurring in bacteria, the biology of plasmids must be considered. You may recall that most bacteria have two types of genetic elements (DNA): a chromosome and one or more types of plasmids. Plasmids store genetic information that may, under the proper conditions, be phenotypically expressed. However, it is currently believed that plasmids do not carry genes for essential metabolic activities; instead, the plasmid genes are for other more specialized features. For example, plasmids may carry genes for one or more of the following abilities: (1) to mate and serve as a donor for genetic exchange; (2) to be resistant to chemicals, such as heavy metals, that are normally toxic to microorganisms; and (3) to degrade complex organic chemicals, such as aromatic hydrocarbons found in petroleum. Plasmids have veterinary significance, because some pathogens can transfer genes that code for virulence to normally nonpathogenic strains.

Plasmid Biology. Plasmids are covalently closed, circular, double-stranded molecules of DNA that probably exist inside the cell in a supercoiled state and seem to be present in almost all bacteria examined (Fig. 3–12). Plasmids are usually less than one two-hundredth the size of the bacterial chromosome, although wide variation in plasmid sizes exists even within a single bacterial cell. Plasmid DNA replicates in the same way as chromosomal DNA; this involves initiation at a single point and bidirectional replication of each separate strand around the circle. However, plasmid and chromosomal DNA replicate independently of one another, and plasmid DNA replication is probably under a different type of control. There are usually multiple copies of each plasmid in the bacterial cell, although the copy number seems to depend upon the type of cell and the environment in which it is growing.

Plasmid Transfer by Conjugation. Conjugation between similar bacteria is a mating process that requires cell-to-cell contact and results in transfer of genetic material from one cell (the donor) to another cell (the recipient). The genetic material transferred may be a plasmid or part of the donor's chromosome that has been mobilized by a plasmid.

Most of what is currently known about conjugation comes from studies of gram-negative bacteria, so the following applies only to this type of bacterial cell.

Cells capable of donating DNA via conjugation carry a plasmid that (in part) codes for the ability to be a donor, and this is called a conjugative plasmid. In gram-negative (but not gram-positive) bacteria, the conjugative plasmid codes for production of a "sex" pilus and for some other proteins needed for DNA transfer. Although it is not clearly understood, it appears that the distal end of the sex pilus on the donor makes contact with an appropriate recipient cell. The pilus then retracts, pulling the two cells together until a conjugation bridge is formed, through which the DNA can pass between the donor and recipient cells. Although the recipient cell lacks the sex pilus, it must have some sort of specific recognition factor, so that tight bonding may be made with the distal end of the donor's sex pilus.

In order for DNA transfer to occur, DNA synthesis must also occur. Current evidence suggests that this synthesis occurs at or near the conjugation bridge, and that one of the DNA strands inserted into the recipient cell is from the donor and the other is newly made (Fig. 3–13). The "rolling circle" model (devised to explain DNA synthesis in certain phages) seems to best explain how this is done. Initiation of plasmid DNA synthesis may be triggered by cell-to-cell contact, and this may open

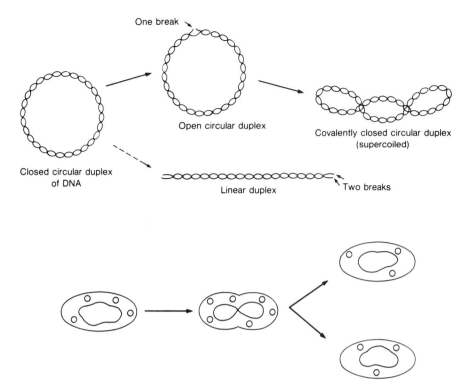

Figure 3–12. Molecular architecture, relative size, and copy numbers of bacterial plasmids. Plasmids are covalently closed, circular, double-stranded, and supercoiled molecules of DNA that are about one two-hundredth the size of the bacterial chromosome. More than one type of plasmid and several copies of the same plasmids may be present in a single cell.

one strand on the donor's plasmid. As this opened strand (the 5′ end) passes through the conjugation bridge, DNA synthesis simultaneously occurs at two places: along the newly unraveled strand, and along the closed complementary strand of the original plasmid. Once the new plasmid is made and fully transferred into the recipient cell, it is covalently closed (circularized) and supercoiled. With this mechanism, the donor cell duplicates its plasmid at the same time transfer occurs, so both the donor and recipient eventually have a complete copy of this plasmid.

Note that conjugative plasmids not only contain genes that allow for conjugation to take place, but they also contain other types of genetic information. Thus, each cell that receives a conjugative plasmid during conjugation not only becomes capable of donating genetic material but it will also receive other genes (such as those that code for antibiotic resistance). This process is so efficient that almost every cell that forms a conjugating pair will acquire new genetic information, and this (along with indiscriminate use of antibiotics) helps to explain how bacterial populations become resistant to antibiotics with such speed. Under proper conditions, the rate of spread of a conjugative plas-

mid through bacterial culture can be exponential and resemble a bacterial growth curve.

Conjugative transfer of plasmids may occur between two strains of the same species, such as between a chloramphenicol-resistant strain of *E. coli* and a chloramphenicol-sensitive strain. Plasmids may also be transferred among different but related bacteria, such as those within the family *Enterobacteriaceae* (from *E. coli* to strains of *Shigella* or *Salmonella*).

Studies of conjugation in *Enterococcus faecalis* suggest that the mechanism of conjugation in gram-positive bacteria is different from that of the well-studied gram-negative bacteria. For example, conjugation between strains of *S. faecalis* does not require a sex pilus. Instead, potential recipient cells release soluble molecules (called pheromones), and these molecules stimulate plasmid-containing cells to produce a substance on their outer surface that allows donor and recipient cells to aggregate. It appears that plasmids are transferred from cell to cell within these aggregates.

Veterinary Significance of Plasmids

Antibiotic Resistance. The emergence of bacteria resistant to several antibiotics is of considerable

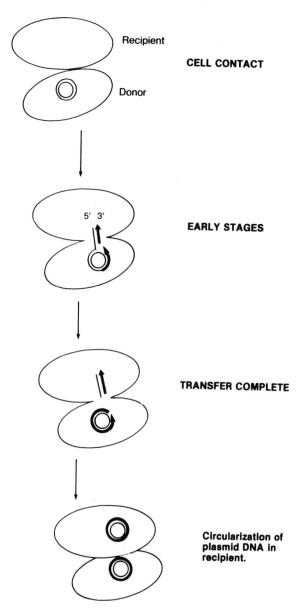

Recipient

CELL CONTACT

Donor

5′ 3′

EARLY STAGES

TRANSFER COMPLETE

Circularization of plasmid DNA in recipient.

Figure 3–13. Replication and transfer of a plasmid during conjugation. Replication occurs along with transfer, so that conjugation does not leave the donor cell devoid of the transferred plasmid and its genetic material.

nickel, and cobalt, and these genes are frequently present on the same plasmids that carry genes for antibiotic resistance. At present, it appears that most R factors are conjugative plasmids, that is, they also carry genes that code for sex-pilus production and other proteins required for conjugation between gram-negative bacteria.

It appears that antibiotic-resistant strains of bacteria that are induced or spontaneously arise in the laboratory almost invariably involve mutations within chromosomal DNA. In most cases, resistance produced by mutated chromosomal DNA arises because of a modification in the target of antibiotic action, such as modifications in the cell wall or ribosome that make the mutants resistant to antibiotic attack.

On the other hand, the majority of drug-resistant strains isolated from patients contain drug-resistant plasmids, and these R factors genetically alter the cell in another way. Plasmid-mediated resistance is usually caused by the introduction of new genes that code for the production of new enzymes that inactivate the drug itself. For example, cells having resistance to the aminoglycoside antibiotics (kanamycin, neomycin, streptomycin, and spectinomycin) make an enzyme that chemically modifies the antibiotic (by acetylation, adenylation, or phosphorylation), and the modified drug lacks antibiotic activity. In penicillin resistance, the plasmid codes for the production of penicillinase (a β-lactamase), an enzyme that cleaves the β-lactam ring of the penicillin molecule, thus rendering it inactive. In the case of chloramphenicol resistance, a gene on the plasmid codes for an enzyme that acetylates the antibiotic, thereby destroying its antibacterial activity.

Toxins and Other Virulence Factors. Research with the gram-negative, enteropathogenic *E. coli* suggests that the ability of pathogenic bacteria to attach and grow at a specific site in the host and to produce toxins may be carried by genes on a plasmid. Specific recognition and attachment of *E. coli* to the epithelial lining of the intestine require that this bacterium produce a protein on its surface. In addition, the synthesis of two toxins (a hemolysin and an enterotoxin) is coded for by plasmid genes. At present it is not clear why these virulence factors are plasmid-coded and others reside on the chromosome, nor is it understood how many other virulence factors are plasmid-related among the gram-negative bacteria.

The common gram-positive bacterium *Staphylococcus aureus* produces a number of substances that add to its virulence, such as coagulase, enterotoxin, fibrinolysin, hemolysin, and a yellow pigment. The

medical importance and is correlated with the increasing use of antibiotics for the treatment of infectious diseases. A variety of plasmids (sometimes called R factors or resistance-transfer factors) carry *multiple* antibiotic resistance genes on a single plasmid. Those most commonly observed carry resistance to four antibiotics (chloramphenicol, streptomycin, the sulfonamides, and tetracycline), but some have fewer or more resistant genes on one plasmid. Plasmids are also known that have resistance to kanamycin, penicillin, and neomycin. Some plasmids also contain genes that allow the bacterium to be resistant to metals such as mercury, genes that code for production of these substances are found on plasmids. Each of these substances contributes to the evasiveness, invasiveness, and survival—and therefore the pathogenicity—of *S. aureus.*

At the present time, much research is being conducted on the significance of plasmids in determining bacterial virulence.

Bacteriocins. Many bacteria produce substances called bacteriocins that kill or inhibit growth of closely related bacteria such as different strains of the same species. This very limited spectrum of activity can be useful to the clinical microbiologist. For example, if all of the *Proteus mirabilis* strains isolated from surgical wounds of patients in the same ward have the same bacteriocin type, they probably originated from the same source and may have had a common means of transmission.

Bacteriocins are usually proteins and frequently have a high molecular weight. Often, the terms used to refer to these large, protein molecules reflect the type of bacteria that produce them. For example, bacteriocins produced by *Escherichia coli* and other enteric bacteria are called colicins, and those produced by staphylococci are called staphylococcins.

The ability to produce most if not all of the known bacteriocins is attributed to genes residing on plasmids, but bacteriocin-producing cells either lack the ability to conjugatively transfer these plasmids or they only transfer these plasmids at very low frequency. This helps the clinical microbiologist, because the production and susceptibility of bacteria to bacteriocins is very strain-specific. Therefore, this stable characteristic can be used by the microbiologist to specifically identify bacterial strains and to study the origin and transmission of these virulent bacterial strains.

GENETIC ENGINEERING THROUGH GENE MANIPULATION

Genetic engineering refers to the application of basic principles of microbial genetics in the isolation, manipulation, and expression of genetic material. At present, genetically engineered bacteria are used in two rather different ways: (1) to increase the quantity of microbial products; and (2) to express inserted genes of animal or plant origin such that the bacterial cell produces a protein normally produced only by an animal or plant cell. The first and oldest application of genetic engineering uses genetic manipulation to increase the yields of desirable microbial products. This may be done by increasing the number of gene copies on the chromo-some, or by altering the gene such that production of the gene product is no longer tightly regulated by the cell.

The second use of genetic engineering is more recent and has received more attention in the popular press. In that application, animal or plant genes are first removed from the chromosome. These genes are then inserted into a bacterial plasmid, and that genetically altered plasmid is placed back into the same bacterial cell. This genetically altered bacterium will now produce a protein whose synthesis is directed by the animal or plant genes. Molecules of DNA that contain unrelated segments are referred to as "recombinant DNA." Hence the phrase "recombinant-DNA technology" is often used in place of "genetic engineering."

What follows is a brief introduction to the second application of genetic engineering and the ways in which genetic engineering may affect the future practicing veterinarian. For a more complete treatment of the basic principles of genetic engineering, the reader is referred to Brock, et al. (1994, Chapter 8).

Plasmids as Cloning Vectors

The microbial geneticist frequently uses the word "clone" to refer to a population of identical bacteria having the same type of recombinant DNA. The term "cloning vector" is used to refer to the complete DNA molecule or virus that can bring about replication of that foreign DNA fragment in the cell. The "host" is the bacterium that contains the genetically reconstructed cloning vector.

A good cloning vector must have the following characteristics: (1) it will self-replicate in the host; (2) its DNA can be easily separated from the host and purified; and (3) it must contain regions of the DNA that are not essential for vector replication and can be removed from the vector and replaced with the foreign DNA fragment. In addition, it is very desirable if the cloning vector is a small piece of DNA that is able to enter the cell and replicate to a high copy number (many copies per cell). It is also desirable that the vector be stable in the host and that it directs a high product yield from the foreign gene. To date, the most useful cloning vectors are certain bacterial viruses and plasmids. However, the following discussion will be limited to the use of plasmids as cloning vectors.

The host for replication of the cloning vector must also be chosen with care. A desirable host is fast-growing, genetically stable, not pathogenic, and able to grow in an inexpensive culture medium. In addition, the desirable host must be transformable, that is, one must be able to make the potential host artificially competent so that it will take up the DNA used as the cloning vector. The methods used to accomplish the insertion of this DNA are the same as those discussed in the previous section on transformation.

Optimum expression of the foreign DNA on the cloning vector is extremely important. Therefore, the plasmid cloning vector must not only contain the proper foreign genes but it should also have adequate regulatory sequences, so that expression of the foreign genes is under control of the microbiologist. It is ideal to grow host cells to a high population density while the cloned genes on the plasmid are repressed, then add an inducer to allow maximum expression of the cloned foreign genes. For this reason, regulatory sequences are usually inserted along with and adjacent to the cloned genes. For example, constructing plasmid vectors that contain the regulatory components for the *lac* operon (promoter, regulator, and operator) to control synthesis of the foreign DNA is one way to provide a suitable regulatory switch. When this is done, cells are grown in the absence of the inducer, lactose (see Fig. 3–7), so that the switch regulating the adjacent foreign genes is turned off. When the cells reach maximum numbers, the inducer (lactose) is added to start expression of the foreign genes. Production of high levels of several mammalian proteins (e.g., up to 15,000 molecules of human interferon per *E. coli* cell) are achieved using these expression vectors.

Steps in Constructing a Plasmid Cloning Vector

The overall process of constructing a plasmid cloning vector is shown in Figure 3–14. First, a plasmid (preferably one that already has a high copy number) is isolated from a bacterium that will later serve as an acceptable host. Cells are gently lysed, and the plasmid fraction is collected by ultracentrifugation. After separation of the various plasmids by size (molecular weight) and purification of a single plasmid type, this potential cloning vector is ready for gene manipulation.

Second, the plasmid DNA is cut open using purified, site-specific enzymes called restriction endonucleases.

Third, the animal or plant gene is precisely described, so that it may be either removed (as shown in Fig. 3–14) or artificially constructed (as most often is the case). If the gene is removed from the chromosome, the same types of restriction endonucleases are used, so that a similarly sized fragment is cut, having ends complementary to those on the cut plasmid. Alternatively, the eucaryotic gene may be artificially constructed in one of at least two ways: (1) the specific mRNA for that protein is isolated, and then an enzyme called reverse transcriptase is used to construct a DNA molecule from the sequence of bases on the mRNA; or, with more difficulty, (2) the desired gene product (protein) is purified, the amino acid sequence determined, an mRNA molecule constructed that will code for synthesis of this protein, and, finally, reverse transcriptase is used to construct the complementary DNA sequence (gene). Regardless of the method used, the foreign gene is now ready to be inserted into the cut plasmid.

Fourth, the broken ends of the foreign DNA are attached to the homologous broken ends of the plasmid DNA with an enzyme called DNA ligase. This creates a recombinant plasmid that is part bacterial and part foreign (eucaryotic) DNA. Note that some time during this process, the regulatory switch, such as that obtained from the *lac* operon, is also added to this recombinant plasmid.

Fifth, host bacteria are made artificially competent (e.g., by applying excessive calcium ions, or by temperature-shock treatment, or electroporation), and the DNA is forced into the cells. Unlike the transformation phenomenon, however, it appears that the entire double-stranded DNA molecule is taken in, and there is no subsequent integration into the cell's chromosome. This newly introduced, genetically engineered vector remains as an extra-chromosomal self-replicating unit and now constitutes part of the host cell's genomic material.

Sixth, the host is now grown in such a way that the expression of the eucaryotic gene is regulated for maximum expression. Often, "fusion proteins" are made, either (1) to make the protein more stable inside the cell, that is, to make it more resistant to the protein-degrading enzymes normally present inside the bacterial cell; or (2) to allow the protein to be exported to the outside, where it can be more easily isolated and purified. Fusion proteins contain a short, procaryotic, amino acid sequence at one end of the protein fused to the desired eucaryotic amino acid sequence at the other. Sometimes the intracellular accumulation of excessive quantities of fusion proteins is toxic to the cell, so additional genes must be added to the engineered plasmid to assure that this eucaryotic gene product can get out of the cell and be released into the medium. After the fusion protein is released from the cell, the procaryotic portion may be chemically cut away, and then the eucaryotic part may be purified and readied for use.

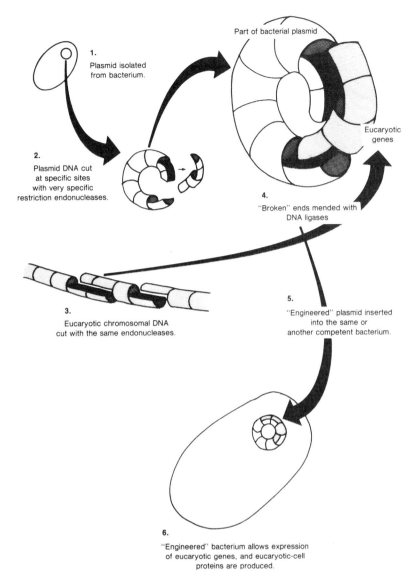

1. Plasmid isolated from bacterium.

2. Plasmid DNA cut at specific sites with very specific restriction endonucleases.

Part of bacterial plasmid

Eucaryotic genes

4. "Broken" ends mended with DNA ligases

3. Eucaryotic chromosomal DNA cut with the same endonucleases.

5. "Engineered" plasmid inserted into the same or another competent bacterium.

6. "Engineered" bacterium allows expression of eucaryotic genes, and eucaryotic-cell proteins are produced.

Figure 3–14. Steps in constructing a plasmid cloning vector. This process is commonly used in the field known as genetic engineering.

Veterinary Significance of Genetically Engineered Plasmids

The potential application of genetically engineered procaryotic cells for the production of animal proteins is staggering. Not only are these processes much less expensive and time-consuming than conventional methods of production, but the bacterially produced proteins are also easier to purify. Therefore, when administered to the animal, they cause fewer side reactions than proteins isolated from animal tissue. At present, genetically altered bacterial cells are producing: human, porcine, and bovine growth hormone (for treatment of growth defects); human insulin (for the treatment of diabetes); human interferon (an antiviral agent); human serum albumin (for transfusion applications); parathyroid hormone (for calcium reg-

ulation); urokinase (for treating blood clotting disorders); and viral proteins (such as coat proteins from cytomegalovirus, hepatitis B virus, influenza virus, and foot-and-mouth disease virus for vaccine production).

One of the most useful veterinary applications of genetically altered bacteria is the production of effective vaccine proteins. Effective vaccines may be made to protect the animal against procaryotic, eucaryotic, or viral pathogens. For simplicity's sake, only virus vaccines will be discussed further.

Virus vaccines for animal use commonly contain either killed or live, attenuated virus. With both types, there is a danger that the vaccine may contain virulent virus particles. In contrast, genetically engineered vaccines may contain only viral coat (capsid) proteins that serve as antigens to stimulate the immune response. Thus, it is desirable to produce the viral coat protein and use only this as the vaccine, so that the potentially dangerous use of live or killed suspensions may be avoided. Safe vaccines composed only of viral coat protein can be made by genetically altered bacteria that have been "engineered" to produce the viral coat protein. Generally, viral DNA is isolated from purified viral suspensions and then fragmented with endonucleases. The fragments are then inserted into an appropriate vector (usually a plasmid) using DNA ligases, and the recombinant plasmid is artificially transferred into the host bacterium. The purified protein produced by these bacteria is then used as a vaccine.

In 1981, the U.S. Department of Agriculture announced the first vaccine produced by genetically altered bacteria (*E. coli*); this was the capsid protein for the virus causing foot-and-mouth disease (FMD) of cattle, sheep, hogs, and other animals. Although strict vigilance has prevented an outbreak in the U.S. since 1929, the disease is still a serious problem in Asia, Africa, South America, and southern Europe. The vaccines in use prior to the development of the *E. coli*-produced vaccine presented many problems. For example, the older vaccines had to be refrigerated, and that presented problems with their use in developing countries. Also, each older vaccine protected against only one type of virus. Since the virus readily mutates, the usefulness of any one vaccine was limited. Nevertheless, an estimated 500 million doses were administered annually, which made it the most widely used antiviral vaccine.

From FMD data made available in 1981, it appeared that the capsid protein was first made inside the genetically altered bacterial cell as a fusion protein that contained about equal parts of viral and bacterial protein. This fusion protein could be physically removed from the bacterial cell and cleaved by cyanogen bromide. This treatment released a small-molecular-weight polypeptide (capsid protein) that protected steers from challenge with virulent FMD virus. The fusion protein was produced in large quantity by the genetically altered *E. coli* (about 10^6 molecules per cell). This meant that one liter of culture medium could produce about 10,000 doses of effective vaccine (purified protein).

Because of the economic advantages of using bacteria to produce pure viral proteins and the safety value of avoiding killed or attenuated viral strains for vaccines, one might logically expect that genetically altered bacterial strains will soon be producing many other vaccines for veterinary use. It is also likely that proteins of animal origin will soon be produced for therapeutic use in domestic animals as is now being done for use with humans.

Another development in the use of genetically engineered bacteria is for the production of either bovine or porcine somatotropin, a growth-regulating hormone that stimulates protein synthesis, and, therefore, muscle development. One industrial process for the bacterial production of porcine somatotropin (pST) is characterized by the production of 3 grams of pST per liter of culture medium, which represents about 40% of the total protein made by the bacterium. Research to date indicates: (1) that injected pST is completely metabolized by the animal (no residue found); (2) its use (by injection or implantation) stimulates weight gain and causes a 24% improvement in feed efficiency; and (3) the animal has about 30% less backfat.

It seems likely that future research will provide us with more examples of genetically altered bacteria that will be used to make other animal proteins for agricultural use or for the manufacture of safer animal vaccines.

FURTHER READING

Brock, T.D., Madigan, M.T., Martinko, J.M., and Parker, J.: Biology of Microorganisms. 7th Ed. Englewood Cliffs, N.J., Prentice-Hall, 1994.

Drlica, K.: Understanding DNA and Gene Cloning: A Guide for the Curious. 2nd Ed. New York, John Wiley & Sons, Inc., 1992.

Freifelder, D.: Microbial Genetics. Boston, Jones and Bartlett Publishers, Inc., 1987.

Hardy, K.: Aspects of Microbiology 4: Bacterial Plasmids. 2nd Ed. American Society for Microbiology, 1986.

Isaacson, R.E., (ed.): Recombinant DNA Vaccines: Rationale and Strategy. New York, Marcel Dekker, Inc., 1992.

Neidhardt, F.C., Ingraham, J.L., and Schaechter, M.: Physiology of the Bacterial Cell: A Molecular Approach. Sunderland, MA, Sinauer Associates, 1990.

Pelczar, M.J., Jr., Chan, E.C.S., and Krieg, N.R.: Microbiology: Concepts and Applications. New York, McGraw-Hill, Inc., 1993.

Watson, J.D., Gilman, M., Witkowski, J., and Zoller, M.: Recombinant DNA. 2nd Ed. New York, W.H. Freeman and Co., 1992.

4

Sources and Transmission
of Infectious Agents

The microorganisms causing diseases in animals (including humans) are derived from the following sources: (1) animals (including humans)—by far the most important; and (2) inanimate nature—relatively less important.

The various organisms that can cause disease have natural habitats to which they are well adapted. Most organisms that have the potential to cause disease in animals are associated with those animals. Some organisms will usually only grow and multiply in certain host species. Some disease-causing organisms are transmissible from animals to humans and vice versa.

There are a large number of microorganisms living in water, soil, and decaying vegetation. The great majority of these are incapable of causing disease in animals, but a few have the capacity to grow and multiply in animal tissue. Some only cause disease when the host's defenses are impaired. When disease is caused by organisms that are uncommon pathogens, the term opportunistic infection is frequently used.

ANIMAL SOURCES

THE ANIMAL'S OWN ORGANISMS

All animals have what is called a normal flora (microbiota). It consists of the bacteria, viruses, and fungi that live in or upon the normal animal without producing disease. Included in this normal flora are a number of potential pathogens.

When considering the normal flora, it should be kept in mind that the kinds and numbers of bacteria and other organisms present in and upon an animal species vary greatly with different individuals and different circumstances. The intestinal flora of the adult animal differs significantly from that of the young animal. The flora is influenced by nutrition, climate, age, and geographic location. The technical methods employed to recover pathogenic organisms may give a distorted idea of the kinds and numbers of organisms present. The gram-negative, nonspore-forming bacteria are the most populous in the large intestine, but this fact is often obscured because the methods used in the clinical laboratory do not necessarily support the growth of these bacteria.

The normal floras of the various domestic animal species have not been studied as thoroughly as those of humans and of the mouse. The little information available and first-hand experience in the veterinary diagnostic laboratory indicate a considerable similarity, in the broad sense, between the normal flora of humans and mice and that of domestic animals. However, it should be kept in mind that there are significant differences in the flora of the alimentary tract, depending on whether the animal is predominantly herbivorous, omnivorous, or carnivorous.

While considering the normal flora in general, it should be kept in mind that it plays an important role in the nutrition of animals, particularly in the herbivores. The normal microbial flora has a protective value in that it tends to exclude other non-resident bacteria, including those that are potentially pathogenic. For example, the presence in the teat canal of *Corynebacterium bovis* may help protect the udder from bacterial infection. Disturbances in the normal flora caused by prolonged antibiotic administration may result in overgrowth and infection by various bacteria and fungi such as staphylococci and *Candida albicans*. Reduction of the gastrointestinal flora of experimental animals by treatment with streptomycin renders them more susceptible to *Salmonella* infection. The selective growth of *Clostridium difficile* in humans caused by antibiotic treatment may result in pseudomembranous colitis.

Some of the kinds of bacteria that can be expected to occur normally in and upon domestic animals follow.

Mouth, Nasopharynx. Micrococci; *Staphylococcus*; alpha- and beta-hemolytic streptococci; *Bacteroides*; lactobacilli; fusiform bacilli; *Actinomyces*; gram-negative cocci; coliforms and *Proteus* spp.; spirochetes; mycoplasmas; *Pasteurella* spp.; diphtheroids; yeasts, including *Candida albicans*; and *Haemophilus*.

Stomach. In monogastric animals the stomach is sterile or contains fewer than 10^3 organisms per ml. Most of the organisms that enter the stomach with food are killed by the hydrochloric acid or removed by forward peristalsis.

Duodenum, Jejunum, Ileum. Only small numbers of bacteria are present in the duodenum and jejunum of humans. There are small numbers in the ileum, with increasing numbers toward its termination. The same probably applies to most of the domestic animals.

Large Intestine. *Escherichia coli*; *Klebsiella*; *Enterobacter*; *Pseudomonas* spp.; *Proteus* spp.; enterococci; staphylococci; clostridia: *Cl. perfringens*, *Cl. septicum*, and others; gram-negative anaerobes; spirochetes; and lactobacilli. The gram-negative non-spore-forming bacteria make up more than 90% of the fecal bacteria. One gram of feces contains about 10^{11} bacteria.

Trachea, Bronchi, Lungs. Few if any bacteria and fungi reside permanently in these structures.

Vulva. Diphtheroids; micrococci; coliforms and *Proteus* spp.; enterococci; yeasts; gram-negative anaerobes. The same kinds of organisms and others can be recovered from the prepuce of the male.

Vagina. The numbers and kinds of bacteria vary with the reproductive cycle and age. The cervix and anterior vagina of the healthy mare have few bacteria. Some of the organisms recovered from the vagina are alpha- and beta-hemolytic streptococci; coliforms; *Proteus* spp.; diphtheroids; lactobacilli; mycoplasmas; and yeasts and fungi.

Lactobacilli metabolize epithelial glycogen to produce lactic acid. The consequent low vaginal pH inhibits colonization by other bacteria.

Skin. By virtue of their habits and environment, animals frequently possess a large and varied bacterial and fungal flora on their hair and skin. *Staphylococcus* spp. occur commonly, as do micrococci, diphtheroids, propionibacteria and *Pityrosporum*. Of the many other organisms isolated, it may be difficult to determine which make up the resident flora and which are "transients."

Milk. Micrococci, staphylococci, nonhemolytic streptococci, mycoplasmas, and diphtheroids, including *Corynebacterium bovis*, are frequently shed from the apparently normal mammary gland. Some reside in the teat canal.

We have mentioned a number of commensal organisms that are potential pathogens. A number of organisms also exist that are not part of the normal flora and, when present in or upon an animal, almost always are associated with latent or overt disease. These organisms, for example *Brucella* spp., certain *Mycobacterium* spp., and *Bacillus anthracis*, are sometimes called obligate pathogens.

ANIMALS INCUBATING A DISEASE

The incubation period is that period from the time of infection until clinical signs appear. During this period the animal appears healthy but may be infectious, i.e., capable of discharging disease-producing organisms. Examples are many of the respiratory diseases caused by viruses, *Pasteurella* spp., and *Haemophilus* spp., in which the organisms may be expelled in saliva or droplets. In intestinal diseases pathogenic organisms may be shed in the feces in the incubative stage.

ANIMALS WITH OVERT DISEASE

Ordinarily the largest numbers of organisms are shed when the animal displays clinical signs of disease. The route by which they are shed depends upon the location of the disease. We have mentioned respiratory and intestinal routes of shedding of infectious organisms. They may also be released from the skin in such diseases as dermatophytosis (ringworm) and dermatophilosis and via the urine or genital secretions if infections involve these systems. The extent and duration of the shedding of organisms varies with different diseases. In the acute diseases such as anthrax, it is usually short, while in chronic diseases such as tuberculosis, it may be long. Some diseases such as actinomycosis are sporadic in their occurrence and are not considered transmissible. Sporadic endogenous infections (those caused by the animal's own organisms) such as actinomycosis, bacterial endocarditis, and meningitis are often not transmissible to other animals.

CONVALESCENT CARRIER ANIMALS

The causative organisms are usually shed for varying periods after clinical recovery from a disease. In respiratory infections some of the causative organisms—e.g., pasteurellas and mycoplasmas—may be shed by way of droplets during expiration for some time after apparent recovery. Likewise in salmonellosis, the salmonella organisms may be shed for weeks in the feces, although the animal is clinically normal. These animals are referred to as *convalescent carriers,* and the state is often referred to as the *carrier state.* The number of organisms shed will diminish with time, but the period of "excretion" may vary from a week to several months. Not all recovered animals are necessarily shedders. In some diseases such as salmonellosis and fowl cholera, a chronic carrier state tends to develop. In some severe diseases such as anthrax in cattle, there usually is no convalescent or chronic carrier state. In recovered strangles and hemorrhagic septicemia the period of the carrier state is usually relatively short.

CONTACT CARRIERS OR SUBCLINICAL INFECTIONS

Animals may acquire pathogenic organisms from other animals with infectious disease without contracting the disease themselves. In most groups of animals exposed to infectious disease there will often be some that acquire the organisms but do not develop clinical disease. The number of such animals depends upon the disease, the virulence of the organism, and the animal's immune state. Such animals are referred to as *contact or subclinical carriers.* This carrier state may be temporary, lasting only a few days, or chronic, lasting weeks or months. Such contact carriers are seen in diseases such as strangles in horses and erysipelas and salmonellosis in swine. The term *convalescent carrier* is sometimes used for those recovered animals that still carry the pathogen. These subclinical carrier states represent a threat to other animals and are a means whereby the disease is perpetuated. Such states can only be detected, sometimes with difficulty, by demonstration of the organisms, usually by cultural procedures; this is the case in salmonellosis and Johne's disease. In epizootic bovine infertility it has been necessary to use "test mating" to detect infected or carrier bulls. The suspected bulls are bred to susceptible heifers to see whether

or not they infect them. Some of the more severe diseases such as anthrax and rinderpest of cattle result in very few if any contact carriers.

INANIMATE SOURCES

Organisms such as some species of *Clostridium, Proteus, Klebsiella,* and *Pseudomonas aeruginosa* exist in the free-living state in the soil, where they derive their sustenance from decaying vegetation. Those just mentioned may also inhabit the intestine as commensals and be shed in the feces. Less common free-living organisms such as species of *Acinetobacter, Aeromonas, Chromobacterium,* and *Flavobacterium* on rare occasions will cause disease in humans and animals. However, most only cause disease under special circumstances. *Pseudomonas aeruginosa* may infect wounds and tissues damaged by burns. *Proteus* can cause urinary tract infections, and *Klebsiella* strains can produce severe mastitis in cows. Impaired defenses and numbers of organisms (dosage) are important in such infections.

The spores of clostridia, which occur widely in soil and feces, gain entrance to wounds and cause such gas gangrene type diseases as blackleg and malignant edema, or tetanus. Other clostridia such as *C. botulinum,* which is also soilborne, cause poisoning as a result of the production of a potent exotoxin in contaminated food. Certain toxin-producing strains of *C. perfringens,* which occur in soil and animal feces, produce toxins in the intestines that may result in severe toxemia.

A number of ordinarily saprophytic fungi have the capacity to produce disease in animals. They cause such sporadic diseases as sporotrichosis, histoplasmosis, and coccidioidomycosis. The occurrence of the last two is dependent upon the geographic distribution of the fungi in the soil.

TRANSMISSION

Infecting agents are most frequently transmitted to new hosts by direct or indirect contact. The direct process refers to spread by contact with the infecting organisms on the infected host, i.e., contact with discharges on the animal that have emanated from the skin or various body openings. The other means of direct contact is by coitus. In most diseases the indirect process is most often responsible. This means that the organisms shed or excreted by the host are carried in or upon various vehicles such as water, milk, food, litter, air, or dust. Such contaminated inanimate objects as food, water, litter, bedding, mangers, and kennels are referred to collectively as *fomites.* Other indirect means of spread are by contaminated medical, surgical, and dental instruments; syringes and needles (these may be responsible for equine infectious anemia, and anaplasmosis); speculums; and dressings.

Various arthropods such as ticks, mites, lice, flies, and mosquitoes act as vectors for infectious diseases. Some agents are transmitted in a purely mechanical manner while others are actually inoculated by biting insects, as in tularemia. In several diseases the infecting agent may multiply in the vector. For example, *Yersinia pestis*, which causes plague, multiplies in the salivary gland of the flea.

Organisms enter the host by one of the following portals of entry:

1. Inhalation and infection via the respiratory tract.
2. Ingestion and infection via the alimentary tract.
3. Inoculation or infection through the skin or mucous membranes by simple contact, injection (e.g., biting insect, contaminated hypodermic syringe or needle), or wound infection.
4. Via the genital tract as a result of coitus. Also by means of contaminated instruments, catheters, and semen from artificial insemination centers.
5. By means of transplacental infection.
6. Via the umbilicus.

Most organisms produce infections only if they enter by way of a particular portal. For example, enteropathogenic *E. coli* gain entrance to the intestine through the upper digestive tract but not through the skin. *Staphylococcus aureus*, on the other hand, readily enters the skin but rarely causes infection as a result of ingestion. Some organisms such as *Brucella* species may enter the host through several portals—the skin and oral or genital tract mucous membranes. The lesions produced by the invading organism may involve tissues and organs remote from the site of entry. Although the mode of infection of the swine erysipelas organism may be ingestion, the lesions are not associated with the alimentary tract.

Infection Via the Respiratory Tract

This is the common mode of infection in respiratory diseases, although these infections can also be acquired by direct contact and from fomites. The source of the organisms is generally the secretions of the respiratory tract of another animal. The infections are acquired as a result of the inhalation of contaminated air. The organisms are trapped on the moist mucous membranes of the nasopharynx

and lower respiratory tract. This is the way that diseases such as pasteurella pneumonias, viral pneumonias, and tuberculosis are transmitted. The spores of a number of fungi, such as *Histoplasma capsulatum*, that infect via the respiratory tract are acquired from the soil by inhalation.

Droplet Infection

Few or no organisms are shed into the air from the nose or mouth in normal breathing. However, large numbers of organisms are expelled during coughing and sneezing. Many of these organisms are derived from the mouth and oropharynx.

In coughing the vast majority of particles emanate from the respiratory tract in the form of droplets. It is estimated that in humans a vigorous cough may release five or six thousand droplets, while a vigorous sneeze may liberate as many as a million droplets.

The majority of the droplets expelled are less than 100 μm in diameter. These evaporate rapidly, leaving *droplet nuclei* suspended in the air for many hours. These consist of dried secretions that may contain organisms. Eventually they fall to the ground or other surroundings, resulting in their contamination. Droplets with a diameter of 100 μm or more have a very short trajectory and fall a very short distance from the host animal.

Of the droplets generated from saliva at the front of the mouth, many do not contain the infecting agent and many are sterile. It should be kept in mind that only a small proportion of the droplet nuclei contain pathogens. However, it often takes only a few organisms to initiate some diseases.

Dust-borne Infections

Many respiratory infections are probably acquired by the following indirect process: (1) the infected animal contaminates itself and its environment with secretions and infected droplets; and (2) the organisms dry on whatever they contaminate to be dispersed into the air subsequently in the form of dust. The inhalation of these infectious dust particles constitutes an important mode of infection in respiratory diseases. The success of the method depends to a considerable extent on the capacity of the organisms to withstand the effects of drying. This mode of infection is responsible for the transmission of such diseases as psittacosis (transmitted through dried infectious feces) and tuberculosis.

Infection by Ingestion

Organisms causing intestinal diseases gain entrance to the alimentary tract after being swallowed, e.g., salmonellas and enteropathogenic *E. coli. Mycobacterium bovis* may enter by this route and cause disease involving the intestine. The preformed exotoxins of *Clostridium botulinum* and *Staphylococcus aureus* are conveyed to the intestine in food. *C. perfringens* organisms giving rise to enterotoxemia may gain entrance to the body by ingestion. A number of infecting agents, such as *Brucella abortus*, enteroviruses, and *Coxiella burnetii*, may enter through the intestinal wall but produce their effects elsewhere. In intestinal disease the feces are the principal source of the pathogens.

Animals may become infected with intestinal pathogens as a result of direct contact with the feces-contaminated host or, more commonly, by contact with fomites such as contaminated feed, milk, bedding, surroundings (stable, mangers), and water. Because of the habits of animals, with the consequent frequent exposure to feces, intestinal diseases usually spread rapidly.

INFECTION RESULTING FROM INOCULATION

Contact

Some diseases are spread by agents that can penetrate apparently undamaged skin or mucous membranes. *Brucella abortus*, *Bacillus anthracis*, and *Francisella tularensis* have this capacity. In animals, disease is spread in this manner most often by means of fomites such as infected litter and bedding, saddles, milker's hands, and milking machines rather than by direct contact. Included among the diseases that may be spread by these direct and indirect means are skin abscesses, pyoderma, poxvirus diseases, ringworm, the various viral papillomatoses, and dermatophilosis.

Wounds

Many organisms gain entrance to the underlying tissues through breaks in the continuity of skin or mucous membranes. In animals, wounds have numerous causes, including accidents, surgical operations (especially docking and castration), calving, goring, biting, and wounds due to nail punctures and bullets or shots. The sources of organisms that lodge in wounds are various. Tetanus results from the contamination of wounds by spores from the soil or feces. *Staphylococcus aureus* and *Actinomyces pyogenes*, which are carried in the nasopharynx of many animals, frequently infect wounds. Soilborne nocardia introduced during non-aseptic treatment of the udder may produce a severe mastitis. Other soil and fecal-borne organisms that infect wounds, resulting in gas gangrene, are *C. septicum* and *C. perfringens*. In surgery involving the stomach or intestine, incisions may become infected with such enteric organisms as *E. coli* and *Bacteroides* spp., sometimes leading to peritonitis.

Injection

As mentioned previously, infectious agents may be injected via the bites of arthropods or insects, or they may be injected mistakenly or carelessly by humans. Diseases such as equine infectious anemia and anaplasmosis, to mention only two, may be transmitted by contaminated hypodermic needles and surgical instruments. These two diseases are also spread by biting insects. The equine viral encephalitides are spread by mosquitoes, and Rocky Mountain spotted fever is initiated by the bite of an infected tick. Tularemia is spread mainly by ticks and plague by fleas. The hog louse appears to be an important disseminator of swine pox virus.

INFECTION VIA THE GENITAL TRACT

Infectious agents may enter the genital tract to set up infections at various times but most frequently after parturition and at estrus. A number of important diseases are transmitted from male to female during coitus, e.g., bovine genital campylobacteriosis, brucellosis, equine vesicular exanthema, and infectious pustular vulvovaginitis. *Corynebacterium renale*, a cause of bovine pyelonephritis, may gain entrance to the urinary tract from the genital tract.

TRANSPLACENTAL INFECTION

The fetuses of several animal species become infected and frequently are stillborn or aborted as a result of transplacental infection. In some diseases, such as brucellosis, *Campylobacter* abortion, and mycotic abortion, the disease process is mostly confined to the placenta, but the organisms can be recovered from the fetal stomach contents and various organs. Lesions within the fetus itself may be minimal. Abortion resulting from *Listeria* infection occurs, and this organism may be recovered from the stomach contents and various organs. The fetus may be profoundly affected by the infecting agent, e.g., a cerebellar hypoplasia may result from infection with the hog cholera virus, and extensive fetal damage occurs in chlamydial abortion of sheep and cattle.

INFECTION VIA THE UMBILICUS

Infection of the newborn may be prenatal, e.g., an extension of cervicitis or placentitis, or postnatal, in which the common modes of infection are ingestion, inhalation, or via the umbilicus. The umbilicus frequently becomes infected if the navel is not properly cared for immediately after birth. The young of all the domestic species are prone to infections that start from the umbilicus, but lambs are particularly susceptible. A variety of organisms enter via the umbilicus, e.g., *Erysipelothrix rhusiopathiae, Salmonella, Klebsiella,* pyogenic streptococci, *Actinomyces pyogenes,* and *Actinobacillus equuli.*

The disease manifestations are variable, depending upon the virulence of the organism and the resistance of the newborn. First there is bacteremia, which, in severe infections, may proceed to septicemia and death. More often, however, the bacteremia results in organisms being disseminated to organs, lymph nodes, and joints, where disease processes develop. A number of names are applied to what are collectively called the neonatal pyosepticemias. They include navel ill, omphalitis, joint ill, omphalophlebitis, pyemic arthritis, and polyarthritis.

Nosocomial Infections

These are hospital-acquired infections. A number of infectious agents, including bacteria, fungi, and viruses, may be transmitted within the veterinary hospital or clinic. Latent infections or carrier states may flare up into serious infections as a result of various stresses, and the agents involved may spread to and threaten other patients. In addition to stress, dosage of organisms, confinement, and immunosuppression may contribute to occurrence and spread. Although most nosocomial infections result from frankly pathogenic organisms, some involve opportunistic microbes considered to be part of the normal flora. *Salmonella* infections are a major nosocomial problem in many veterinary clinics, particularly the larger ones. Canine infectious tracheobronchitis (kennel cough) is a troublesome nosocomial infection in veterinary hospitals. These infections can only be prevented and controlled by careful attention to effective sanitation and management practices.

FURTHER READING

Beck-Nielsen, S.: Nosocomial (hospital-acquired) infection in veterinary practice. J. Am. Vet. Med. Assoc., *175*:1304, 1979.

Greene, C.E.: Environmental factors in infectious disease. *In* Infectious Diseases of the Dog and Cat. Edited by C.E. Greene. Philadelphia, W.B. Saunders Co., 1990.

Jones, R.L.: Control of nosocomial infections. *In* Current Veterinary Therapy IX. Edited by R.W. Kirk. Philadelphia, W.B. Saunders Co., 1985.

Lippert, A.C., Fulton, R.B., and Parr, A.M.: Nosocomial infection surveillance in a small animal hospital intensive care unit. J. Am. Anim. Hosp. Assoc., *24*:627, 1988.

Mims, C.A.: The Pathogenesis of Infectious Disease. 3rd Ed., New York, Academic Press, 1987.

Schaechter, M.: Normal microbial flora. *In* Mechanisms of Microbial Disease. 2nd Ed. Edited by M. Schaechter, et al. Baltimore, Williams & Wilkins, 1993.

Thomas, C.G.A.: Medical Microbiology. 5th Ed. London, Bailliere Tindall, 1983.

Thrusfield, M.: Veterinary Epidemiology. Boston, Butterworths, 1986.

Willett, H.P.: Normal flora and opportunistic infections. *In* Zinsser Microbiology, 20th Ed. Edited by W.K. Joklic, et al. Norwalk, CT, Appleton & Lange, 1992.

Youmans, G.P., Paterson, P.Y., and Sommers, H.M.: The Biologic and Clinical Basis of Infectious Diseases. 3rd Ed. Philadelphia, W.B. Saunders Co., 1985.

5

Host-Parasite Relationships

Microorganisms, on the basis of their habitat and mode of living, may be classified as saprophytes or parasites. A small number, such as species of *Candida, Proteus, Klebsiella,* and *Pseudomonas,* can exist as either saprophytes or as parasites (commensals). Some important parasitic states and kinds of pathogens are defined below.

Saprophytism. Organisms in this state live on dead or decaying organic matter. They ordinarily are not parasites of animals, although on occasion they can cause disease. For example, brooder pneumonia is caused by the fungus *Aspergillus fumigatus,* which may be present in large numbers on food or litter. Some of the clostridia live in the soil as well as in the intestine.

Parasitism. This is a general term that denotes a state in which an organism lives on or within another living organism. The parasite does not necessarily harm the host; in fact, the most successful parasites achieve a balance with the host that ensures the survival of both. Among the parasites found on and within domestic animals and humans are bacteria, protozoans, fungi, mycoplasmas, rickettsiae and viruses. A relatively small number of the parasitic microbes have the potential to cause disease.

Some terms that describe different parasitic states are given below.

Commensalism. This is a parasitic state in which the organism lives in or upon the host without causing disease. The organism benefits from this relationship, while the host may or may not. Most of the bacteria in the alimentary tract, both aerobic and anaerobic, are commensals. The term *potential pathogen* is used to denote an organism

that is ordinarily a commensal, but under certain circumstances, such as the lowering of the host's resistance or an increase in the organism's virulence, can cause disease. For example, *Staphylococcus aureus* may cause bovine mastitis as a result of damage to the udder, and *Pasteurella haemolytica* may cause pneumonia in young cattle fatigued and weakened by shipment and cold. Most commensals do not have the potential to cause disease.

Symbiosis. This is a state whereby an organism lives in or upon the host in a mutually beneficial relationship. Good examples of symbiosis are the microfloras of the cecum of rabbits and of the rumen of ruminants, which are provided food and shelter while enabling the host to utilize cellulose. Microbial symbiosis is not common in animals, and the term has little use in the discussion of infectious diseases of animals.

Opportunistic Pathogen. This term describes organisms that are generally harmless commensals in their normal habitats but can cause disease when they gain access to other sites or tissues. For example, non-enterotoxin-producing strains of *E. coli* from the intestine that cause urinary tract infections have been termed opportunists. As indicated below, many saprophytic bacteria and fungi can also cause opportunistic infections.

Impairment of the host's defenses is the principal factor leading to opportunistic infections caused by normally harmless commensals. Lowered antimicrobial defense can be congenital or acquired, for example, as a result of immunosuppressants used in cancer therapy and organ transplantation. The type of defense impairment, e.g., of humoral or cell-mediated immunity, will often determine which organisms result in opportunistic infections. A wide variety of ordinarily harmless bacteria and fungi have been incriminated in opportunistic infections. More than 200 species of saprophytic bacteria have been considered causes of opportunistic infections in humans. Among the fungi involved in infrequent opportunistic infections in animals are *Penicillium, Aspergillus,* and *Candida* spp. *Pseudomonas aeruginosa* and *Acinetobacter* spp. are frequent opportunists in animals.

Obligate Pathogen. This denotes an organism that almost always causes disease when it encounters animals or humans. Examples include *Brucella abortus, Yersinia pestis, Mycobacterium bovis* and *Bacillus anthracis.*

The terms that follow are frequently used in the discussion of infectious diseases.

Pathogenicity. This is the capacity of the organism to produce disease. Variation in this capacity is referred to in terms of virulence.

Virulence. This is a measure of the degree of pathogenicity. For example, pathogenic strains of *Streptococcus equi* may vary in their capacity to produce disease in the horse. All may cause disease, but some may cause more severe disease than others.

Infectivity. This is the capacity of the organism to become established in the tissues of the host. It involves the ability to penetrate the tissues, to survive the host's defenses, and to multiply and disseminate within the animal.

Toxigenicity. This is the capacity of certain organisms to produce exotoxins. For example, there are both toxigenic and nontoxigenic strains of *Clostridium perfringens;* only the former cause disease.

If the host-parasite relationship is kept in balance or equilibrium, no apparent disease results and the infection is asymptomatic. In such diseases as tuberculosis and brucellosis, a delicate equilibrium may be established that is easily upset. Disease results when the parasite cannot be kept in check and a combination of damage done to the host and the host's adaptive reactions results in the phenomenon we recognize as infectious disease.

The two principal determinants of the outcome of the host-parasite relationship are the virulence of the parasite and the resistance of the host. In natural disease the relative significance of each in the development of the disease is difficult to estimate.

For the sake of discussion, it is convenient to treat the roles of the parasite and the host separately.

PATHOGENIC PROPERTIES OF BACTERIA

Bacteria cause disease by two basic mechanisms: (1) invasion of tissues; and (2) production of toxins. Those specific characteristics that contribute to the pathogenicity of microorganisms are frequently referred to as virulence factors.

INVASIVENESS

Invasive bacteria can be classed as intracellular parasites and as extracellular parasites.

Intracellular Parasites

Facultative Intracellular Parasites. These parasites are not confined to cells, but they can survive and in some instances multiply in phagocytic cells. These cells may also destroy the parasites and prevent or ultimately eliminate an infection. For example, *Brucella abortus* and *Mycobacterium bovis* may be eliminated by macrophages in this manner. When a balance is established between the bacterium and the phagocyte, usually macrophages, the bacteria may survive in this intracellular state of relative equilibrium for months or years, as evidenced by *Salmonella, Brucella,* and mycobacteria.

Obligate Intracellular Parasites. Chlamydia, rickettsiae, and the viruses are obligate intracellular parasites in that they can only propagate within cells.

Extracellular Parasites

Extracellular organisms damage tissues while they are outside phagocytes and other cells. They do not have the capacity to survive for long periods in phagocytic cells. When phagocytized, these organisms, e.g., *Klebsiella* and *Pasteurella* spp., are destroyed.

Antiphagocytic Capsules

These surface structures, found principally on extracellular bacteria, consist of hydrophilic gels, usually polysaccharides, that protect the organisms from ingestion by phagocytic cells. Examples include mucoid forms of *Pasteurella multocida, Enterobacter aerogenes,* and *Bacillus anthracis.*

Extracellular Enzymes

Some bacteria produce substances that are not toxic directly but that do play an important part in the development of disease:

1. *Coagulase,* produced by *Staphylococcus aureus,* clots fibrin, thus protecting the bacteria.
2. *Hyaluronidases,* produced by many bacteria, are thought to aid in the spread of organisms

by breaking down the ground substance (hyaluronic acid) of tissues.

3. *Collagenase* produced by some strains of *Clostridium perfringens;* it aids in the spread of this organism by breaking down the collagen of tissues.

Other extracellular enzymes are streptokinase (a fibrinolysin) and streptodornase (a DNase), produced by streptococci. Others will be dealt with under specific pathogens.

Adsorption or Adherence to Surfaces

Although the adsorption of viruses to epithelial cells has been studied extensively, it is only recently that the adsorption and adherence to cell surfaces by pathogenic bacteria with consequent colonization, penetration, or both have been investigated.

Most bacteria and fungi that live in or on their hosts adhere at least temporarily to host cells in order to colonize and grow. Consequently most of these organisms possess surface components called *adhesins* or *ligands* that enable them to adhere specifically to host cells via corresponding receptors on the surface of these cells. Microbial adhesins include components of outer membranes, capsules, and pili (fimbriae). Most adhesins in microorganisms thus far studied are glycoproteins or lipoproteins. The host cell receptors frequently are sugars such as mannose.

It has been shown that pili of enteropathogenic strains of *Escherichia coli* are involved in adherence and colonization of the mucous membrane of the small intestine. Pili may also be involved in the adherence of *Monaxella bovis, Bordetella* spp., and many other gram-negative bacteria. Strains of *Mycoplasma pneumoniae* that have lost their capacity to adhere are also found to have lost their virulence. The adsorption of some bacteria to mucous membranes may be caused by a physicochemical attraction, e.g., hydrophilicity or hydrophobicity, that depends on certain surface compounds associated with the capsules of virulent organisms. These compounds may be lost on in vitro cultivation.

The phenomenon of adherence of bacteria is now receiving a great deal of attention. Its study may have important practical implications, as suggested by the development of an *Escherichia coli* pilus vaccine to prevent scours in swine.

General Comments

Great variation exists in the extent of invasiveness of microorganisms. At one end of the scale are the exotoxin producers, such as the tetanus bacillus, which are noninvasive. At the other end are organisms such as *Yersina pestis* and *Bacillus anthracis,* the plague and anthrax bacilli, which are highly invasive. Organisms such as some *Pasteurella* spp., streptococci, and *Haemophilus* spp. are in between and have only a moderate capacity to invade.

How do we know that a particular organism is pathogenic? The traditional criteria used are Koch's postulates:

1. The organism must be regularly isolated from cases of the disease.
2. It must be grown in vitro in pure culture.
3. Such a culture should produce the typical disease when inoculated into a susceptible animal species.
4. The same organism must be isolated from the experimentally induced disease.

Although these postulates have been met for many diseases, they have not been fulfilled for all, e.g., some human viral diseases (because viruses are frequently very host-specific), diseases such as leprosy and Tyzzer's disease (in which the causal agent has not been grown on lifeless media), and diseases associated with stress with a complex etiology such as pneumonic pasteurellosis (shipping fever) of cattle.

TOXIGENICITY

Exotoxins

Most of the weakly or noninvasive bacteria that cause disease produce exotoxins. These are protein substances that are liberated from intact and lysed cells. They vary greatly in their toxicity, from the extremely potent botulinum toxin to the relatively weak toxin of *Actinomyces pyogenes*. They are almost all antigenic, eliciting specific protective antitoxic antibodies. The various disease-producing clostridia are notable for their production of exotoxins. Some of these toxins can be converted to nontoxic immunizing agents called toxoids by treatment with formalin.

Some of the bacteria other than clostridia that produce exotoxins are enteropathogenic *Escherichia coli, Yersinia pestis,* several *Corynebacterium* species, the highly invasive *Bacillus anthracis,* some strains of *Pasteurella multocida,* and *Staphylococcus aureus*. It is of interest that the toxin of *Corynebacterium diphtheriae* and the erythrogenic toxins of *Streptococcus pyogenes* are only produced by lysogenic strains of these species. In these bacteria the toxin-producing characteristic is coded for by bacteriophage DNA.

A number of exotoxins are encoded by plasmid genes. Examples are the tetanus neurotoxin, the enterotoxin of *E. coli*, and staphylococcal enterotoxin.

Unlike the endotoxins, the clinical and experimental effects of the different exotoxins vary greatly with particular bacterial species. They are described in the discussion of the specific diseases.

Endotoxins

Some properties of endotoxins are as follows:
1. They are produced by gram-negative bacteria, both pathogenic and nonpathogenic species, and they are released during growth and upon lysis.
2. They were originally described as phospholipid-polysaccharide-protein complexes (somatic O antigen). However, their biologic and immunologic properties reside with the lipopolysaccharide portion. The terms endotoxin and lipopolysaccharide are often used synonymously. Their chemical structure is described in Chapter 1.
3. They are a major part of the cell wall of gram-negative bacteria.
4. They are heat-stable, with molecular weights between 100,000 and 900,000.
5. Their toxicity resides in the lipid portion, while their specific antigenic determinants are the sugars that constitute the side chains of the lipopolysaccharide. They do not form toxoids.
6. They are less specific and potent in their cytotoxic effects than exotoxins.
7. They are weak antigens, although they may have an adjuvant effect with other antigens.
8. Potency differs among species.

Although many biologic effects have been ascribed to endotoxins, their role in the pathogenesis of bacterial diseases is poorly understood and largely conjectural. Part of their injurious effect is thought by some investigators to be immunologic in nature. It is suggested that a state of immunologic sensitivity may be involved. It has been noted that germ-free animals are less susceptible to the toxic effects of endotoxins.

Among the effects of endotoxins observed clinically and experimentally are fever, leukopenia, hypoglycemia, hypotension and shock, intravascular coagulation, Shwartzman reaction, adjuvancy, and activation of complement components leading to acute inflammatory reactions. Endotoxins may have an effect on the clotting system, leading to the kind of intravascular coagulation seen in gram-negative septicemias. Thrombocytopenia with lysis of platelets and the release of histamine, serotonin, and bradykinin may lead to the kind of cardiovascular changes that are seen in endotoxemia, including shock. The tumor necrosis factor-alpha (cachexin) is produced by macrophages stimulated by endotoxin. TNF-α binds to various tissues and alters their metabolism. It may damage blood capillaries resulting in increased permeability with loss of large amounts of fluids. Blood pressure may fall sufficiently to produce shock. Endotoxemia occurs in gram-negative bacterial sepsis and hemorrhagic septicemia.

The amount of endotoxin can be determined by the limulus lysate assay. Endotoxin reacts with proteins from horseshoe crab amebocytes to produce a gel. It is a remarkably sensitive test that detects nanogram amounts of endotoxin.

NONSPECIFIC MECHANISMS OF HOST RESISTANCE

Nonspecific mechanisms of host resistance are sometimes referred to as innate immunity. It is well known that great differences in susceptibility to infectious agents exist among domestic animal species. Some of the important features of innate resistance or immunity are discussed below.

The Skin

The skin provides a generally effective barrier. Some microorganisms, such as *Brucella abortus* and *Francisella tularensis*, can penetrate skin. Others enter and cause infections of sweat and sebaceous glands and hair follicles. The glands secrete acidic, antibacterial substances that contain fatty acids. Young animals are thought to be more susceptible to dermatophytes because they have a lower concentration of fatty acids on the skin than adult animals. Lysozyme, an enzyme that breaks down the cell walls of bacteria, is present on the skin. This mucolytic enzyme splits sugars off the glycopeptides of the cell wall of many gram-positive bacteria, leading to lysis.

Mucous Membrane

Mucus covers the surface of the various tracts of the body. Bacteria are caught by the mucous film and are readily phagocytized. The phagocytes carry the bacteria via lymph channels to the lymph nodes, which act as barriers. The cilia of the respiratory tract are constantly moving bacteria and mucus to the natural orifices. Both mucus and tears contain the protective enzyme lysozyme.

Hair in the nares is protective, as is the cough reflex. Saliva, stomach acid, and proteolytic enzymes have an antibacterial action. The acid pH of the vagina caused by lactobacilli has a limiting and stabilizing influence on the vaginal flora. The normal flora of mucous membranes is a rather stable ecosystem that resists the intrusion of alien bacteria. Disturbance of the flora by antibiotic therapy may allow establishment and multiplication of disease-producing organisms, e.g., staphylococci resulting in staphylococcal enteritis or *Candida albicans* resulting in mycotic gastritis or enteritis.

Phagocytosis

Microorganisms entering organs and tissues such as the lungs, lymphatics, bone marrow, and bloodstream may be engulfed by various phagocytic cells. Among these are the polymorphonuclear leukocytes and the wandering and fixed macrophages of the reticuloendothelial system. Phagocytosis may be nonspecific in the absence of antibody, but specific when antibodies to the offending microorganism are available. Phagocytes may kill the engulfed microorganisms. Alternatively, however, the microorganisms may survive and in some instances actually multiply in the phagocytic cell (intracellular parasites).

The phagocytic vacuole is called the phagosome. Lysosomal granules provide the hydrolytic enzymes, including lysozyme, that aid in the destruction of microorganisms. Macrophages may be specifically activated by immunologically active T-lymphocytes.

Reticuloendothelial System

This system refers to the macrophages found in blood (monocytes) and the fixed macrophages (histiocytes) found in lymphoid tissue, spleen, liver, bone marrow, and other tissues. They engulf and remove particulate matter and microorganisms from the blood and lymph, and infected areas. Included in the system are the macrophages lining the blood sinuses of the liver (Kupffer cells), those lining the lymph sinuses, histiocytes found in tissues, and the alveolar macrophages in the lungs.

Resistance of Tissues

Various constituents of tissues have an inhibitory effect on microorganisms; thus some tissues are more readily invaded than others. The interferon produced by tissues in response to viral infection has antiviral properties.

Most healthy tissues inhibit the multiplication of microorganisms. This resistance can be impaired by depression of the inflammatory response by x-rays, corticosteroids, leukemic disease, and antineoplastic drugs. Injury resulting from foreign bodies, trauma, and disturbances in fluid and electrolyte balance may predispose to infection.

Natural Antibodies

These are immunoglobulins that react with a wide range of organisms and antigens to which the animal has not been exposed or immunized. Low levels are found in germ-free animals. Examples include ABO blood group system isohemagglutinins and Forssman's antibodies.

Inflammatory Response

Pathogenic microorganisms, like other damaging agents, elicit inflammatory responses of varying kinds and severity. The changes elicited are complex, and some of the phenomena involved include increased vascular permeability, edema, increased blood flow, infiltration of phagocytic cells, fluid exudation, fever, pain, and swelling. Many of these changes are brought about by the inflammatory mediators, serotonin, histamine, various kinins, prostaglandins, leukotrienes, interleukin-1, C3a and C5a (complement), platelet-activating factor, and products from fibrinogen breakdown. The nature and function of these inflammatory mediators are discussed in detail by pathologists and immunologists.

Fever

Fever is frequently observed as a manifestation of the inflammatory response. It is the cardinal symptom or sign of infectious disease. Fever results from influences on the thermoregulatory centers in the brain.

The lipopolysaccharides released from phagocytes that have engulfed gram-negative bacteria cause macrophages to produce a small protein called interleukin-1, which was formerly called endogenous pyrogen. Interleukin-1 is carried by the blood to the hypothalamus. There it stimulates the temperature control center to release prostaglandins that reset the thermostat in the hypothalamus to a higher temperature, thus causing a fever. Aspirin reduces fever by inhibiting the production of prostaglandins.

Fever of Unknown Origin

In cases of fever of unknown origin in animals, the most frequent causes are probably undetected infections and neoplasms. Other causes may be endocrine disturbances and hypersensitivity reactions.

CONDITIONS AND FACTORS INFLUENCING INFECTIONS

Species, Sex, and Age. There are great differences in susceptibility to infectious agents among animal species. Likewise, there are differences in susceptibility between male and female of the same species. Age is also an important factor. Generally speaking, infectious diseases in both animals and humans are more severe at the extremes of life. The importance of species, sex, and age as they relate to particular infections are discussed later under specific infectious agents.

Stress. The term stress is frequently used to summarize various factors and circumstances that contribute to the development of an infectious disease or diseases. Although both mental and physical disturbances lead to the stress reaction, the latter are probably most important in animals.

Among the more common disturbances leading to stress are fatigue, exposure to extremes of cold and heat, crowding, wounds, transport, change in feed, and weaning. The stress of transport may activate latent infection, e.g., that caused by *Chlamydia psittaci* in birds. A number of physical disturbances contribute to the development of shipping fever (bovine pneumonic pasteurellosis). For example, viral or mycoplasmal infection of the respiratory tract may seriously damage the epithelium and ciliary activity, thus predisposing to bacterial colonization and infection.

If the disturbances are severe enough, a coordinated response originating in the cortex and hypothalamus is initiated; this involves either the autonomic nervous system or the pituitary-adrenal axis. Corticosteroids and catecholamines are released in an effort to counter the deleterious effects of the disturbance. Corticosteroids in large amounts depress the inflammatory reaction and have pronounced effects on lymphoid tissues, causing lymphocyte destruction and thymic involution with possible aggravation of infection.

Circulatory Disturbances. Such disturbances may be local, causing ischemia or congestion and edema; or general, as occurs in shock. They interfere with the mobilization and functioning of phagocytic cells. Mechanical obstruction of the biliary or urinary tracts can have similar effects, thus contributing to infections.

Nutritional Deficiency. There has long been an association between famine and pestilence. Poorly fed animals are more susceptible to a variety of infections. Vitamin A deficiency results in the loss of integrity of epithelium. Other nutritional deficiencies may lead to diminished phagocytic capacity, reduction of the efficiency of the reticuloendothelial system, weakened antibody response, lowered production of lysozyme and interferon, undesirable changes in microbial flora, and alterations of the endocrine system.

Extremes of Temperature and Humidity. There is experimental evidence that animals are less resistant to bacterial infections if they are maintained at a low temperature for extended periods. Environmental stresses—including cold and intemperate weather—no doubt contribute to the occurrence of bovine pneumonic pasteurellosis (shipping fever). High humidity, with an increase in infectious droplets, may contribute to an increase in respiratory disease in groups of animals. Production of corticosteroids by stressed animals is anti-inflammatory and immunosuppressive, thus contributing to or aggravating the infectious process.

Genetic Effects. There is evidence of genetic resistance to bovine mastitis. Leghorns are more resistant to Marek's disease than some other breeds. Some varieties of rabbits are more resistant to myxomatosis as a consequence of the highly susceptible strains having been selected out by the disease. Defects in the immune system frequently have a genetic basis, e.g., combined T and B cell deficiency contributing to fatal adenoviral infections in Arab foals; disseminated histoplasmosis in dogs with thymic hypoplasia; and agammaglobulinemia in humans and animals that are especially prone to bacterial infections.

Chronic Infections. Chronic infections may predispose animals to more severe infection often caused by so-called secondary invaders, e.g., the pasteurellas in shipping fever pneumonia in cattle. Some viral infections such as influenza may suppress resistance to certain bacterial infections.

Physical Fatigue. It is widely held that extreme fatigue predisposes to infection, presumably because it contributes to stress.

Hormonal Imbalance. Diabetics and animals receiving adrenal steroids are known to be abnormally prone to infections.

Acute Radiation Injury. This injury may result in damage to the bone marrow with consequent granulocytopenia and thus a lowering of the host's resistance.

Chemotherapy. Prolonged antibiotic administration leads to alteration, suppression, or elimination of normal microbial flora. The term superinfection is frequently used for infections caused by "alien" organisms that replace the normal flora as a result of prolonged chemotherapy. An example is staphylococcal enteritis.

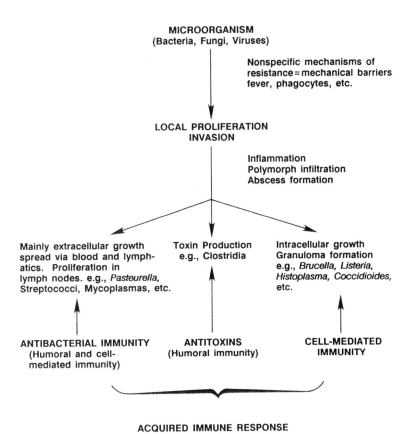

Figure 5–1. Progress of infection and various defense mechanisms (Adapted from: Weir, D.M.: Immunology. 5th ed. New York, Churchill Livingstone, 1983)

SPECIFIC MECHANISMS OF HOST RESISTANCE

Nonspecific resistance has already been discussed. Immunity is classified as follows:

Immunity
{
Natural Immunity
Acquired Immunity
}
{
Passive Immunity
Active Immunity
}

Immunology is of such importance in veterinary medicine that it is taught as a separate discipline.

It involves the study of the immune responses to foreign material (antigens). The essential function of the immune system (but not the only one) is defense against infectious agents. The immune system is of paramount importance in this regard. For purposes of general orientation, the progress of infection as it relates to immunological defense mechanisms is summarized in the outline in Figure 5–1.

Acquired immunity consists of passive immunity and active immunity. Passive immunity, which lasts for only a few weeks, results from the acquisition of "immune cells" or antibodies that have been produced in another animal, or acquired by the fetus or the newborn from the mother.

Active immunity results from the immune response mounted by the host. It consists of cell-mediated immunity and humoral immunity. The immune response of the former is dependent upon certain cells, whereas the latter is mediated by antibodies. The three important features of cell-mediated and humoral responses are recognition of foreign material or "non-self," specificity, and memory.

SOME TERMS USED IN THE DISCUSSION OF INFECTIOUS DISEASES

Axenic. This term is used to denote animals that have been raised in a germ-free atmosphere and are consequently germ-free. These animals are remarkably susceptible to infectious agents. They have a retarded development of antibody-producing organs and are consequently deficient in immunoglobulins. The absence of normal flora influences the responsiveness of the host to infectious agents.

Carrier. When this term is used in connection with a microbe, it indicates that it is present on or within an animal, generally as a commensal. There is usually no evidence of disease. A pig may carry *Salmonella choleraesuis* without showing any clinical signs of disease.

Carrier Rate. This denotes the percentage of animals carrying a certain organism. For example, the carrier rate of *Pasteurella* spp. in the mouths of cats may be as high as 60%.

Disease. Any disturbance of the structure or function of constituents of the animal organism. Some make a distinction between infection and disease. Because these terms are mostly used synonymously, such a distinction is not recommended.

Endogenous Infection. An infection produced or originating from within the animal, e.g., infections due to *Fusobacterium necrophorum*.

Enzootic. The habitual presence of an animal disease in a certain geographic area. The word *endemic* has the same meaning but is usually applied to human beings; however, it may also be used for animals.

Epidemiology. This is the study of the factors and mechanisms that govern the spread of disease within a population or community. Microbiology is particularly important in epidemiology, as most of the diseases studied are caused by microorganisms.

Special methods have been developed to identify precisely the particular variety or type of microorganism involved in a disease outbreak. Such identification enables the epidemiologist to trace the spread of various infectious agents. The well known epidemiologic typing methods include the antibiogram, biotyping, serotyping, bacteriocin typing, and bacteriophage typing. Among the more recent molecular typing methods are plasmid analysis, restriction endonuclease analysis of chromosomal DNA, ribotyping, and electrophoresis of various proteins.

Epizootic. A disease attacking a large number of animals within a short time span and usually spreading rapidly, e.g., foot-and-mouth disease. Epidemic may be used as a synonym for epizootic.

Exogenous Infection. An infection produced or originating external to the animal, e.g., anthrax.

Gnotobiotic. This term is used to describe animals whose flora and fauna are known because they have previously been defined and established. In order to maintain their gnotobiotic status, they must be kept in isolation to prevent the addition of alien organisms.

Incidence (in Epidemiology). A measurement of only the new cases of a disease occurring during a given period.

Infectivity. The capacity to become established in the tissues of the host.

Invasive. This term is sometimes used to describe an organism's capacity for entering and spreading within tissues.

Latent and Inapparent Infections. Persisting subclinical infections. There is frequently a latent state in tuberculosis.

Mixed Infections. More than one microbial agent may be associated with a disease. For example, shipping fever pneumonia in cattle may involve a bacterium, a virus, and a mycoplasma. It may be difficult to determine or estimate the relative importance of each.

Natural History of Disease. The usual course of infectious disease from the beginning to the end if there is no treatment.

Pathogenicity. The capacity of an infectious agent to cause disease in a susceptible host.

Prevalence (in Epidemiology). A measurement of all cases of disease existing at a given time.

Primary Agent of Disease. A microbial agent that can initiate disease on its own, e.g., *Brucella abortus*.

Secondary Invader. A microbial agent that invades or establishes itself in tissues that have been infected by a primary agent.

Specific Pathogen-Free Animals. Animals that have been derived from stock established from caesarian-delivered animals. Swine thus derived may be maintained free of *Bordetella bronchiseptica*, *Salmonella* species, transmissible gastroenteritis virus, and *Mycoplasma hyopneumoniae*.

Specific Pathogen-Free Flocks. Flocks established from eggs free of known pathogenic agents, including mycoplasmas. They are used to provide eggs and chickens for research and for the initiation of other similar flocks.

Virulence. The degree of pathogenicity of a microorganism.

FURTHER READING

Britton, G., Marshall, K.M. (eds.): Adsorption of Microorganisms to Surfaces. New York, John Wiley & Sons, 1980.
Joklik, W.K., et al. (eds.): Zinsser Microbiology. 20th Ed. Norwalk, CT, Appleton-Lange, 1992.
Mims, C.A.: The Pathogenesis of Infectious Diseases. 3rd Ed. New York, Academic Press, 1987.
Myrvik, Q.N., and Weiser, R.S.: Fundamentals of Medical Bacteriology and Mycology. 2nd Ed. Philadelphia, Lea & Febiger, 1988.
Roitt, I.M.: Essential Immunology. 7th Ed. London, Blackwell Scientific Publications, 1991.
Roth, J.A. (ed.): Virulence Mechanisms of Bacterial Pathogens. Washington, American Society for Microbiology, 1988.
Silverstein, S.C., and Steinberg, T.H.: Host-Parasite Relations in Bacterial Infections. In Microbiology. Edited by B.D. Davis, et al. 4th Ed. Philadelphia, J.B. Lippincott Co., 1990.
Tizzard, I.R.: Veterinary Immunology: An Introduction. 4th Ed. Philadelphia, W.B. Saunders Co., 1992.
Youmans, G.R., Paterson, P.Y., and Sommers, H.M. (eds.): The Biologic and Clinical Basis of Infectious Diseases. 3rd Ed. Philadelphia, W.B. Saunders Co., 1985.

6

Antimicrobial Drugs

Chemotherapy, a term that originated with Paul Ehrlich, refers to the treatment of infectious diseases by administering drugs that are inhibitory or lethal to the infecting agents. Such a drug must exhibit a selective toxicity directed at the causative organism rather than the host. Drugs that are highly toxic to both organism and host are obviously unsatisfactory.

Although chemotherapeutic drugs were known before Ehrlich's time, he was the first to deliberately seek new antimicrobial compounds. When he found a compound that showed at least limited activity for an organism, he would synthesize closely related compounds in order to find more effective ones. Organic chemists are still using this approach. In 1907, after trying many compounds for their activity against the spirochetes of syphilis, Ehrlich found that the arsenical compound arsphenamine was selectively toxic for *Treponema pallidum*. This was the first of a long series of drugs to be synthesized in the laboratory.

A number of years later, Domagk (1935) showed that the red dye Prontosil was effective in the treatment of streptococcal infections. Later it was shown that its antibacterial activity was due to sulfanilamide derived from Prontosil. The success of this drug stimulated a search for related compounds and resulted in the synthesis of a host of effective compounds of the sulfonamide group.

Although Ehrlich is rightly considered the father of modern chemotherapy, a number of drugs were developed for various diseases prior to his time. Paracelsus (16th century) used mercury compounds for the treatment of syphilis. By the 19th

century the natives of South America had found that quinine was an effective treatment for malaria.

Antibiotics

An antibiotic is defined as an antimicrobial substance produced by a living microorganism. Pasteur and Joubert (1877) first reported that common airborne contaminants had a lethal effect on a culture of *Bacillus anthracis*. Similar observations were made over the years, and Fleming (1929) observed that a fungus, *Penicillium notatum*, when present on a culture plate, strongly inhibited the growth of staphylococci. In fact, he carried out a crude plate susceptibility test. This discovery was not exploited until 1940, when Chain, Florey, and associates succeeded in obtaining preparations from *Penicillium* that had high antibacterial activity but low toxicity for humans and animals. The remarkable therapeutic efficacy of penicillin against a variety of diseases was soon demonstrated.

After the discovery of penicillin, an extensive search for antibiotics began. The richest source of these drugs was found to be species of *Streptomyces*. Other sources of useful antibiotics have been bacteria, actinomycetes, and certain fungi. Some semisynthetic penicillins, e.g., methicillin, ampicillin, carbenicillin, and others, are derived from naturally produced 6-amino-penicillanic acid. The chemical structures of some important antibiotics are shown in Figure 6–1.

MECHANISM OF ACTION OF ANTIMICROBIAL DRUGS

Antimicrobial drugs are divided into two classes, based upon their general effects on bacterial populations.

81

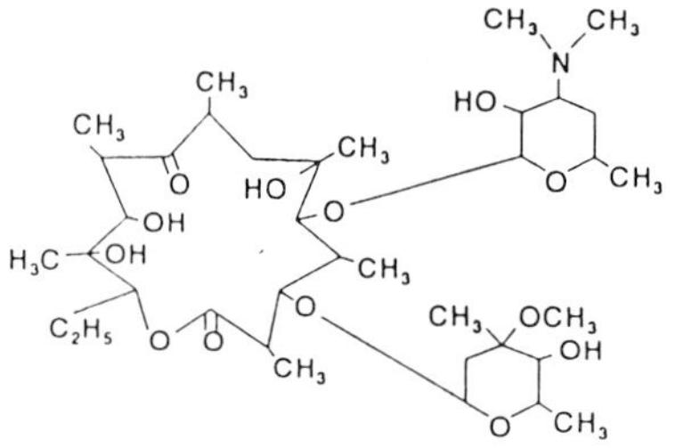

Erythromycin

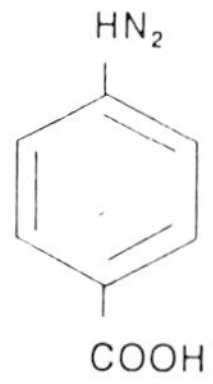

PABA

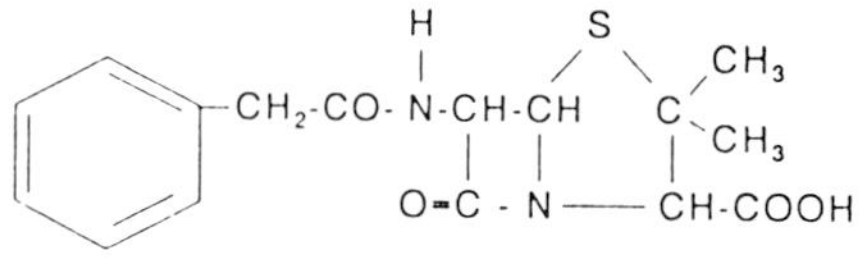

Penicillin G

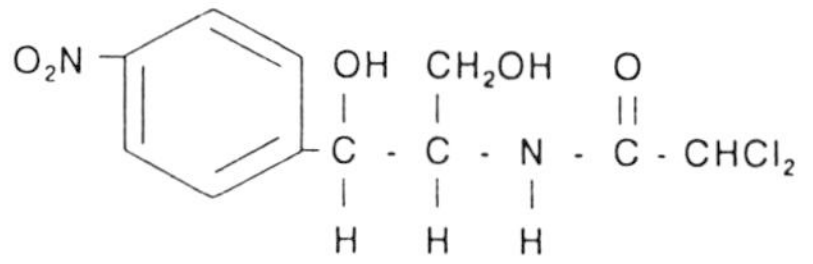

Chloramphenicol

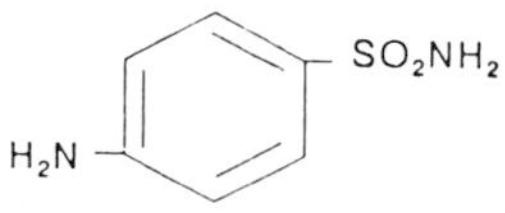

Sulfanilamide

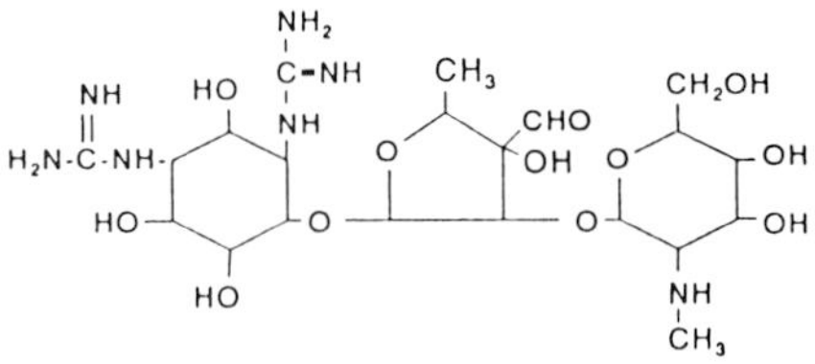

Streptomycin

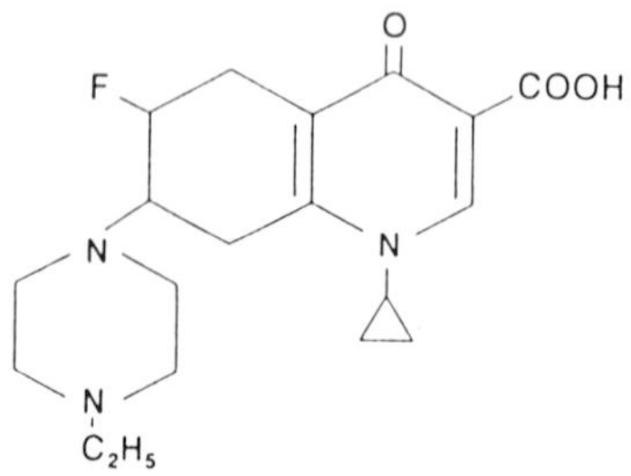

Enrofloxacin

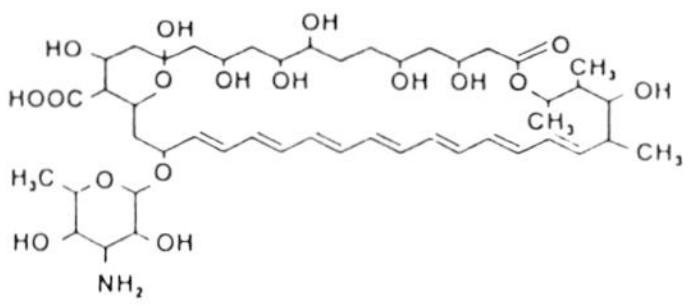

Amphotericin B

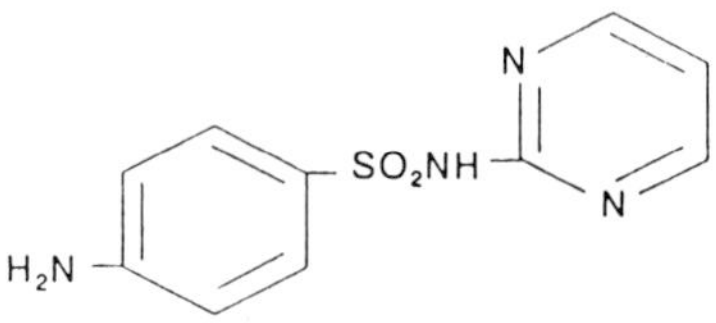

Sulfadiazine

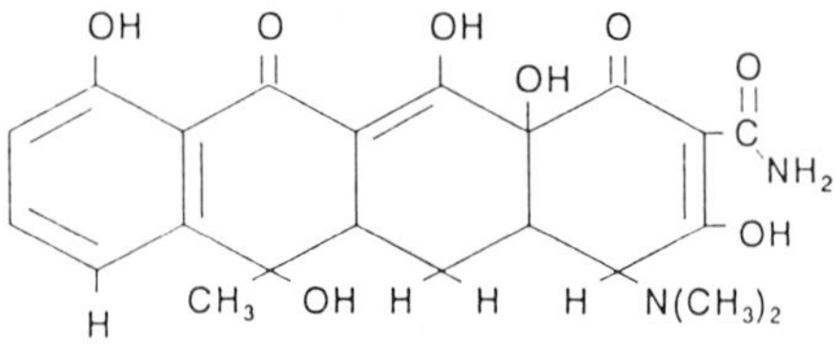

Tetracycline

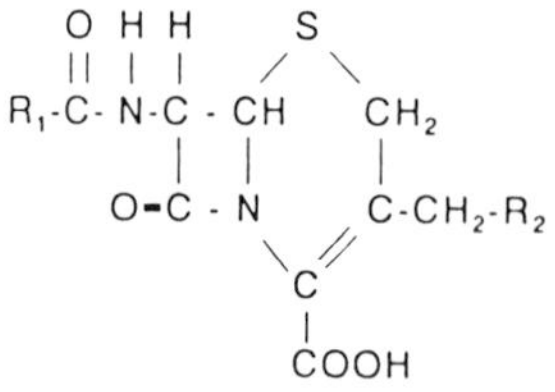

Cephalosporin nucleus

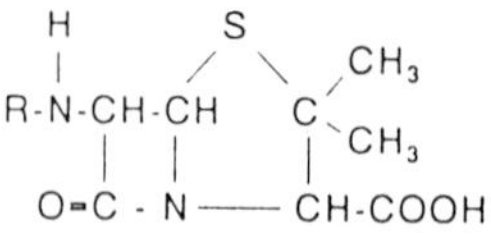

Penicillin nucleus

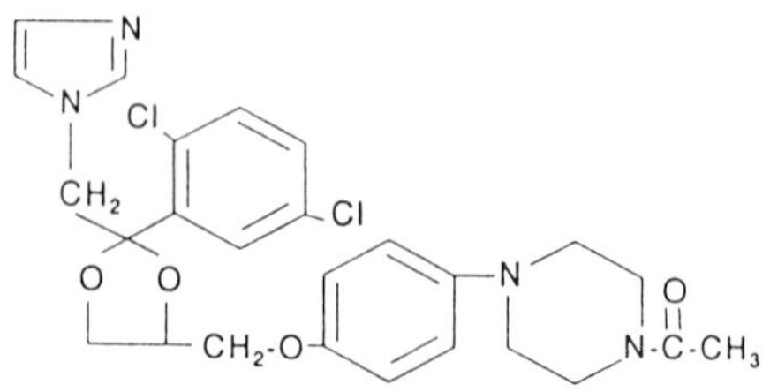

Ketoconazole

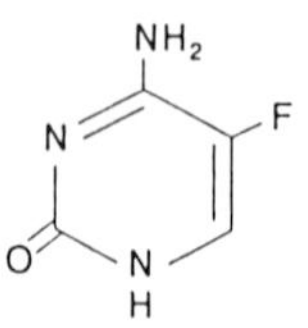

5-Fluorocytosine

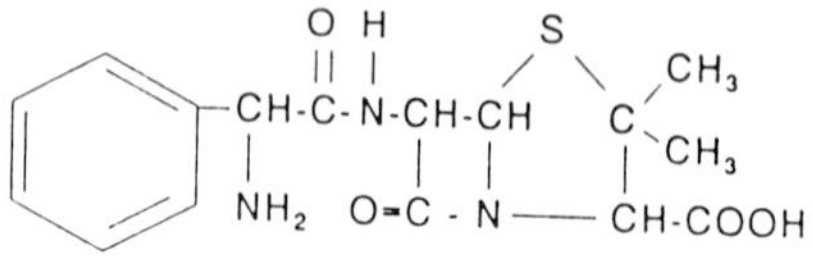

Ampicillin

Figure 6–1. Structures of drugs representing important groups of antimicrobial agents.

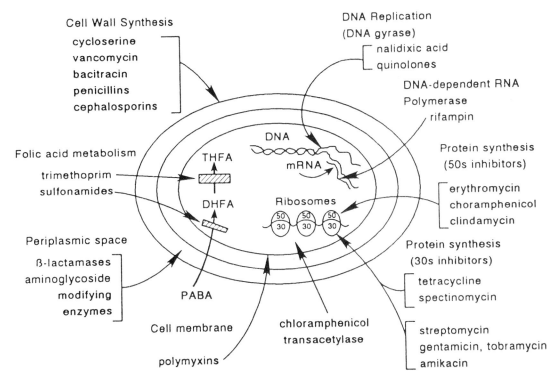

Figure 6–2. Sites of action of various antimicrobial agents. mRNA = messenger RNA; tRNA = transfer RNA; PABA = para-aminobenzoic acid; DHFA = dihydrofolic acid; THFA = tetra hydrofolic acid. (Courtesy of H.C. Neu, Science, 257:1064, 1992.)

1. *Bactericidal* drugs. These have a rapid lethal action. Examples are penicillin, streptomycin, the cephalosporins, polymyxin, and neomycin. In high concentrations erythromycin may be bactericidal.
2. *Bacteriostatic* drugs. These inhibit the growth of organisms. Examples are tetracyclines, sulfonamides, and chloramphenicol. They depend upon the immune system to kill and remove the bacteria.

In practice, this classification is not always clear-cut. Most drugs are, in varying degrees, both bactericidal and bacteriostatic. The way in which they act depends upon the drug, its concentration, and factors such as the type, quantity, and growth state of the organism. For example, penicillin is strongly bactericidal against rapidly growing organisms but has little effect on organisms in a stationary state. Intracellular bacteria may be dormant in macrophages and thus are not destroyed by antimicrobial drugs.

The major antimicrobial drugs are grouped according to their mechanism of action (Fig. 6–2).

INHIBITION OF GROWTH BY ANALOGUES

Sulfonamides

As mentioned earlier, these compounds are bacteriostatic, i.e., they inhibit growth but do not kill.

They are effective against growing and proliferating bacteria but not against dormant ones.

Unlike animal cells, for many bacteria para-aminobenzoic acid (PABA) is an essential metabolite in the synthesis of folic acid, which in turn is required in the synthesis of purines. Sulfonamides are structural analogues of PABA and thus can compete with it, resulting in the formation of nonfunctional analogues of folic acid. Some bacteria, like some animal cells, cannot synthesize folic acid but require it for growth. These organisms are not inhibited by sulfonamides.

An excess of PABA, such as that released during extensive tissue destruction, counteracts the inhibiting action of sulfonamides. For this reason, PABA may be added to culture media when attempting to isolate bacteria from animals that have been treated with sulfonamides. Another competitive inhibitor of PABA is *para* aminosalicylic acid (PAS). It is used in conjunction with isoniazid or streptomycin in the treatment of tuberculosis.

Sulfonamides may be given with the synthetic compound trimethoprim or other closely related compounds to produce sequential blocking that results in enhanced activity. Trimethoprim, which is not a growth analogue, blocks the formation of folic acid by inhibiting the action of dihydrofolic acid reductase. The reductase is essential for the formation of tetrahydrofolate from dihydrofolate.

The presence of thimidine interferes with the activity of trimethoprim and sulfonamides.

Trimethoprim + sulfadiazine (Tribrissen) has the following spectrum of activity:

Very Susceptible	Susceptible	Moderately Susceptible	Not Susceptible
Escherichia	*Staphylococcus*	*Moraxella*	*Mycobacterium*
Streptococcus	*Neisseria*	*Nocardia*	*Leptospira*
Proteus	*Klebsiella*	*Brucella*	*Pseudomonas*
Salmonella	*Fusiformis*		*Erysipelothrix*
Pasteurella	*Corynebacterium*		
Shigella	*Clostridium*		
	Bordetella		

Trimethoprim is also combined with other sulfonamides, e.g., sulfadoxine and sulfamethoxazole. Many sulfonamides are available and their use depends to some extent on their physicochemical characteristics, particularly their solubility. Although mutant resistance occurs with sulfonamides most resistance is due to an R factor (see Chapter 3).

Sulfones

The sulfones are structural analogues of para-aminobenzoic acid and their mode of action is similar to the sulfonamides. The sulfones are relatively toxic and have a limited antimicrobial spectrum. Their actions include suppression of nonspecific inflammation. Dapsone is the most widely used sulfone. It is used in the treatment of human leprosy and mycobacterial infections in dogs and cats, including feline leprosy.

Inhibition of Cell Wall Synthesis

The peptidoglycan of bacterial cell walls is unique. Thus it is not surprising that a number of antimicrobial drugs that inhibit the synthesis of these glycopeptides are effective clinically. Synthesis of peptidoglycan is inhibited at several points, depending upon the drugs.

Penicillins

Penicillin inhibits the synthesis of cell walls of growing susceptible bacteria. The bacterial protoplasm increases and eventually bursts the cytoplasmic membrane, resulting in lysis and death. If the bacteria are growing in a medium of high osmotic tension, cell-wall-deficient forms called protoplasts (gram-positive) or spheroplasts (gram-negative) with intact cytoplasmic membranes are formed. Penicillin inhibits the enzyme responsible for the cross-linking between the layers of peptidoglycan. Although penicillins are most active against the gram-positive organisms, they are also active against a number of gram-negative ones.

Of the many different penicillins derived from *Penicillium*, only several are of value in treatment. Two that are widely used are penicillin G (benzylpenicillin), which is administered intramuscularly, and penicillin V (phenoxymethyl penicillin), which is resistant to acid decomposition and can therefore be given orally. Procaine is used in penicillin preparations to delay absorption.

Semisynthetic Penicillins

The origin of semisynthetic penicillins has been referred to previously. They have the important advantage of being resistant to the penicillin-destroying enzyme penicillinase (β-lactamase). Certain penicillins, e.g., cloxacillin, oxacillin, and methicillin, can bind the penicillin-destroying enzyme β-lactamase produced by some gram-negative bacteria, e.g., *Pseudomonas aeruginosa*. Thus they can protect simultaneously administered hydrolyzable penicillins, such as ampicillin, from being destroyed. Ampicillin is acid-resistant and more active against gram-negative bacteria than the natural penicillins, but it is somewhat less active against gram-positive organisms. Carbenicillin and ticarcillin have an even broader spectrum of activity against gram-negative bacteria.

The combination of clavulanic acid with amoxicillin (augmentin) or ticarcillin (timentin) is active against β-lactamase-producing gram-positive or gram-negative bacteria. Clavulanic acid is a naturally occurring weak antimicrobial agent produced by a *Streptomyces* and known to inhibit β-lactamase activity. It acts synergistically with certain penicillins.

Two additional types of resistance to penicillin are thought to occur. One results from the failure of β-lactam antibiotic to activate autolytic enzymes in the cell wall. The other is attributed to the absence in bacteria of some penicillin receptors and occurs as a result of chromosomal mutation.

Although remarkably low in toxicity, the penicillins are occasionally allergenic.

Cephalosporins

The original antibiotics in this group were derived from a *Cephalosporium* mold. They have a nucleus that chemically resembles the nucleus of penicillin. Their mode of action is similar to that of penicillin, and they are bactericidal with low toxicity. Cephalosporins have the following characteristics: (1) resistance to penicillinase in varying degrees; (2) they are not as allergenic as penicillin; and (3) they have a broad spectrum of activity and can be used against staphylococci (including penicillin-resistant strains), streptococci (although enterococci are resistant), and a wide range of gram-negative bacteria.

Some of the oral cephalosporins in use are cephradine, cephaloglycin, cephalexin, and cefadroxil. The parenteral cephalosporins include cephaloridine, cephalothin, cephapirin, cephalonidine, cephradine, cefadroxil, cefoxitin, and cefamandole.

Many cephalosporins have been developed, a number of which are not available in the United States. The older cephalosporins (cephalothin, cefazolin, cephapirin, cephradine, cephadroxil, and cephalexin) are referred to as first generation cephalosporins. These are active against most gram-positive bacteria and have limited activity against gram-negative bacteria. The second generation cephalosporins (cefamadole, cefonicid, ceforanide, cefotiam, cefuroxime, cefotitan, cefoxitin, and cefaclor) are active against most gram-positive bacteria and have a broader spectrum of activity against gram-negative organisms. The third generation cephalosporins (cefotaxime, ceftiofur, cefixime, ceftazidime, ceftizoxime, cefoperazone, and cefmenoxine) have limited activity against gram-positive bacteria but are effective against most gram-negative organisms. Not all of the cephalosporins have been listed above.

Cycloserine

This antibiotic, recovered from a streptomycete, is a structural analogue of D-alanine, and it interferes with the formation of the D-alanine–D-alanine portion of the cell wall pentapeptide. It is bactericidal, producing protoplasts that lyse. Its antimicrobial spectrum is fairly broad, and includes coliform bacteria, *Proteus*, and mycobacteria. However, its use is limited by its neurotoxic effects.

Bacitracin

Bacitracin is a polypeptide produced by a strain of *Bacillus subtilis*. It interacts with the bacterial cell membrane to prevent the transfer of structural cell wall units. It is bactericidal and acts principally against gram-positive organisms. High toxicity precludes its systemic use, but it is useful for topical application. It is often combined with such drugs as polymyxin and neomycin.

Vancomycin

This antibiotic is derived from a streptomycete. Its mode of action and spectrum of activity are similar to those of bacitracin. Although rather toxic (it may cause nerve deafness, thrombophlebitis, and kidney damage), it is used in emergencies to treat serious staphylococcal infections.

INHIBITION OF PROTEIN SYNTHESIS

Aminoglycosides (aminocyclitols)

All drugs in this group of antibiotics, derived from *Micromonospora* spp. (gentamicin, sisomicin, and netilmicin) or from *Streptomyces* spp. (streptomycin, neomycin, tobramycin, spectinomycin, and kanamycin), have similar structures and modes of action. They bind to the smaller (30S) of the two ribosomal subunits, resulting in the miscoding of proteins and inhibition of peptide elongation.

Streptomycin. This drug is bactericidal and is active against gram-negative bacteria, mycobacteria, and some gram-positive organisms. Resistance to streptomycin is encountered frequently and may be caused by mutation or R factors. It is not absorbed from the gut and is normally administered intramuscularly. When combined with tetracycline it is very useful in the treatment of brucellosis and plague.

Streptomycin sulfate has replaced the more toxic dihydrostreptomycin. Prolonged high blood levels of streptomycin can result in severe disturbances of hearing and vestibular function.

Neomycin and Kanamycin. These drugs are closely related structurally and have similar activity and complete cross-resistance. They are stable and both are poorly absorbed from the intestinal tract but readily absorbed if given intramuscularly. Both are excreted in the urine. Kanamycin is less toxic than neomycin and consequently is used systemically.

Both drugs are bactericidal for many gram-negative species. In animals neomycin is used most frequently to treat intestinal infections, metritis, and bovine mastitis. Neomycin also is used with other drugs in topical preparations.

Both drugs may cause renal damage and nerve deafness.

Gentamicin. Gentamicin resembles neomycin and is mainly active against many gram-negative organisms, including *Pseudomonas aeruginosa*, and some gram-positive species. It is included in topical preparations with other drugs.

It may be nephrotoxic and ototoxic.

Tobramycin. Tobramycin resembles gentamicin chemically and pharmacologically.

Spectinomycin. This drug somewhat resembles the aminoglycosides in structure and site of action. It has been used mainly to treat infections caused by gram-negative bacteria and mycoplasmas.

Amikacin. Amikacin is a derivative of kanamycin and resembles gentamicin. It is active against many gram-negative organisms that are resistant to tobramycin and gentamicin.

Sisomicin and netilmicin. These are recently introduced broad-spectrum aminoglycosides.

Resistance to Aminoglycosides. There are several mechanisms of resistance to aminoglycoside antibiotics: 1. Impaired ribosomal binding: For example, in some *E. coli* and *Pseudomonas aeruginosa* strains, a single step mutation prevents the binding of the aminoglycoside to the ribosome. This is not considered an important mechanism of resistance. 2. Impaired transport: This involves impairment of transport across the cell membrane. Because transport is oxygen dependent, this non-plasmid-mediated resistance occurs more frequently with anaerobes. 3. Aminoglycoside-altering enzymes: This type of resistance may be either plasmid or chromosome mediated and is encountered with both gram-negative and gram-positive bacteria. Three different enzymes may be involved in the destruction of the drug. Several other mechanisms of resistance of minor importance have been described.

Tetracyclines

Drugs in this group are derived from streptomycetes. The three naturally occurring tetracyclines are chlortetracycline, oxytetracycline, and demethylchlortetracycline. A number of antibiotics have been derived semisynthetically from these, e.g., tetracycline, methacycline, doxycycline, and minocycline. They act by binding to the 30S ribosomal subunit, causing inhibition of the function of tRNA. They are bacteriostatic and their mode of action is reversible. Trade names of the more common tetracyclines are Achromycin (tetracycline), Aureomycin (chlortetracycline), and Terramycin (oxytetracycline).

The tetracyclines are broad-spectrum antibiotics that are active against a wide range of gram-positive and gram-negative organisms, including rickettsiae, chlamydiae, and mycoplasmas. Organisms that are resistant to penicillin are often susceptible to the tetracyclines. Also, they are often of value in treating mixed infections. In animals they may be conveniently administered in feed or water.

Superinfection with *Candida albicans* or *Staphylococcus aureus* can be a complication after treatment with the tetracyclines. Although they are of relatively low toxicity, liver damage has been encountered in pregnant women administered the drugs. In addition, it has been found that tetracyclines may inhibit the growth of bones and teeth in the fetus and in infants. Long-term administration should be avoided in children and presumably in young animals.

Other drugs in this group include clomocycline, doxycycline, demeclocycline, minocycline, lymecycline, and rolitecycline. The antibacterial activity of drugs among the tetracycline group is similar, but they differ slightly in their duration of action and rates of absorption and excretion.

Resistance to the tetracyclines depends for the most part on decreased penetration of the drug into bacteria that were previously susceptible. Plasmid-mediated resistance (R factor) is widespread and results in either reduced uptake or efflux of the drug from bacteria. General cross-resistance exists among the tetracyclines.

Chloramphenicol (Chloromycetin)

This is a broad-spectrum drug derived from a streptomycete. It is bacteriostatic and acts by specifically binding to the larger 50S ribosomal subunit, thus inhibiting protein synthesis. It is a very effective drug in animals, although its use in food-producing animals is restricted in the United States and Canada.

In rare instances, prolonged administration results in severe or even fatal depression of bone marrow function, leading to aplastic anemia. Because of this its use in humans is reserved for very serious infections such as typhoid fever. Veterinarians have found chloramphenicol to be a relatively safe drug for a variety of infections in companion animals.

Chloramphenicol resistance, which is plasmid mediated, is due to the destruction by the bacterial enzyme chloramphenicol acetyltransferase.

Erythromycins (Macrolides)

The macrolide antibiotics contain a macrocyclic lactone ring to which one or more sugars are attached. They are derived from streptomycetes and inhibit protein synthesis by binding to the 50S ribosomal subunit. Erythromycin and tylosin are the most useful of the macrolides. Related drugs are spiramycin, oleandomycin, and leucomycin.

The macrolides are effective against gram-positive bacteria including staphylococci, streptococci, clostridia, corynebacteria and *Listeria*. Some gram-negative bacteria, including *Pasteurella*, *Campylobacter*, and *Haemophilus*, are susceptible, as well as mycoplasmas, *Chlamydia* and *Rickettsia*.

Resistance may be plasmid mediated or chromosomal (mutant) in origin. With gram-negative bacteria it involves the inability to penetrate, and with gram-positive bacteria it involves alteration of the receptor site on the ribosome. The resistance caused by modified ribosomes crosses to clindamycin and lincomycin, suggesting that the site of action of these two non-macrolide drugs is similar to that of erythromycin.

Tylosin

Tylosin inhibits protein synthesis by preventing the translocation of the aminoacyl-tRNA on the 50S ribosomal subunit. It displays partial or complete cross-resistance with erythromycin. Tylosin is relatively water-insoluble and is administered in feed to treat intestinal infections and systemically for some gram-positive, gram-negative, and mycoplasmal infections, e.g., various pneumonias, chronic respiratory disease of chickens, and infectious sinusitis of turkeys. Tylosin has been widely used as a feed additive for promoting growth in poultry and livestock. However, recently the drug has been taken off the market as a feed additive for swine, for safety reasons.

Tilmicosin

Tilmicosin, a macrolide, is derived from tylosin and is active against some gram-negative and gram-positive bacteria. This new injectable drug is being used to treat bovine pneumonic pasteurellosis associated with *Pasteurella haemolytica*.

Clindamycin and Lincomycin (Lincosamides)

Lincomycin is derived from a streptomycete and clindamycin is a chlorine-substituted derivative of lincomycin. They resemble erythromycin in mechanism of action, spectrum of activity, and possession of ribosomal receptors. They are active against a number of gram-positive species and several gram-negative bacteria that are penicillin-resistant. Clindamycin is useful in the treatment of some infections caused by *Bacteroides* and other anaerobes.

Clindamycin has been implicated in human antibiotic-associated colitis due to *Clostridium difficile*. This organism, which is clindamycin-resistant, gains prominence in the colon when other members of the colonic flora are diminished. The pseudomembranous colitis caused by the necrotizing toxin of *C. difficile* can be fatal.

Tiamulin

Tiamulin is a semisynthetic derivative of the antibiotic pleuromutilin, a diterpenoid-like compound initially isolated from the Basidiomycetes, *Pleurotus mutilus* and *P. passeckerianus*. It inhibits protein synthesis by binding to the 50S ribosomal subunit. The drug is primarily used in livestock and poultry feed and drinking water. It is effective against a number of porcine diseases including swine dysentery, enzootic pneumonia, swine pleuropneumonia, and *Streptococcus suis* infections.

IMPAIRMENT OF MEMBRANE FUNCTION

The polypeptide antibiotics polymyxin B and colistin (polymyxin E) are derived from *Bacillus polymyxa*. They damage the membranes of gram-negative species especially, resulting in a loss of osmotic control, which in turn causes leakage of potassium ions and other vital bacterial components and ultimately death. Polymyxin is poorly absorbed from the intestinal tract and is rather toxic (renal damage). Unlike most other bactericidal drugs, it kills resting as well as multiplying cells. It is used for bovine mastitis, enteritis in young calves, and serious infections such as those due to *Pseudomonas aeruginosa*. It is used with other antibiotics in topical preparations.

Polymyxins are large molecules that diffuse poorly in agar media and therefore result in small inhibition zones in disc susceptibility tests. The tube dilution test shows greater susceptibility.

INHIBITION OF NUCLEIC ACID SYNTHESIS

Quinolones

Quinolones, H-quinolones, and quinolone-carboxylic acid derivatives are closely related synthetic compounds that possess activity against a wide range of gram-positive and gram-negative aerobic bacteria. The quinolones, such as enrofloxacin, ciprofloxacin, clinoxacin, and norfloxacin, inhibit bacterial DNA-gyrase, leading to a reduction in supercoiling of chromosomal DNA around an RNA core. The loosely coiled DNA then is degraded quickly into small nonfunctional fragments by the action of exonucleases. The quinolones, which are bactericidal, often have significant antibacterial activity at very low concentrations when compared to other classes of antimicrobial agents with similar spectra of activity. They are also known to interrupt bacterial membrane integrity.

Bacterial resistance to quinolones has been recognized infrequently and is not considered a significant clinical problem. Plasmid-mediated resistance has not been reported. Resistance appears to be due to either modified DNA-gyrase or to failure of entry of the drug. Enrofloxacin is the only quinolone that has been approved for veterinary use in the United States. Nalidixic acid, which is related to the quinolones, is used in human urinary tract infections caused by some gram-negative bacteria. Obligate anaerobes are resistant to most quinolones. Although injectable forms are available, quinolones are commonly administered orally.

Rifampin

This is a semisynthetic derivative of the *Streptomyces*-derived antibiotic rifamycin. It inhibits DNA-dependent RNA polymerase activity, which is responsible for the synthesis of cellular RNA. Rifampin is given orally and is active against a wide range of gram-positive and gram-negative bacteria, chlamydiae, and poxviruses. It has been used effectively in combination with other drugs in the treatment of tuberculosis.

Novobiocin

This drug, derived from a streptomycete, is readily absorbed from the intestinal tract, but its effectiveness is limited because it binds to protein. It is bacteriostatic and acts by inhibiting the synthesis of DNA and teichoic acid at the cell membrane. Although active against gram-positive cocci and some gram-negative organisms in vitro, it is only used in combination with other drugs in the treatment of serious staphylococcal infections.

Frequent side-effects, such as impaired renal function, vomiting, and jaundice, are encountered in humans.

ADDITIONAL CHEMOTHERAPEUTIC AGENTS

The Nitrofuran Derivatives

These synthetic compounds are strongly bactericidal in vitro for many gram-positive and gram-negative bacteria. Most are very insoluble, and some, such as nitrofurazone, are used in topical preparations. For safety reasons, nitrofurans have been withdrawn from the market for use other than in topical preparations. They are thought to be potential carcinogens.

The nitrofurans are thought to inhibit a variety of enzyme systems of bacteria and also damage DNA but their precise mechanism of action is not known. They were widely used in veterinary practice, and little toxicity was encountered.

Mandelamine (Methenamine Mandelate)

Like nalidixic acid, this drug is used as a "urinary antiseptic." It is most useful to suppress bacteria in the urine of animals and humans with chronic urinary tract infections. It requires a urinary pH lower than 5.5 to be effective. At this pH and below, it is hydrolyzed to ammonia and formaldehyde. This compound has no antibacterial activity by itself.

Sodium Arsanilate and Arsanilic Acid

These compounds are used in the treatment of swine dysentery. Their value may result from action against *Serpulina hyodysenteriae*.

Para-Aminosalicylic Acid (PAS)

This synthetic compound has a mode of action similar to that of sulfa drugs. It inhibits bacterial growth by inhibiting folic acid synthesis. It has largely been supplanted by ethambutol in the treatment of tuberculosis.

Ethambutol

This synthetic complex alcohol has tended to replace *para*-aminosalicylic acid in the treatment of tuberculosis. It is active only against mycobacteria. The mechanism of action is thought to be inhibition of the incorporation of mycolic acid into the cell wall.

Isoniazid

This inexpensive, relatively nontoxic compound is very effective in the treatment of tuberculosis. It acts by inhibiting the synthesis of mycolic acids. There is some evidence that it may also be of value in the treatment of nocardial mastitis and actinobacillosis of cattle.

Carbapenems

Imipenem is the first carbapenem developed for clinical use. This broad-spectrum, semisynthetic antibiotic is a derivative of thienamycin, which is produced by *Streptomyces* spp. These antibiotics work by inhibiting cell wall synthesis. They are resistant to most plasmid- or chromosomally-mediated β-lactamases.

ANTIMYCOTIC AGENTS

Antimycotic agents, including the polyene antibiotics such as amphotericin B and nystatin, are discussed in Chapter 31.

SUSCEPTIBILITY TESTS

Two kinds of tests are carried out in the laboratory: disc susceptibility and tube susceptibility.

Disc Susceptibility Test

Resistant strains are now so prevalent that it is recommended that all clinical isolates be tested for susceptibility.

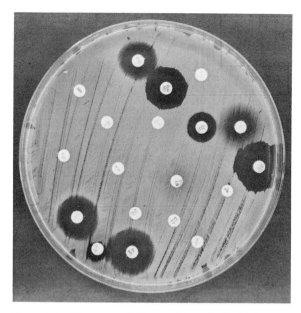

Figure 6–3. Disc susceptibility test. The antimicrobial agents incorporated in the discs diffuse into the agar, inhibiting the bacterial growth (clear zones).

The plate or disc procedure is routinely used in veterinary diagnostic laboratories (Fig. 6–3). It involves the uniform inoculation of a plate containing a suitable medium with a standardized amount of organism of the culture to be tested. Paper discs impregnated with the various antimicrobial drugs are then applied, appropriately spaced, with a dispenser. After incubation, usually 24 hours, the size of the zones of inhibition is measured, and based upon values that have been established, a culture is reported as being susceptible or resistant. Some laboratories report zones between susceptible and resistant as intermediate.

Most laboratories now use the Kirby-Bauer procedure, which employs high potency discs and Mueller-Hinton agar in large Petri dishes. The zones of inhibition described as susceptible, intermediate, and resistant relate to blood concentration and therapeutic efficacy in humans. Mueller-Hinton agar is free of PABA. If PABA is present in the medium, it will inactivate or inhibit the activity of the sulfonamide disc, thus yielding an erroneous result. PABA should only be used in media for isolation purposes.

Direct susceptibility tests employing clinical material such as pus and urine as inocula are not recommended. The inoculum is not standardized and may contain several different organisms.

Appropriate modifications in the routine Kirby-Bauer procedure are made for fastidious organisms and anaerobes. Blood, serum, and nicotinamide adenine dinucleotide (NAD) or yeast extract may

have to be added in order to grow such organisms as *Haemophilus* species, *Actinobacillus pleuropneumoniae*, *Actinomyces pyogenes*, and some streptococci.

The Tube Susceptibility Test

This procedure is more complicated than the disc susceptibility test and is only rarely carried out in veterinary diagnostic laboratories. The aim of the test is to determine the *minimum inhibitory concentration* (MIC) of the drug. This is accomplished by adding a standardized inoculum of organisms (pure culture) to a series of tubes containing increasing concentrations of the drug being tested (Fig. 6–4). After incubation, the results are recorded. The MIC is defined as the highest dilution (i.e., the least amount of the drug) that prevents growth. For the drug to be effective clinically, the MIC must be well below the peak blood concentration of the drug expected under recommended dosage schemes.

The minimum bactericidal concentration (MBC) can be determined by plating loopfuls from the three successive tubes not showing evidence of growth onto a suitable agar medium. The plate showing no growth indicates the tube with no growth and thus the MBC.

MICs are not commonly conducted in veterinary diagnostic laboratories, but the availability of automated instruments for the performance of MICs may hasten their use in the larger laboratories.

Serum Bactericidal Test

This is essentially the same as the MIC test except that the drug is present in the patient's serum. This test is rarely carried out in veterinary laboratories. The standardized inoculum of organisms is added to the dilutions of serum. After incubation, the test is read and the *serum bactericidal concentration* is defined as the highest dilution of serum that prevents growth.

E-Test

The E-test, a variant of the disc diffusion test, allows the qualitative determination of MICs. The test system consists of a plastic strip containing a gradient of antimicrobial agent to one side and an interpretive scale on the other side. The strip is placed on the surface of an agar plate containing a uniform lawn of the test organism. The strip is incubated at 37° C for 24 hours. The MIC is determined by reading the scale at the point where the zone of inhibition intersects the strip. Results of these tests appear to agree well with the standard agar dilution method.

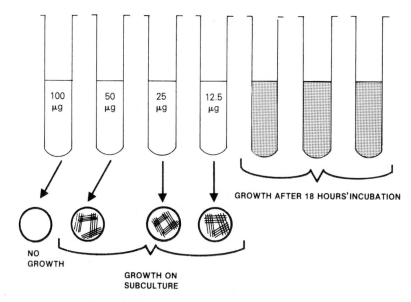

Figure 6–4. Tube susceptibility test for determining the minimum inhibitory concentration (MIC). Those tubes without evidence of growth (turbidity) are plated out to determine the minimum bactericidal concentration (MBC).

MINIMUM INHIBITORY CONCENTRATION = 12.5 µg/ml

MINIMUM BACTERICIDAL CONCENTRATION = 100 µg/ml

Automated Systems

A variety of new automated and semiautomated systems have been introduced in recent years for susceptibility testing of bacteria. Some contain components for rapid identification of bacteria. These systems are capable of providing qualitative (susceptible, intermediate, or resistant) and quantitative (MIC) information in a relatively short period of time. These same-day procedures are more expensive to perform than the traditional tests. The high initial equipment cost and the ongoing cost of reagents make these systems almost prohibitive for many veterinary laboratories; however, some veterinary laboratories are using them.

Of a number of these systems, the Sensititre system is the one most widely used for veterinary pathogens. It provides microdilution susceptibility plates containing various antimicrobial agents for full range MICs and breakpoints. The test plates may be read with a fluorimeter after 5 hours, or 18 to 24 hours incubation. The Sensititre system makes available custom susceptibility plates to meet the needs of a particular laboratory.

DRUG RESISTANCE

Many organisms have the ability to produce mutants that are resistant to most of the drugs to which they would ordinarily be susceptible in the wild state. The use of subinhibitory levels of antibiotics contributes to the survival and multiplication of resistant mutants. The amount of resistance, and the time it takes to develop, depend upon the organism and the drug.

Some organisms, such as *Streptococcus agalactiae* and other pyogenic streptococci, lack the capacity to produce resistant mutants. The development of resistance by *Staphylococcus aureus* in response to penicillin and the tetracyclines is usually slow, occurring in small steps over a considerable period of time and exposure. However, many resistant strains now exist. On the other hand, resistance of the tubercle bacillus to streptomycin may develop to a high level in a single-step manner.

Resistance is specific in that an organism will become resistant to a particular antibiotic. Cross-resistance only occurs among closely related drugs such as the different tetracyclines, aminoglycosides, and so forth. Resistance to one drug may be followed by resistance to another drug, and thus strains emerge that are resistant to a number of drugs. In addition to this type of chromosomal resistance, multidrug resistance due to R factors is encountered. This is referred to briefly further on, and in detail in Chapter 3.

MECHANISMS OF DRUG RESISTANCE

Some of the mechanisms of drug resistance known are:

1. Adoption by the organism of an alternative metabolic pathway in order to bypass the inhibited reaction; e.g., those bacteria resistant

Table 6–1. Guide to the Selection of Antimicrobial Drugs in the Absence of Susceptibility Tests

Organism	First-Choice Drugs	Alternative Drugs
Pyogenic streptococci	Penicillin	Ampicillin, erythromycin, cephalosporins
Staphylococcus aureus, S. intermedius	Synthetic penicillins: methicillin, cloxacillin, augmentin*, enrofloxacin	Erythromycin, cephalosporins
Clostridia	Penicillin	Tetracyclines, erythromycin
Erysipelothrix rhusiopathiae	Penicillin	Tetracyclines, erythromycin
Listeria monocytogenes	Penicillin, ampicillin, tetracyclines	Chloramphenicol
Corynebacteria	Penicillin, erythromycin	Tetracyclines, erythromycin
Nocardia asteroides	Sulfadiazine, sulfisoxazole	Tetracyclines, streptomycin
Actinomyces bovis A. viscosus	Penicillin, sulfonamides	Erythromycin, tetracyclines
Enterobacteriaceae in general *Escherichia coli* *Salmonella* spp. *Proteus* spp.	Neomycin, tetracyclines, chloramphenicol, ampicillin, apramycin, enrofloxacin	Cephalosporins, streptomycin
Pasteurella multocida	Tetracyclines, penicillin, ceftiofur	Sulfonamides, erythromycin, ampicillin
Pasteurella haemolytica	Tetracyclines, ceftiofur, tilmicosin	Sulfonamides, erythromycin, chloramphenicol
Haemophilus spp.	Ampicillin, ceftiofur	Tetracyclines, cephalosporins, sulfonamides
Bordetella bronchiseptica	Sulfonamides, erythromycin	Tetracyclines
Pseudomonas aeruginosa	Gentamicin, tobramycin, enrofloxacin	Carbenicillin
Serpulina hyodysenteriae	Tylosin, arsanilic acid, sodium arsanilate, mecadox	Lincomycin, streptomycin, tetracyclines
Mycoplasmas	Tylosin, tetracyclines, erythromycin	
Campylobacter spp.	Streptomycin (with or without penicillin)	Tetracyclines
Acinetobacter spp.	Kanamycin	Gentamicin, polymyxin
Bacteroides spp.	Penicillin, clindamycin, chloramphenicol	Tetracyclines, ampicillin
Fusobacterium necrophorum	Penicillin	Tetracyclines, sulfonamides
Actinobacillus equuli A. lignieresii	Streptomycin, tetracyclines	Erythromycin
A. pleuropneumoniae	Penicillin, oxytetracycline	Tiamulin
Leptospires	Penicillin, streptomycin	Tetracyclines, erythromycin

* Amoxicillin with clavulanic acid.

to sulfonamides adapt to using preformed folic acid.

2. Production of an enzyme that destroys the antibiotic; e.g., penicillinase (β-lactamase) from *Staphylococcus aureus* and other bacteria; or production of enzymes by some bacteria that inactivate drugs by acetylation, adenylation, or phosphorylation.

3. Change in permeability or decreased uptake of the drug by the cell or some special part of the cell, such as occurs in bacteria resistant to tetracyclines and polymyxins.

4. Altered structural target for the drug; e.g., erythromycin-resistant organisms have an altered protein on the 50S subunit of the bacterial ribosome.

DEVELOPMENT OF RESISTANCE DURING TREATMENT

Mutation

Resistant mutants may emerge during treatment. The occurrence and establishment of resistant mutants vary with different drugs. Selection of mutants is favored by underdosage, prolonged administration, and the presence of a "closed" focus of infection, such as is found in an abscess.

The drugs listed below are grouped roughly according to the likelihood that resistant mutants will emerge during treatment.

Frequent: sulfonamides, streptomycin, nalidixic acid, rifamycin.

Less frequent: erythromycin.

Table 6–2. Antimicrobial Agents for Routine Susceptibility Testing*

Companion and Equine	Food Animal	Mastitis	Avian	Ocular	Anaerobes
Amikacin	Ampicillin	Ampicillin	Amikacin	Bacitracin	Ampicillin
Ampicillin	Amoxicillin	Cephalothin	Bacitracin	Carbenicillin	Augmentin
Augmentin	Apramcyin	Erythromycin	Chloramphenicol	Cephalothin	Carbenicillin
Carbenicillin	Ceftiofur	Penicillin	Clindamycin	Chloramphenicol	Cephalothin
Cephalothin	Cephalothin	Penicillin/ Novobiocin	Enrofloxacin	Enrofloxacin	Chloramphenicol
Chloramphenicol	Clindamycin	Pirlimycin	Erythromycin	Erythromycin	Clindamycin
Clindamycin	Enrofloxacin	Oxacillin	Gentamycin	Gentamycin	Metronidazole
Enrofloxacin	Erthromycin	Tetracycline	Neomycin	Neomycin	Penicillin
Erythromycin	Gentamycin		Penicillin	Polymyxin B	Tetracycline
Gentamycin	Mecadox		Streptomycin	Tetracycline	Ticarcillin
Kanamycin	Neomycin		Sulfadimeth- oxine	Tobramycin	
Methicillin	Penicillin		Sulfaquinoxaline		
Neomycin	Spectinomycin		Sulfathiazole		
Penicillin	Streptomycin		Tetracycline		
Tetracycline	Sulfachlorpyridazine		Tribressen		
Ticarcillin	Sulfadimethoxine		Triple Sulfa		
Timentin	Tetracycline				
Tribressen	Tilmicosin				
Triple Sulfa	Tribressen				
	Triple Sulfa				
	Tylosin				

* List may differ from laboratory to laboratory.

Infrequent: tetracyclines, penicillin, cephalosporins, chloramphenicol.

Superinfection

This term is frequently used to describe the infection that is caused by "alien" organisms such as *Candida albicans* as a result of the alteration or suppression of the normal flora by prolonged antibiotic administration. The disturbance of the normal flora in animals does not ordinarily cause more than occasional intestinal upsets and diarrhea. However, prolonged administration of antibiotics affecting gram-negative intestinal organisms may cause a deficiency or diminution in the amounts of vitamin K, biotin, riboflavin, pantothenate, and pyridoxine available to the host. Supplementation with vitamins, particularly vitamin B complex, is used in humans.

The term is also used to describe the replacement of the original infecting agent with a new strain of the same species that is resistant, or a resistant strain of another species. *Pseudomonas aeruginosa* and *Acinetobacter* are not infrequently encountered as "replacement" strains.

Infectious Drug Resistance

Transferable multiple drug resistance caused by R factors occurs most commonly in members of the Enterobacteriaceae. This type of resistance, i.e., the whole multiple pattern, is transferable among strains of the same species and among strains of closely related species, e.g., from a *Salmonella* to an *Escherichia coli.* Transfer of this kind can be readily demonstrated in vitro and no doubt also occurs in vivo. It is now very widespread, and strains are commonly encountered that are resistant to as many as four drugs, e.g., streptomycin, a tetracycline, penicillin, and a sulfonamide. It seems likely that the great increase in infectious drug resistance has resulted from the practice of routinely adding antibiotics to animal feeds.

The genetics of drug resistance are discussed in Chapter 3.

SUGGESTIONS ON THE USE OF ANTIMICROBIAL DRUGS

The suggestions that follow are based in part on those provided by Thomas.* When selecting and using antimicrobial drugs, the possibility of the emergence of resistant organisms should always be kept in mind.

---

*Thomas, C.G.A.: Medical Microbiology. 5th Ed. London, Balliere Tindall, 1983.

Table 6–3. Group, Action, and Primary Spectrum of Important Antimicrobial Drugs

	Family	Action Static	Action Cidal	Primary Spectrum Gram negative	Primary Spectrum Gram positive	
Ampicillin		−	+	+	+	Inhibit cell wall synthesis
Carbenicillin		−	+	+	−	
Cloxacillin		−	+	−	+	
Methicillin	Penicillin	−	+	−	+	
Nafcillin		−	+	−	+	
Oxacillin		−	+	−	+	
Penicillin G		−	+	−	+	
Gentamicin		−	+	+	−	Inhibition of ribosomal function (protein synthesis)
Kanamycin		−	+	+	+	
Neomycin	Aminoglycoside	−	+	+	+	
Streptomycin		−	+	+	+	
Spectinomycin		−	+	+	+	
Tobramycin		−	+	+	+	
Erythromycin		+	−	−	+	Inhibition of ribosomal function (protein synthesis)
Oleandomycin	Macrolide	+	−	−	+	
Tylosin		+	−	+	+	
Tilmicosin		+	−	+	+	
Bacitracin		−	+	−	+	Inhibition of cell wall synthesis, impairment of membrane function
Polymycin B	Polypeptide	−	+	+	−	
Colistin		−	+	+	−	
Vancomycin	Glycopeptide	−	+	−	+	Inhibition of peptidoglycan synthesis
Cephalothin		−	+	+	+	Inhibition of cell wall synthesis
Cephalexin	Cephalosporin	−	+	+	+	
Cephaloridine		−	+	+	+	
Ceftiofur		−	+	+	+	
Sulfadiazine		+	−	+	+	Competitive inhibition preventing folic acid formation
Sulfamerazine		+	−	+	+	
Sulfadimethoxine	Sulfonamide	+	−	+	+	
Sulfasoxazole		+	−	+	+	
Chloramphenicol		+	−	+	+	Inhibition of ribosomal function
Tetracyclines	Tetracycline	+	−	+	+	Inhibits ribosomal function
Rifampin	Rifamycin	+	−	−	+	Interferes with RNA synthesis
Nitrofurantoin	Nitrofurans	−	+	+	+	Mechanism uncertain, inhibits bacterial enzymes and damages DNA
Nalidixic acid	Quinolones	−	+	+	+	Inhibits bacterial DNA gyrase
Enrofloxacin		−	+	+	+	
Methenamine mandelate		−	+	+	+	Liberates formaldehyde in acid urine
Paraamino salicyclic acid		+	−	Mycobacteria		Similar to sulfa, inhibits folic acid synthesis

1. Antimicrobial drugs should not be employed for mild, inconsequential infections. The harm done through possibly selecting out resistant organisms may outweigh the benefit derived from treatment.
2. They should only be used prophylactically for individuals and in contact animals if a real risk of severe infection exists, as, for example, in blackleg in cattle or fowl cholera.
3. One should not be less thorough in surgical asepsis or in the control of cross-infection because of the availability of many antibiotics.
4. Treatment should be based on a definite clinical and microbiologic diagnosis. Although treatment may have to be started before the laboratory report is received, it should be modified if indicated.
5. The laboratory report is not a directive for treatment. The choice of the best drug to use

should be made after considering a number of factors. In general, it is poor practice to use a broad-spectrum antibiotic if the infecting agent is sensitive to a more specific one. All antimicrobial drugs are potentially toxic and some are actually dangerous, so very serious consideration should be given to their administration.

6. When antimicrobial drugs are administered, they should be given in full therapeutic doses for an adequate period. This will vary with the disease. The period ordinarily should not be less than 3 to 5 days, but in some diseases such as nocardiosis, treatment will have to be continued for weeks. However, because of the danger of superinfection, the use of some drugs, such as the tetracyclines, should not be unnecessarily prolonged. If there is no response or poor response to treatment, it is possible that a resistant population of organisms has developed. In such cases specimens should be forwarded to the laboratory for additional susceptibility testing. Special attention may have to be given to animals in which abscesses and mixed infections are involved.

7. In some instances it is advisable to consider the simultaneous use of two drugs. Only drugs that act synergistically should be given together.

8. As a general rule, only those antimicrobial drugs that are not suitable for systemic use should be used topically or locally. This reduces the likelihood of the development of drug allergy and reserves the use of systemic drugs for serious infections.

9. Regulations are in place that set withdrawal times for various microbial drugs prior to slaughter. These range from 24 hours to 30 days and must be taken into account in the selection of drugs for treatment.

Table 6–1 is provided to assist in the selection of antimicrobial agents in the absence of susceptibility tests. Table 6–2 lists antimicrobials for routine susceptibility testing. Table 6–3 summarizes information on the action and spectrum of major groups of drugs.

COMBINATIONS OF ANTIMICROBIAL AGENTS

In some circumstances, such as the inaccessibility of the infecting agent, mixed infections, and very serious unresponsive infections, it may be advantageous to use a combination of two drugs that act synergistically. The combinations that are generally synergistic consist of pairs of drugs that are bactericidal. Antagonism is usually observed when a bactericidal drug such as penicillin, which kills rapidly multiplying organisms, is used with a bacteriostatic drug such as a tetracycline. Although they are bacteriostatic, the sulfonamides do not appear to antagonize penicillin, perhaps because their action is slow. Because the bactericidal action of polymyxin is exerted on resting cells as well as on multiplying cells, it is not antagonized by bacteriostatic drugs.

In treating mixed infections with two drugs, it is advisable to select drugs that have rather different spectra of activity, thus broadening the overall antibacterial spectrum. The simultaneous use of two drugs has the following theoretical advantage. Considering the rate of mutation of bacteria to resistance, the probability of an organism becoming resistant to two antimicrobial drugs being used for treatment is very low. When three drugs are used, as, for example, in the treatment of tuberculosis, the probability of a mutant emerging that is resistant to all three drugs is extremely low.

FURTHER READING

Balows, A. (ed.): Current Techniques for Antibiotic Susceptibility Testing. Springfield, Il, Charles C Thomas, 1974.

Chengappa, M.M.: Antimicrobial Agents and Susceptibility Testing. *In* Diagnostic Procedures in Veterinary Bacteriology and Mycology. Edited by G.R. Carter and J.R. Cole, Jr. 5th Ed. New York, Academic Press Inc., 1990.

Eisenberg, M.S., Furukawa, C., and Ray, G.G.: Manual of Antimicrobial Therapy and Infectious Diseases. Philadelphia, W.B. Saunders Co., 1980.

Eliopoulos, G.M., and Eliopoulos, C.T.: Antibiotic combinations: should they be tested? Clin. Microbiol. Rev. 1:139, 1988.

Garrod, L.P., Lampert, H.P., and O'Grady, F.: Antibiotic and Chemotherapy. 5th Ed. London, Churchill Livingstone, 1976.

Klastersky, J. (ed.): Clinical Use of Combinations of Antibiotics. New York, John Wiley & Sons, 1975.

Lorian, V. (ed.): Antibiotics in Laboratory Medicine. 2nd Ed. Baltimore, Williams & Wilkins, 1986.

Paynes, M.A.: The Rational Use of Antibiotics on Dairies. Vet. Med. 88:160, 1993.

Pratt, W.B.: Chemotherapy of Infection. New York, Oxford University Press, 1977.

Prescott, J.F., and Baggot, J.D. (eds.): Antimicrobial Therapy in Veterinary Medicine. 2nd Ed. Ames, Iowa State University Press, 1993.

Smith, H.: Antibiotics in Clinical Practice. 3rd Ed. Baltimore, University Park Press, 1977.

Smith, I.M., Donata, S.T., and Rabinovitch, S.: Antibiotics and Infections. Flushing, NJ, Spectrum Publishing, Inc., 1974.

Yao, J.D.C., and Moellering, R.C., Jr.: Antimicrobial Agents. *In* Manual of Clinical Microbiology. 5th Ed. Edited by A. Balows, et al. Washington, D.C. American Society for Microbiology, 1991.

7

Sterilization and Disinfection

Sterilization and disinfection are of great importance to the practicing veterinarian. The sterilization of dressings, surgical instruments, and syringes is a commonplace procedure, as is the disinfection of kennels, infected premises, and contaminated footwear. So that such operations can be carried out effectively, an understanding of the general principles of sterilization, disinfection, and antisepsis is necessary.

Sterilization. This is the process whereby all viable microorganisms are eliminated or destroyed. The criterion of sterilization is the failure of the organisms to grow if a growth-supporting medium is supplied. The limiting requirement of sterilization is destruction of the bacterial spore, the most resistant form of microbial life.

Disinfection. Disinfection involves the destruction of pathogenic organisms associated with inanimate objects, usually by physical or chemical means. All disinfectants are effective against the vegetative (growing) forms of organisms but not necessarily against their spores.

Antisepsis. Antisepsis involves the inactivation or destruction by chemical means of microbes associated with the animal. Antiseptic agents may be bactericidal or bacteriostatic. Bacteriostatic means the inhibition of multiplication or growth, which, unlike the bactericidal effect, may be reversible. For ordinary purposes, the terms disinfectant and antiseptic are used synonymously.

PHYSICAL METHODS

Moist Heat

Heat is used to destroy microorganisms in four different ways.

Boiling

Boiling water or steam (common instrument, sterilizer) at 100° C is widely used in veterinary practice for preparing syringes, needles, and instruments for minor surgery. This process kills vegetative forms of microorganisms and viruses in 5 minutes. Many spores are also killed at 100° C in this same period, but many of the more resistant spores, e.g., those of *Clostridium tetani* and the common *Bacillus* species, can survive boiling for as long as several hours. Thus, although boiling kills most pathogenic bacteria, boiling is not sterilization as the term is defined.

Steam Under Pressure (Autoclave)

The most resistant spores are killed by a temperature of 121° C for 15 minutes. This temperature is obtained at sea level by steam at a pressure at 15 lb/in² in excess of atmospheric pressure. The autoclave, which is a metal cylinder designed to contain steam under pressure, is an essential piece of equipment in microbiology laboratories and operating rooms. Many veterinarians have small autoclaves for the sterilization of instruments, dressings, solutions, and surgical packs. In order to obtain a temperature of 121° C, all air must first

95

be blown out. In the large, modern, high-vacuum autoclaves, 98% of the air is removed by a powerful pump. Air is removed in two stages in the down-ward-displacement autoclaves. Steam is admitted at the top of the chamber and residual air is driven out at the bottom.

The killing power of steam is attributable to the fact that when it condenses on the item being steri-lized, it liberates a large amount of latent heat. The shrinkage resulting from condensation—a thin film of moisture on the surface of the load—draws in fresh steam and thus more heat. As this process con-tinues, the steam penetrates and surrounds the vari-ous items, producing a high uniform temperature.

The following points should be kept in mind when using the office autoclave:

1. Air and condensate must be removed for ef-fective sterilization.
2. The required temperature of 121° C must be maintained.
3. All mechanisms, such as gauges and timers, must be in proper working order.
4. Packs should be properly prepared. They should not be too large nor should the wrap-pings be impervious. Volumes of fluid should not be too large. The load should be arranged to allow for penetration of steam.
5. The effectiveness of the autoclave can be tested by affixing heat-sensitive tape to the packs being sterilized. Paper strips impreg-nated with spores of *Bacillus stearothermophi-lus* also can be used to test the autoclave. If the autoclave is functioning effectively, the spores will be killed.

The high-vacuum autoclaves used in clinics and hospitals should be operated strictly according to directions provided by the manufacturer. Pres-sures, temperatures, and times of each sterilization cycle must be recorded, and routine checks must be made of temperatures and sterilizing effectiveness.

Steaming (Tyndallization)

This process has been replaced largely by filtra-tion. It involves placing the media or solutions in flowing steam for 1 hour on each of 3 successive days. The period between steaming allows the spores to germinate and thus to be killed at the next exposure. Tyndallization requires a medium or so-lution that is sufficiently nutritious to promote ger-mination of spores in the intervals between steam-ing. Bacteriologic media qualify in this respect.

Pasteurization

This process, which involves the heating of milk to the point that all potential human pathogens are killed, has greatly reduced the incidence of brucellosis and tuberculosis in humans over the years. The occasional outbreaks of group A (*Strep-tococcus pyogenes*) streptococcal disease spread by milk also have been eliminated.

In the slow method of pasteurization, milk is held at 62.78° C for 30 minutes and in the flash method at 71.67° C for 15 seconds. A few heat-resistant vegetative bacteria (thermoduric) and spores survive. The milk is rapidly cooled after pasteurization to discourage growth of the re-maining viable organisms.

ULTRAVIOLET LIGHT

Direct sunlight kills unprotected vegetative or-ganisms fairly rapidly, but spores are resistant. The bactericidal activity of sunlight is caused by the ultraviolet portion of the spectrum. Glass is imper-vious to this radiation. Sunshine is no doubt of great importance in the destruction of pathogenic organisms contaminating fields, pastures, and other areas used by livestock.

Ultraviolet (UV) light is a nonionizing or low-en-ergy radiation with a wavelength in the range of 2500 angstroms. Ultraviolet light from mercury lamps is widely used in inoculating hoods, op-erating theaters, animal quarters, and other areas to reduce airborne infections. It acts most efficiently at temperatures from 27° to 40° C. Ultraviolet radia-tion acts by causing errors in the replication of DNA. Its mutagenic activity on living cells is well known.

IONIZING RADIATION

This form of radiation has an energy content much higher than that of ultraviolet light and con-sequently has a strong disinfectant action. Gamma rays emitted from cobalt-60 are used commercially to sterilize disposable syringes, needles, pipettes, surgical sutures, dressings, bone grafts, plastic arte-rial prostheses, catheters, plastic Petri dishes, and other heat-sensitive items. Unfortunately, when ionizing radiation is used on foods, flavors may be affected, and when it is used on such items as drugs, hormones, and enzymes, potency may be reduced.

FILTRATION

Filtration has been used for decades to sterilize bacteriologic media, serum, injection solutions, and other solutions containing heat-sensitive sub-stances. A pore size of 0.45 μm or less removes almost all bacteria from solutions. Membrane filters composed of cellulose esters and plastic polymers have largely supplanted other kinds of filters. The porosities of these membrane filters range from 0.1 μm to 10 μm. The coarse sizes are used for clarification prior to using the smaller pore sizes. Those filters commonly used to remove bacteria do not hold back viruses or mycoplasmas. Filters with a porosity of about 0.3 μm are used to filter air in rooms and operating theaters.

CHEMICAL AGENTS

Chemical agents act more selectively on microorganisms than do the physical methods, such as heat and radiation. This review emphasizes the antiseptics and disinfectants that are now in use by veterinarians. The goal should be the selection of the best agent for a particular situation and task.

In assessing an antiseptic or disinfectant, Thomas* has listed the following important considerations:

1. *Organisms killed.* Spores are highly resistant compared with vegetative forms, and only a few disinfectants, e.g., halogens, mercuric chloride, formalin, and ethylene oxide, are effective in the concentrations usually used. Mycobacteria are more resistant than most other vegetative organisms. Phenolic and alcoholic compounds are recommended for this group. Generally speaking, viruses are more resistant than vegetative bacteria. Halogens, oxidizing agents, and formalin are active against many viruses. Quaternary compounds and dyes are not.

2. *Organisms inhibited.* Organisms should be killed rather than merely inhibited. The quaternary compounds employed in high dilutions are bacteriostatic rather than bactericidal. Such agents as formaldehyde, ethylene oxide, and chlorine are clearly bactericidal.

3. *Rate of action.* The rate of action differs greatly among the various chemical agents. Some act rapidly, whereas others are completely effective only after some minutes or even hours. Disinfectants have an optimum pH range, and all are more active at higher temperatures. Growing and multiplying cells are more readily poisoned than are those in a resting or stationary state. All disinfectants are to some extent inhibited in their activity by organic matter, such as that found in feces, pus, exudates, discharges, and blood. Mercury salts, halogens, and quaternaries are especially inhibited by organic matter. In the disinfection of premises, stables, and kennels, the power of penetration of dirt, grease, and organic matter is important. Soaps and surface-active agents assist penetration.

4. *Side effects.* Other limiting considerations are toxicity, possession of an irritating vapor, undesirable staining properties, and destructive effects on instruments and fabrics. Antiseptics or disinfectants used on or around animals should be relatively nontoxic to tissues.

5. *Additional considerations.* Disinfectants should be reasonable in price and maintain their potency for long periods of time. They should be soluble in water and stable in aqueous solution.

THE PHENOL COEFFICIENT

This value expresses the capacity of a disinfectant to kill bacteria when compared with phenol. In the official test, a broth culture is diluted 1:10 with different concentrations of the test compound. The end point is the lowest concentration that yields sterile loopful samples after incubation for 10 minutes at 20° C. The compound is generally recommended for use at five times this concentration. For example, a phenol coefficient may be stated to be 40, which means its killing power is 40 times that of phenol. The three organisms used in the official test are *Salmonella typhi* (gram-negative), *Staphylococcus aureus* (gram-positive), and *Pseudomonas aeruginosa* (gram-negative).

Although of some value, the phenol coefficient does not take into account such considerations as toxicity for tissues, inactivation by organic matter, corrosive properties, and other factors relating to particular situations.

USE-DILUTION TEST

This test is sometimes used to evaluate a disinfectant. In this procedure, the test bacteria are added to broth tubes containing increasingly strong concentrations of the test disinfectant. After incubation, the growth, or absence of such, is recorded. The result is used to rate the disinfectant.

Special tests are used to evaluate the fungicidal efficacy of disinfectants.

MAJOR GROUPS OF CHEMICAL DISINFECTANTS*

Some of the properties of the common classes of disinfectants are listed in Table 7–1.

*Thomas, C.G.A.: Medical Microbiology. 5th Ed. London, Balliere Tindall, 1983.

*Modified from Wilson, M.E., and Mizer, H.E.: Microbiology in Patient Care. 2nd Ed. New York, Macmillan, 1974.

Table 7–1. Some Properties of the Common Classes of Disinfectants

	Disinfectant Class					
	Quaternary Ammonium Compounds	Phenolics	Sodium Hypochlorite	Iodophors	Glutaraldehyde	Chlorhexidine
Example	Roccal	Staphene	Clorox	Betadine	Cidex	Nolvasan
Bactericidal	2–3+	3+	3+	3+	3+	2–3+
Mycobactericidal	0–1+	2–3+	3+	2–3+	2–3+	0–1+
General virucide	0–1+	0	3+	2–3+	3–4+	0
Lipophilic or lipophilic-like viruses	2–3+	2–3+	3+	2+	3–4+	2–3+
Sporicidal at room temperature	0	0–1+	2+	0–1+	2–3+	0
Fungicidal	2–3+	2–3+	2+	3+	2–3+	0–1+
Effective in the presence of organic material	0–1+	2–3+	0–1+	0–1+	2+	0–1+
Effective in the presence of soaps	0	3+	2+	3+	3+	0
Effective in hard water	2–3+	2–3+	2+	2+	3+	1–2+
Most effective pH range	alkaline	neutral	acid	neutral	alkaline	alkaline

4+, very high activity; 3+, high activity; 2+, moderate activity; 1+, slight activity; 0, no activity.
Adapted from Kowalski, J.J., and Mallmann, W.L.: Is your disinfection practice effective? J. Am. An. Hosp. Assoc., 9:3, 1973.

GROUP: SOLUBLE ALCOHOLS

Ethyl (C₂H₅OH)
Isopropyl (CH₃CHOHCH₃)

Mode of Action. Protein coagulation and dissolution of membrane lipids.

Dilution. 70 to 90%.

Recommended for. Thermometers (add 0.2 to 1% iodine); instruments; skin preparations; hands; spot disinfection.

Advantages. Rapidly bactericidal; tuberculocidal; active against enveloped and nonenveloped viruses.

Limitations. Not sporicidal; not active against fungi; inactivated by organic material; corrodes metals unless reducing agent added (e.g., 2% sodium nitrite); drying to skin; bleaches rubber tile.

GROUP: STERILIZING GASES

Ethylene Oxide

Mode of Action. Substitution of the cell alkyl groups for labile hydrogen atoms.

Proprietary Products. Carboxide, Cryoxide, Steroxide.

Dilution. Gas; exposure time 4 to 18 hours.

Recommended for. Blankets, pillows, mattresses; lensed instruments; rubber goods, thermolabile plastics; books; papers.

Advantages. Active against bacteria, fungi, and viruses; harmless to most materials; sterilizes.

Limitations. Requires special equipment; used in human hospitals for large-volume sterilization.

GROUP: DISINFECTANT GAS

Formaldehyde

Mode of Action. Same as ethylene oxide.

Proprietary Product. Bard-Parker Formaldehyde Germicide; glutaraldehyde is similar to formaldehyde in range of activity.

Dilution. Gas, or full-strength solution.

Recommended for. Gas: cabinet and incubator disinfection; solution: transfer forceps, instrument soak.

Advantages. Active against bacteria, fungi, and viruses; vapor disinfection of delicate instruments; sporicidal, noncorrosive.

Limitations. Requires long period for effective disinfection; odorous; toxic to skin and mucous membranes; inactivated by organic material.

GROUP: HALOGENS

Chlorines
Iodines

Mode of Action. Inactivate by oxidizing free sulfhydryl groups; active against bacteria, fungi, and viruses.

Chlorines. Hypochlorites or hydrochlorous acid derivates (HClO).

Proprietary Products. Hypochlorites, such as Clorox, Purex, and other bleaches; HClO: Warexin.

Dilution. Hypochlorites: strongest concentration recommended by manufacturers; if dry, mix to thin paste. Warexin: used in 1.5% aqueous solution.

Recommended for. Floors; plumbing fixtures; spot disinfection; fabrics not harmed by bleaching; Warexin for dishes but not silverware.

Advantages. Tuberculocidal unless highly diluted (Warexin limited).

Limitations. Bleach fabrics; corrode metals; unstable in hard water; must be freshly prepared; tarnish silver. Chlorine is inactivated by organic material.

Iodines. Tincture or aqueous solution (2 to 5%). Iodophors consist of iodine combined with surface-active agents. They act rapidly and have low toxicity for tissue.

Proprietary Products. Wescodyne; Betadine; Iobac; Klenzade; Micro-Klene; Virac.

Dilution. Tincture: full strength. Wescodyne: 77 ppm (90 ml or 3 oz to 5 gal water), or 450 ppm to kill tubercle bacilli; tincture = 10% Wescodyne in 50% ethyl alcohol. Other iodophors: see manufacturer's recommendations.

Recommended for. Tincture: skin preparations; thermometers (see Soluble Alcohols). Wescodyne: thermometers, utensils, rubber goods, dishes; tincture: used for spot disinfection, or for single presurgical scrub. Betadine: presurgical skin preparation. Others: many designed for specific purposes, including milking and dairy operations, e.g., Iosan.

Advantages. Iodophors are cleaning and disinfecting; nonstaining; leave residual antibacterial effect; and are tuberculocidal as tinctures. Loss of germicidal activity is indicated by fading color.

Limitations. Tincture of iodine stains and is irritating to tissues. Iodophors are somewhat unstable and are inactivated by hard water; may corrode metals; drying to skin as tinctures.

GROUP: PHENOLICS
Saponated Creosol
Semisynthetic Phenols

Mode of Action. Protein coagulation. They destroy selective permeability of cell membranes, resulting in leakage of cell constituents.

Proprietary Products. Synthetics: Amphyl, Lysol, O-Syl, Staphene, Vesphene, Tergisyl, Armisol.

Dilution. Creosol, 2% for 30 minutes; 5% if hard water. Amphyl, 0.5 to 1% (also available as spray). Lysol, 1%. O-Syl, 2.5%. Staphene, 0.5 to 2%. Vesphene, 1 to 2%. Tergisyl, 2%.

Recommended for. Creosol: equipment, linen, excreta. Amphyl: instruments. Lysol: laundry rinse for blankets, linens. O-Syl, Staphene, Vesphene: floors, walls, equipment. Tergisyl, Armisol: environmental uses.

Advantages. Not inactivated by organic matter, soap, or hard water (except creosol); residual effect if allowed to dry on surfaces; high detergency.

Limitations. Phenolics are not sporicidal and only weakly effective against nonenveloped viruses. Creosol must be used in soft water and is slow acting; Lysol and creosol both have odors that may be objectionable.

GROUP: QUATERNARY AMMONIUM COMPOUNDS
Cationic Detergents

Mode of Action. See under Detergents.

Proprietary Products. Zephiran, Roccal, and many others.

Dilution. 1:1000 to 1:5000 aqueous.

Recommended for. Cleaning and disinfection of instruments, utensils, and rubber goods; also for milking and dairy operations. Instrument soak (except for those with cemented lenses), lacquered catheters, synthetic rubber goods, and aluminum instruments.

Advantages. Low tissue toxicity.

Limitations. Not tuberculocidal; limited viricidal activity; must be diluted with distilled water; is inactivated by protein, soap, and cellulose fibers.

GROUP: SOAP OR DETERGENT ADDITIVES
Anionic Detergents

Because of recent restrictions in use, formulations of products listed may be altered.

Mode of Action. See under Detergents.

Proprietary Products. Hexachlorophene (G-11): Bar soaps—Gamophen. Liquid detergents—Septisol, pHisoHex, Hex-O-San, Surofene. Hand creams—Septisol antiseptic skin cream. Tetrachlorosalicylanilide: Bar soap—Coleo, Dial.

Dilution. Septisol, 2%, pHisoHex, 3%; others as recommended by manufacturer.

Recommended for. Skin disinfection, but note limitations.

Advantages. Good cleansers and have prolonged antibacterial action.

Limitations. Not sporicidal, not tuberculocidal, have slow action; limited viricidal activity; toxic if used continuously and absorbed into the body in increasing quantities (especially through delicate skin of infants); should be rinsed off after use on skin.

ADDITIONAL DISINFECTANTS

Salts. Organic mercury compounds, such as mercurochrome and thimerosal, are less toxic than other mercuric compounds but they have only slight bactericidal activity. Mercuric chloride and silver nitrate are used as antiseptics in a dilution of 1:1000.

Alkalis. Lye (NaOH) solutions are used in veterinary medicine for disinfecting stables and premises, as indicated later in this section.

Hydrogen Peroxide. This oxidizing agent, available as a 3% aqueous solution, is useful for cleaning and disinfecting wounds and as a mouthwash in humans and animals with septic stomatitis.

Soaps. Soaps have only slight bactericidal activity but they are effective in the mechanical removal of organisms. However, the act of washing appears to bring the resident flora to the surface of the skin of the hands, resulting in increased bacterial counts. For this reason, the germicides hexachlorophene and tetrachlorosalicylanilide are added to soap.

DETERGENTS

Detergents concentrate at the cell membrane and probably act by disrupting the normal function of the membrane.

Anionic Detergents. These include the natural soaps. They are used as cleaning agents, and because they have little bactericidal activity, they are combined with phenolic compounds.

Cationic Detergents. These include the many quaternary ammonium compounds, e.g., Zephiran and Cetavolon. Because of their surface-active properties, they are excellent cleansing agents for skin, burns, wounds, and inanimate objects. They are more active against gram-positive than gram-negative organisms. In high dilutions they are bacteriostatic, but spores, viruses, mycobacteria, and *Pseudomonas aeruginosa* are relatively resistant. This class of detergents is neutralized by soaps and anionic detergents.

Biguanide Compounds. Chlorhexidine (Hibitane, Nolvasan) is the most commonly used disinfectant of this group. It is bactericidal in high dilutions, but viruses (except lipophilic ones), spores, and mycobacteria are relatively resistant. It is combined with a quaternary ammonium compound to increase its germicidal activity. This combination, called Nolvasan, is used widely by veterinarians for preoperative treatment of skin, surgical scrub, obstetric procedures, and milking and dairy operations.

Dialdehydes. Glutaraldehyde (Cidex) is the most widely used compound of this group. It has one of the widest spectrums of any disinfectant, being bactericidal, viricidal, fungicidal, and sporicidal. A 2% aqueous solution buffered to pH 7.5 to 8.5 is useful for disinfecting surgical instruments, cystoscopes, and anesthetic equipment, although heat sterilization is preferable. Spores are killed within 3 hours and vegetative bacteria in 10 minutes.

MISCELLANEOUS NOTES

Merthiolate (1:10,000) is used as a preservative in serum and in biologic products. Actidione is used in Sabouraud agar to depress the growth of common saprophytic fungi. Formalin (0.3 to 0.5%) is used to kill bacteria in bacterins. Gentian violet, potassium tellurate, malachite green, brilliant green, and selenite F are incorporated in a variety of media to inhibit the growth of undesirable bacteria. Thallium acetate is incorporated in mycoplasma media to inhibit growth of gram-negative bacteria. Beta-propiolactone is used to sterilize grafts, vaccines, bacterins, and sera.

Sodium nitrite (0.2%) should be added to alcohol, formalin, formalin-alcohol, iodophor, and quaternary ammonium solutions to prevent corrosion. Sodium bicarbonate (0.5%) is added to phenolic solutions to prevent metallic corrosion.

Disinfectants in the Control of Bovine Mastitis. Disinfectants play a major role in the control and prevention of mastitis. The various procedures and some of the disinfectants commonly used are:

	Procedures	*Solutions Used*
1.	Predipping teats before udder preparation.	Iodophores, naturally occurring antimicrobial proteins
2.	Dipping teats after milking.	Chlorhexidine, iodophores, sodium hypochlorite, naturally occurring antimicrobial proteins, quaternary ammonium compounds
3.	Disinfectant washes for udder preparation.	Iodophores, quaternary ammonium compounds
4.	Washing hands of milker.	Chlorhexadine, iodophores
5.	Backflushing the teat cups between cows.	Iodophores
6.	Storing teat cup lines.	None, store dry

DISINFECTANTS RECOMMENDED FOR SELECTED ANIMAL DISEASES

Disinfection in regard to important diseases is dealt with in detail in *A Guide for Accredited Veterinarians* (U.S.D.A.) and is carried out under the supervision of State-Federal and Accredited Veterinarians. A table is provided in the *Guide* for the preparation and use of the recommended disinfectants. Some general directions relating to disinfection from the *Guide* follow.

Employees supervising the official disinfecting of farm buildings, other facilities, and transportation equipment exposed to diseases of animals are required to use federally permitted disinfectants.

First, remove all animals or birds and feed and water containers from the premises (car, boat, truck, coop, or crate). Remove all litter and manure from floors, walls, and surfaces of barns, pens, stalls, chutes, and other facilities and fixtures occupied or traversed by diseased animals or birds. After thorough cleaning is accomplished, saturate all surfaces with the disinfectant solution.

Immerse in the disinfectant solution all halters, ropes, and other types of equipment used in handling or restraining animals or birds, as well as the forks, shovels, and scrapers used in removal of litter and manure.

Ventilate buildings, cars, and other closed conveyances, and do not house livestock or poultry or employ equipment until treatment has been absorbed, set, or dried. All treated feed racks, mangers, troughs, automatic feeders, fountains, and waterers must be thoroughly scrubbed with detergents and rinsed with potable water prior to use. Cresylic disinfectants are permitted for nonfood use only. They must not be applied directly to animals and poultry or milking parlors or milk houses because of current federal regulations for food use.

Table 7–2. Recommended Disinfectants and the Diseases for Which They Are Used

Disinfectants	Diseases
Cresylics	Brucellosis, hog cholera, tuberculosis, swine erysipelas, shipping fever
Sodium Carbonate (soda ash)	Foot-and-mouth disease, vesicular exanthema
Lye (sodium hydroxide)	Anthrax, blackleg, foot-and-mouth disease, vesicular exanthema
Sodium orthophenylphenate (e.g., Lysol)	Tuberculosis, infectious laryngotracheitis

Some disinfectants and the diseases for which they are used are given in Table 7–2.

FURTHER READING

Anonymous: A Guide for Accredited Veterinarians. Publication of the Animal and Plant Health Inspection Service. Hyattsville, MD, U.S. Department of Agriculture, 1989.

Block, S.S.: Disinfection, Sterilization and Preservation. 3rd Ed. Philadelphia, Lea & Febiger, 1983.

Greene, C.E.: Environmental control of microbes. *In* Clinical Microbiology and Infectious Diseases of the Dog and Cat. 2nd Ed. Edited by C.E. Greene. Philadelphia, W.B. Saunders Co., 1990.

Huber, W.G.: Antiseptics and disinfectants. *In* Veterinary Pharmacology and Therapeutics. 5th Ed. Edited by N.A. Booth and L.E. McDonald. Ames, IA, Iowa State University Press, 1982.

Lowbury, E.J.L., Ayliffe, G.A.J., Geddes, A.M., and Williams, J.D.: Control of Hospital Infection: A Practical Handbook. New York, John Wiley, 1975.

Lowler, D.F.: Disinfection of animal environments. *In* Current Veterinary Therapy X. Edited by R.W. Kirk. Philadelphia, W.B. Saunders Co., 1989.

Roberts, R.B. (ed.): Infection and Sterilization Problems. Boston, Little, Brown, 1972.

8

Outline of Procedures for the Bacteriologic and Mycologic Examination of Clinical Specimens

The term "clinical specimens" denotes those materials, e.g., tissues, blood, urine, skin scrapings, and body fluids, taken from animals for diagnostic purposes. In the diagnosis of microbial diseases, such materials must reach the diagnostic laboratory with as little change as possible from their original state. Suspension of microbial multiplication is usually accomplished by maintaining the specimens at refrigerator temperature until they reach the laboratory. On occasion, it may be advisable to freeze specimens.

Obviously the diagnostic microbiology laboratory can function most effectively when the correct specimens are selected and properly submitted. Most diagnostic laboratories supply veterinary practitioners with instructions on the selection, packing, and shipment of specimens. The submission form provides space for information on the origin and nature of the specimen, the clinical history, and the disease or diseases suspected.

Just prior to death of the animal and shortly thereafter, a number of intestinal bacteria may invade the host's tissues. The significance of these organisms, some of which are potential pathogens, is difficult to assess when tissues have been taken even a short time after death. Live, sick animals

presented for necropsy are usually the best source of specimens. In all instances, the importance of fresh tissues taken as soon as possible after death cannot be overemphasized.

In the interest of protecting laboratory personnel, persons submitting specimens should inform the laboratory if they are submitting specimens from suspected zoonotic diseases, such as tuberculosis, brucellosis, tularemia, and avian chlamydiosis.

In order to underscore the importance of the correct selection and submission of clinical specimens, some instructions relating to particular diseases are provided in the following section.

SPECIMENS FOR BACTERIOLOGIC AND MYCOLOGIC EXAMINATIONS

Preservation and Shipment of Tissues, Feces, Milk, and Urine. Place tissues in plastic bags or leakproof jars. Portions of intestines should be packed separately. If there are no apparent lesions and an infectious disease is suspected, portions of liver, lung, kidney, spleen, intestine, and lymph nodes should be submitted. Specimens taken at the margin of diseased and normal tissue are preferred. Specimens can be conveniently shipped in a Styrofoam box or ice chest containing a generous amount of ice. Dry ice with plenty of insulation is preferred for longer preservation. Small specimens may be shipped in an insulated container with an ice pack.

Brains sent for examination should be halved longitudinally. One half is refrigerated or frozen over dry ice, and the other is placed in 10% buffered formalinized saline for histopathologic examination. Tissues packed in formalin should not be frozen.

Swabs. Swabs are of value for the submission of infectious material to the laboratory. On conventional cotton swabs, many bacteria are susceptible to desiccation during shipment; therefore the swab must be placed in a nonnutritional transport medium. The survival rate of many pathogenic bacteria is significantly increased by good transport media. Special swabs are required for swabbing the cervix of cows and mares. These can be prepared by attaching absorbent cotton to the end of an 18- to 24-inch-length wire with a rubber band. Several convenient swab systems utilizing a transport medium are available commercially.

Feces. Fecal specimens should be obtained directly from the rectum. Because of contamination, "ground droppings" should be avoided.

Milk. Milk should be collected from animals aseptically in sterile screw-capped or stoppered vials. Examinations may be negative if samples are taken during treatment.

Urine. Urine should be collected aseptically by midstream, catheter, or bladder tap. In collecting urine for bacteriologic examination, the aim should be to limit to a minimum normal flora and environmental bacteria. Because urine can support the growth of bacteria, it should be refrigerated immediately and certainly not left at room temperature for longer than 1 hour. The actual number of bacteria present in the urine at the time of collection indicates whether a urinary tract infection exists. If the urine is to be examined for leptospira by dark-field, 1.5 ml of 10% formalin should be added to 20 ml of urine. Leptospira disintegrate shortly after collection unless fixed in formalin solution.

Blood Culture. Optimally, 3 to 4 blood samples, 5 to 10 ml each, should be cultured in a liquid or biphasic medium during a 24-hour period. Many convenient blood culture systems are available commercially.

DISEASES REQUIRING SPECIAL CONSIDERATION

The specimens required for diagnostic purposes for most microbial diseases will be evident from discussions in Parts II and III. Some of the diseases that require special consideration with regard to specimens are mentioned in the following sections. This information is provided here to emphasize the importance of the correct selection and submission of clinical specimens to the diagnostic laboratory.

Clostridial Infections (Blackleg, Malignant Edema)

Fresh, affected tissue is especially important because clostridia rapidly invade tissues after death. The muscle tissue involved may be difficult to locate.

Enterotoxemia (Clostridia)

Several ounces of fresh small-intestinal contents are required. They can be submitted in a jar or plastic bag, or a section of affected intestine may be tied off and submitted. This material should be dispatched to the laboratory as soon as possible.

Campylobacteriosis (Cattle and Sheep)

To enable isolation and cultivation, semen, fetal stomach, or cervical mucus should reach the laboratory within 5 hours. If this is not possible, the material should be frozen over dry ice. Failing recovery of live organisms, dead *Campylobacter* can be recognized by negative staining and by a fluorescent antibody (FA) procedure.

Porcine Campylobacteriosis

Six to eight inches of severely affected fresh ileum is submitted. The putative causal organisms often can be seen in mucosal scrapings stained by the modified acid-fast technique.

Anthrax

Cotton swabs are soaked in exuded blood, or blood is taken from a superficial ear vein. Because the organism may not be present in the blood of horses and swine, swabs should be taken from exudates and the cut surface of hemorrhagic lymph nodes.

Johne's Disease

For the demonstration and culture of *Mycobacterium paratuberculosis*, the most suitable specimens are 1 or 2 feet of the terminal sections of the ileum with the ileocecal junction (ileocecal valve) and a similar length of the adjacent cecum, flushed free of intestinal content. Several mesenteric lymph nodes of the ileocecal region should be included also. In the live animal, 10 to 20 g of feces are submitted for culture.

Tuberculosis

The directions are those recommended by the Agricultural Research Service, United States Department of Agriculture. The affected tissue and adjacent lymph nodes should be submitted.

If no lesions are observed but the mycobacteriologic examination is justified, lymph nodes should be selected to represent the head, thorax, and abdomen.

One half of the tissue specimen, about 10 g, should be sent in saturated sodium borate for culture, and one half should be placed in 10% buffered formalin solution for histopathologic study. When infection is discovered by incising a lymph node, that node and one adjacent to it (unincised) should be submitted.

The bottles containing specimens should be placed in a refrigerated polystyrene container and dispatched to the laboratory.

Dermatophytosis (Ringworm)

Scrapings or epilations should be taken at the edge of active lesions. Submit in a cotton-plugged test tube or paper envelope. Saprophytic fungi frequently proliferate rapidly in a sealed tube because of the moisture.

Anaerobes

Some anaerobes, particularly some of the gram-negative nonspore-formers, are sensitive to oxygen. Special commercial transport systems are available for the submission of materials suspected of containing significant anaerobes. Some laboratories provide tubes with rubber stoppers containing oxygen-free gas for the submission of swabs. Liquid material can be submitted in syringes devoid of air bubbles. Unless suitable specimens are delivered to the laboratory promptly, culturing for anaerobes rarely provides useful information.

Other Diseases

Other diseases that require special consideration are brucellosis, contagious equine metritis, and mycoplasmosis. Specimens for their diagnosis are referred to in Part II.

EXAMINATION OF CLINICAL SPECIMENS

The procedures to be followed in processing clinical specimens depend largely on the disease or organisms suspected. Thus, an adequate clinical history with suggestions by the veterinarian as to the disease or diseases suspected is extremely important.

The various steps that are followed in the bacteriologic examination of most specimens are outlined in Figure 8–1. Of particular importance is the direct microscopic examination of the specimen.

Direct Examination

The materials most frequently submitted for examination are tissues, feces, swabs, milk, urine, pus, discharge, fetal stomach contents, cervical mucus, and skin scrapings. The microbiologist carries out a direct examination for the agent suspected by the veterinarian or veterinary pathologist. These examinations are dealt with in this book under the appropriate pathogen or disease. The examination of stained smears and wet mounts should be routine with most materials. The findings may aid in the selection of appropriate culture media. When indicated, fluorescent antibody procedures are carried out on smears of tissues, fluids, or exudates.

Procedures Followed in Bacteriologic Examinations

The examination of clinical specimens for the purpose of isolating and identifying bacteria and fungi of possible pathogenic significance is referred to as diagnostic or clinical bacteriology and mycology. This part of veterinary microbiology is traditionally taught in laboratory exercises that accompany the lecture course and thus will only be alluded to briefly here.

The steps listed in Figure 8–1 are followed in the routine processing of specimens. The considerations listed at the top of the chart determine the selection of the primary media. Occasionally a strong presumptive diagnosis can be made on the basis of a direct examination (smear or wet mount), e.g., in actinobacillosis, actinomycosis, blastomycosis, or nocardiosis. If gram-negative bacteria are involved, the results of inoculation of triple sugar iron agar slants at Step 3 (Fig. 8–1) may be particularly useful. The fluorescent antibody procedure is used to identify some organisms in clinical materials, e.g., *Clostridium chauvoei* and *C. septicum,* and also in cultures, e.g., *Listeria monocytogenes* and *Francisella tularensis.*

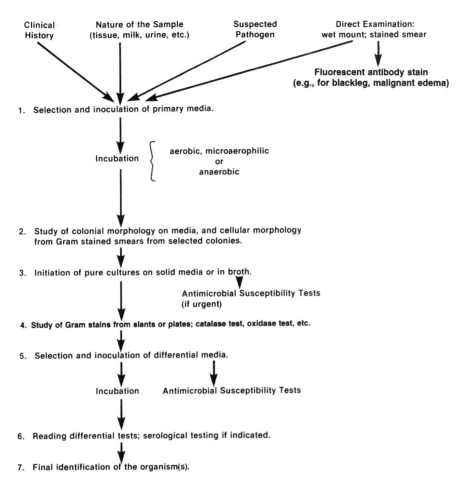

Figure 8–1. Steps usually followed in the isolation and identification of bacteria from clinical specimens.

Experienced veterinary microbiologists first determine the Gram stain reaction and microscopic morphology (e.g., coccus, rod) of the unknown organism. This, along with the history and animal origin, often suggests the probable genus or family to which the organism belongs. With this knowledge certain differential tests can be carried out to confirm the generic, and eventually the species, identification. Tables listing the differential characteristics of organisms of veterinary significance are provided in this and other texts.

In urgent cases, antimicrobial susceptibility tests may be performed before the organism is finally identified. The direct inoculation of clinical material for antimicrobial susceptibility is not recommended because the culture may be mixed and the number of organisms inoculated is not standardized.

Many laboratories have replaced the classic multistep procedures previously referred to with semiautomated or automated commercial systems for identification of bacteria and yeasts. Most of these systems involve miniaturization of conventional methods. Some have a computer-generated

identification data base. Other automated identification systems employ fatty acid profiles, measurement of growth or metabolism, and enzymatic profiling. Systems that employ miniaturized methods, such as Sensititre and Vitek, are used most frequently in veterinary diagnostic laboratories.

The veterinary clinician should interpret the bacteriologic findings. The microbiologist can help in this regard by indicating the amount of growth of a particular organism. This may be stated as few colonies, very light growth, moderate or heavy growth, or moderate growth of a pure culture. Interpretation may be particularly difficult if several different organisms are isolated. This illustrates the importance of a veterinary practitioner's familiarity with the normal flora, commensals, and pathogens of domestic animals.

Recent years have seen the development of various molecular methods of identification for the clinical microbiology laboratory. Because of their expense and the current limited availability of useful reagents, these methods thus far have had limited veterinary application. The available methods include genetic probes, restriction enzyme analysis of chromosomal DNA, Southern blots, ribotyping, and the polymerase chain reaction. The principles of these methods are described in Chapter 3. Their application is referred to under specific infectious agents.

Practice Microbiology

Some veterinarians carry out diagnostic microbiologic procedures in their clinics. Well-trained veterinary personnel using primary media and appropriate commercial rapid identification kits and systems can at least tentatively identify some of the more common pathogens. Examinations for bovine mastitis and canine urinary tract infections can be carried out effectively. The isolation and tentative identification of dermatophytes and the performance of antimicrobial susceptibility tests are well within the capacity of many clinics.

FURTHER READING

Anonymous: Diagnostic Reference Manual. Ames, IA, National Veterinary Services Laboratories, 1990.

Biberstein, E.L., and Zee, Y.C. (eds.): Review of Veterinary Microbiology. Boston, Blackwell Scientific Publications, 1990.

Carter, G.R. and Cole, J.R., Jr. (eds.): Diagnostic Procedures in Veterinary Bacteriology and Mycology. 5th Ed. New York, Academic Press, 1990.

Greene, C.E. (ed.): Clinical Microbiology and Infectious Diseases of the Dog and Cat. 2nd Ed. Philadelphia, W.B. Saunders Co., 1990.

Isenberg, H.D., Washington II, J.A., Doern, G.V., and Amsterdam, D.: Specimen collection and handling. *In* Manual of Clinical Microbiology. 5th Ed. Edited by A. Balows, et al. Washington, D.C., American Society for Microbiology, 1991.

Jarrett, J.A. (ed.): The Veterinary Clinics of North America. Philadelphia, W.B. Saunders Co., 1984.

Jones, R.L.: Clinical microbiology. *In* Clinical Textbook for Veterinary Technicians. Edited by D.M. McCurnin. Philadelphia, W.B. Saunders Co., 1985.

Part II

BACTERIA

9

Streptococcus

The streptococci are gram-positive, nonmotile (few exceptions), nonspore-forming cocci occurring singly, in pairs, or in chains. Most are facultatively anaerobic and some are strictly anaerobic. They are catalase- and oxidase-negative, and fermentative.

HABITAT

The streptococci are widely distributed in nature and as commensals in animals. More than 37 species are listed in *Bergey's Manual of Systematic Bacteriology*, Vol. 2. Potentially pathogenic and nonpathogenic species may be present on the skin and on the mucous membranes of the genital, upper respiratory, and digestive tracts.

CLASSIFICATION

They can be divided into six principal categories based on growth characteristics, type of hemolysis, and biochemical activities. These categories are: pyogenic streptococci, oral streptococci, enterococci, lactic streptococci, anaerobic streptococci, and other streptococci. Most of the disease-producing streptococci are in the pyogenic category. The last category, other streptococci, represents those that cannot be placed in one of the other five categories.

Another important way in which the streptococci are classified is into Lancefield groups, which are designated by the capital letters A, B, C, etc. This grouping is based on serologic differences in a carbohydrate substance in the cell wall called component C. The antigenic determinants are amino sugars. A precipitin test is employed using extracts containing component C and specific grouping sera that are usually prepared in rabbits. Other serologic procedures, such as latex agglutination, coagglutination, and fluorescent antibody tests, also can be used to identify Lancefield groups. Nonserologic procedures have been developed and used to recognize one or more of Lancefield's groups. These procedures are based primarily on biochemical activities.

Some of the Lancefield groups may be further divided by means of the agglutination test. There are at least 70 types of group A, *Streptococcus pyogenes*, based on serologic differences in the M protein, as recognized by the agglutination procedure. They are designated by Arabic numbers. M proteins are responsible for type-specific immunity.

More than one species may be in a group, and species may be identified by their biochemical activities.

Strains are also categorized according to the type of hemolysis:

1. Alpha-hemolysis: partial hemolysis often revealed as a zone of green discoloration around the colony; hemolysis with an inner zone of unhemolyzed cells.
2. Beta-hemolysis: clear, colorless zone caused by complete hemolysis.
3. Gamma-hemolysis: no detectable hemolysis.
4. Alpha-prime-hemolysis: a small zone of partially lysed red blood cells (RBCs) lying adjacent to the colony followed by a zone of completely lysed RBCs extending farther into the

medium. It can be confused easily with beta-hemolysis.

MODE OF INFECTION AND TRANSMISSION

Infections may be endogenous or exogenous. Exogenous infections are usually acquired by inhalation or ingestion. Aerosol, direct contact, or fomites are the most common modes of spread. Human carriers and infected subjects are the important reservoirs of *S. pyogenes*.

PYOGENIC INFECTIONS IN GENERAL

The bacteria that most frequently result in the production of pus are the staphylococci, streptococci, and some corynebacteria. A pyogenic infection is characterized by the production of pus. When pyogenic bacteria invade a tissue, such as the mucous membrane of the pharynx, they evoke an inflammatory response characterized by vascular dilation and a marked exudation of plasma and neutrophils. In response to chemotaxis, the neutrophils move toward the bacteria and engulf many of them. After phagocytosis, the bacteria may be digested, but some bacteria are resistant to the lysosomal enzymes and multiply within the neutrophils. Some produce toxins that kill the phagocytic cells, and enzymes liberated from the dead neutrophils bring about partial liquefaction of the dead tissue and phagocytic cells. The liquefied mass becomes visible as thick, usually yellow, pus. The viscous consistency of pus is attributable to a considerable amount of deoxyribonucleoprotein from the nuclei of dead cells.

PATHOGENESIS

Various disease processes result from streptococcal infections, and their development depends on various factors, such as portal of entry, animal species, and streptococcal species. Three diseases illustrating somewhat different pathogenesis are strangles of horses, jowl abscesses of swine, and streptococcal arthritis. Although usually localized, streptococcal infections may become septicemic or bacteremic, resulting in death or foci of infection in various locations. As in many microbial diseases, the severity of the infection depends on the immune status of the animal.

Surface M protein and to a lesser degree surface hyaluronic acid are considered to be major virulence factors in streptococci. The capacity of streptococci to spread within tissue and cause damage results at least partially from DNase, hyaluronidase, streptolysins O and S, NADase, M protein, leukotoxins, and cell wall mucopeptide complex.

Protein X, a surface protein of *Streptococcus agalactiae*, is frequently associated with strains recovered from cases of bovine mastitis. This protein behaves as a target of opsonins and, therefore, is possibly an important protective antigen against *S. agalactiae* mastitis. Bovine complement S (vitronectin) is thought to be important in the adherence of *S. agalactiae* to bovine epithelial cells.

EXTRACELLULAR PRODUCTS

Group A streptococci produce more than 20 extracellular products. No doubt many of these are produced by pyogenic animal streptococci. Some of the better known are the following.

Hemolysins. Streptolysins O and S are responsible for beta-hemolysis; each is produced under certain conditions. Antibody to streptolysin O is a good indicator of present or past infection. Streptolysin O is oxygen sensitive, but streptolysin S is not; both are toxic for neutrophils and macrophages. Streptolysin O, a protein, elicits neutralizing antibodies, whereas streptolysin S, a peptide, is nonantigenic.

Streptokinase (Fibrinolysin). This enzyme activates plasminogens to become plasmin (protease), thus leading to the digestion of fibrin clots. This process prevents the buildup of fibrin clots that may contain and protect organisms. Several antigenically distinct forms exist. It elicits neutralizing antibodies in many streptococcal infections.

DNases A, B, C, and D (streptodornase). These extracellular enzymes assist in the production of substrates for growth. Antibody to DNase B is used in the serodiagnosis of group A human infections. These enzymes reduce the viscosity of fluid containing DNA. Streptococcal pus may be thin because of this enzyme.

Hyaluronidase. A correlation probably exists between the production of this enzyme and virulence, e.g., in streptococcal cellulitis. Hyaluronidase promotes the spread of infection in tissues. Convalescent serum is rich in neutralizing antibodies.

Erythrogenic Toxins (Types A, B, and C). These are low-molecular-weight proteins. A group A erythrogenic toxin is responsible for the rash in scarlet fever. These toxins produce neutralizing antitoxins used in the human "Dick Test."

NADases. These enzymes, which kill phagocytes, are produced by some group A streptococci.

Proteinase. This enzyme, which has broad substrate specificity, is produced by some group A streptococci.

Lipoproteinase, Amylase, and Esterase. These enzymes attack host-derived substrates.

PATHOGENICITY

S. pyogenes. (Group A) Principal cause of streptococcal disease in humans. May rarely cause bovine mastitis with possible dissemination to humans. It occasionally causes lymphangitis in foals.

S. agalactiae. (Group B) This streptococcus and *Staphylococcus aureus* are the most important and frequent causes of bovine mastitis. *Streptococcus agalactiae* is an obligate pathogen that can be eliminated from herds. Infection is spread by the milker's hands or by contaminated teat cups. *S. agalactiae* also causes mastitis in sheep and goats. Five to 20% of women are cervical carriers of group B streptococci that are identical or closely related to *S. agalactiae*. Group B streptococci are carried by about one third of pregnant women as part of the flora of the intestine and/or the vagina. These streptococci may cause septicemia, meningitis, pneumonia, and death in newborn infants. Major vaginal colonization provides the principal reservoir of these streptococci for neonatal infections that follow parturition. These streptococci may also cause opportunistic infections in adult diabetic and alcoholic persons. This species has been associated with several canine neonatal deaths and kidney and uterine infections in cats.

S. dysgalactiae. (Group C) Bovine mastitis; polyarthritis of lambs.

S. equisimilis. (Group C) Associated with strangles, wound infections, genital infections, and mastitis in the horse; cause of various infections in swine, cattle, dog, and fowl; and a rare cause of human infections.

S. equi. (Group C) Strangles and other infections of the horse; genital and udder infections in the mare.

S. zooepidemicus. (Group C) Primary cause of genital infections in the mare, epididymitis in stallions, and navel infections in foals. This streptococcus is associated with cervicitis, metritis, and mastitis in cattle; arthritis, abortion, and septicemia in swine; fibrinous pleuritis, pericarditis, and pneumonia in lambs; mastitis in goats; and fatal septicemia in chickens.

S. bovis. (Group D) Alimentary tract of ruminants. This organism has been recognized as a probable cause of lactic acidosis and other gastric disorders in ruminants. *S. bovis* causes endocarditis, meningitis, and septicemia in humans.

S. equinus. (Group D) Alimentary tract of horses.

Enterococcus faecalis, E. faecium, and E. durans. (Group D. Formerly: *Streptococcus faecalis*, *S. faecium*, *S. durans*) These *Enterococcus* spp. are common inhabitants of the intestinal tract of animals and humans. *E. faecalis* may cause urinary infections in various animals and endocarditis in chickens.

Streptococcus suis. (Groups D, R, S). Frequently causes meningitis, septicemia, pneumonia, and arthritis in pigs of all ages. Other conditions in pigs, such as local abscesses, endocarditis, encephalitis, polyserositis, and peritonitis, are less frequently seen. It is also associated with abortion in sows. Based on capsular polysaccharide antigens, more than 28 serotypes of *S. suis* have been recognized plus type 1/2, which has antigens of types 1 and 2. *S. suis* may cause meningitis, arthritis, septicemia, diarrhea, and deafness in humans.

S. uberis. (Groups C, D, E, P, U) Serologically heterogeneous; causes bovine mastitis; found in the vagina and tonsils of cattle.

S. porcinus. (Groups E, P, U, V) Causes abscesses of mandibular, pharyngeal, and other lymph nodes in pigs; sometimes called jowl abscesses or cervical lymphadenitis.

S. avium. (Group Q) Recovered from chickens, animals, and humans. Its significance is not known.

S. pneumoniae. (Group: none. Synonym: *Diplococcus pneumoniae*). This species resembles the other streptococci except that it occurs principally as pairs of cocci rather than as chains. It is made up of more than 84 serotypes that are identified on the basis of serologic differences in capsular antigens. It is found as a commensal in the upper respiratory tract of humans and less commonly of animals. Most of the infections are caused by less than 10 different serotypes. Lobar pneumonia, empyema, sinusitis, and conjunctivitis are among the important diseases caused by *Streptococcus pneumoniae* in humans. It is an important cause of pneumonia in guinea pigs and has been implicated in respiratory infections in calves, horses, dogs, goats, monkeys, rabbits, and rats. There are several reports of bovine mastitis caused by pneumococci; septicemia and septic arthritis have been reported in the domestic cat.

S. intestinalis. (Group: none) It is recovered from the colon and feces of pigs; its significance is not known.

S. canis. (Group G) It causes genital, skin, and wound infections in dogs.

Additional groups of streptococci.

Group G: Mastitis in cows; lymphadenitis in cats.

Group M: Various infections in dogs and humans.

Group N: Formerly *Lactococcus lactis, Streptococcus lactis*. Present in milk and dairy products.

Table 9–1. *Differential Characteristics of Important Streptococci from Animals*

	Group	He-mol-ysis	Treha-lose	Sorbi-tol	Manni-tol	Sali-cin	Lac-tose	Raffi-nose	Inu-lin	Escu-lin	Sodium Hip-purate	6.5% NaCl	Category
S. pyogenes	A	β	+	−	V	+	+	−	−	−	−	−	Pyogenic
S. agalactiae	B	α,β,γ	+	−	−	(+)	+	−	−	−	+	−	Pyogenic
S. dysgalactiae	C	α,β,γ	+	−	−	−	+	−	−	−	−	−	SIS
S. equisimilis	C	β	+	−	−	(+)	V	−	−	−	−	−	SIS
S. equi	C	β	−	−	−	+	+	−	−	−	−	−	Pyogenic
S. zooepidemicus	C	β	−	+	−	+	+	−	−	−	−	−	Pyogenic
S. bovis	D	α	V	−	V	+	+	+	+	+	−	−	Other
S. equinus	D	α	V	−	−	(+)	−	+	+	+	−	−	Other
E. faecalis	D	α,β,γ	+	+	+	+	+	−	−	+	V	+	Enterococci
S. uberis	C,D,E,P,U	α,γ	+	+	+	+	+	−	+	+	+	(+)	Other
S. suis	D,R,S	α	+	−	−	+	+	(+)	(+)	+	−	−	SIS
S. pneumoniae		α	+	−	−	V	+	+	+	(+)	−	−	Pyogenic
S. porcinus	E,P,U,V	β	+	+	+	+	(+)	−	−	+	−	+	SIS
S. canis	G	β	V	−	−	+	+	−	−	−	V	−	Other
E. avium	Q	α,γ	+	+	+	+	+	−	−	+	V	(+)	Enterococci

Adapted from Carter, G.R., and Cole, Jr., J.R.: Procedures in Veterinary Bacteriology and Mycology. 5th Ed. San Diego, Academic Press, 1990.

(+), majority of strains positive; V, variable reactions; SIS, species incertae sedis.

Viridans streptococci. These are widespread commensals that are frequently isolated from clinical specimens. They are alpha hemolytic, not soluble in bile, do not usually split esculin, do not grow in 6.5% NaCl, and not groupable.

Anaerobic streptococci. These bacteria are found as commensals in the alimentary and upper respiratory tracts. Because so little effort has been made to isolate anaerobes from infections in animals, their real significance is not known. They may occur alone or in mixed infections, and it seems likely that they will be found, as in humans, in infections associated with operative procedures or wounds involving the gastrointestinal or genitourinary tract.

Nutritionally variant streptococci. These streptococci, which have special nutritional requirements, are isolated from a variety of clinical specimens taken from horses, cattle, and sheep. Whether or not these streptococci have a significant role in the disease processes in animals is not clear. In humans, nutritionally variant streptococci are most commonly recovered from patients with subacute bacterial endocarditis. In addition, these streptococci have been implicated in such infections as postpartum or postabortal sepsis, cirrhosis, pancreatic abscesses, otitis media, otitis externa, and conjunctivitis.

SPECIMENS

These vary with the disease. Among the infectious materials submitted are: pus (strangles), joint fluid (arthritis), milk (mastitis), organs, blood (septicemia), and meningial swabs (*S. suis* infections).

DIRECT EXAMINATION

Organisms can be demonstrated in smears stained with Gram stain and in milk with Newman's stain. If the medium in which they are grown is liquid, characteristic chains may be seen.

ISOLATION AND CULTIVATION

The pathogenic strains grow best on serum or blood-enriched media; blood agar is preferred. Colonies are about 1 mm in diameter, round, smooth, glistening, and look like dewdrops. Hemolysis may or may not be present, depending on various factors, including the kind of blood used. Colony varieties are mucoid (hyaluronic acid), matt (much M protein, virulent), and glossy (little M protein, low virulence).

IDENTIFICATION

If the streptococci are found to be in the pyogenic group by the tests in Table 9–1, they are more apt to be of pathogenic significance. Tests for the lactic streptococci are usually only carried out when examining milk samples. Most pyogenic streptococci associated with infections are beta-hemolytic. Some exceptions are listed in Table 9–1. The significance of an isolate is determined by culture purity, type of lesions, and clinical findings. To save time, susceptibility tests may be conducted before precise identification is determined.

Precise identification is based on biochemical reactions and the characteristics listed in Tables 9–1 and 9–2. Lancefield grouping by the precipitin or other tests is not routinely carried out. Several commercial systems are available for identification of

Table 9–2. *Differential Characteristics of Streptococci Recovered from Intramammary Infections*

| Organism | Lancefield Group | CAMP test | Hydrolysis of | | Acid Produced in Broth Containing | | Reduction of 0.1% MBM† |
			Esculin*	Sodium Hippurate	Inulin	Raffinose	
S. agalactiae	B	+	–	+	–	–	–
S. dysgalactiae	C	–	V	–	–	–	–
S. uberis	C, D, E, P, U	–/+	+	+	+	–	–
Enterococci‡	D	–	+	V	–/+	–/+	+
S. bovis	D	–	+	–	V	+	–
Strep. species	–	–	+	–	–	–	–

*Tested in Difco tryptose blood agar base containing either 5% defibrinated blood or 5% serum, 0.05% esculin, and 0.01% ferric citrate.
†Methylene blue milk.
‡*E. faecalis* and *E. faecium*
–/+, most strains negative; V, variable.
Adapted from Microbiological Procedures for Use in the Diagnosis of Bovine Mastitis. Washington, D.C., National Mastitis Council, Inc., 1981.

streptococcal groups and species. They are based on differential biochemical and serologic characteristics.

The CAMP test may be used for the presumptive recognition of *S. agalactiae*. It involves the completion of the partial hemolysis (beta toxin zone) of *Staphylococcus aureus* when *Streptococcus agalactiae* is streaked at right angles to the *Staphylococcus* streak on blood agar. The CAMP test may be conducted in a medium that contains beta toxin of *S. aureus* to screen for *Streptococcus agalactiae*. The incorporation of esculin into the medium makes possible the presumptive recognition of *S. agalactiae*, *S. dysgalactiae*, and *S. uberis* (Fig. 9–1). Identification of group A streptococci can be made easily by placing a bacitracin disc (0.02 units) on a diffusely inoculated plate. A zone of inhibition is present with a group A Streptococcus.

Edward's medium containing esculin, crystal violet, and thallium acetate is used for the rapid presumptive identification of the important mastitis streptococci. It inhibits gram-negative bacteria and staphylococci.

RESISTANCE

None of the pathogenic streptococci is particularly resistant to the usual chemical disinfectants. Many species survive for weeks in soil, clothing, bedding, food, stalls, milking machines, and milk containers.

IMMUNITY

Animals infected with streptococci often develop a hypersensitivity of the delayed type. The role of this reaction in streptococcal disease is not known. It has been suggested that immune complexes may be responsible for purpura hemorrhagica in the horse after *S. equi* infection. Immunity to

streptococcal infections is considered to be primarily humoral. Protection is type-specific and considered to depend upon antibodies to M protein.

A *S. equi* bacterin is available to prevent strangles, and a vaccine consisting of predominantly M protein has been developed to reduce the undesirable reactions that sometimes result from the use of strangles bacterins. A live attenuated strain of group E *(S. porcinus)* is used to vaccinate pigs against jowl abscesses. Bacterins containing various serotypes of *S. suis* are available.

TREATMENT

Penicillin is the preferred drug; resistant pyogenic strains are rare, although there have been some reports of plasmid-mediated resistance to tetracyclines and chloramphenicol. Sulfamerazine and sulfamethazine are useful. Other drugs that may be used are erythromycin, the cephalosporins, lincomycin, and the tetracyclines. Antibiotic resistance is most commonly encountered among the enterococci. All group A throat infections in humans should be treated for at least 10 days with therapeutic levels of penicillin to prevent rheumatic fever and glomerular nephritis.

Most viridans streptococci are susceptible to penicillin, but many enterococci are resistant. Enterococci are usually susceptible to ampicillin.

PUBLIC HEALTH SIGNIFICANCE

S. pyogenes (group A) may infect the bovine udder and be disseminated to humans in milk. On occasion, animal pyogenic streptococci may infect humans. Although women frequently carry group B streptococci, there is no evidence that these bacteria are acquired from milk. *S. suis* has been reported to cause meningitis, arthritis, septicemia, diarrhea, and ear infections in women, slaughter house

114

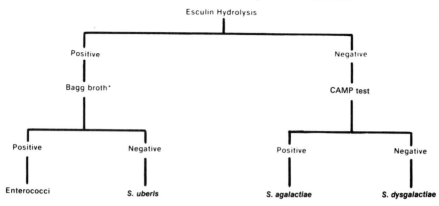

Presumptive Identification of Streptococci from Milk

Buffered azide glucose glycerol broth

Figure 9–1. Presumptive identification of important streptococci from milk samples.

workers, and farmers. *S. bovis* has been identified as a cause of endocarditis, meningitis, and septicemia. Recent studies have also linked increased levels of *S. bovis* with human colon cancers.

Streptococcus pneumoniae

SYNONYM: *Diplococcus pneumoniae*

This species resembles the other streptococci except that it occurs principally as pairs of cocci rather than as chains. It is made up of many serotypes that are identified on the basis of serologic differences in capsular antigens. They are found as commensals in the upper respiratory tract of humans and less commonly of animals.

PATHOGENICITY

Most of the infections are caused by serotypes 12 to 18. Lobar pneumonia, empyema, sinusitis, and conjunctivitis are among the important diseases caused by *Streptococcus pneumoniae* in humans. It is an important cause of pneumonia in guinea pigs and has been implicated in respiratory infections in calves, horses, dogs, goats, monkeys, rabbits, and rats. There are several reports of bovine mastitis caused by pneumococci.

ISOLATION, CULTIVATION, AND IDENTIFICATION

S. pneumoniae grows well on blood agar. It appears as small round colonies with elevated edges and is alpha-hemolytic. It is gram-positive, and paired cocci are seen in stained smears. It is bile-soluble and inhibited by optochin; other biochemical tests are used for definitive identification (see Table 9–1).

IMMUNITY

In humans, immunity is considered essentially humoral. A vaccine consisting of specific polysaccharides of more than 20 types is available to protect humans.

FURTHER READING

Anonymous: Microbiological Procedures for Use in the Diagnosis of Bovine Mastitis. 2nd Ed. Washington, D.C., National Mastitis Council, Inc., 1981.

Durack, D.T.: The streptococci. *In* Mechanisms of Microbial Disease. Edited by M. Schaechter, et al. Baltimore, Williams & Wilkins, 1993.

Erickson, E.D.: Streptococcosis. J. Am Vet. Med. Assoc. *191*:1391, 1987.

Gottschalk, M., et al.: Description of 14 new capsular types of *Streptococcus suis*. J. Clin. Microbiol. 27:2633, 1989.

Hardie, J.M.: Genus *Streptococcus*. *In* Bergey's Manual of Systematic Bacteriology, Vol. 2. Edited by P.H.A. Sneath. Baltimore, William & Wilkins, 1986.

Krantz, G.E., and Dunne, H.W.: An attempt to classify streptococci isolates from domestic animals. Am. J. Vet. Res. *26*: 951, 1965.

Myrvik, Q.N., and Weiser, R.S.: *Streptococcus*. *In* Fundamentals of Medical Bacteriology and Mycology. 2nd Ed. Philadelphia, Lea & Febiger, 1988.

Patterson, M.J., and Batool-Hafeez, A.E.: Group B streptococci in human disease. Bact Rev. *40*:774, 1976.

Perch, B., Pederson, K.B., and Henricksen, J.: Serology of capsulated streptococci pathogenic for pigs: New serotypes of *Streptococcus suis*. J. Clin. Microbiol. *17*:993, 1983.

Rouff, K.L.: Nutritionally variant streptococci. Clin. Microbiol. Rev. *4*:184, 1991.

Skinner, F., and Quesnel, L. (eds.): Streptococci. New York, Academic Press, 1978.

Storch, G.: The pneumococcus and bacterial pneumonia. *In* Mechanisms of Microbial Disease. Edited by M. Schaechter, et al. Baltimore, Williams & Wilkins, 1993.

Wanamaker, L.W., and Matsen, J.M. (eds.): Streptococci and Streptococcal Diseases. New York, Academic Press, 1972.

Windsor, R.S.: Streptococcal infection in young pigs. *In* The Veterinary Annual. Edited by C.S.G. Grunsell and F.W.G. Hill. Bristol, England, Scientechnica, 1978.

10

Staphylococcus

Principal Characteristics of Staphylococci

Staphylococci are gram-positive cocci occurring in pairs, short chains, and clusters. They are aerobic and facultatively anaerobic (most species), usually catalase-positive, oxidase-negative, nonmotile, nonspore-forming, and fermentative.

There are now 27 species in the genus *Staphylococcus*, including the 19 species listed in the current *Bergey's Manual of Systematic Bacteriology*, Vol. 2, and 8 recently described species. *S. hyicus* ss. *chromogenes* has been elevated to the rank of a separate species, *S. chromogenes*.

Important animal pathogens are *S. aureus, S. intermedius,* and *S. hyicus. S. epidermidis,* a common commensal of the skin and mucous membranes of humans and animals, is usually nonpathogenic, but occasionally causes mastitis, abscesses, and skin infections in animals. *S. saprophyticus* occurs in nature and is usually not pathogenic for animals. It can cause urinary tract and wound infections in humans.

Other *Staphylococcus* spp. recovered from animals are listed in Table 10–1. For the most part they are harmless commensals.

Staphylococcus aureus

Habitat

Commensal of the skin and mucous membranes, especially of the upper respiratory and digestive tracts.

The various human *Staphylococcus* spp. demonstrate considerable habitat preference, e.g., head,

*Table 10–1. Some Less Well-Known **Staphylococcus** spp. Recovered from Animals*

S. kloosi	Carnivora, pigs
S. arlettae	Goats, poultry
S. equorum	Horses
S. gallinarum	Poultry
S. delphini	Dolphins
S. chromogenes	Cattle
S. caprae	Goats
S. lentus	Goats, sheep (skin)
S. sciuri	Rodents, other mammals
S. caseolyticus	Milk, dairy products
S. felis	Cats (infections)
S. simulans	Cats (infections)

ears, anterior nares (*S. aureus*), and skin areas. No doubt animal staphylococci exhibit similar niche preferences.

Extracellular Products

Some of the substances thought to be involved in the production of staphylococcal infections follow. Not all these products can be classified as toxic, but data indicate that some of the enzymes are virulence enhancers. Some of these enzymes are able to increase the invasive powers of the organism and possibly protect it from body defense mechanisms. For the most part, their effects have been demonstrated experimentally in rabbits and mice.

Coagulase. Clotting of plasma; converts prothrombin to thrombin, which converts fibrinogen to fibrin. Almost all strains of *S. aureus* produce coagulase; occasional mutants do not. Coagulase-negative staphylococci produce a localized lesion like that of coagulase-positive strains. As a result, the role of coagulase in virulence has been questioned.

Enterotoxins A, B, C1, C2, C3, D, E. These toxins are extracellular proteins composed of single polypeptide chains of about 30 kd. There are 7 distinct serologic types of toxin. Approximately 50% of *S. aureus* strains produce 1 or more enterotoxins. These toxins are highly heat-resistant (100° C, 30 min). A favorable milieu, such as custards, raw milk, cream, ice cream, meat gravy, fish, cheese, or oysters, is required for their production. Clinical signs in humans are nausea, vomiting, and diarrhea within 1 to 6 hours. In contrast, *Salmonella* food poisoning takes effect in 24 to 48 hours. Enterotoxins in the food can be detected by an agar gel precipitin test or by a radioimmunoassay.

Hemolysins α, β, γ, and δ (hemotoxins, cytolysins). All are antigenically distinct. Erythrocytes from various species differ in susceptibility. The alpha and beta toxins are potent hemolysins. The alpha toxin is most active against rabbit erythrocytes and is responsible for the inner clear zone of hemolysis. This toxin causes spasms of smooth muscle and is dermonecrotizing and lethal. The beta toxin is sphingomyelinase C and is responsible for the outer partial zone of hemolysis. It is most active against sheep erythrocytes. The gamma toxin has a narrow hemolytic spectrum and is inhibited by agar and cholesterol. The delta toxin has a broad hemolytic spectrum and is inhibited by phospholipids. The mode of action of gamma and delta toxins and their roles in pathogenesis are not well understood.

Lipase. Degrades protective fatty acids on skin. Lipase-positive strains tend to cause abscesses of skin and subcutis.

Staphylokinase. Degrades fibrin clots by converting plasminogen to the fibrinolytic enzyme plasmin.

Leukocidin. Kills granulocytes and macrophages; it is composed of two heat-labile interacting proteins.

Exfoliative toxins A and B (Exfoliatin). Causes cleavage of desmosomes in the stratum granulosum of the epidermis. The toxins are specific for the epidermis; intraperitoneal inoculation results in exfoliation in mice. The toxins are potent mitogens that act on T- and B-lymphocytes. These toxins are usually, but not exclusively, produced by organisms of phage group II.

Toxic shock syndrome toxin. Produced by strains that cause human toxic shock syndrome. Approximately 15% of *S. aureus* strains produce this toxin.

Hyaluronidase. This enzyme is known as "spreading factor"; it degrades hyaluronic acid. Its significance in disease production is not clear.

Penicillinase. Splits the β-lactam ring of penicillin.

Lysostaphin. This lytic enzyme is produced by *S. simulans* and is active against staphylococci but not micrococci.

Protein A. Is present as a surface component on most strains of virulent *Staphylococcus aureus*. It has the unique ability to bind to the Fc region of IgG and thus may have a role in pathogenesis. The useful serologic procedure coagglutination depends on protein A. When specific IgG antibody is added to staphylococci possessing protein A followed by homologous antigen, coagglutination is produced.

Slime. Several *Staphylococcus* spp., including *S. aureus*, produce a surface mucoid substance or slime that is thought to contribute to adhesiveness.

Other Toxins and Enzymes: Collagenase, acid and alkaline phosphatases, catalase, proteases, nuclease, pyrogenic exotoxin, and elastase may be produced.

Several products of staphylococci that may be helpful in the identification of species, but not listed in Table 10–2, are phosphatase production, ornithine decarboxylase activity, acetoin production, β-galactosidase activity, and urease production.

Antigenic Nature

Antigenic structure is complex and heterogeneous. The cell wall of *S. aureus* has three major components: peptidoglycan, teichoic acids, and protein A. These components have been useful in the taxonomic differentiation of *Staphylococcus* spp. and *Micrococcus* spp. Teichoic acids are species specific. Protein A is antiphagocytic and makes up the major protein portion of the cell wall. Protein A may be linked to the peptidoglycan layer or may be partially released into the surrounding medium.

The polysaccharide capsule of some strains of *Staphylococcus aureus* is antiphagocytic. The ability to produce capsule, however, does not appear to be a prerequisite for virulence. Eleven serologic types of *S. aureus* have been recognized in humans and animals on the basis of capsular polysaccharide antigens. Capsule type 5 is predominant in bovine milk, whereas capsule type 8 is predominant in caprine and ovine milk.

The cell wall of all *S. aureus* strains contains a species-specific polysaccharide A. The antigenic component of this polysaccharide is the N-acetyl glucosaminyl ribitol unit.

Pathogenesis

Endogenous infections are probably most frequent, but exogenous infections also occur. Transmission is usually by direct contact or by fomites.

Strains of this widespread commensal have the capacity to invade tissues, producing abscesses, pustules, various other pyogenic infections, and on occasion bacteremia and septicemia.

The inflammatory response to infection mobilizes neutrophils to the site of infection, which leads to the pyogenic response. This leads to abscess formation followed by rupture of skin and drainage of pus at the surface. The extracellular products of *S. aureus*, referred to earlier, are involved in the development of these infections. Both capsules and protein A of staphylococci are thought to be strongly antiphagocytic. Delayed hypersensitivity is thought to play a role in local tissue damage in staphylococcal infections. As stated earlier, leukocidin, hemolysins, and other enzymes and toxins of *S. aureus* damage blood cells, macrophages, epithelial cells, and other types of cells in the body. Extracellular products of *S. aureus* may function to permit survival of the organisms on the skin and invasion of tissues. For example, lipases may protect the bacteria from the bactericidal action of lipids on the skin.

Enterotoxins of *S. aureus* are the major factors in the pathogenesis of food poisoning in humans. These toxins are thought to stimulate the emetic center in the brain. In general, staphylococcal infections occur in animals and humans when normal host defenses are lacking or impaired.

Pathogenicity

Botryomycosis is characterized by infrequent chronic granulomatous lesions involving the udder of the mare, cow, and sow and the spermatic cord of horses. Suppurative wound infections and septicemia in all animals. Pyoderma, especially of dogs (more commonly *S. intermedius*) and horses. Pyemia in lambs, especially from tick-bite wounds; also lameness and bacteremia in lambs.

Mastitis in the cow, goat, sow, and ewe. Staphylococcal bovine mastitis can be acute, but most frequently is chronic and subclinical. It is common and of great economic importance. Gangrenous mastitis caused by alpha-toxin is seen in postparturient cows.

Various pyogenic infections of the skin of many animals; subcutaneous abscesses, cellulitis in horses, and various pyogenic infections in rabbits.

Staphylococcal arthritis and septicemia in turkeys.

Urinary tract infections in humans and animals.

Staphylococcal enterocolitis, seen principally in humans after prolonged antibiotic therapy, e.g., after intestinal surgery.

Impetigo involving the sow's udder as a result of piglets biting.

In humans, osteomyelitis, sinusitis, mastitis, furuncles, carbuncles, endocarditis, toxic shock syndrome, pneumonia, tonsillitis, and impetigo. Nosocomial infections. Food poisoning.

Specimens

Pus, usually provided on swabs; affected tissue; milk samples.

Isolation, Cultivation, and Identification

S. aureus and other staphylococci grow well on common laboratory media. Selective media are available for *S. aureus*, e.g., mannitol salt agar. Blood agar is preferred for primary isolation. Colonies appear in 24 hours and are up to 4 mm in diameter, round, smooth, and glistening; they may have "gold" pigmentation. Double-zone hemolysis is especially characteristic. Bovine red cells are best for demonstrating the hemolysis of *S. aureus*.

Smears disclose clumps of gram-positive cocci. Presumptive identification is made on the basis of the double zone of hemolysis and cultural and morphologic features. Definitive identification is based on coagulase production and the other characteristics listed in Table 10-2. Although staphylococci are sensitive to lysostaphin, micrococci are not. Rapid miniaturized commercial systems are available for identifying most staphylococci encountered in clinical specimens. A latex agglutination test is available for the rapid identification of *S. aureus*.

Phage Typing

Some strains of *S. aureus* can be identified by their susceptibility to one or several staphylococcal phages, e.g., strain 80/81 (penicillin-resistant) is susceptible to lysis by phages 80 and 81; this variety has been important in human nosocomial infections. Phage typing is of value in the study of the epidemiology of staphylococcal infections. There are a number of phage types. Animal staphylococcal types are usually different from human types.

A number of phage culture lysates are used in the typing procedure. A single drop of each lysate is added to a plate confluently inoculated with the organism to be tested; it is incubated overnight at 30° C and then is observed for zones of lysis. The pattern of lysis indicates the type. Sources of error

Table 10–2. *Differential Characteristics of Staphylococci and Micrococci*

	S. aureus	S. epidermidis	S. intermedius	S. hyicus	S. saprophyticus	Micrococci
Oxidase	–	–	–	–	–	+
Coagulase	+	–	+	V	–	–
Hemolysis (beta)	+	–	+	–	–	–
Pigment	+	–	–	–	V	V
Maltose	A	A	(+)	–	A	–
Purple agar base	A	A	A	–	NT	NT
Mannitol	A	–	V	–	V	NT
DNase	+	–	+	+	–	–
Novobiocin	S	S	S	S	R	S
Glucose (O-F)	F	F	F	F	–	O

(+), delayed positive reaction; V, variable reactions; A, acid; NT, not tested; S, susceptible; R, resistant; F, fermentation; O, oxidation.

include the fact that staphylococci may be lysogenic for the phages used and that some harbor as many as five different temperate phages.

Resistance

Staphylococci are susceptible to common disinfectants. Pus is protective, and organisms remain viable in dried pus for weeks. This consideration is important in clinics.

Unlike many other vegetative bacterial forms, some staphylococci can survive a temperature of 60° C for 30 minutes. They are resistant to disinfectants including phenolic compounds. Their resistance to high salt concentration is taken advantage of in the selective medium mannitol salt agar.

Immunity

Strains of *S. aureus* possessing capsular and certain surface antigens are most immunogenic. Bacterins and toxoids are employed. They are considered to be of questionable value in the prevention of bovine mastitis. Autogenous bacterins have given variable results.

Hypersensitivity to staphylococci probably plays a role in aggravating infections; thus, dogs should be desensitized with pyoderma when using an autogenous bacterin. The delayed hypersensitivity reaction, however, may have a beneficial effect on the host in that the reaction tends to localize the infection and thus to prevent systemic spread of organisms. Immunity is both cell mediated and humoral; the latter is antibacterial as well as antitoxic. Humoral antibodies are thought to be important for protection. Opsonization may play a key role in humoral immunity by promoting phagocytosis by neutrophils.

Treatment

Antimicrobial susceptibility tests should be conducted on isolates considered significant. Penicillin is the drug of choice if strains are susceptible. Penicillin-resistant strains 80/81 of human origin have been found in cattle and dogs; resistance is attributable to penicillinase (β-lactamase), an enzyme that hydrolyzes the β-lactam ring of penicillin. Plasmid-based penicillin resistance may be transferred by transduction. New synthetic (penicillinase-resistant) penicillins are of value, e.g., methicillin, oxacillin, and nafcillin. Tetracyclines, bacitracin, nitrofurans, and erythromycin may be effective. Trimethoprim-sulfamethoxazole, vancomycin, cephalosporins, and clindamycin have been effective against *S. aureus* infections. Newer drugs, such as Augmentin (amoxicillin and clavulanic acid) and enrofloxacin, have been shown to be effective in staphylococcal infections in animals. Surgical drainage may be indicated.

Treatment may be ineffective because of abscesses and because *S. aureus* can survive in phagocytes.

ADDITIONAL *STAPHYLOCOCCUS* SPP.

Although *S. aureus* is the most significant species, the species described in the following sections are of considerable significance. Their isolation, cultivation, identification, and treatment are generally similar to those described in *S. aureus*.

The staphylococcal species listed in Table 10–1 are not routinely identified in diagnostic laboratories because additional differential procedures are required.

Staphylococcus epidermidis

This species is found commonly on the skin of humans and, to a lesser extent, as a commensal on the skin and hair of many animals. It is an occasional opportunist of low pathogenicity. Among the infections attributed to *S. epidermidis* are low-grade bovine mastitis, suture abscesses, and abscesses in various sites, including wounds.

S. epidermidis is coagulase negative. Colonies are nonhemolytic and unpigmented but otherwise resemble those of *S. aureus*. It is identified definitively by the criteria listed in Table 10–2.

Staphylococcus intermedius

S. intermedius is similar to *S. aureus* in many ways. Colonies are grey-white, smooth, nonpigmented, glistening, and beta hemolytic on blood agar. Many strains of this species were identified previously as *S. aureus*, especially the strains recovered from dogs. *S. intermedius* possesses two different teichoic acid antigens in its cell wall, poly(C) and poly(P). Dog strains possess poly(P); pigeon strains possess poly(C). Protein A is not present in this species.

S. intermedius produces coagulase and hemolysins (alpha, beta, and delta). Important differential characteristics are listed in Table 10–2. These organisms are normal inhabitants of the nasopharynx and skin of dogs, raccoons, foxes, and mink. This species also has been recovered frequently from other animals, including cats, cattle, horses, and pigeons, in which its significance is not always clear. *S. intermedius* causes a variety of infections in dogs, including pyoderma, otitis externa, mastitis, eye infections, urinary tract infections, folliculitis, and furunculosis. It also causes mastitis in cows.

Staphylococcus hyicus

S. hyicus, formerly known as *S. hyicus* subspecies *hyicus*, is an important swine pathogen. Colonies are creamy white, glistening, nonpigmented, nonhemolytic, convex, and circular on blood agar. It produces DNAse, including the heat-stable nuclease. Coagulase and fibrinolysin are produced by some strains (Table 10–2). Protein A and enterotoxins are produced, but they are not identical to those of *S. aureus*. It does not produce alpha-, beta-, or delta-hemolysins.

A cytotoxin produced by *S. hyicus*, however, has some properties similar to the delta-hemolysin of *S. aureus*. In addition, *S. hyicus* produces an exfoliative toxin that causes exfoliation in chickens, some laboratory animals, dogs, and cats.

S. hyicus is closely related to *S. epidermidis* antigenically. Lysogeny has been demonstrated among avian strains of *S. hyicus*. This organism occurs frequently on the skin of pigs and on the skin and nares of healthy poultry. In addition, it can be found less frequently on the skin and in the milk of cattle, in animal products, and in slaughter house effluents. It causes exudative epidermitis or "greasy pig disease" in swine. The disease is highly contagious and varies in severity from one group of pigs to another. It also has been implicated in septic arthritis of pigs, abortion in sows, seborrheic dermatitis of a pygmy goat, dermatitis of donkeys and horses, and skin and udder infections of cattle. Strains of *S. hyicus* recovered from bovine mastitis milk appear to lack protein A.

Public Health Significance

Human beings may become infected with *S. aureus*, *S. hyicus*, and possibly other staphylococci of animal origin.

Micrococci

The micrococci (genus *Micrococcus*) are a large group consisting of at least nine species. They resemble the staphylococci morphologically, but differ biochemically (Table 10–2). In contrast to staphylococci, the micrococci have neither teichoic acids nor glycine in the interpeptide bridge of the peptidoglycan. Cytochromes also differ among these genera. Micrococci are gram-positive to gram-variable, aerobic, oxidase positive, catalase positive, and usually nonmotile. *M. agilis* is the only motile species. They occur singly and in clusters of varying size, and are usually pigmented.

They split sugars by oxidation, in contrast to staphylococci, which ferment sugars. Staphylococci can be distinguished readily from micrococci in the laboratory because staphylococci are resistant to bacitracin and susceptible to furazolidone.

Planococci

These motile, nonpathogenic cocci occur singly or in pairs, triads, or tetrads. They are found in sea water and are rarely encountered in clinical specimens.

Stomatococci

These nonmotile, capsulated, nonpathogenic cocci occur in clusters. They are considered normal inhabitants of the mouth and upper respiratory tract of humans.

FURTHER READING

Allaker, R.P., Whitlock, M., and Lloyd, D.H.: Cytotoxic activity in *Staphylococcus hyicus*. Vet. Microbiol. 26:161, 1991.
Biberstein, E.L., et al.: Antimicrobial sensitivity patterns in *Staphylococcus aureus* from animals. J. Am. Vet. Med. Assoc. *164*:1183, 1974.

Carrol, P.J., and Francis, P.G.: The basic phage set for typing bovine staphylococci. J. Hyg. *95*:665, 1985.

Cohen, J.O.: Staphylococcosis. J. Am. Vet. Med. Assoc. *190*:150, 1987.

Devriese, L.A., et al.: *Staphylococcus hyicus* (Sompolinsky 1953) comb. nov. and *Staphylococcus hyicus* subsp. *Chromogenes* subsp. nov. Int. J. Syst. Bact. *28*:482, 1978.

Devriese, L.A., and Thelissen, M.: *Staphylococcus hyicus* in donkeys. Vet. Rec. *118*:76, 1986.

Devriese, L.A., Poutrel, R., Kilpper-Bälz, R. and Schlerfer, K.H.: *Staphylococcus gallinarium* and *Staphylococcus caprae*, two new species from animals. Int. J. Syst. Bacteriol. *33*:480, 1983.

Easmon, C.S.F., and Adlam, C. (eds.): Staphylococci and Staphylococcal Infections. Vols. 1 and 2. Orlando, FL, Academic Press, Inc., 1983.

Iandolo, J.J.: Genetic analysis of extracellular toxins of *Staphylococcus aureus*. Ann. Rev. Microbiol. *43*:375, 1989.

Igimi, S., Kawamura, S., Takahashi, E., and Mitsuoka, T.: *Staphylococcus felis*, a new species from clinical specimens from cats. Int. J. Syst. Bacteriol. *39*:373, 1989.

Kenny, K., et al.: Production of enterotoxins and toxic shock syndrome toxin by bovine mammary isolates of *Staphylococcus aureus*. J. Clin. Microbiol. *31*:706, 1993.

Kibenge, F.S.B., Rood, J.I., and Wilcox, G.E.: Lysogeny and other characteristics of *Staphylococcus hyicus* isolated from chickens. Vet. Microbiol. *8*:411, 1983.

Markel, M.D., Wheat, J.D., and Jang, S.S.: Cellulitis associated with coagulase-positive staphylococci in race horses: nine cases (1975-1984). J. Am. Vet. Med. Assoc. *189*: 1600, 1986.

Novick, R.P.: Staphylococci. *In* Microbiology. 4th Ed. Edited by B.D. David, et al. Philadelphia, J.B. Lippincott Co., 1990.

Phillips, Jr., W.E., and Kloos, W.E.: Identification of coagulase-positive *Staphylococcus intermedius* and *Staphylococcus hyicus* subsp. *hyicus* isolates from veterinary clinical specimens. J. Clin. Microbiol. *14*:671, 1981.

Poutrel, B., Boutonnier, A., Sutra, L., and Fournier, J.M.: Prevalence of capsular polysaccharide types 5 and 8 among *Staphylococcus aureus* isolates from cow, goat, and ewe milk. J. Clin. Microbiol. *26*:38, 1988.

Sato, H., et al.: Susceptibility of various animals and cultured cells to exfoliative toxin produced by *Staphylococcus hyicus* subsp. *hyicus*. Vet. Microbiol. *28*:157, 1991.

Schamber, G., and Alstad, A.D.: Isolation of *Staphylococcus hyicus* from seborrheic dermatitis in a pygmy goat. J. Vet. Diagn. Invest. *1*:276, 1989.

Schleifer, K.H., Kilpper-Bälz, R., and Devriese, L.A.: *Staphylococcus arlettae* sp. nov., *S. equorum* sp. nov., and *S. kloosii* sp. nov.: Three new coagulase-negative staphylococci from animals. Syst. Appl. Microbiol. *5*:501, 1984.

Talan, D.A., et al.: *Staphylococcus intermedius* in canine gingiva and canine inflicted human wound infections: Laboratory characterization of a newly recognized zoonotic pathogen. J. Clin. Microbiol. *27*:78, 1989.

Tally, F.P.: Staphylococci: abscesses and other diseases. *In* Mechanisms of Microbial Diseases. Edited by M. Schaechler, et al. Baltimore, Williams & Wilkins, 1993.

Varaldo, P.E., et al.: *Staphylococcus delphini* sp. nov., a coagulase-positive species isolated from dolphins. Int. J. Syst. Bacteriol. *38*:436, 1988.

White, S.D., et al.: Occurrence of *Staphylococcus aureus* on the clinically normal canine hair coat. Am. J. Vet. Res. *44*:332, 1983.

11

Corynebacteria and Rhodococcus

The genus *Corynebacterium* has included several species that recently have been assigned to new genera after taxonomic studies. Two of these species, *Corynebacterium equi* and *C. suis*, have been transferred to the genera *Rhodococcus* and *Eubacterium*, respectively. For convenience *Rhodococcus equi* is discussed in this chapter. *Eubacterium* is dealt with in Chapter 16. The important species formerly known as *Corynebacterium pyogenes*, now *Actinomyces pyogenes*, is discussed in Chapter 26.

Principal Characteristics of the Corynebacteria

The corynebacteria are gram-positive, small, pleomorphic rods with club-shaped swellings at one or both ends. They are nonmotile (except for some plant pathogens) and nonspore-forming. Most are aerobic or facultatively anaerobic, catalase-positive, and fermentative.

Historical

Corynebacterium diphtheriae was shown to be the cause of human diphtheria by Löffler in 1884. It does not cause disease in animals.

General

Members of this genus, other than *C. diphtheriae*, are commonly called "diphtheroids." According to *Bergey's Manual of Systematic Bacteriology*, Vol. 2, the genus *Corynbacterium* is restricted to bacteria with meso-diaminopimelic acid, an arabano-galactan polymer, and certain short-chain mycolic acids in their cell wall. By chemotaxonomic criteria, the genus is most closely related to the genera *Nocardia*, *Rhodococcus*, and *Mycobacterium*.

Some of the pathogenic and saprophytic species have been reclassified. More than 30 species and unnamed varieties have been identified, many of which are parasites on humans and animals. Some that occur in animals are commensals that have not been speciated. Nonpathogenic diphtheroids are frequently recovered from clinical specimens.

Corynebacterium diphtheriae strains may produce a potent toxin that has been studied extensively. The capacity to produce toxin depends on the infection of the bacteria by a temperate phage. The toxin is only produced when the concentration of iron in the medium is low.

The cell wall of some species is weaker at the ends, resulting in a club-like shape. During division, the daughter cells can remain attached on one side, resulting in L and V arrangements that are referred to, when in groups, as "Chinese letters." Many corynebacteria possess metachromatic granules that are thought to be reserves of phosphate. They are readily stained with methylene blue. The various corynebacteria vary considerably in colonial appearance.

Resistance

Corynebacteria are susceptible to common disinfectants.

Corynebacterium renale Group

Three immunologic types of *C. renale*, viz., I, II, and III, have been recognized for some years.

Table 11–1. *Differentiation of* Corynebacterium renale, C. pilosum, *and* C. cystitidis

Characteristic	C. renale	C. pilosum	C. cystitidis
Colony color	yellow	yellow	whitish
Growth in broth at pH 5.4	+	–	–
Acid from:			
xylose	–	–	+
starch	–	+	+
Nitrate reduction	–	+	+
Casein digestion	+	–	–
Hydrolysis of Tween 80	–	–	+
Original designation	C. renale type I	C. renale type II	C. renale type III

Taxonomic studies, including DNA and phenotypic analysis, have shown that these types differ sufficiently to warrant species names. Type I becomes *C. renale*, type II *C. pilosum*, and type III *C. cystitidis*. They can be distinguished by biochemical tests (Table 11–1).

C. renale, which causes bovine and less frequently ovine pyelonephritis, ureteritis, and cystitis, is the most important of the three species. Because it has received the most study, most of the information that follows applies to this species.

Habitat

C. renale has been recovered from the normal bovine female and male genital tracts. *C. pilosum* has been recovered from the bovine genital tract and urine, but it is an infrequent cause of bovine pyelonephritis and cystitis. It seems likely that all species can be carried in the male genital tract with impunity.

Mode of Infection

With all species, infection is transmitted venereally and by contaminated urine. The adherence of *C. renale*, and probably of *C. pilosum* and *C. cystitidis*, to the mucous membrane of the urogenital tract may be facilitated by pili.

Pathogenicity and Pathogenesis

C. renale causes cystitis, ureteritis, and pyelonephritis in cows and kidney abscesses in swine. Cystitis and pyelonephritis have been reported in the bitch, and enzootic posthitis in castrated male sheep also has been attributed to *C. renale* and *C. pilosum*. Posthitis is thought to result from the inflammation caused by the ammonia resulting from urease produced by *C. renale*.

C. cystitidis and *C. pilosum* also cause cystitis and pyelonephritis in cows.

The infection is ascending and involves the bladder, ureter(s), and one or both kidneys in a severe pyogenic inflammatory process. The bladder wall, ureters, and kidney are greatly thickened and enlarged. Hemorrhage, necrosis, and ulceration are extensive, and abscesses may be found throughout the kidney. The urine is purulent and blood stained.

Direct Examination

Gram-stained smears from purulent urine disclose clumps of short, pleomorphic, gram-positive rods. Definitive diagnosis depends on isolation and identification.

Isolation and Identification

Carefully collected urine samples are usually plated on blood agar and incubated aerobically at 37° C. Young colonies are initially small, but the colony characteristics of each species vary somewhat. Those of *C. renale* become opaque and ivory colored as they enlarge. The colonies of *C. pilosum* resemble those of *C. renale*, but tend to be cream colored to yellow. Those of *C. cystitidis* tend to be semitransparent to white. All three species produce urease.

The final identification of the *C. renale* group is based on the characteristics listed in Table 11–2. Differentiation of the three species is based on the criteria of Table 11–1.

Antigenic Nature and Immunity

The classification of *C. renale* into type I (*C. renale*), type II (*C. pilosum*) and type III (*C. cystitidis*) was based on the recognition of different surface antigens by agar diffusion precipitin tests. The protein of the pilus is antigenic and distinct for each species.

Although various serologic procedures have been used to detect antibodies in these infections, none has been found to be of practical value. As in other urinary tract infections, corynebacteria in cows with upper urinary tract involvement are coated with antibody (IgG). The immune response in these infections is not sufficient to effectuate recovery.

*Table 11–2. Differentiation of Some Important Corynebacteria and **Rhodococcus equi***

	Cata-lase	Hemol-ysis	Casein hydrol-ysis	Nitrate reduction	Urease	Acid Production			
						Glucose	Maltose	Lactose	Sucrose
C. pseudotu-berculosis	+	+	−	V	+	+	V	V	V
C. renale group	+	−	+	V	+	+	V	V	−
C. bovis	+	−	−	−	−	−	−	−	−
C. kutscheri	+	V	−	+	+	+	+	−	+
R. equi	+	−	−	+	+	−	−	−	−

V, variable.

Treatment

There are reports of successful treatment of *C. renale* infections with large doses of penicillin, although remissions are frequent. Treatment is most satisfactory if it is begun early in the disease. Effectiveness of treatment should be monitored by urine culture.

Corynebacterium pseudotuberculosis

Synonym: *Corynebacterium ovis*

C. pseudotuberculosis resembles somewhat *C. diphtheriae* and is susceptible to some of the phages used to type *C. diphtheriae*. When lysogenized with the *tox*⁺ phage, *C. pseudotuberculosis* synthesizes diphtheria toxin.

Habitat

It may occur on the normal skin and mucous membranes. Survival in the environment is brief.

Mode of Infection

The organisms most commonly enter abrasions resulting from shearing and injuries. Occasionally, infections occur as a result of inhalation or ingestion.

Pathogenicity

C. pseudotuberculosis causes caseous lymphadenitis in sheep and goats, and abscesses and chronic lymphadenitis in wild ruminants, camels, and rarely in cattle and humans. In horses and mules, mainly in warm climates, it produces ulcerative lymphangitis. Folliculitis and pectoral abscesses in horses and purulent arthritis in lambs have been reported.

Pathogenesis

C. pseudotuberculosis is a facultative intracellular parasite. When infection spreads, it does so via the lymphatics. The pus is green, frequently caseous, and may be arranged in onion-like concentric layers in lymph nodes.

A relatively weak exotoxin, phospholipase D is considered an important virulence factor. It produces hemolysis, dermal necrosis in rabbits, and lethality in some laboratory animals. Antibodies to it are protective. A surface lipid has been found that protects organisms from phagocytosis and contributes to abscessation.

Ulcerative lymphangitis in horses and mules, and rarely in cattle, appears as nodules, most often involving the superficial lymphatics around the fetlocks. The organism enters via injuries, and the disease is frequently chronic and long lasting.

Slowly developing abscesses of the pectoral, lower abdominal, and inguinal regions of horses have frequently yielded *C. pseudotuberculosis*. These infections, which have been reported mainly from California, may be complications of habronemiasis and dermatitis caused by the horn fly.

Isolation and Cultivation

This gram-positive, pleomorphic rod grows well on blood agar aerobically at 37° C. Colonies are initially small, but after several days of incubation they enlarge to 3 to 4 mm in diameter, become dry and crumbly, and turn cream to orange in color. Complete hemolysis is usually seen on blood agar.

Identification

Definitive identification is based on the differential biochemical characteristics listed in Table 11–2. Cultures from horses and cattle have been reported to reduce nitrate, whereas those from sheep and goats seldom do.

On blood agar, *C. pseudotuberculosis* inhibits the staphylococcal beta-toxin but results in a synergistic hemolysis with *Rhodococcus equi*.

Antigenic Nature and Immunity

Two serotypes, 1 and 2, have been identified. The first is recovered most frequently from sheep and goats, whereas serotype 2 has been mainly found in cattle and buffaloes. Differences in restriction endonuclease analyses and nitrate reduction have been noted between equine strains and those from sheep and goats.

Corynebacterium pseudotuberculosis is a facultative, intracellular parasite, and consequently, the cellular immune response is particularly important. Some protective immunity is elicited by the exotoxin phospholipase D.

Autogenous (flock) bacterins have been used in an attempt to control outbreaks of caseous lymphadenitis, but their value is questionable. Because of the importance of cell-mediated immunity, attenuated live vaccines may have value.

An enzyme-linked immunosorbent assay employing phospholipase D as antigen has been developed to detect infected or carrier animals.

Treatment

Although *C. pseudotuberculosis* is susceptible to many antimicrobial agents, including penicillin, tetracyclines, erythromycin, and chloramphenicol, the nature of the lesion and the intracellular location preclude their effectiveness. Culling and segregation and sanitary measures during shearing and dipping are considered helpful.

Public Health Significance

Infrequent human infections arise from contact with animals and are characterized by a chronic or subacute lymphadenitis.

Rhodococcus

Rhodococcus belongs in the order Actinomycetales and consists of 16 species, most of which, if not all, are thought to be soil-borne. They all produce pink to red pigment, and only one species, *R. equi*, is an important animal pathogen. *R. sputi* has been recovered from mesenteric lymphadenitis in swine.

Principal Characteristics of Rhodococci

They are gram-positive, variably acid-fast organisms that assume coccoid and bacillary forms. They grow aerobically, are nonfermentative, and are catalase and urease positive.

Rhodococcus equi

Synonym: *Corynebacterium equi*

Habitat

Rhodococcus equi is soil-borne and often is present in manure. It is present in the intestine of many horses and persists for long periods in the manure and litter of stables.

Mode of Infection

Infection may result from direct contact with, or inhalation of, contaminated soil, manure, infectious secretions, or feces.

Pathogenicity and Pathogenesis

The principal disease is suppurative bronchopneumonia in foals and is characterized by large pulmonary abscesses. It is a common cause of submandibular and cervical lymphadenitis of swine and an infrequent cause of abscesses of the lungs and lymph nodes of various animals and humans. It occasionally causes abortion in mares and necrotizing enterocolitis and subcutaneous abscesses in foals. Abscesses probably derived from wounds, and sometimes spread hematogenously, have been reported in cats. Infections in dogs are rare.

The route of infection in bronchopneumonia is thought to be via the respiratory tract. Dosage and repeated exposure are probably important, as suggested by the fact that equine infections are more prevalent if premises are heavily laden with *R. equi*.

The organism is a facultative intracellar parasite that is able to survive in macrophages. After an initial granulomatous response, it then culminates in suppurative pneumonia with large abscesses. Toxin has not been demonstrated; however, a phospholipase and a cholesterol oxidase produced by this species are thought to have an important role in pathogenesis.

Direct Examination

Gram-positive, usually coccoid, occasionally rod-shaped organisms are seen in pus.

Isolation and Cultivation

The organism grows well on blood agar aerobically at 37° C. In 48 hours colonies are smooth, mucoid, translucent, and 3 to 5 mm in diameter. On some media, colonies have a salmon to red pigment, but on blood agar colonies appear grayish-white.

Identification

Identification is based on the characteristic cellular and colonial morphology with the differential characteristics listed in Table 11–2.

A phenomenon resembling the CAMP reaction can be used to identify *R. equi*. "Partial hemolysins" from *R. equi* enhance the hemolysis of the phospholipase D of *Corynebacterium pseudotuberculosis* or the beta-hemolysin of *Staphylococcus aureus*.

Antigenic Nature and Immunity

Rhodococcus equi possesses a large polysaccharide capsule that is antigenically diverse. More than 10 different capsular serotypes have been identified from different animal and geographic sources. Capsular serotypes 1 and 2 were predominant in North American horses.

Although antibody to *R. equi* is found in the sera of normal horses and can be elicited by inoculation of killed organisms, most protection seems to depend on a cell-mediated response. Autogenous bacterins have not been effective in preventing the disease. Adult horses are generally immune to infection.

Treatment

R. equi is susceptible to penicillin, lincomycin, rifamycins, erythromycin, neomycin, gentamycin, and streptomycin. Because of the suppurative nature of the lesions, treatment is usually effective only if started early. Large doses of penicillin or one of the rifamycins given for several weeks have been effective. Also effective is a combination of one of the previously mentioned drugs with erythromycin.

Public Health Significance

Human infections caused by *R. equi* are infrequent. Most common are those occurring in immunocompromised adults, some AIDS-related, with deficient cell-mediated immunity. The disease is usually a subacute necrotizing pneumonia, although abscesses, osteomyelitis, peritonitis, and septicemia have been reported.

Other Species

Corynebacterium bovis

This organism differs significantly from bona fide members of the genus *Corynebacterium* and ultimately will be moved to another genus.

It is a commensal found in the reproductive tract of some cows and bulls and on the squamous epithelium of the teat duct of as many as 20% of the quarters of cows. Although it is not considered a cause of mastitis, the slight inflammation it causes is thought to aid in protecting the udder from infection.

C. bovis is a lipophilic organism that grows best in the presence of unsaturated long-chain fatty acids. Although it grows well on enriched media, colonies are more prevalent on the fatty areas of plates inoculated with milk. The morphology is

characteristic of the genus, and identification is based on the criteria listed in Table 11–2.

Corynebacterium kutscheri (C. murium)

This organism culturally resembles *C. pseudotuberculosis*. It causes an important, although infrequent, disease of mice and rats characterized by caseous tuberculosis-like focal lesions in the lungs and other organs.

Morphologically *C. kutscheri* is indistinguishable from other corynebacteria. Identification is based on the differential characteristics listed in Table 11–2.

Corynebacterium minutissimum

C. minutissimum has been reported from docking wounds in lambs, inflammation of interdigital spaces ("scald"), and scabs on the brisket. A superficial infection of the axillary and pubic regions in humans, called erythrasma (scaly plaques), is recognized, as are infrequent bacteremia and endocarditis.

Corynebacterium parvum (now renamed *Propionibacterium parvum*)

A nonpathogenic anaerobe used for its adjuvant properties in tumor therapy.

Corynebacterium ulcerans

C. ulcerans, which resembles in some respects *C. diphtheriae*, has been recovered from bovine mastitis. Like *C. pseudotuberculosis*, it produces phospholipase D, and some strains produce small quantities of diphtheria toxin.

FURTHER READING

Barton, M.D., and Hughes, K.L.: Ecology of *Rhodococcus equi*. Vet. Microbiol. *9*:65, 1984.

Barton, M.D., and Hughes, K.L.: *Corynebacterium equi*: A review. Vet. Bull. *50*:65, 1980.

Brooks, B.W., and Barnum, D.A.: The susceptibility of bovine udder quarters colonized with *Corynebacterium bovis* to experimental infection with *Staphylococcus aureus* or *Streptococcus agalactiae*. Can. J. Comp. Med. *48*:146, 1984.

Brown, C.C., and Olander, H.S.: Caseous lymphadenitis in goats and sheep: a review. Vet. Bull. *57*:1, 1987.

Coyle, M.B., and Lipsky, B.A.: Coryneform bacteria in infectious diseases: Clinical and laboratory aspects. Clin. Microbiol. Rev. *3*:227, 1990.

Egen, N.B., et al.: Purification of the phospholipase D of *Corynebacterium pseudotuberculosis* by recycling isoelectric focusing. Am. J. Vet. Res. *50*:1319, 1989.

Elissalde, G.S., and Renshaw, H.W.: *Corynebacterium equi*: An interhost review with emphasis on the foal. Comp. Immunol. Microbiol. Infect. Dis. *3*:433, 1980.

Elliot, G., Lawson, G.H., and Mackenzie, C.P.: *Rhodococcus equi* infection of cats. Vet. Rec. *118*:693, 1986.

Giddens, W.E., Jr., Keahey, K.K., Carter, G.R., and Whitehair, C.K.: Pneumonia in rats due to infection with *Corynebacterium kutscheri*. Pathol. Vet. *5:*227, 1968.

Goodfellow, M., and Alderson, G.: The Actinomycete-genus, *Rhodococcus*: A home for the "rhodochrous" complex. J. Gen. Microbiol. *100:*99, 1977.

Hart, R.J.C.: *Corynebacterium ulcerans* in humans and cattle in North Devon. J. Hyg. *92:*161, 1984.

Hiramune, T., Inui, S., Muras, N., and Yanagawa, R.: Virulence of three types of *Corynebacterium renale* in cows. Am. J. Vet Res. *32:*237, 1971.

Krech, T., and Hollis, D.G.: *Corynebacterium* and related organisms. *In* Manual of Clinical Microbiology. 5th Ed. Edited by A. Balows. Washington, D.C., American Society for Microbiology, 1991.

Leamaster, B.R.: Efficacy of *Corynebacterium pseudotuberculosis* bacterin for the immunologic protection of sheep against development of caseous lymphadenitis. Am. J. Vet. Res. *48:*869, 1987.

Miers, K.C., and Ley, W.B.: *Corynebacterium pseudotuberculosis* infection in the horse: Study of 117 clinical cases and consideration of etiopathogenesis. J. Am. Vet. Med. Assoc. *177:*250, 1980.

Muckle, C.A., and Gyles, C.L.: Characterization of strains of *Corynebacterium pseudotuberculosis*. Can. J. Comp. Med. *46:*206, 1982.

Prescott, J.F.: *Rhodococcus equi*: an animal and human pathogen. Clin. Microbiol. Rev. *4:*20, 1991.

Prescott, J.F.: Capsular serotypes of *Corynebacterium equi*. Can. J. Comp. Med. *45:*130, 1981.

Prescott, J.F., and Muckle, C.A.: *Corynebacterium. In:* Pathogenesis of Bacterial Infections in Animals. Edited by C.L. Gyles and C.O. Thoen. Ames, IA, Iowa State University Press, 1986.

Songer, J.G., et al.: Biochemical and genetic characterization of *Corynebacterium pseudotuberculosis*. Am. J. Vet. Res. *49:*223, 1988.

Tkachuk-Saad, O., and Prescott, J.: *Rhodococcus equi* plasmids: isolation and partial characterization. J. Clin. Microbiol. *29:*2696, 1991.

Tsukamura, M., et al.: Mesenteric lymphadentitis of swine caused by *Rhodococcus sputi*. J. Clin. Microbiol. *26:*155, 1988.

Yager, A.: The pathogenesis of *Rhodococcus equi* pneumonia in foals. Vet. Microbiol. *14:*225, 1987.

Yanagawa, R., and Honda, E.: *Corynebacterium pilosum* and *Corynebacterium cystitidis*, two new species from cows. Int. J. Syst. Bact. *28:*209, 1978.

12

Listeria

PRINCIPAL CHARACTERISTICS OF *LISTERIA*

They are small, motile, gram-positive rods that are catalase-positive, oxidase-negative, mesophilic, facultatively anaerobic, fermentative, and non-spore-forming.

The taxonomy of the genus *Listeria* has undergone considerable change in recent years.

Currently, two genomically distinct groups are recognized. The first group includes the following species:

L. murrayi **and** *L. grayi.* These are nonpathogenic and rarely isolated. Their natural habitat is probably soil and vegetation.

The other group includes the following:

L. monocytogenes. This is the principal pathogen of the genus for animals and humans.

L. ivanovii. This is the only species other than *L. monocytogenes* that is naturally pathogenic for animals, including humans. It can cause abortion in sheep and cattle and is pathogenic for mice experimentally. Little is known at present about the extent of infections caused by this species. There is a carrier state in normal animals and humans.

L. innocua. This recently recognized variety has been isolated from soil, plants, and human and animal feces.

L. welshimeri. This species has been recovered from soil and decaying vegetation.

L. seeligeri. It has been recovered from soil, vegetation and animal feces.

L. denitrificans does not belong in the genus *Listeria.* It has been moved to the genus *Jonesia.*

Listeria monocytogenes

Historical

The organism was first recovered by Murray, Webb, and Swann in 1926 from guinea pigs and rabbits showing hepatic necrosis.

Habitat

Listeria monocytogenes has been recovered from the soil. It has been found in the feces (many enteric carriers), genital secretions, and nasal mucus of apparently healthy animals and in silage. Organisms multiply when pH of silage rises above 5.5.

In recent years, *L. monocytogenes* has been recovered from raw and processed foods, including meat, seafood, vegetables, and dairy products. Although not yet proved, some believe that *L. monocytogenes* is a saprophytic, soil-borne organism.

Mode of Infection

The modes of infection of the neural and visceral forms are considered to be different. In the neural form, infection is via branches of the trigeminal nerve or probably via the eye, nose, and oropharynx; in the visceral form, ingestion is the mode of infection. Most infections are thought to be exogenous.

Pathogenicity

The disease is referred to as listeriosis or listerellosis, and the neural form is sometimes called "circling disease."

The neural form of the disease is most common in ruminants. It is seen in cattle and sheep, particularly in winter and early spring; all ages are susceptible. Outbreaks occur in feedlots. The occurrence of the disease has been associated with feeding of silage that may contain large numbers of *L. monocytogenes*. An increase in iron consumption resulting from eating silage is thought to contribute to listeriosis. Central nervous system (CNS) signs include unilateral ataxia and meningitis. Microabscesses are found, principally involving the brain stem.

Keratoconjunctivitis and ophthalmitis have been described in cattle and sheep.

Abortions occur in cows and ewes, but without the neural manifestations of the disease. The organism can be recovered from the aborted fetus and uterus. A case of equine abortion caused by *L. monocytogenes* serotype 4 has been reported.

The neural form of the disease occurs in the horse, but it is infrequent. Both the neural and abortion forms have been reported in llamas.

In chickens and turkeys, it usually takes a septicemic form. Necrotic foci of the liver and myocardium are seen. Cases of the neural form of listeriosis in broiler chickens have been reported in recent years.

A visceral or septicemic form of the disease with liver necrosis is seen in the rabbit, guinea pig, chinchilla, reindeer, antelope, and other species. Several cases of neural listeriosis have been encountered in the dog.

Pathogenesis

The neural form of the disease is seen most frequently in ruminants. The visceral form is seen most often in monogastric animals, and spread appears to be hematogenous after ingestion. Organisms are intracellular (macrophages) in both forms. As with other intracellular bacteria, a granulomatous reaction leads to focal areas of necrosis in the liver in this disease. Organisms replicate in phagocytic cells and slowly destroy many of them. A monocytosis-producing agent (a glyceride) has been extracted from *L. monocytogenes*. Monocytosis is only seen in monogastric animals.

L. monocytogenes produces a heat-labile, antigenic, mouse-lethal hemolysin known as listeriolysin O. It is thought to act by disrupting membranes of the phagocytic vacuole and liposomes, thus contributing to intracellular survival. Virulence appears to depend mainly on the hemolysin, and all virulent strains of *L. monocytogenes* produce it.

Specimens

Neural form: pons and medulla.
Visceral form: portions of affected organs.
Abortion: fetus and fetal membranes.

Isolation and Cultivation

The organism is frequently difficult to recover from the brain in neural listeriosis, presumably because the organisms are intracellular and present in small numbers. If no growth is obtained initially, ground brain stored at refrigerator temperature ("cold enrichment") should be recultured weekly for as many as 12 weeks before it is discarded as negative. The organism is able to grow at refrigerator temperatures, thus the value of cold enrichment. It is more difficult to recover from the bovine brain, in which the number of organisms is fewer than that in the sheep and goat brain. Cultural procedures may be indicated by the finding of microscopic lesions characteristic of listeriosis in the brain or brain stem.

The organism grows well on ordinary media but is routinely isolated on blood agar. Primary growth is stimulated by 5 to 10% carbon dioxide. Smooth colonies are approximately 2 mm in diameter, round, entire, glistening, and bluish by transmitted light; narrow zones of beta-hemolysis are evident.

Small gram-positive rods occurring singly, in pairs, or in short chains are seen in stained smears. Morphologically they may resemble some diphtheroids and streptococci. A characteristic tumbling motility is noted at room temperature.

Identification

The organism somewhat resembles *Erysipelothrix rhusiopathiae*. Three important distinguishing features of *Listeria monocytogenes* are: (1) it is catalase-positive; (2) it is motile at room temperature; and (3) experimental infections in guinea pigs are fatal. See Table 12–1 for differentiation of the various species.

A fluorescent-labeled globulin is available for the identification of *L. monocytogenes*. It is most satisfactorily employed with organisms from cultures. False-positive results have been reported.

L. monocytogenes monoclonal antibodies have made possible an effective fluorescent conjugate for use with food specimens and cultures. Several DNA probes have been developed to detect *L. monocytogenes* in enrichment cultures of foods.

L. grayi, *L. innocua*, and *L. murrayi* are not betahemolytic, pathogenic for mice, or positive in the Anton test. *L. ivanovii* is pathogenic for mice.

The CAMP test (see Chapter 9, Streptococcus) is helpful in the differentiation of *L. monocytogenes*, *L. innocua*, and *L. ivanovii*. Results with the CAMP tests are as follows:

with *Staphylococcus aureus* streak:
Listeria innocua −, *L. ivanovii* −, *L. monocytogenes* +

Table 12–1. *Differential Characteristics of* Listeria spp. *and* Erysipelothrix rhusiopathiae

	Umbrella Motility (25° C)	Beta-Hemolysis	Coagulase	CAMP-Test with		Acid Production		
				S. aureus	R. equi*	Mannitol	Rhamnose	Xylose
L. monocytogenes	+	+	–	+	–	–	+	–
L. ivanovii	+	++	–	–	+	–	–	+
L. innocua	+	–	–	–	–	–	V	–
L. welshimeri	+	–	–	–	–	–	V	+
L. seeligeri	+	+	–	+	–	–	–	+
L. murrayi	+	–	–	–	–	+	V	–
L. grayi	+	–	–	–	–	+	–	–
E. rhusiopathiae	–	–	+	–	–	–	–	–

*Rhodococcus equi.
V, variable reactions.

with *Rhodococcus equi* streak:

Listeria innocua –, *L. ivanovii* +, *L. monocytogenes* –

Experimental Animals. Mice, rabbits, and guinea pigs are susceptible. A keratoconjunctivitis (Anton test) is produced by *L. monocytogenes* within 24 hours after the instillation of organisms into the eyes of guinea pigs and rabbits.

Antigenic Nature and Serology

On the basis of heat-stable somatic (O) and heat-labile flagellar (H) antigens, 4 principal serologic groups and 11 serotypes have been identified. They bear no relation to the host species or the clinical syndrome from which they are recovered. Serotype 4b is the predominant strain in Canada and the United States. Most infections are caused by three serotypes: 1/2a, 1/2b, and 4b. Numbers indicate O antigens and letters H antigens. Serologic tests have not been of value in the diagnosis or control of listeriosis.

Resistance

Pasteurization (62° C for 30 min; 71.6° C for 15 to 30 sec) destroys *L. monocytogenes*. It is remarkably resistant to drying, can survive for months in food, straw, soil, and shavings, and is susceptible to common disinfectants.

Immunity

For the most part, immunity depends on the T-cell-mediated activation of macrophages by lymphokines. The role of the humoral response is not clear. Immunization has not been widely practiced. Autogenous bacterins have given inconclusive results. Studies in experimental animals confirm that much of the immunity in listeriosis is cell-mediated. In view of this, live attenuated vaccines may be of value. Live attenuated vaccine containing serovars 1/2 and 4b has been used successfully against listeriosis in sheep.

Public Health Significance

Infections in humans are frequently opportunistic, involving mainly immunocompromised and immunologically immature individuals. As in animals, infections involve the reticuloendothelial system. In humans, *L. monocytogenes* causes meningitis and encephalitis; uterine infections with abortion, still births, and a neonatal septicemic form called granulomatosis infantiseptica; valvular endocarditis; febrile pharyngitis; and septicemia.

The possible sources for human infections are soil (contaminated dust), animals, contaminated milk, cheese, meat, some vegetables, and human carriers. Infections are frequently associated with the use of corticosteroids, radiation therapy, and other underlying diseases.

Several cases of bovine mastitis caused by this organism have been reported. Unpasteurized cow's milk yielding the organism is a potential source of human infections. There may be human genital and enteric carriers.

Treatment

Treatment is usually of little value, particularly in sheep and goats, after neurologic signs are seen. The drugs of choice are chloramphenicol and the tetracycline antibiotics, given at maximum dosage. Cephalosporins are not recommended because of their limited penetration of the meninges. Treatment may be of some use in cattle, but relapses may occur. Sulfonamides, penicillin, and tetracyclines may be used prophylactically and therapeutically. Erythromycin and ampicillin have been the drugs of choice in the human disease. The cure rate is low in the immunocompromised host.

FURTHER READING

Alexander, A.V., et al.: Bovine abortions attributable to *Listeria ivanovii*: Four cases (1988–1990). J. Am. Vet. Med. Assoc. 200:711, 1992.

Barlow, R.M., and McGorum, B.: Ovine listerial encephalitis: Analysis, hypothesis and synthesis. Vet. Rec. *116*:233, 1985.

Bille, J., and Doyle, M.P.: *Listeria* and *Erysipelothrix. In* Manual of Clinical Microbiology. 5th Ed. Edited by A. Balows. Washington, D.C., American Society for Microbiology, 1991.

Charlton, K.M., and Garcia, M.M.: Spontaneous listeric encephalitis and neuritis in sheep. Light microscope studies. Vet. Pathol. *14*:297, 1977.

Cooper, G., et al.: Listeriosis in California broiler chickens. J. Vet. Diagn. Invest. *4*:343, 1992.

Emerson, F.G., and Jarvis, A.A.: Listeriosis in ponies. J. Am. Vet. Med. Assoc. *152*:1645, 1968.

Fleming, D.W., et al.: Pasteurized milk as a vehicle of infection in an outbreak of listeriosis. N. Engl. J. Med. *312*:404, 1985.

Gellin, B.G., and Broom, C.V.: Listeriosis. J. Am. Vet. Med. Assoc. *261*:1313, 1989.

Gronstol, H.: Listeriosis in sheep. *Listeria monocytogenes* in sheep fed hay or grass silage during pregnancy. Immunological state, white blood cells, total serum protein and serum iron. Acta Vet. Scand. *21*:1, 1980.

Jaton, K., Sahl, R., and Bille, J.: Development of polymerase chain reaction assays for detection of *Listeria monocytogenes* in clinical cerebral spinal fluid samples. J. Clin. Microbiol. *30*:1931, 1992.

Killinger, A.H., and Mansfield, M.E.: Epizootiology of listeric infection in sheep. J. Am. Vet. Med. Assoc. *157*:1318, 1970.

Ladds, P.W., Dennis, S.M., and Njoku, C.O.: Pathology of listeric infection in domestic animals. Vet. Bull. *44*:67, 1974.

McLaughlin, B.G., Greer, S.C., and Singh, S.: Listeria abortion in llama. J. Vet. Diagn. Invest. *5*:105, 1993.

Menguad, J., et al.: Identification of the structural gene encoding the 5H-activated hemolysin of *Listeria monocytogenes*: listeriolysin O is homologous to streptolysin O and pneumolysin. Infect. Immun. *55*:3225, 1987.

Nieman, R.E., and Lorber, B.: Listeriosis in adults: A changing pattern. Report of eight cases and review of the literature, 1968–1978. Rev. Infect. Dis. *2*:207, 1980.

Rocourt, J., and Grimont, P.A.D.: *Listeria welshimeri* sp. nov. and *Listeria seeligeri* sp. nov. Int. J. Syst. Bact. *33*:866, 1983.

Rocourt, J., Wehmeyer, U., and Stackebrandt, E.: Transfer of *Listeria denitrificans* to a new genus, *Jonesia* gen. nov., as *Jonesia denitrificans* comb. nov. Int. J. Syst. Bact. *37*:266, 1987.

Rocourt, J., Wehmeyer, U., Cossart, P., and Stackebrandt, E.: Proposal to retain *Listeria murrayi* and *Listeria grayi* in the genus *Listeria*. Int. J. Syst. Bact. *37*:296, 1987.

Seeliger, H.P.R.: Serovariants of *Listeria monocytogenes* and other *Listeria* species. Acta Microbiol. Acad. Sci. Hung. *22*:179, 1975.

Wexler, H., and Oppenherm, J.D.: Isolation, characterization and biological properties of an endotoxin-like material from the gram-positive organism *Listeria monocytogenes*. Infect. Immun. *23*:845, 1979.

13

Erysipelothrix

The genus *Erysipelothrix* is in the same family as the genera *Listeria* and *Lactobacillus* and contains only one species, *Erysipelothrix rhusiopathiae*. This species is an important pathogen of mainly swine and poultry.

Principal Characteristics of *Erysipelothrix*

Erysipelothrix organisms are small, nonmotile, gram-positive rods. They are nonspore-forming, catalase-negative, mesophilic, facultatively anaerobic, and fermentative.

Erysipelothrix rhusiopathiae

SYNONYM: *ERYSIPELOTHRIX INSIDIOSA*

Historical

The organism was first described adequately by Löffler in 1886 and first recovered in the United States in 1892.

Habitat

E. rhusiopathiae is found on the mucous membranes of normal swine and some other animals. It may also be present in the slime on the bodies of freshwater and saltwater fish and crustacea. The organism has been thought to live and multiply during the warm months in alkaline soil throughout the world, however, recent work suggests that it may survive for only several weeks in soil and that carrier pigs are the primary reservoir of the organism.

Mode of Infection and Transmission

Erysipelas is worldwide in distribution and is acquired by direct contact with infected pigs and fomites. The mode of infection is thought to be by ingestion. The organism occurs in the surface slime of freshwater and saltwater fish and consequently may be transmitted in fish meal.

Pathogenesis and Pathogenicity

Toxins have not been demonstrated. Hyaluronidase, coagulase, and neuraminidase are produced by some strains and may be related to virulence. Neuraminidase cleaves alpha-glycosidic linkages in neuraminic acid, a mucopolysaccharide on the surface of the host's cells.

The organisms regularly invade the bloodstream, and the type of disease that develops probably depends to a considerable extent on the immune status of the individual.

Swine. Pigs are most susceptible in the 3- to 18-month age range. Erysipelas is enzootic and of considerable economic significance in certain regions. The several forms of disease seen include the acute form, the skin or urticarial form, the arthritic form, and the cardiac form (endocarditis). These various forms may occur separately, in a sequence, or together. In the acute septicemic form, the course is short and the mortality is high. Reddish or purple rhomboidal blotches, scabs, and sloughing are seen in the skin form. Lesions are probably the result of thrombus formation following Arthus-type reactions (immune complexes). The arthritic form is usually seen in older pigs; it is characterized by a marked periarticular fibrosis resulting in part from an allergic reaction to the bacteria and their fragments that may persist in joints.

Sheep. Post-dipping lameness is a laminitis resulting from an extension of a focal cutaneous infection in the region of the hoof. Nonsuppurative polyarthritis is seen in lambs. The organisms gain entry via the unhealed navel and wounds. This form of the disease also may be seen in calves.

Fowl. Turkeys, chickens, ducks, geese, and many game and wild birds are susceptible. Erysipelas is an important economic disease of growing turkeys. The acute disease is characterized by septicemia, and the organism may be recovered from all tissues.

Dogs. A number of cases of valvular endocarditis have been reported in dogs. The organism may be recovered in blood cultures.

Cattle. Infrequent occurrences of polyserositis, septicemia, and arthritis have been reported.

Marine Mammals. Serious and fatal infections are encountered in cetaceans (dolphins, porpoises) and pinnipeds (sea lions, walruses).

Specimens

Acute or Septicemic Form. Blood and blood smears from live animals, and liver, spleen, and coronary blood of necropsied animals.

Chronic Form. Affected tissues, e.g., heart, skin, and joint fluid. The organism may be difficult to obtain from advanced skin and joint lesions.

Isolation and Cultivation

E. rhusiopathiae grows readily on media enriched with serum or blood. Five to 10% CO_2 stimulates growth. Selective media are available to aid in the isolation of *E. rhusiopathiae* from contaminated specimens.

Two kinds of colonies are seen. Smooth colonies are small and round; rough colonies are larger, with irregular borders. Rough colonies are obtained more frequently from chronic infections. Growth is slight after 24 hours of incubation but is readily apparent after 48 hours. Alpha hemolysis (greenish) is usually seen around young colonies.

Gram-stained smears from smooth colonies reveal slender gram-positive rods resembling those of *Listeria* species. Smears from rough colonies disclose highly pleomorphic and filamentous forms. Characteristic organisms can be demonstrated from the blood and tissues of infected animals.

Identification

Erysipelothrix rhusiopathiae most closely resembles *Listeria* species. Important features that differentiate it from *Listeria* are its nonmotile and catalase-negative characteristics. Most strains (>99%) are coagulase positive, whereas *Listeria* and *Corynebacterium* spp. are coagulase negative. Evidence of H_2S near the stab line in TSI agar medium is highly characteristic of *Erysipelothrix rhusiopathiae*. (See also Table 12–1.)

Experimental Animals. Mice are susceptible to infection and usually die within 4 days after intraperitoneal inoculation. Guinea pigs are resistant to infection. Pigs can be infected by applying virulent organisms to scarified skin.

Antigenic Nature and Serology

Employment of agglutination procedures has allowed identification of groups or types, designated A, B, and N, on the basis of differences in somatic antigens. Type A strains are the principal cause of the acute disease in swine, whereas types B and N are associated with the chronic disease. Some researchers have used numbers rather than letters to designate serologic varieties based on differences in peptidoglycans. Based on peptidoglycan antigens, at least 22 different serotypes (designated 1 to 22) have been recognized. The numeric system is preferable to the alphabetic system. Serotypes A and B correspond to serotypes 1 and 2. The various serologic varieties are closely related immunologically. Serotypes 1 (subtypes 1a and 1b) and 2 were recovered most frequently from tonsils and acute disease of swine.

The protective antigen is thought to be a glycolipoprotein that does not confer serologic specificity. Serologic tests are of little value in diagnosis.

Resistance

The organism is remarkably resistant for a non-spore-former. It survives drying at room temperature for several months. Moist organisms survive for years; one broth culture remained viable for 17 years. The organism survived boiling for 2 hours in pork 6 inches thick. It survives for long periods in smoked and unsmoked meats and in cadavers. Disinfectants, except for phenolic compounds, are quite effective against it.

Immunity

Immunity is mainly humoral. The formation of immune complexes and the occurrence of hypersensitivity reactions are responsible in part for some of the lesions seen.

Passive. Hyperimmune antierysipelas serum is no longer widely used. It is prepared in horses and cattle. It may be used therapeutically during an outbreak and to protect in-contact pigs. Protection is of short duration.

Active. Avirulent living vaccines are fairly widely employed. One of these is administered orally. Bacterins, usually prepared from serotype 2 and consisting of formalin-killed cultures adsorbed on alumina gels, are widely employed and generally protect pigs until market age. They are also of value in preventing the disease in turkeys. A lysate bacterin developed originally in France is licensed in the United States. The immunizing antigen is present in culture filtrate.

Treatment

Penicillin is the drug of choice for swine and turkeys; it may be combined with antiserum. Erythromycin, cephalosporins, and clindamycin are used in human patients who are allergic to penicillin.

Public Health Significance

Erysipeloid is the name given to *E. rhusiopathiae* infection in humans. It is usually an occupational disease of veterinarians, packing house workers, butchers, and fish handlers. Cooks are occasionally infected from fish and contaminated meat and poultry. The organism usually enters via the skin (intact or broken), and after 1 to 5 days of incubation, a painful erythematous swelling develops at the site of entry. Infection is usually localized and most frequently involves the hand or fingers. The course is usually about 3 weeks; occasionally more severe systemic complications occur. Several cases of septicemia, valvular endocarditis, and septic arthritis have been reported. Erysipeloid responds well to penicillin.

FURTHER READING

Blood, D.C., and Radostits, O.M.: Veterinary Medicine. 7th Ed. London, Balliere Tindall, 1989.

Chandler, D.S., and Craven, J.A.: Persistence and distribution of *Erysipelothrix rhusiopathiae* and bacterial indicator organisms on land used for disposal of piggery effluent. J. Appl. Bacteriol. 48:367, 1980.

Dreyfuss, D.J., and Stephens, P.R.: *Erysipelothrix rhusiopathiae*-induced septic arthritis in a calf. J. Am. Vet. Med. Assoc. 197:1361, 1990.

Galan, J.E., and Timoney, J.F.: Cloning and expression of protective antigen of *Erysipelothrix rhusiopathiae*. Infect. Immun. 58:3116, 1990.

Grieco, M., and Sheldon, C.: *Erysipelothrix rhusiopathiae*. Ann. N.Y. Acad. Sci. 174:523, 1970.

Hariharan, H., et al.: An investigation of bacterial causes of arthritis in slaughter hogs. J. Vet. Diagn. Invest. 4:28, 1992.

Jones, T.D.: Aspects of the epidemiology and control of *Erysipelas insidiosa* polyarthritis of lambs. In The Veterinary Annual. Edited by C.S.G. Grunsell and F.W.B. Hill. Bristol, Scientechnica, 1978.

Kircsera, G.: Proposal for the standardization of the designations used for serotypes of *Erysipelothrix rhusiopathiae* (Migula) Buchanan. Int. J. Syst. Bact. 23:184, 1973.

Kluge, J.P., and Perl, S.: *Erysipelothrix rhusiopathiae* septicemia-polyserositis and streptococcal encephalitis in a calf. J. Vet. Diagn. Invest. 4:196, 1992.

Roboli, A.C., and Farrar, E.W.: *Erysipelothrix rhusiopathiae*: An occupational pathogen. Clin. Microbiol. Rev. 2:354, 1989.

Rosenwald, A.S., and Corstvet, R.E.: Erysipelas. In Diseases of Poultry. 8th Ed. Edited by M.S. Hofstad. Ames, IA, Iowa State University Press, 1984.

Takahasi, T., et al.: Serotypes of *Erysipelothrix rhusiopathiae* strains isolated from slaughtered pigs affected with chronic erysipelas. Jpn. J. Vet. Sci. 46:149, 1984.

Takahasi, H., et al.: Serotype, antimicrobial susceptibility, and pathogenicity of *Erysipelothrix rhusiopathiae* isolates from the tonsils of apparently healthy slaughter pigs. J. Clin. Microbiol. 25:536, 1987.

Tesh, M.J., and Wood, R.L.: Detection of coagulase activity in *Erysipelothrix rhusiopathiae*. J. Clin. Microbiol. 26:1058, 1988.

Timoney, J.F., Jr., and Berman, D.T. *Erysipelothrix* arthritis in swine. Bacteriologic and immunologic aspects. Am. J. Vet. Res. 31:1411, 1970.

Wood, R.L.: Swine erysipelas—a review of prevalence and research. J. Am. Vet. Med. Assoc. 184:944, 1984

Wood, R.L., and Harrington, R., Jr.: Serotypes of *Erysipelothrix rhusiopathiae* isolated from swine and from soil and manure of swine pens in the United States. Am. J. Vet. Res. 39:1833, 1978.

14

Clostridium

Principal Characteristics

Clostridia are large, gram-positive (young cultures) rods. Most are motile (*C. perfringens* is an exception), anaerobic (some are microaerophilic), spore-forming, fermentative, and catalase-negative.

Historical

Bollinger (1875) is usually given credit for first describing a pathogenic *Clostridium*, viz., *C. chauvoei*. Other species were also described quite early, but *C. haemolyticum* was not characterized until 1926 by Vawter.

General

More than 100 species of clostridia have been described. Only a few cause diseases in man and animals. These can be divided into four major groups according to the kind of disease they produce.

1. The histotoxic clostridia cause a variety of tissue (often muscle) infections frequently following wounds or other trauma. Examples are blackleg and malignant edema.
2. The hepatotoxic clostridia produce their toxins in the liver, thus resulting in the diseases bacillary hemoglobinuria and black disease.
3. The enterotoxigenic clostridia produce mainly enterotoxemia and food poisoning, although they are occasionally histotoxic.
4. The neurotoxic clostridia cause disease by the production of the potent exotoxins (neurotoxins) of tetanus and botulism.

Habitat

Clostridia are free-living saprophytes distributed widely in the soil. They persist in ecologic niches with a suitably low oxidation-reduction potential. Some species are more prevalent in some geographic areas. Several species commonly occur in the intestinal tract.

Mode of Infection

Although most important clostridial infections are acquired by ingestion or via wounds, some arise endogenously.

Ingestion. Blackleg (cattle), botulism (food), enterotoxemia, bacillary hemoglobinuria, and black disease are acquired by ingestion.

Wounds. *C. tetani, C. chauvoei* (sheep), *C. septicum*, and other gas gangrene (myonecrosis) organisms infect wounds.

Morphology

The disease-producing clostridia are motile (except for *C. perfringens*) and nonencapsulated. They are relatively large rods with rounded ends, occurring singly, in short chains, or as long filaments. Endospores may be located centrally, subterminally, or terminally.

Cultivation

Most grow well on blood agar, in cooked meat medium, and in thioglycolate broth in an atmosphere devoid of oxygen. Oxygen is toxic in varying degrees to the clostridia. Some species are aerotolerant, whereas others, such as *C. novyi*, are particularly sensitive to oxygen. Colonies are 1 to 3 mm in diameter, round or slightly irregular, slightly raised, granular, and transparent or translucent with fine filamentous margins. Special media are employed for toxin production.

RESISTANCE

The endospores of clostridia are resistant to physical influences and disinfectants. In this respect they are similar to the spores produced by *Bacillus anthracis,* e.g., 30 minutes of boiling may be required to kill the spores of *Clostridium botulinum;* 121° C in an autoclave for 20 minutes is lethal.

Clostridium chauvoei

Synonym. *Clostridium feseri.*

Disease. *C. chauvoei* causes blackleg.

Occurrence. *C. chauvoei* is widespread, but is more prevalent in certain geographic areas. It is found in the intestine and in normal tissues of some animals, including the livers of some apparently normal dogs and cattle. It is not as common in the soil as are some other clostridia.

Toxins.
1. Alpha toxin: hemolysin, necrotoxin.
2. Beta toxin: deoxyribonuclease.
3. Gamma toxin: hyaluronidase.
4. Delta toxin: hemolysin.

Pathogenesis. In blackleg, *C. chauvoei* is thought to enter the animal by ingestion or to be endogenous. The pathogen is carried by the blood to damaged muscle tissue, where it multiplies if conditions are anaerobic. *C. chauvoei* may enter wounds along with other organisms. The mixed infection and necrotic tissue provide an anaerobic milieu for *C. chauvoei,* which multiplies and produces its exotoxins and other metabolites. Bacteremia usually occurs late in the disease.

Pathogenicity. Blackleg in ruminants: cattle (usually 4 months to 2 years)—ingestion; may be endogenous; sheep and goats—wounds. The lesion is not always easy to find; it is dry, dark, has gas bubbles, and a rancid odor. There may be a bacteremia.

Immunity. Formalinized whole-broth cultures, usually alum precipitated, are used to produce life-long immunity. Protection is both antibacterial and antitoxic. A soluble heat-labile protective antigen is associated with the alpha toxin. Recovery from disease renders animals immune for life. A double bacterin contains *C. chauvoei* and *C. septicum.* Some products contain *C. novyi* type A, or *C. sordellii,* or both.

C. chauvoei is antigenically heterogeneous, although cross-protection among strains is considerable.

Clostridium septicum

Disease. *C. septicum* causes malignant edema.

Occurrence. It occurs worldwide and is found in the intestine and soil.

Toxins.
1. Alpha toxin: lethal, lecithinase, necrotizing and hemolytic.
2. Beta toxin: a deoxyribonuclease and leukocidal.
3. Gamma toxin: hyaluronidase.
4. Delta toxin: a hemolyzing and necrotizing factor.

Pathogenicity. The pathogenesis of *C. septicum* infection is similar to that of gangrene caused by *C. chauvoei.*

It affects horses, cattle, sheep, pigs, and occasionally other animals in the form of malignant edema or gas gangrene. The common portals of entry are wounds and compound fractures. A large expanding swelling involving skeletal muscles pits on pressure, is gelatinous and red, and has little gas.

In sheep, the disease braxy is associated with eating frozen succulent feed. It produces necrotic lesions and hemorrhagic edema of the abomasal and duodenal walls. It is mainly a European disease, although several cases have been reported in the United States.

In chickens, it produces gangrenous dermatitis.

Immunity. *C. septicum* is included in some multiple-component bacterins. The species is antigenically heterogeneous.

Clostridium haemolyticum

Synonym. *Clostridium novyi,* type D.

Disease. *C. haemolyticum* causes bacillary hemoglobinuria.

Occurrence. *C. haemolyticum* is probably worldwide wherever liver flukes occur. In the United States, it is found predominantly in the mountain valleys of Nevada, Montana, and several other western states, as well as along the Gulf of Mexico. Apparently it is not abundant in either the intestine or soil. Subclinical infections may occur in some animals, which may serve as carriers that shed organisms via the intestinal tract.

Toxins. Toxins include beta toxin, a phospholipase C, which is lethal, necrotizing, and in addition causes lysis of erythrocytes in vitro as well as in vivo. Other minor toxins are produced.

Pathogenicity. Infection with *C. haemolyticum* is limited to cattle and sheep, in which it causes bacillary hemoglobinuria or "red water." The mode of infection is by ingestion, with the organism probably reaching the liver hematogenously. Liver flukes result in infarction of branches of the portal vein. The organism can germinate and grow in the damaged anaerobic tissue, where it produces its toxin. The infarct is usually 5 to 20 cm in diameter. The disease does not appear in areas where conditions are not favorable for the flukes or the snails.

Death is apparently brought about by lysis of erythrocytes by the toxin, and the animal perishes of anoxia. The disease appears to be produced by a single enzyme, phospholipase C, acting upon a single substrate, the lecithoprotein complex of the surface of the erythrocyte.

Immunity and Control. The disease may be controlled by elimination of liver flukes through destruction of the carrier snails.

Formalized alum precipitated whole-broth cultures are used to produce an active immunity. Immunity is considered to be more antibacterial than antitoxic and is of relatively short duration. Animals at risk should be vaccinated every 6 months.

Strains are antigenically homogeneous.

Clostridium novyi

Synonym. *Clostridium oedematiens.*

The three types are: Type A—Gas gangrene: worldwide in man, cattle, and sheep; big head in rams. Type B—Black disease: has been reported in Oregon, Colorado, Montana; worldwide. Type C—Osteomyelitis in water buffaloes (Indonesia).

Occurrence. Worldwide where liver flukes occur. It has been identified in sheep in Colorado and Montana.

Toxins. Numerous exotoxins are produced, including some with lethal and necrotizing properties. Types A and B differ antigenically and with respect to their toxins. Serum protection tests in animals distinguish them.

Pathogenicity. Type A, which causes gas gangrene, is found in mixed infections with *C. chauvoei, C. septicum,* or *C. sordellii.* It is also seen in "big head," a disease of rams characterized by significant swelling of the head and neck that is edematous in nature. Damage caused by butting allows entrance of the organism into the subcutis of the head. "Big head" may be caused by other clostridia.

Type B causes black disease or infectious necrotic hepatitis in sheep and occasionally cattle. The mode of infection is oral, with the organism being carried to the liver via the blood. This is a localized infection of the liver, initiated by local tissue destruction resulting from the migration of young liver flukes. Toxin is produced in the local lesion and absorbed into the circulating blood, eventually producing death. Recovery is rare. Intense congestion of the blood vessels of the skin may result in blackening of the pelt. Cutaneous edema resulting from impairment of the heart may be present; it is usually sterile.

Type B *C. novyi* produces alpha and beta toxins. The beta toxin, like the beta toxin of *C. haemolyticum,* is phospholipase C. The alpha toxin is phage mediated.

Immunity and Control. Elimination of liver flukes by destruction of snails is required.

Formalinized bacterin and toxoid are of value. Type A is included in some bacterins for the prevention of gas gangrene infections.

Clostridium perfringens

Synonym. *Clostridium welchii.*

Disease. *C. perfringens* causes enterotoxemia.

Occurrence. *C. perfringens,* type A, is probably more widespread than any other potentially pathogenic bacterium. It is present in air, soil, dust, and manure and in water of lakes, streams, and rivers. It has been isolated from vegetables, milk, cheese, canned food, fresh meat, shellfish, and mollusks. It is constantly present in the intestinal contents of humans and animals and in their environment. Types B, C, D, and E strains are found less commonly in the intestinal tracts of animals.

Toxins and Antigens. *C. perfringens* produces at least 12 different toxins and antigens, some of which have important roles in the production of the various disease manifestations. The species is divided into types A to E on the basis of immunologic differences in the four major lethal necrotic toxins, alpha, beta, epsilon, and iota, as determined by protection tests in animals. The alpha toxin referred to later is the principal lethal toxin. Among the substances produced are lethal, necrotizing toxins, proteinase, hemolysins, collagenase, hyaluronidase, and deoxyribonuclease.

Some of the more important toxins and antigens are as follows:

Alpha. This is the principal lethal toxin (a phospholipase C) produced in varying amounts by all types of *C. perfringens.* In addition to being lethal, hemolytic, and necrotizing, it possesses the ability to split lecithin or lecithin-protein complexes.

Beta. This toxin is produced by strains of types B and C. In addition to its lethal properties, it is responsible for inflammation of the intestine and the partial loss of the mucosa. These properties are associated with the types causing enteritis in cattle, sheep, and humans.

Epsilon. Epsilon toxin is produced by strains of types B and D as a protoxin that is only slightly toxic, if at all. The protoxin is then converted to toxin by proteolytic enzymes, such as trypsin and pepsin, as well as those produced by the microorganism itself (kappa and lambda). This toxin is necrotizing and highly lethal.

Theta. Theta is a lethal, hemolytic, necrotizing toxin produced by strains of types A, B, C, D, and E.

Iota. This toxin is produced only by type E strains. Like epsilon, it is formed as a protoxin and is subsequently activated by proteolytic digestion.

Kappa. Kappa is a proteolytic enzyme that breaks down collagen. This toxin, produced by all types, is principally responsible for the softening and "pulping" of affected muscles.

Lambda. Lambda is a proteolytic enzyme produced by strains of types B and E and by some strains of type D. It differs from kappa in that it is without activity on native collagen, but it does attack gelatin, casein, and hemoglobin.

Mu. It has the property of hydrolyzing hyaluronic acid. It is produced by most strains of types A and B, and some of types C and D.

Nu. This toxin, which has the property of a deoxyribonuclease, is produced by all types except B. It is not considered important in disease production.

Enterotoxin. This toxin (MW 34,000) is produced primarily by type A strains; other types may or may not produce it. Toxigenic type A strains rank third behind *Salmonella* and *Staphylococcus aureus* as the cause of food poisoning in humans in the United States.

Pathogenicity.

Type A. Most widespread. Wound infection, gas gangrene, and food poisoning in humans (diarrhea: 6 to 24 hours after eating meat; not serious). These strains are especially heat resistant. Enterotoxemia has been reported in nursing lambs ("yellow lamb") and horses. This type has been recovered from the genital tract of breeding dogs with and without reproductive problems. It also causes ruminal and abomasal tympany and abomasal ulceration in neonatal calves, and necrotic enteritis and gangrenous dermatitis in fowls.

Type B. Type B causes dysentery in newborn lambs, which is primarily an enterotoxemia with significant enteritis and extensive ulceration. It does not occur in the United States or Australia.

This type also causes enterotoxemia in calves, sheep, goats, and foals.

Type C. Type C produces struck, an acute intoxication in adult sheep in England and Wales, and hemorrhagic enteritis in neonatal calves, foals, lambs, and young pigs. It is also responsible for enteritis necroticans, a serious disease of humans.

Type D. Type D causes enterotoxemia, "overeating disease," or "pulpy kidney" disease in sheep and goats of all ages, but particularly in feedlot sheep. It is a problem in lambs in feedlots. It is a true toxemia with little evidence of enteritis. Epsilon toxin is apparently produced in the upper intestine, and the protoxin is activated by tryptic enzymes.

Type E. Type E is found in uncommon enterotoxemia (dysentery) of lambs and calves.

Immunity and Control. Good management and feeding practices are important in prevention.

Immunity is primarily antitoxic rather than antibacterial. Immunization is practiced principally in sheep. Formalinized whole-broth cultures prepared from strains of type C and type D are used to produce an active immunity. Immunity may not last for more than 6 to 12 months unless booster injections are given.

In addition, antitoxins derived from horses that have been hyperimmunized against toxins produced by types B, C, and D *C. perfringens* are available. Passive immunization is protective for no longer than 2 to 3 weeks.

Toxoids and bacterins are used to protect against types B, C, and D enterotoxemia of lambs. Ewes are given 2 doses of toxoid 6 weeks before lambing. Lambs may be immunized with bacterin or toxoid during the first week of life if ewes were not immunized, and prior to entering feedlots.

C. perfringens antigens are sometimes included in multivalent clostridial bacterins.

Clostridium tetani

Occurrence. Spores of *C. tetani* are found throughout the world. It may be part of the normal flora of the soil, especially in the eastern part of the United States. It is less common west of the Mississippi River. It frequently has been isolated from the intestinal tract. It is probably not more common in horse manure. The horse, however, is more subject to hoof injuries and quite susceptible to tetanus.

Toxins. Two toxic substances are produced: a hemolysin (tetanolysin or cytotoxin) and a potent lethal toxin (tetanospasmin or neurotoxin). The hemolysin is responsible for areas of hemolysis around colonies on blood agar plates, whereas neurotoxin is responsible for the characteristic signs of tetanus.

Neurotoxin (tetanospasmin), which is a protein (MW 150,000), is highly toxic when injected parenterally; however, it is harmless if administered by mouth. Animals vary in their susceptibility to the toxin. Horses and humans are the most susceptible. One milligram of pure toxin contains about 100 million mouse-lethal doses.

Toxin is elaborated at the site of infection and passes directly to major nerves and then to the spinal cord; it may also travel via blood and lymph. The toxin binds almost irreversibly to the gangliosides of nerve cells, and as a result, antitoxin is ineffective. All strains produce only one antigenic type of neurotoxin. Once in the cord, it ascends to the medulla. The toxin acts at the inhibitory synapse, where it blocks the normal function of the inhibitory transmitter.

Pathogenesis and Pathogenicity. Spores usually germinate in dirty and neglected wounds with some necrosis (lowered oxidation reduction potential); infection is usually mixed. Toxin is elaborated at the wound site after spores germinate. Docking and castration wounds, umbilical infections (tetanus neonatorum), parturition (puerperal tetanus), dehorning, and ringing are among the circumstances that can contribute to tetanus.

Tetanus is sometimes described as ascending or descending based on the movement and distribution of the toxin. Descending tetanus is the most common form seen in horses and humans. The first sign to appear in horses involves the nictitating membrane followed by involvement of the muscles of the fore and hind limbs.

Humans and horses are most susceptible, followed by pigs. Cattle and sheep are next; it is rare in dogs; cats and poultry are resistant.

Tetanus is characterized clinically by convulsive contractions of voluntary muscles. In fatal cases, muscles throughout the body become involved. When death occurs, it results from spasms of muscles involved in respiration. In nonfatal tetanus, the spasms that involve fewer muscles gradually regress.

Immunity. Immunity can be considered almost totally antitoxic.

Strains possess different heat-stable and heat-labile antigens, and 10 serotypes have been reported on the basis of flagellar antigens.

Toxoid is of value and is widely used in horses. Antitoxin is employed prophylactically but is of questionable value therapeutically. Recovery from tetanus does not usually confer permanent immunity because so little toxin is produced.

Treatment and Prophylaxis. If indicated, surgical debridement of the wound or probable site of infection should be carried out. Antitoxin and penicillin are administered for prophylaxis. Toxoid may be administered at another site.

There is no effective and specific treatment for tetanus. Administration of antimicrobial drugs and antitoxin is of limited or no value. Active immunization with toxoid should be carried out. Nursing care with appropriate tranquilizers and sedation to prevent tetanic seizures is important. Mortality may be as high as 50% in generalized tetanus in humans and horses.

Clostridium botulinum

Occurrence. Spores of *C. botulinum* are frequently encountered in the soil. Ordinarily it does not take up residence in the intestine. Some cases of infant botulism have occurred, however, in which the toxin has been produced in the stomach or intestine. The type of *C. botulinum* may vary from one geographic area to another.

Toxins. Like other clostridial toxins, the exotoxins of *C. botulinum* are heat-labile proteins (100° C for 10 minutes).

Eight types of neurotoxin (A, B, Cα, Cβ, D, E, F, and G) have been identified on the basis of antigenic differences. The toxins have been purified and are the most potent toxic substances known. One milligram of neurotoxin contains more than 120 million mouse lethal doses. Less than 1μg of toxic polypeptide preparation is lethal for man.

The toxins, usually produced in foods, are absorbed from the intestinal tract. The toxin is released when the organisms die and undergo lysis. Unlike most other toxins, they are resistant to peptic and tryptic digestion. After absorption, the toxin is transported to susceptible neurons via the bloodstream. It appears to be specifically directed to the peripheral nerves and does not affect other body cells. It does not abolish conduction in the motor nerves but rather prevents the passage of impulses from the nerve to the muscle. The action may be concerned with inhibition of the release of acetylcholine. There is no evidence that the toxin affects the nerve cells of the brain. Paralysis is ascending, and death is caused by circulatory failure and respiratory paralysis, as a result of the action of the toxin on motor nerves.

Pathogenicity. The principal media for the production of botulinum toxins are various spoiled foods, e.g., canned vegetables, forage, meat, and fish. The toxin also may be produced in animal carcasses that dogs, chickens, and other animals may eat. Botulism in mink (types A, B, and C) has been traced to spoiled meat, including whale meat. There are considerable differences in the potency of the various types of toxin.

Type C botulism occurs in cattle, sheep, turtles, chickens ("limberneck"), and wild fowl, particularly water fowl that have eaten rotting vegetation. Forage (spoiled oat, hay, silage) poisoning of horses has been claimed to be type C botulism. Type Cα primarily affects birds and turtles. Type Cβ toxicosis is seen mainly in cattle, sheep, and horses.

Type D botulism causes "lamziekte" or "loin disease" in cattle with pica (phosphorus deficiency) in South Africa, Texas, South America, and probably other regions. The toxin is produced in bones and tissues of dead animals as a result of the growth of *C. botulinum* in carcasses. Hungry animals eat toxin-containing bones and tissue. The disease is seen most frequently during droughts, when the pasture is poor. Sheep are also susceptible to this toxin type.

Types A, B, E, and F have been reported most commonly in humans. Type E toxin is greatly potentiated by tryptic digestion in the intestinal tract. Rare cases of type B botulism have been reported in cattle and horses. A disease called shaker foal syndrome has been attributed to types A and B.

Type G outbreaks have not been reported.

Wounds and infant botulism occasionally occur in humans. In infants, the toxin is produced in the gastrointestinal tract.

Many clinical diagnoses of botulism are not confirmed in the laboratory.

Immunity. As in tetanus, immunity is almost totally antitoxic. Immunization is not widely practiced in the United States. Toxoids have been used principally in cattle and mink, with success in some parts of the world. Bivalent or trivalent antitoxins are available for prophylactic use. They are of questionable value after clinical signs have appeared.

Control. This involves avoiding spoiled or otherwise suspicious food. Cooking at 100° C for 10 minutes destroys the toxin.

Treatment and Prophylaxis. Treatment of botulism requires early tracheotomy and intravenous administration of antitoxin. Animals that have consumed toxin and have not developed clinical signs should, if feasible, be given the appropriate antitoxin.

Other Clostridia

C. spiroforme. The organism is considered to be the cause of spontaneous and antibiotic-associated diarrhea and colitis in rabbits and guinea pigs. Naturally occurring enterocolitis has been reported in foals and swine.

C. bubalorum. This clostridium is closely related, if not identical, to *C. novyi* type B and has been associated with osteomyelitis in buffaloes in Indonesia.

C. sordellii (bifermentans). *C. sordellii* has been reported to cause gas gangrene in cattle and enterotoxemia in cattle and foals.

C. colinum. This species is the cause of an acute or chronic ulcerative enteritis of quail, young turkeys, grouse, partridge, and other game birds.

C. difficile. *C. difficile* is responsible for pseudomembranous colitis in humans and ileocecitis in laboratory animals on prolonged antibiotic regimens. It causes hemorrhagic necrotizing enterocolitis in swine and foals. Chronic diarrhea in dogs also has been reported. Two antigenically different toxins, A (enterotoxin) and B (cytotoxin), have been identified. Toxin B is more potent than A; both are cytotoxic and found in fecal specimens.

C. sporogenes. Although ordinarily a nonpathogen, *C. sporogenes* occurs occasionally along with other bacteria in clostridial gas gangrene, causes enterotoxemia in rabbits, and is possibly involved in the causation of cerebrocortical necrosis (polioencephalomalacia) of ruminants by virtue of its production of thiaminase in the intestine and rumen.

C. villosum. This organism has been isolated from fight wounds and pyothorax in cats. It is probably part of the normal oral flora of the cat.

LABORATORY DIAGNOSIS

GAS-GANGRENE-TYPE DISEASES (ANAEROBIC MYOSITIS)

Specimens. Should be from affected muscles and should be fresh. Because clostridia of the type that cause gas gangrene invade tissues from the intestine shortly after death, isolation or demonstration of these organisms is not always significant. This is especially so with *C. septicum* and *C. perfringens.*

C. chauvoei. Isolation and identification. Animal inoculation: guinea pigs die within 48 hours; however, rabbits are resistant. A reliable direct fluorescent antibody (FA) procedure is available for identification of organisms in tissues or cultures.

Table 14–1. *Neutralization Reactions between* **Clostridium perfringens** *Toxins and Antitoxins*

Type	Major Lethal Toxins	Antitoxins				
		A	B	C	D	E
A	Alpha	+	+	+	+	+
B	Alpha, beta, epsilon	–	+	–	–	–
C	Alpha, beta	–	+	+	–	–
D	Alpha, epsilon	–	+	–	+	–
E	Alpha, iota	–	–	–	–	+

+, toxin neutralized mice protected.
–, no neutralization mice die.

C. septicum. Isolation and identification. Animal inoculation: lethal for guinea pigs; rabbits are susceptible. Long chains of filaments are seen in impression smears from the tissues of guinea pigs and rabbits. An FA procedure similar to that for *C. chauvoei* is available.

Other clostridia that occasionally cause gas gangrene, such as *C. novyi*, type A (FA available), *C. sordellii*, and *C. perfringens*, type A, are isolated and identified by conventional procedures.

BACILLARY HEMOGLOBINURIA AND BLACK DISEASE

Specimens. These should be taken from affected liver tissue.

C. haemolyticum. Isolation and identification. An FA procedure is available.

C. novyi type B. Isolation and identification. The FA procedure does not distinguish between types. This type is also difficult to isolate.

CLOSTRIDIAL ENTEROTOXEMIA

Specimens. Fresh, small intestinal contents. Refrigerate.

C. perfringens. In cases of enterotoxemia, many large gram-positive organisms usually are seen in smears from the small intestine.

First, determine if the intestinal content is toxic for mice intravenously. If it is, mice are injected with mixtures of sterile (filtered) or antibiotic-treated intestinal contents and *C. perfringens* type sera. The tests also may be carried out in the skin of guinea pigs. The type of *C. perfringens* involved is determined by the protection pattern observed (Table 14–1).

Isolation and identification can also be carried out. All toxigenic strains of *C. perfringens* produce the lethal alpha toxin (phospholipase C), which can be identified by the Nagler reaction. The Nagler reaction is an opalescence shown in a special medium produced by the neutralization of the toxin by antitoxin. The type is determined by animal protection tests using toxin produced (if toxic) in a broth culture. Not all strains are toxigenic. *C. perfringens* produces few spores unless grown on special media and is nonmotile. Although characteristic, stormy fermentation in milk is not specific

Table 14–2. *Differentiation of Important Clostridia*

		Egg Yolk Agar					Fermentation				Principal
	Spores	Lecithinase	Lipase	Milk	Gelatin Hydrolysis	Indole	Glucose	Maltose	Lactose	Sucrose	Fermentation Products
C. perfringens	ST	+	–	S	+	–	+	+	+	+	A, B
C. chauvoei	ST	–	–	C	+	–	+	+	+	+	A, B
C. septicum	ST	–	–	C	+	–	+	+	+	–	A, B
C. novyi, A	ST	+	+	CG	+	–	+	+	–	–	A, P, B, V
C. novyi, B	ST	+	–	( )	+	( )	+	+	–	–	A, P, B, V
C. haemolyticum	ST	–	–	AC	+	( )	+	–	–	–	A, P, B, V
C. sordellii	ST	+	–	CD	+	+	+	+	–	–	A, F, P, IB, IV, IC
C. bifermentans	ST	+	–	CD	+	+	+	+	–	–	A, F, P, IB, IV, IC
C. sporogenes	ST	–	+	D	+	–	+	+	–	–	A, P, IB, IV, V, IC
C. histolyticum	ST	–	–	CD	+	–	–	–	–	–	A
C. botulinum:											
Group 1	ST	–	+	(C)(D)	+	–	+	+	–	–	A, P, IB, B, IV, V, IC
Group 2	ST	–	+	(C)	+	–	+	+	–	–	A, B
Group 3	ST	( )	+	(C)(D)	+	–	+	( )	–	–	A, P, B
C. tetani	T	–	–	( )	+	( )	–	–	–	–	A,P,B
C. difficile	ST	–	–	–	+	–	+	–	–	–	A, B, IC, IV, IB
C. colinum	ST	–	–	–	–	–	+	+	–	+	A, F, P

A, acid (milk); A, acetic acid (fermentation product); B, butyric; C, curd; D, digestion; F, formic; G, gas; IB, isobutyric; IC, isocaproic; IV, isovaleric; P, propionic; S, stormy fermentation; ST, subterminal; T, terminal; V, valeric; ( ), variable.

for *C. perfringens*. DNA probes specific for genes that are responsible for toxins currently are being evaluated. A latex test for detecting type A enterotoxin is available commercially.

TETANUS

Specimens. Material from wound site.

C. tetani. Diagnosis is usually based on clinical signs. Isolation of the organism is not usually attempted. Organisms cannot always be demonstrated. Not all cultures of *C. tetani* are toxin producers. Characteristic "drumstick" spores (terminal) are produced. Swarming is seen in agar cultures.

BOTULISM

Specimens. Suspected food, meat, forage, urine, and serum.

C. botulinum. Extracts of food or forage are inoculated into guinea pigs or mice to determine whether or not toxin is present. If this material is toxic, protection tests are carried out using the extract and type antitoxins in guinea pigs or mice to determine the type involved. Food is fed to the test species. The organism often can be recovered from food and typed.

If the level of toxin is high in an animal, it sometimes can be demonstrated in urine and serum by mouse inoculation.

IDENTIFICATION OF CLOSTRIDIA IN GENERAL

The determination of the metabolic end products produced in glucose broth by gas chromatography is helpful in the final identification of some species. Criteria of the kind listed in Table 14–2 are also used.

TREATMENT

Penicillin and broad-spectrum antibiotics are effective if given early in the gas gangrene diseases and bacillary hemoglobinuria. In blackleg, all cattle of a susceptible age in a group or herd should be treated. Treatment is of little value in the enterotoxemias and black disease.

FURTHER READING

Abbitt, B., et al.: Catastrophic losses in a dairy herd attributed to type D botulism. J. Am. Vet. Med. Assoc., *185*:798, 1984.

Berkhoff, H.A.: *Clostridium colinum* sp. nov., nom rev., the causative agent of ulcerative enteritis (quail disease) in quail, chickens, and pheasants. Int. J. Syst. Bacteriol. *35*:155, 1985.

Berry, A.P., and Levett, P.N.: Chronic diarrhea in dogs associated with *Clostridium difficile* infection. Vet. Rec. *118*:102, 1986.

Blackwell, T.E., et al.: Differences in signs and lesions in sheep and goats with enterotoxemia induced by intraduodenal infusion of *Clostridium perfringens* type D. Am. J. Vet. Res. *52*:1147, 1991.

Borriello, S.P., and Carman, R.J.: Association of iota-like toxin and *Clostridium spiroforme* with both spontaneous and antibiotic-associated diarrhea and colitis in rabbits. J. Clin. Microbiol. *17*:414, 1983.

Divers, T.J., et al.: *Clostridium botulinum* type B toxicosis in a herd of cattle and a group of mules. J. Am. Vet. Med. Assoc. *188*:382, 1986.

Durakhashan, H., and Lauerman, C.H.: Some properties of the beta toxin produced by *Clostridium haemolyticum* strain IRP135. Comp. Immunol. Microbiol. Infect. Dis. *4*:307, 1981.

Hatheway, C.L., and McCroskey, L.M.: Examination of feces and serum for diagnosis of infant botulism in 336 patients. J. Clin. Microbiol. *25*:2334, 1987.

Holdeman, L.V., Cato, E.P., and Moore, W.E.C.: Anaerobic Laboratory Manual. 4th Ed. Blacksburg, VA, Anaerobe Laboratory, Polytechnic Institute and State University, 1977 (Updated 1987).

Jones, R.L., et al.: Hemorrhagic necrotizing enterocolitis associated with *Clostridium difficile* infection in four foals. J. Am. Vet. Med. Assoc. *193*:76, 1988.

Kinde, H., et al.: *Clostridium botulinum* type C-intoxication associated with consumption of processed alfalfa hay cubes in horses. J. Am. Vet. Med. Assoc. *199*:742, 1991.

Laird, W.J., et al.: Plasmid associated toxigenicity of *Clostridium tetani*. J. Infect. Dis. *142*:623, 1980.

Lamana, C., and Sakaguchi, G.: Botulinal toxins and the problem of nomenclature of simple toxins. Bacteriol. Rev. *35*:242, 1971.

Love, D.N., et al.: Isolation and characterization of bacteria from pyothorax (empyaema) in cats. Vet. Microbiol., *7*:455, 1982.

Lyerly, D.M., Krivan, H.C., and Wilkins, T.D.: *Clostridium difficile:* Its disease and toxins. Clin. Microbiol Rev. *1*:1, 1988.

MacLennan, J.D.: The histotoxic clostridial infections of man. Bacteriol. Rev. *26*:177, 1962.

Niilo, L.: *Clostridium perfringens* in animal diseases: a review of current knowledge. Can. Vet. J. *21*:141, 1980.

Oakley, C.L., and Warrack, G.H.: Routine typing of *Clostridium welchii*. J. Hyg. *51*:102, 1953.

Perrin, J., et al.: *Clostridium difficile* associated with typhlocolitis in an adult horse. J. Vet. Diagn. Invest. *5*:99, 1993.

Roberts, T.A., Keymer, I.F., Borland, E.D., and Smith, G.R.: Botulism in birds and mammals in Great Britain. Vet. Rec. *91*:11, 1972.

Smith, L.D.S.: The Pathogenic Anaerobic Bacteria. 3rd Ed. Springfield, IL, Charles C Thomas, 1984.

Smith, L.D.S.: Botulism. Springfield, IL, Charles C Thomas, 1977.

Sterne, M., and Battey, I.: Pathogenic Clostridia. London, Butterworths, 1975.

Sutter, V.L., et al.: Wadsworth Anaerobic Manual. 4th Ed. St. Louis, Star, 1985.

Thomas, R.J., Rosenthal, D.V., and Rogers, R.J.: *Clostridium* type B vaccine for prevention of shaker foal syndrome. Aust. Vet. J. *65*:78, 1988.

Weinstein, L.: Tetanus. N. Engl. J. Med. *289*:1293, 1973.

Wierup, M.: Equine intestinal clostridiosis. An acute disease in horses associated with high intestinal counts of *Clostridium perfringens* type A. Acta Vet. Scand. (Suppl.) *62*:1, 1977.

Williams, B.M.: Black disease of sheep: Observations on the disease in mid-Wales. Vet. Rec. *74*:1536, 1962.

Witchel, J.J., and Whitlock, R.H.: Botulism associated with feeding alfalfa hay to horses. J. Am. Vet. Med. Assoc. *199*:471, 1991.

15

Bacillus

PRINCIPAL CHARACTERISTICS

Species of the genus *Bacillus* are gram-positive (old cultures decolorize easily) large rods. They are aerobic (some are facultatively anaerobic), spore-forming, mostly catalase-positive, and fermentative or respiratory or both. Some do not attack sugars and most are motile.

There are many species. They are ubiquitous, occurring widely in the soil, air, dust, and water. They are among the most common laboratory contaminants. If clinical specimens, such as bovine milk samples, are not collected carefully, they are often contaminated with *Bacillus* species.

B. anthracis is the only important pathogen of animals and humans in the genus. Infrequent infections have been attributed to *B. cereus*, but animal disease caused by other species is rare.

Bacillus anthracis

HISTORICAL

Discovery of the bacillus that causes anthrax is credited to Davaine and Rayer (1863–1868). Koch fulfilled his postulates with *B. anthracis* in 1876–1877.

DISTRIBUTION

B. anthracis is found worldwide where anthrax spores are located. Anthrax organisms sporulate with greater frequency in low-lying marshy areas with a soil pH higher than 6. Apparently vegetative forms grow poorly if at all in the soil. Some regions of the Mississippi and Missouri River valleys har-

bor spores, and flooding disseminates them. Outbreaks have occurred, however, in other locations in the United States as well. Animals may become infected from contaminated soil, water, bone meal, oil cake, tankage, offal, carion birds, and wild animals.

MODE OF INFECTION

The microorganism is acquired by ingestion, inhalation, wounds, scratches, and through the skin. Mechanical transmission of *B. anthracis* by blood-feeding insects has been reported in humans.

PATHOGENESIS

In the past, death was attributed to the plugging of capillaries by the bacilli. Neither endotoxin nor exotoxin had been demonstrated, although it was apparent that animals died of toxemia. Exotoxin subsequently was found in the plasma of dead or dying animals.

The anthrax toxin is a complex consisting of three protein components, I, II, and III. Component I is the edema factor, component II the protective antigen, and component III the lethal factor. Components I and II cause edema with low mortality; however, when component III is included, there is maximum lethality. Only encapsulated, toxigenic strains are virulent. The unique capsular polypeptide (poly D-glutamic acid) is antiphagocytic but does not elicit protective antibodies. The three components act synergistically to produce the toxic effects seen in anthrax. When virulent strains are grown in media containing serum or bicarbonate or both, they produce capsules and the colonies appear mucoid. In the absence of serum or bicarbonate, they fail to produce capsules and the colonies are rough. Virulent strains harbor two large plasmids that code for the capsule and the exotoxin.

The spores usually enter through the skin or mucous membranes and germinate at the site of entry. In the septicemic form, the vegetative bacilli spread via the lymphatics to the bloodstream. Death is attributed to respiratory failure and anoxia caused by the toxin. In the more localized form, as seen in swine, the infection may principally involve the lymph nodes of the head and neck. Large numbers of bacilli are shed from the orifices of animals during the terminal stage.

PATHOGENICITY

The organism is generally classed as an obligate pathogen. Peracute, acute, subacute, chronic, and cutaneous forms of the disease are seen. The more acute infections occur in cattle, sheep, horses, and mules. The cutaneous form is occasionally seen in horses and cattle when wounds or abrasions become infected.

Swine. The disease is usually subacute and may result in pharyngitis with extensive swelling and hemorrhage of the mouth and throat. An intestinal form with gastroenteritis also occurs. Chronic infection with localization in the tonsils and lymph nodes of the cervical region is frequent.

Dogs and Cats. A rare infection resembling that seen in swine.

Humans. Depending on the portal of entry, the forms seen in humans are pulmonary anthrax, malignant carbuncle or pustule (>90% of cases), and intestinal anthrax.

DIRECT EXAMINATION

To prevent sporulation, diseased animals should not be opened. Cremation or deep burial (at least 6 feet) in lime (calcium oxide) is recommended for disposal.

Smears from tissues or blood are made and stained with Gram, Giemsa's, or Wright's stain; the capsule stains a reddish-mauve. The finding of large, square-ended, gram-positive rods suggests the possibility of anthrax. It should be kept in mind that clostridial organisms are frequently found in the blood and tissues shortly after death. They can be eliminated in the differential diagnosis because they are not capsulated and because they fail to grow aerobically.

SPECIMENS

Septicemic form (cattle, sheep, horses, and possibly other species): swabs from exuded blood or blood taken by syringe. Blood smears may also be submitted.

Localized form (swine): swabs from the cut surface of hemorrhagic lymph nodes or fluid aspirated from affected lymph nodes are preferred.

ISOLATION AND CULTIVATION

If tissues are submitted, a composite suspension is prepared with a Ten Broeck grinder or mortar and pestle using sterile physiologic saline or broth as a diluent.

The organism grows well on all laboratory media. Guinea pigs and mice are inoculated from suspensions or blood and usually begin to die within 24 hours; large capsulated rods can be demonstrated in smears from the spleen and blood.

Colonies appear in 24 hours. They look rough, flat, and grey, and usually are nonhemolytic. Some are called Medusa-heads or "judge's wig"-type colonies; the wavy edge of the colony resembles a tangled mass of curly hair. Colonies are rough, smooth, and mucoid; the rough variant, which consists of capsulated organisms, is the most virulent.

Other *Bacillus* species, especially *B. cereus*, resemble *B. anthracis*.

IDENTIFICATION

Identification of *B. anthracis* is based on the following:

1. Pathogenic for guinea pigs and mice.
2. Characteristic colony morphology; gram-positive rods; spore-formers. Spores centrally located.
3. Nonmotile and aerobic. Most other "anthracoids" are motile.
4. Virulent cultures encapsulated; square ends.
5. *B. anthracis* isolates produce rough colonies in the absence of increased CO_2, but develop mucoid colonies on bicarbonate or serum-enriched media in an atmosphere of 5% CO_2.

B. anthracis may be distinguished from *B. cereus* as follows:

B. anthracis	B. cereus
Nonmotile	Motile*
Salicin utilization: slow or not at all	Rapid
Methylene blue reduction: slow	Rapid
Gelatin liquefaction: slow	Rapid
Slight or no hemolysis	Hemolytic
Penicillin-susceptible (some exceptions)	Not susceptible
Virulent strains: encapsulated	Not encapsulated

*nonmotile strains occur

String of Pearls Test. This test produces characteristic growth showing cell wall impairment of *B. anthracis* in a medium containing penicillin.

Bacteriophage. A preparation of specific phage (gamma phage) is added to a diffusely inoculated plate of suspected *B. anthracis* culture. Only *B. anthracis* is lysed.

Fluorescent antibody may be used to presumptively identify *B. anthracis*.

In addition to the differential characteristics previously listed, *B. cereus* is not capsulated. In the past, most *Bacillus* isolates could not be identified to species. The API 50 CH test strip along with the API 20E test strip now allows identification of as many as 38 species and subspecies.

ANTIGENIC NATURE AND SEROLOGY

Strains appear to be antigenically identical.

RESISTANCE

The endospores of *B. anthracis* are considerably more resistant to physical influences and chemical disinfectants than are vegetative cells. They may survive at least 22 years in dried cultures; they remain viable in soil for many years; and freezing temperatures have little if any effect on them. They are destroyed, however, by boiling for 10 minutes and by exposure to dry heat at 140° C for 3 hours. When used, most chemical disinfectants must be employed in high concentrations over long periods of time. Spores are destroyed by lye in 8 hours; by 5% phenol in 2 days; by 10 to 20% formalin in 10 minutes; and by autoclaving at 121° C for 15 minutes. Mercuric chloride 1:1000 added to heat-fixed smears kills in 5 minutes. Wool, hides, and horse hair from areas where anthrax occurs should be gas sterilized.

TREATMENT

Sick animals should be treated and well animals should be immunized. The organism is susceptible to penicillin, tetracyclines, gentamycin, streptomycin, enrofloxacin, erythromycin, and chloramphenicol; the first two are commonly used. Treatment in humans is effective in the cutaneous infection but not usually in the pulmonary form.

IMMUNITY

Protective immunity is thought to be largely antitoxic.

Active immunity can be produced in several ways:

1. Attenuated two-stage spore vaccine: Pasteur strains grown to sporulate. No longer used.
2. Avirulent spore vaccine: Sterne's noncapsulated strain gives good protection and has replaced Pasteur's spore vaccine.
3. Several nonliving vaccines containing "protective antigen" have been developed to protect workers at high risk.

CONTROL

In most states and countries, all suspected cases of anthrax must be reported to government veterinary officials.

PUBLIC HEALTH SIGNIFICANCE

Necropsies on animals must be performed with great care, particularly if there is a likelihood that death was caused by anthrax.

Infections most often result from spores entering injuries to the skin. Cutaneous anthrax (malignant pustule) accounts for more than 95% of the human disease. Some sources of spores for humans are soil, hair, hides, wool (wool sorter's disease), feces, milk, meat (inadequately cooked), and blood products.

The skin lesion is usually solitary, painless, seropurulent, necrotizing, hemorrhagic, and ulcerous. It leaves a black eschar, which accounts for the name malignant pustule.

The disease is seen most frequently in farmers, herdsmen, butchers, veterinarians, and tannery and slaughterhouse workers. Failure to diagnose human anthrax correctly can result in death.

ADDITIONAL *Bacillus* SPECIES

B. cereus has been incriminated as a cause of gangrenous bovine mastitis and abortion in cows and ewes. In humans, it has been implicated in food poisoning. Spores germinate in various foods, including fried rice, meats, desserts, sauces, and soups, where an enterotoxin or an emetic toxin may be produced. Two syndromes, the emetic and the diarrheal, are seen. The emetic type is caused by a heat-stable toxin and the diarrheal form by a heat-labile toxin.

B. subtilis is claimed to cause occasional conjunctivitis, iridocyclitis, septicemia, endocarditis, respiratory infections, and food poisoning in humans.

B. licheniformis has been implicated as a cause of bovine, ovine, and porcine abortions in a number of herds. It occasionally causes septicemia, peritonitis, and food poisoning in humans.

B. stearothermophilus spores are used to test the efficacy of autoclaving and other sterilizing procedures.

FURTHER READING

Ezzel, J.J., and Abshire, T.G.: Immunological analysis of cell-associated antigens of *Bacillus anthracis.* Infect. Immun. 56:349, 1988.

Fish, D.C., and Lincoln, R.E.: Biochemical and biophysical characterization of anthrax toxin. Fed. Proc. 26:1534, 1967.

Fox, M.D., et al.: Anthrax in Louisiana, 1971: Epizootiologic study. J. Am. Vet. Med. Assoc. 163:446, 1973.

Fox, M.D., et al.: An epizootiologic study of anthrax in Falls County, Texas. J. Am. Vet. Med. Assoc. 170:327, 1977.

Green, B.D., et al.: Demonstration of a capsule plasmid in *Bacillus anthracis.* Infect. Immun. 49:291, 1985.

Hambleton, P., Carman, J.A., and Melling, J.: Anthrax: the disease in relation to vaccines. Vaccine 2:125, 1984.

Hunter, L., Corbett, W., and Grindem, C.: Anthrax. J. Am. Vet. Med. Assoc. 194:1028, 1989.

Ivins, B.E., and Welkos, S.L.: Recent advances in development of an improved human anthrax vaccine. Eur. J. Epidemiol. 4:12, 1988.

Jackson, S.G.: Rapid screening test for enterotoxin-producing *Bacillus cereus.* J. Clin. Microbiol. 31:972, 1993.

Kaufmann, A.F., Fox, M.D., and Kalb, R.C.: Anthrax in Louisiana, 1971. An evaluation of the Sterne strain anthrax vaccine. J. Am. Vet. Med. Assoc. 163:442, 1971.

Kirkbride, C.A., et al.: Porcine abortion caused by *Bacillus* sp. J. Am. Vet. Med. Assoc. 188:1060, 1986.

Lincoln, R.J., Walker, J.S., Klein, F., and Haines, B.W.: Anthrax. Adv. Vet. Sci. 9:327, 1964.

Logan, N.A.: *Bacillus* species of medical and veterinary importance. J. Vet. Microbiol. 25:157, 1988.

Mikesell, P., et al.: Plasmids, Pasteur, and anthrax. Am. Soc. Microbiol. News 49:320, 1983.

Sterne, M.: Distribution and economic importance of anthrax. Fed. Proc. 26:1493, 1967.

Turnbull, P.C.B., and Kramer, J.M.: Bacillus. *In* Manual of Clinical Microbiology. 5th Ed. Edited by A. Balows. Washington, D.C., American Society for Microbiology, 1991.

Van Ess, G.B.: Ecology of anthrax. Science 172:1303, 1971.

Whitford, H.W.: Factors affecting the laboratory diagnosis of anthrax. J. Am. Vet. Med. Assoc. 173:1467, 1978.

Wohlgemuth, K., Bicknell, E.J., and Kirkbride, C.A.: Abortion in cattle associated with *Bacillus cereus.* J. Am. Vet. Med. Assoc. 161:1688, 1972.

16

Nonspore-forming Anaerobic Bacteria

The nonsporulating anaerobic bacteria constitute a large group of organisms that exist in nature and are present in large numbers, particularly in the intestinal tract of animals.

Many reports dealing with various infections in humans indicate that necrotic and suppurative processes frequently yield nonspore-forming anaerobic bacteria, either alone or with aerobic bacteria. Considerable evidence now shows that such is also the case with certain animal infections.

These bacteria can be isolated from various infectious processes in animals; however, they will not be recovered unless proper isolation techniques are used. Most of these infections are caused by one or more species of several of these anaerobic bacteria. Infections caused by these anaerobes usually also yield aerobes or facultative anaerobes. Lower tissue oxidation-reduction potential (Eh) favors the growth of these bacteria. Normal tissues have an Eh of +120 to +240 mV, whereas necrotic abscesses have an Eh of −250 to −150 mV. Since anaerobes do not survive in an Eh above −100 mV, they are usually associated with necrotic abscesses.

Knowledge of the extent and importance of infections in animals caused by these anaerobes is lacking mostly because they are difficult and expensive to isolate (e.g., because of oxygen sensitivity) and identify, and also because the infections are usually sporadic rather than multiple in occurrence. Improved procedures and techniques for the isolation and identification of members of this group have spurred much interest in this neglected area of veterinary bacteriology.

It should always be kept in mind that isolation of such organisms does not necessarily mean they are of pathogenic significance, any more than does the isolation of aerobic organisms necessarily mean they are significant.

Most of the disease-producing nonspore-forming, anaerobic, gram-negative bacteria causing disease in humans and animals are in the family Bacteroidaceae. This family also contains many species that are not pathogenic. Several of the more important and better-known species are listed here, as are some of the anaerobic gram-positive bacteria occasionally recovered from clinical specimens and infectious processes.

FAMILY BACTEROIDACEAE

Thirteen genera are listed in this family in *Bergey's Manual of Systematic Bacteriology*, Vol. 1. The correct taxonomic position of some of these genera is still questionable. Only two well-known genera, *Bacteroides* and *Fusobacterium*, are of veterinary significance. All are gram-negative rods that occur as normal flora of the intestinal tract, oropharynx, lower genitourinary tract, and skin of animals and humans.

Bacteroides

B. fragilis. This rod is isolated from the feces of humans and animals; it is the most important of

146

this group in humans. It occasionally causes intestinal infections in foals, pigs, calves, and lambs.

B. melaninogenicus. (*Prevotella melaninogenica*). It causes infections in humans and animals.

B. serpens. This species cause infections in humans.

B. nodosus. *B. nodosus* is responsible for contagious foot rot in sheep.

B. pneumosintes. This organism causes infections in humans.

B. corrodens (ureolyticus). *B. ureolyticus* causes infections in humans and animals.

B. asaccharolyticus. This species is implicated as the cause of osteomyelitis in dogs, cats, horses, and cattle.

B. levii. This has been associated with summer mastitis in cattle.

B. salivosus. This organism has been associated with subcutaneous abscesses and empyema in cats.

B. heparinolyticus. This has been associated with oral diseases of horses and cats.

Fusobacterium

F. necrophorum. This species produces many infections in animals and humans.

F. nucleatum. This species is associated with frequent infections in humans. Infections in animals are rare.

GRAM-POSITIVE ANAEROBIC COCCI

Gram-positive anaerobic cocci have been grouped in the following four genera: *Peptococcus*, *Peptostreptococcus*, some species of *Staphylococcus* and *Streptococcus*. *Peptococcus niger*, the only species of the genus, is rarely isolated from animals. In the genus *Peptostreptococcus*, *P. anaerobius* has been isolated from a variety of veterinary clinical specimens, and *P. indolicus* has been implicated as a cause of mastitis in cows. None of the anaerobic streptococci (three species) has been considered an animal pathogen. Aerotolerant streptococci (two species), however, have been recovered from veterinary clinical specimens. Their pathogenic significance is not always clear. The true taxonomic status of these aerotolerant cocci also remains unclear.

NONSPORE-FORMING GRAM-POSITIVE RODS

The most common nonspore-forming gram-positive organism isolated from animal infections currently is *Actinomyces pyogenes* (formerly *Corynebacterium pyogenes*). This species, which is facultatively anaerobic, is reviewed in Chapter 26.

A significant anaerobic pathogen is *Eubacterium suis*, the causal agent of cystitis and pyelonephritis in swine. This organism was formerly known as *Corynebacterium suis*. Boars appear to carry *Eubacterium suis* as normal flora in the preputial diverticulum and serve as the source of infection.

Members of the genus *Lactobacillus* are frequently isolated from animals, but they are not thought to have pathogenic significance. Species of *Propionibacterium* are usually associated with dairy products and the skin. These organisms are rarely recovered from clinical specimens; their clinical significance is not known.

HABITAT

Many of these anaerobes are commensals on mucous membranes of the upper respiratory, genital, and alimentary tracts of animals. They make up more than 90% of the bacteria of the intestinal tract, and they are predominant in the large bowel and in the rumen flora, where they have a vital role in digestion. Numerous species probably have not yet been identified.

INFECTIONS IN WHICH NONSPORE-FORMING ANAEROBES MAY BE INVOLVED

These organisms frequently invade tissues that are damaged and in which some necrosis provides a favorable anaerobic milieu for their growth. They also may be secondary to other primary infections. They are frequently recovered from:

1. Necrotic, gangrenous (often with clostridia), and suppurative processes. They may be foul-smelling.
2. Abscesses in the lung, liver, and brain; pyometritis; infrequently, cystitis and urinary tract infections; some postsurgical abscesses; diarrheal diseases; pneumonia; abortion; septicemias and bacteremias; foot rot of cattle and sheep; cellulitis; periodontal abscesses; guttural pouch infection; chronic sinusitis; and suppurative mastitis and osteomyelitis.

METHODS FOR THE ISOLATION AND CULTIVATION OF ANAEROBES

1. Anaerobic jars—Brewer, Torbal, and GasPak systems. These use catalysts to eliminate oxygen.
2. Anaerobic roll tube technique (Hungate method) using prereduced media. Air is excluded by means of "gassing" the media-lined tubes.
3. Glove box technique using prereduced media. Oxygen is excluded from the glove box. All operations are carried out in the glove box.

4. Media containing reducing agents, e.g., cooked meat media and thioglycolate broth.

Of utmost importance is the exclusion of oxygen from clinical specimens and cultures. Conventional swabs and other specimens not protected from oxygen are not satisfactory. Thus, special precautions must be taken in submitting specimens. Special anaerobic transport systems are available commercially. Fluid material can be submitted in a syringe, and some laboratories provide special tubes with oxygen excluded.

Specimens not in anaerobic transport systems should be kept at room temperature because oxygen absorption is greater at lower temperature. In addition, chilling is known to be harmful to some anaerobes. The maintenance of an anaerobic atmosphere for large specimens or tissue samples is not so critical.

Reference may have to be made to detailed differential tables for the precise identification of many species.

Fusobacterium necrophorum

Synonym. *Sphaerophorus necrophorus.*

Distribution and Mode of Infection. Distribution is worldwide. *Fusobacterium necrophorum* is a commensal in the alimentary tract and on mucous membranes. Infections are endogenous.

Antigens. Four biotypes of *F. necrophorum* have been described. Among them, biotype A is most frequently isolated in pure culture from bovine liver abscesses. Biotype B, which predominates in ruminal contents and ruminal lesions, is usually isolated in mixed infections from liver abscesses. Biotype A is more virulent than biotype B. Biotype AB is rarely isolated from animals, and its pathogenicity is intermediate to that of biotype A and biotype B. Biotype C strains are avirulent and their existence is somewhat questionable. Based on growth patterns, biologic and biochemical characteristics, and DNA analysis, biotypes A and B have been recently elevated to the rank of subspecies *necrophorum* and *funduliforme*, respectively. Although *F. necrophorum* is antigenically heterogeneous, little information is available on its serotypes. Using an immunodiffusion procedure, common antigens have been identified among strains of *F. necrophorum*.

Pathogenesis and Pathogenicity. *F. necrophorum* invades and multiplies in the anaerobic environment provided by damaged tissue. It is frequently a secondary invader. Infections are characterized by a necrotic process and are frequently mixed (e.g., liver abscesses in cattle, where

it is often found with *Actinomyces pyogenes*). Lesions are thought to be caused by, in part, a necrotizing endotoxin and a potent leukotoxin. *Fusobacterium necrophorum* produces a hemolysin, the significance of which is not known. In addition, *F. necrophorum* produces a variety of extracellular products, such as hemolysin, hemagglutinin, adhesins, platelet aggregation factor, proteases, and DNase. The pathogenic significance of these products is not clear. Capsulated strains of *F. necrophorum* are more virulent for mice than are noncapsulated strains.

F. necrophorum may be isolated from numerous infections initiated by a variety of wounds and injuries in all domestic animals. It is a common secondary invader in necrotic stomatitis, pharyngitis, and enteritis. Enteritis is seen most commonly in swine. The general term used for *F. necrophorum* infections is necrobacillosis.

Some of the better-known diseases with which *F. necrophorum* is associated in various animals follow.

Horse. It is usually involved in the infectious process called "thrush," involving the frog of the hoof. Infrequent cases of pneumonia and septicemia also have been reported.

Cattle. It is associated with metritis, cellulitis, mastitis, and calf diphtheria, and is found in necrotic foci in the mouth, larynx, and trachea. It is also seen in necrotic laryngitis in feeder cattle. *F. necrophorum* is the primary cause of liver abscesses and foot rot.

Sheep. It is a frequent secondary invader in lip and leg ulcerations (primary cause is the ulcerative dermatosis virus). In combination with *Actinomyces pyogenes*, it causes foot abscess (ovine interdigital dermatitis) and abortion.

Swine. It is considered the principal cause of "bull nose" resulting from the injury caused by "ringing" boars. It is a secondary invader in swine dysentery.

Fowl. It is involved in avian diphtheria, the primary cause of which is the fowl pox virus.

Human. *Fusobacterium necrophorum* has been recovered from a variety of infections, including abscesses in various organs, thrombophlebitis and oral lesions.

Specimens. Affected tissue and pus from abscesses. Specimens should be cultured immediately, or precautions must be taken to prevent exposure to oxygen. Material can be conveniently collected and submitted in a syringe.

Direct Examination. Gram-stained smears of affected tissues reveal gram-negative rods of variable length with long, characteristically beaded filaments.

Isolation and Cultivation. The organism is a strict anaerobe and grows best on enriched media. Two to four days of incubation are required. Many strains produce some L-forms on initial isolation. L-forms are cell-wall-deficient forms that resemble mycoplasmas in some respects.

Colonies are small, smooth, convex, and whitish-yellow in color, with a narrow zone of alpha- or beta-hemolysis. Initially cultures may be pleomorphic; short rods, long filaments, and "moniliform" bodies may be seen.

F. necrophorum can be recovered frequently in pure culture from bovine liver abscesses. Pus or caseous material is taken aseptically by syringe or pipette and inoculated into previously heated thioglycolate broth.

Identification. Definitive identification is made on the basis of differential characteristics of the kind listed in Table 16–1.

Treatment and Control. Surgical measures should be taken when indicated. Sulfonamides, penicillin, tetracyclines, and erythromycin have been effective against *F. necrophorum*. Susceptibility tests should be carried out. The aminoglycosides are ineffective. Tetracyclines and tylosin in feed have been found effective.

Vaccination against *F. necrophorum* infections has not been very successful. Toxoids have provided some protection in cattle.

Bacteroides nodosus

Synonym. *Fusiformis nodosus.*

General. This organism is a large gram-negative, nonmotile, anaerobic rod. The exact taxonomic position of this organism is not clear. Its placement in the genus *Dichelobacter* has been proposed. It is the primary cause of contagious foot rot of sheep. *Fusobacterium necrophorum* and *Actinomyces pyogenes* are common secondary invaders, and *Treponema penortha*, although present, is not pathogenic. *Bacteroides nodosus* can cause infections of the foot in goats, pigs, and cattle. Virulence appears to be associated with the production of proteolytic enzymes resulting in the breakdown of keratin. The disease is aggravated by moist environmental conditions.

Virulent strains of *B. nodosus* possess pili, which are thought to play a major role in the attachment and colonization of the epidermal matrix of the ovine hoof.

Antigens. Based on pilus antigens, ten (A, B1, B2, B4, C through H) serologically distinctive groups of *B. nodosus* have been identified with an agglutination test or an ELISA.

Direct Examination. Contagious foot rot of sheep can be diagnosed by the demonstration of the characteristic organism in gram-stained smears from typical lesions. Smears are made from material taken well down in the lesion after the horn has been pared away. The rods of *B. nodosus* may be straight or slightly curved and vary from 0.6 to 1.2 μm in length. They do not form spores and are gram-negative. When stained with Löffler's methylene blue, one, two, or more red-staining granules can be seen at either end or along the rod.

Treponema penortha can be seen in large amounts in positive smears as slender filaments displaying loose, irregular curves. The organism is gram-negative and stains faintly compared with the *Bacteroides nodosus* stain.

Isolation and Cultivation. Foot rot can be readily diagnosed by demonstration of the characteristic organisms in smears from typical lesions, and cultural procedures are not usually carried out. The isolation and identification procedures recommended for other gram-negative anaerobes are applicable to *B. nodosus*.

Table 16–1. *Differentiation of Some Important Gram-Negative, Nonspore-Forming Anaerobes*

Tests	Fusobacterium necrophorum	Fusobacterium nucleatum	Bacteroides fragilis	Bacteroides nodosus	Bacteroides melaninogenicus*
Nitrate	+	NK	–	–	–
Indole	+	+	–	–	–
Gelatinase	V	–	–	+	+
Esculin hydrolyzed	–	–	+	–	V
Growth in 20% bile	V	+	+	V	–
Black pigment	–	–	–	–	+
Acid from:					
Glucose	V	V	+	–	+
Lactose	–	–	+	–	+
Maltose	–	–	+	+	–
Sucrose	–	–	+	–	+
Major acid	B,P,A	B,P,A	A,S,P	A,S,P	A,S

*Current name *Prevotella melaninogenica*.
NK, not known; V, variable; B, butyric; A, acetic; P, propionic; S, succinic.

Identification. The necessary differential characteristics are listed in Table 16–1.

Treatment and Control. Foot trimming should be carried out prior to treatment. Formalin, copper or zinc sulfate foot baths and 10% tincture of chloromycetin are used. The organism does not survive for longer than 2 weeks in pastures. Systemic use of penicillin, tetracyclines, tylosin, erythromysin, and streptomycin is of value when accompanied by other control measures.

An oil-adjuvant *B. nodosus* bacterin has been shown to be useful in prevention, but it occasionally causes abscesses at the site of injection. Vaccines containing pilus antigens provide significant protection.

Bacteroides melaninogenicus

This saccharolytic organism, which produces a dark colonial pigment, has been reclassified recently as *Prevotella melaninogenica*. This species has been found in a considerable number of specimens from suppurative processes in cattle, sheep, dogs, and cats. It is frequently associated with *Fusobacterium necrophorum* in foot rot of cattle.

Bacteroides fragilis Group

This group was formerly made up of five subspecies, each of which has now been given species status. All are recovered from clinical specimens. *B. fragilis* is the most common anaerobe causing infections in humans. It is encountered occasionally in various anaerobic infections in domestic animals.

Some strains of *B. fragilis* produce enterotoxin, which causes accumulation of fluid in ligated intestinal loops of lambs and calves. Enterotoxigenic strains have been implicated as the cause of diarrheal diseases in calves, lambs, foals, piglets, and humans.

TREATMENT IN GENERAL OF GRAM-NEGATIVE ANAEROBIC INFECTIONS

Antimicrobial susceptibility tests should be carried out because antibiotic resistance and beta-lactamase production by some *Bacteroides* strains have been reported. If the organism is susceptible, penicillin is recommended. Other useful drugs are gentamicin, chloramphenicol, metronidizole, and clindamycin. Carbenicillin and the related drug ticarcillin, as well as cefoxitin (a cephalosporin), have been used in humans. Newer penicillins and cephalosporins are active against many gram-negative anaerobes. One must keep in mind that anaerobic infections are seldom caused by a single bacterial species. For this reason, a combination of antimicrobial agents is frequently recommended. Examples of such combination therapy include gentamicin-cephalosporin and gentamicin-penicillin.

FURTHER READING

Berg, J.N., and Evans, J.W.: Identification of common antigens in ribosome-rich extracts from *Fusobacterium necrophorum*. Am. J. Vet. Res. 46:127, 1985.

Berg, J.N., Fales, W.H., and Scanlon, C.M.: Occurrence of anaerobic bacteria in diseases of the dog and cat. Am. J. Vet. Res. 40:876, 1979.

Berkhoff, G.A., and Redenbarger, J.L.: Isolation and identification of anaerobes in the veterinary diagnostic laboratory. Am. J. Vet. Res. 38:1069, 1977.

Bulgin, M.S., et al.: Comparison of treatment methods for the control of contagious ovine footrot. J. Am. Vet. Med. Assoc. 189:194, 1986.

Collins, J.E., et al.: Exfoliating colitis associated with enterotoxigenic *Bacteroides fragilis* in a piglet. J. Vet. Diagn. Invest. 1:349, 1989.

Dow, S.W., and Jones, R.L.: Anaerobic infections. Part II. Diagnosis and treatment. The Compendium 9:827, 1987.

Egerton, J.R., et al.: Protection of sheep against footrot with a recombinant DNA-based fimbrial vaccine. Vet. Microbiol. 14:393, 1987.

Elleman, T.C., and Stewart, D.J.: Efficacy against footrot of a *Bacteroides nodosus* 265 (serogroup H) pilus vaccine expressed in *Pseudomonas aeruginosa*. Infect. Immun. 56:595, 1988.

Holdeman, L.V., Cato, E.P., and Moore, W.E.C.: Anaerobic Laboratory Manual. 4th Ed. Blacksburg, VA, Anaerobe Laboratory, Virginia Polytechnic Institute and State University, 1977 (Updated 1987).

Jousimies-Somer, H.R., and Finegold, S.M.: Anaerobic gram-negative bacilli and cocci. In Manual of Clinical Microbiology. 5th Ed. Edited by A. Balows, et al. Washington, D.C., American Society for Microbiology, 1991.

Kirkbride, C.A., Gates, C.E., and Libal, M.C.: Ovine and bovine abortion associated with *Fusobacterium nucleatum*. J. Vet. Diagn. Invest. 1:272, 1989.

Myers, L.L., and Shoop, D.S.: Association of enterotoxigenic *Bacteroides fragilis* with diarrheal disease in young pigs. Am. J. Vet. Res. 48:774, 1987.

Myers, L.L., Shoop, D.S., and Byars, T.D.: Diarrhea associated with enterotoxigenic *Bacteroides fragilis* in foals. Am. J. Vet. Res. 48:1565, 1987.

Nguhiu-Mwangi, J.A., and Gitao, C.G.: Acute cellulitis as a complication of footrot in cattle. Mod. Vet. Pract. 68:110, 1987.

Prescott, J.F.: Identification of some anaerobic bacteria in nonspecific anaerobic infections in animals. Can. J. Comp. Med. 43:194, 1979.

Prescott, J.F., and Chirino-Trejo, M.: Non-sporeforming anaerobic bacteria. In Diagnostic Procedures in Veterinary Bacteriology and Mycology. 4th Ed. Edited by G.R. Carter. Springfield, IL, Charles C Thomas, 1984.

Smith, L.D.S.: The Pathogenic Anaerobic Bacteria. 3rd Ed. Springfield, IL, Charles C Thomas, 1984.

Tan, Z.L., Nagaraja, T.G., and Chengappa, M.M.: Factors affecting the leukotoxin activity of *Fusobacterium necrophorum*. Vet. Microbiol. 32:15, 1992.

Walker, R.L., and MacLachlan, N.J.: Isolation of *Eubacterium suis* from sows with cystitis. J. Am. Vet. Med. Assoc. 195:1104, 1989.

17

Enterobacteriaceae

PRINCIPAL CHARACTERISTICS

Enterobacteria are gram-negative, aerobic, and facultatively anaerobic medium-sized rods. They are oxidase-negative, catalase-positive (there are some exceptions), nonspore-forming, fermentative (often with gas), and usually motile.

CLASSIFICATION

The classification of Enterobacteriaceae has undergone considerable change in recent years. Based on DNA-relatedness studies, the family now consists of 28 genera and more than 82 clearly defined species. Genera and species of Enterobacteriaceae are listed in Table 17–1.

HABITAT

The enterobacteria are worldwide in distribution. There are both potentially pathogenic and nonpathogenic species. Many of the enterobacteria are part of the normal flora of the intestinal tract.

Some species are free-living, occurring in soil and water. Fecal contamination of water is indicated by the presence of *Escherichia coli*. *Klebsiella* (including *K. pneumoniae*), *Enterobacter*, and *Citrobacter* species have been recovered from vegetables and wood products.

MODE OF INFECTION AND TRANSMISSION

This is almost always by ingestion. Fomites are especially important. Some infections are endogenous.

PATHOGENICITY

Clinical manifestations and pathologic changes may be partly the result of endotoxins. The entero-toxins of *Escherichia coli* are important in diarrheal diseases. Salmonellae and shigellae are frankly pathogenic. Such genera as *Proteus*, *Serratia*, *Klebsiella*, and *Enterobacter* are mostly opportunists that produce disease under certain circumstances, e.g., trauma to tissues (mastitis), debilitation, wounds, and malnutrition.

Escherichia

Escherichia coli is recovered from a wide variety of infections in many animal species. It may be a primary or secondary agent. Nursing and young animals are particularly susceptible, and urinary tract infections are frequent.

From the standpoint of pathogenic mechanisms and diseases, four major categories of *E. coli* are recognized (Table 17–2): enterotoxigenic (ETEC), enteropathogenic (EPEC), enteroinvasive (EIEC), and enterohemorrhagic (EHEC). In addition, two less-well-defined *E. coli* categories are recognized in animals and humans (Table 17–2): enteroaggregative and cytotoxin necrotizing factor-positive. The aforementioned categories are represented by different serotypes. Certain serotypes show a host preference and are encountered more frequently in some disease syndromes. Of the four major categories, ETEC is the most common cause of diarrhea in calves, lambs, and pigs. Strains in the other categories cause the less-common diarrheal and other disease syndromes.

Enterotoxins and pilus antigens are the two most prominent virulence factors thus far identified for ETEC. Two enterotoxins, one heat-stable (ST) and one heat-labile (LT), are produced by enterotoxigenic strains of *E. coli*; not all cultures produce

Table 17–1.   *Members of the Family Enterobacteriaceae**

Genus	Species	Genus	Species
Budvicia	aquatica	Providencia	alcalifaciens
Buttiauxella	agrestis		heimbachae
Cedecea	davisae		rettgeri
	lapagei		rustigianii
	neteri		stuartii
Citrobacter	amalonaticus	Rahnella	aquatitis
	diversus	Salmonella	Subgroup 1
	freundii		Most serotypes
Edwardsiella	hoshinae		S. choleraesuis
	ictaluri		S. gallinarum
	tarda		S. paratyphi
Enterobacter	aerogenes		S. pullorum
	agglomerans		S. typhi
	amnigenus		Subgroup 2
	asburiae		Subgroup 3a
	cancerogenus		Arizona group
	cloacae		Subgroup 3b
	dissolvens		Arizona group
	gergoviae		Subgroup 4
	hormaechei		Subgroup 5
	intermedium		Subgroup 6
	nimipressuralis	Serratia	entomophila
	sakazaki		ficaria
	taylorae		liquefaciena
Escherichia	blattae		marcescens
	coli		odorifera
	fergusonii		plymuthica
	hermanii		rubidaea
	vulneri	Shigella	boydii
Ewingella	americana		dysenteriae
Hafnia	alvei		flexneri
Klebsiella	planticola		sonnei
	pneumoniae	Tatumella	ptyseos
	ozaenae	Trabulsiella	guamensis
	rhinoscleromatis	Xenorhabdus	luminescens
	ornithinolytica		nematophilus
	oxytoca	Yersinia	aldovae
	terrigena		bercovieri
Kluyvera	cryocrescens		enterocolitica
	oscorbata		frederiksenii
Leclercia	adecarboxylata		intermedia
Leminorella	grimontii		kristensenii
	richardii		pestis
Moellerella	wisconsensis		pseudotuberculosis
Morganella	morgani		rohdei
Obesumbacterium	proteus		ruckeri
Pragia	fontium	Yokennella	regensburgii
Proteus	mirabilis		
	myxofaciens		
	penneri		
	vulgaris		

*Species of veterinary significance are discussed in the text. Some species are only rarely recovered from clinical specimens.

both of these plasmid-based enterotoxins. The ST is further divided into STa and STb, and the LT is further divided into LT-I and LT-II. The action of ST or LT toxin can be demonstrated in ligated intestinal segments, certain cell cultures, and suckling mice. The enterotoxin producers do not ordinarily invade, but their enterotoxin is adsorbed to epithelial cells. The LT stimulates adenylcyclase, resulting in conversion of ATP to cyclic AMP. Cyclic AMP induces the excretion of Cl^- and inhibits the adsorption of Na^+, causing great fluid losses. The two enterotoxins can be differentiated on the basis of their toxic, immunologic, physical, and chemical characteristics. Some of the properties of the two different enterotoxins are given in Table 17–3.

The letter K ordinarily stands for the surface or envelope antigen of enterobacteria (reviewed further on). In the case of K88 and K99 cultures of ETEC, these terms represent different pilus antigens. K88 cultures of ETEC are associated with diarrhea primarily in swine, and K99 cultures of ETEC with diarrhea primarily in calves.

Table 17–2. Designation and Important Characteristics of Diarrheagenic E. coli

Alpha Designation	Principal Disease	Invasive	Principal Virulence Factors
ETEC (Enterotoxigenic *E. coli*)	Diarrhea in calves, lambs, pigs, and humans.	–	Enterotoxins, Pili/adhesin
EPEC (Enteropathogenic *E. coli*)	Diarrhea in humans.	–	Cytotoxin, Pili/adhesin
EIEC (Enteroinvasive *E. coli*)	Diarrhea in humans.	+	Pili/adhesin?
EHEC (Enterohemorrhagic *E. coli*)	Diarrhea in humans and animals.	–	Verotoxins, Pili/adhesin
EAEC (Enteroaggregative *E. coli*)	Diarrhea in humans.	–	Pili/adhesin?
CNF-PEC (Cytotoxin Necrotizing Factor-positive *E. coli*)	Diarrhea in humans, calves, and pigs	–	Cytotoxin necrotizing factor

Table 17–3. Some Properties of Two Enterotoxins of Escherichia coli

	Heat-Stable (ST)	Heat-Labile (LT)
Calves	Most cases	Few cases
Pigs	Most cases	Most cases
Molecule	Very small; peptide	Large; protein
Heat stability	Resists 121° C/15 min	Destroyed by 60° C/30 min
Antigenicity	Negative	Positive
Antibody neutralization	Generally negative	Positive
Onset time and duration (ligated rabbit ileal loop)	Rapid and short	Slow and long
Adenyl cyclase activation	No	Yes
Guanylate cyclase activation	Yes	No
Tissue culture assay	Negative	Positive
Suckling mouse assay	Positive	Negative

Colonization of the small intestine by enterotoxigenic strains of *E. coli* depends on certain types of pili. Important pilus antigens of *E. coli* associated with diseases in domestic animals are:

Animal species	Pilus antigen
Swine	K88 or F-4
	K99 or F-5
	989P or F-6
	F-41
	Type 1*
Calves	K99 or F-5
	F-41
	Type 1*
Lambs	K99 or F-5
	F-41

*Occasionally.

The pilus antigens of ETEC that cause diarrhea in humans are referred to as colonization factor antigens (CFAs). Currently, the three antigenically distinct CFAs in ETEC are: CFA/I, CFA/II, and CFA/IV. These pilus antigens are antigenically distinct from those that are found on ETECs of animals.

The term enteropathogenic *E. coli* (EPEC) is used rather loosely in veterinary medicine to refer to *E. coli* strains that cause intestinal infection in animals. By definition, EPEC refers to specific serogroups recognized as causing diarrheal syndromes of humans. In animals, these strains attach to small intestinal epithelial cells and cause effacement of the microvilli. Mechanisms by which these strains pro-duce lesions are not fully understood. However, certain plasmid-coded virulence factors are known to be involved. EPEC does not produce LT and ST toxins. EPEC lack the invasiveness of EIEC strains.

As a general rule, the acute infections of neonatal animals characterized by bacteremia or septicemia are caused by invasive strains of *E. coli*; the diarrheal infections are caused by enterotoxin-producing strains. Invasiveness has been recognized as a distinct, but less common, pathogenic mechanism. Invasive *E. coli* (EIEC) strains can penetrate the intestinal epithelium, mainly that of the large intestine. These strains belong to a few serotypes and generally produce watery diarrhea. EIEC strains have both chromosomal and plasmid genes that are essential for virulence. They are not common in farm animals. Invasiveness can be detected by the capacity of a strain to cause keratoconjunctivitis in the eye of a guinea pig (Sereny test), or by its capacity to penetrate cells in tissue culture. Other tests, such as the enzyme-linked immunosorbent assay (ELISA) and DNA probe assay, are also available for the identification of EIEC strains.

Certain strains of *E. coli* (EHEC) produce shiga-like toxins (verotoxins) that are active in vero and HeLa cells. The variant of verotoxin Type 2 is suspected to play a role in the pathogenesis of edema disease in pigs and diarrhea in calves and rabbits. These *E. coli* strains attach to and efface the microvilli of the gut epithelium. They are also referred to as verotoxigenic *E. coli* (VTEC) or attaching and effacing *E. coli* (AEEC). More than 57 serotypes of EHEC have been recognized in humans and animals. EHEC do not synthesize LTs or STs, and they are not enteroinvasive. They colonize the intestinal mucosa by intimate attachment to and effacement of microvilli. Plasmid coded pili and verotoxins are the two most important virulence factors of these strains. Verotoxin types 1 and 2 are synonymous with shiga-like toxins I and II.

EHEC serotype 0157:H7 is the most important serotype associated with hemorrhagic colitis and hemolytic uremic syndrome in humans. In the United States, recent outbreaks of these diseases with some deaths have been traced to consumption of undercooked hamburgers. These EHEC strains are known to be present in the intestines of cattle; meat can be contaminated through contact with feces during slaughter.

Evidence for the presence of enteroaggregative *E. coli* as pathogens in domestic animals is currently lacking. Cytotoxin necrotizing factor-producing *E. coli* are infrequently associated with diarrhea in calves, pigs, and humans. Toxin and pili are thought to be the most important virulence factors of these strains.

Colibacillosis is a general term that denotes an *E. coli* infection characterized by one or more of the following: diarrhea, enteritis, septicemia, or bacteremia. Rota- and coronaviruses, bovine viral diarrhea virus, coccidia, and cryptosporidia may be involved as well.

Cattle. Infection with *E. coli* takes the form of neonatal calf scours or diarrhea occurring during the first 3 weeks of life. Dehydration is caused by enterotoxin(s). Colisepticemia with a course as short as 48 hours or mastitis occurs.

Swine. *E. coli* produces diarrhea in pigs a few days old, and significant dehydration is caused by enterotoxin(s). Hemorrhagic gastroenteritis and edema disease may occur 1 to 2 weeks after weaning. The edema of edema disease has been attributed to verotoxin.

Chickens and Turkeys. Colibacillosis is seen in turkeys and chickens. The organism enters the bloodstream via the respiratory tract and causes acute septicemia. Other conditions associated with colibacillosis in chickens and turkeys include airsacculitis, Hjarre's disease or coligranuloma, and fibrinopurulent serositis. Coligranuloma is a chronic condition characterized by granulomatous lesions in the epithelium of the intestine and other organs.

Lambs. *E. coli* causes diarrhea in lambs similar in pathogenesis to that in calves and pigs. *E. coli*

with K99 pilus antigen is the most common serotype associated with diarrhea in lambs.

Other animals. *E. coli* causes urinary tract infections in dogs and cats, pyometra in bitches, and enteritis in young dogs. Foals are highly susceptible to *E. coli* infection; deaths can reach as high as 25%. *E. coli* also has been implicated in abortions in mares, enteritis in foals, and metritis in mares. Nonenterotoxigenic *E. coli* (attaching and effacing) causes severe enteritis in rabbits.

Edwardsiella

Edwardsiella tarda is recovered occasionally from the intestinal tract of animals and humans. A few opportunistic infections have been reported in humans and animals.

E. tarda has been implicated as the cause of diarrhea, wound infections, and sepsis in animals and humans. *E. tarda* and *E. ictaluri* are common pathogens of catfish.

Enterobacter

Strains of this group, *Klebsiella*, and *E. coli* are referred to as coliforms.

Strains of *Enterobacter* are only occasionally incriminated in animal disease. *E. cloacae* and *E. aerogenes* are opportunistic pathogens. The most common infection they produce is bovine mastitis. *E. sakazaki* is known occasionally to cause meningitis and sepsis in human neonates.

Klebsiella

Klebsiella strains have been recovered from various animal infections, such as pneumonia and suppurative infections in foals; cervicitis and metritis in mares; mastitis in cows; wound infections; urinary infections, particularly in dogs; and septicemia and pneumonia in dogs. Most of the strains recovered from clinical specimens are *K. pneumoniae*. *Klebsiella* organisms are associated with wood products used as bedding for cattle. *Klebsiella* mastitis is more common when cows are kept on such bedding.

Morganella

M. morganii (formerly *Proteus morganii*) is a well-recognized human pathogen. It has been associated with ear and urinary tract infections in dogs and cats.

Proteus

Proteus mirabilis has been implicated in a variety of sporadic infections of dogs, cats, cattle, and fowl. Cystitis and urinary infections are the most common, particularly in dogs and ponies. On occasion,

Proteus species are thought to be involved in diarrhea in young mink, lambs, calves, goats, and puppies. *Proteus* species occasionally are involved in ear infections in dogs and cats.

Providencia

Species of this genus rarely cause animal infections. *P. heimbachae* has been isolated from penguin feces and from an aborted bovine fetus; its significance is not known.

Salmonella

Infection is by the oral route. Unlike the other enteric bacteria, except for *Yersinia,* the salmonellae are frequently facultative intracellular parasites. The invasive strains are taken up by macrophages, and spread is via the lymphatic system, bloodstream, or both. Three principal forms of salmonellosis are described as occurring in humans: enteric fevers, septicemia, and gastroenteritis. The forms seen in animals are principally peracute septicemia, acute enteritis, subacute enteritis, and chronic enteritis. An asymptomatic carrier state is common.

More than 2000 different serovars have been identified, all of which are potentially pathogenic, causing sporadic infections as well as outbreaks of frequently fatal disease.

The classification of the *Salmonella-Arizona* group has undergone several changes in recent years. On the basis of differences in biochemical reactions, antigenic nature, host adaptations, geographic distributions, and DNA-relatedness, the salmonellae have been placed into 7 subgroups. Most serovars that are isolated from clinical specimens of humans and warm-blooded animals are in subgroup 1. Other subgroups contain strains that are usually isolated from the environment and from cold-blooded animals. Strains in subgroup 1 are highly pathogenic; strains in other subgroups are relatively less pathogenic to animals and humans. Based on DNA hybridization studies, the subgroup 3 has been further subdivided into subgroup 3a and subgroup 3b. The *Arizona* serovars are included in subgroups 3a and 3b. This subdivision correlates with differences in the flagellar antigen and the speed of lactose fermentation.

On the basis of biochemical characteristics, salmonellae have been grouped into three species (Table 17–4): *S. choleraesuis, S. typhi,* and *S. enteritidis.* In this classification, *S. enteritidis* includes all the serotypes that are known today. Grouping of all *Salmonella* serotypes under one species also has been suggested recently. For simplicity and convenience, we choose to recognize all the named serotypes of *Salmonella* as species. Thus, *Salmonella* serotype *choleraesuis* is simply written *Salmonella choleraesuis;* likewise, serotype *newport* is written *Salmonella newport.* This classification is used more commonly than the one introduced recently (subgroups 1 to 7). The *Salmonella* serovars can be subdivided into biovars based on differences in biochemical patterns within a serovar, e.g., *S. choleraesuis* biovar *kunzendorf.*

The *Arizona* serovars occur widely in nature. Occasionally they cause severe or fatal infections in chicks, turkey poults, humans, dogs, cats, and other animals. They are frequently recovered from snakes and lizards. The infections are egg transmitted.

Some important diseases caused by the *Salmonella* appear in Table 17–5. It has been generally accepted that endotoxin (lipopolysaccharide) of *Salmonella* contributes significantly to the pathogenesis. In addition, several other virulence factors are known to contribute to the establishment of disease. These factors include adhesion pili, production of colicin, siderophores, enterotoxin, cytotoxin, and porins. Ability to resist the lethal effects of serum complement is also considered an important mechanism by which *Salmonella* establishes itself in a host. Large plasmids, ranging from 30 to 60 megadaltons, have been found to confer strain virulence in *Salmonella.* The virulence trait can be passed easily to other bacteria via plasmids.

Serotypes within a group have a common O antigenic determinant. There are additional groups, but most clinical isolates from humans and animals are found in groups A through O.

Serratia

The one species of significance in infections is *S. marcescens,* which may produce a red pigment. It is responsible for infrequent cases of bovine mastitis and other uncommon sporadic infections in cattle and horses. It also causes septicemia in chickens and is thought to cause infections in geckos and tortoises.

Shigella

Members of this group are not important as causes of disease in domestic animals. All species cause dysentery in humans and other primates. Unlike the salmonellae, they do not cause systemic disease. *Shigella* species are closely related to *Escherichia coli.*

Yersinia

This genus was created for bacteria that were formerly called *Pasteurella pestis, P. pseudotuberculo-*

Table 17–4. Differentiation of the Three Species of Salmonella

	S. choleraesuis	S. enteritidis*	S. typhi
Stern's glycerol fuchsin	–	(+)	–
Simmons' citrate	–	(+)	–
Ornithine decarboxylase	(+)	(+)	–
Gas from glucose	(+)	(+)	–
Dulcitol	(–)	(+)	(–)
Arabinose	–	+	–
Rhamnose	+	(+)	–
Trehalose	–	+	+

*Includes all salmonellae except *S. choleraesuis* and *S. typhi.*
( ), most.

Table 17–5. Important Diseases Caused by Salmonella

Serogroup	Species or Serovars	Disease
A	S. paratyphi A	Paratyphoid fever in humans.
B	S. schottmuelleri	Paratyphoid fever in humans.
	S. typhimurium	Gastroenteritis in humans; most prevalent species causing infection in various animal species.
	S. agona	Various infections in horses and other animals.
	S. abortus-equi	Abortion in mares and jennets.
	S. abortus-bovis	Abortion in cattle.
	S. abortus-ovis	Abortion in sheep.
C₁	S. choleraesuis	Enteritis in pigs; frequent secondary invader in hog cholera; infections in humans.
	S. typhisuis	Infections in young pigs.
	S. montevideo	Infections in cattle and pig primarily.
C₂	S. newport	Infections in humans, various animals, and especially cattle.
D₁	S. enteritidis	Infections in various animals; gastroenteritis in humans.
	S. gallinarum	Fowl typhoid, an acute intestinal disease of young chickens and turkeys.
	S. pullorum	Severe intestinal infections of chicks and poults (pullorum); chronic infections in older fowl.
	S. typhi	Typhoid fever in humans.
	S. dublin	Severe infections in calves.
E₁	S. anatum	Keel disease in ducklings.
	S. muenster	Infections in cattle primarily.

sis, and other closely related bacteria. They are true enterobacteria and did not belong in the genus *Pasteurella. Yersinia pestis* is the cause of plague; *Y. pseudotuberculosis, Y. enterocolitica,* and other closely related species cause infections in humans and animals. The important species are dealt with in some detail further on.

ANTIGENIC NATURE AND SEROLOGY

Escherichia coli

Identification of the serotypes (pilus antigens) of this species is carried out routinely in most veterinary diagnostic laboratories. Serotyping could be of value in identifying serotypes that are frequently enterotoxin producers. The antigens used to designate serotypes are as follows:

1. Somatic or O antigens: designated by Arabic numerals, e.g., 0133.
2. K (surface or envelope) antigens: There are more than 80 K antigens. They are designated by the letter with an Arabic number, e.g., K4.
3. H or flagellar antigens: designated by H followed by an Arabic number, e.g., H2. If there are no flagella, it is designated NM (nonmotile).

An example of a complete designation is 0111:K4:H2.

Salmonella

1. Somatic or O antigens: designated by Arabic numerals; group classification is based on several of these antigens.

2. Flagellar antigens—phase 1: Designated by small letters of the alphabet, more or less specific for the salmonella. Isolates must be in this phase before they can be typed. Phase 2: Designated by Arabic numerals; less specific, and duplicated in other bacterial species.

3. K antigens (capsular or envelope): "Vi" antigen, "M" antigen, and so forth. These antigens may interfere with agglutinability of O antisera.

An example of a complete designation is *S. typhimurium,* 1,4,[5],12:i:1,2. Major antigens are separated by colons, and the components of an antigen are separated by commas.

In most veterinary diagnostic laboratories, the salmonella isolates are examined serologically to determine their group. Group identification is based on the possession of certain somatic or O antigens. Salmonella O antisera are available commercially for each group. The procedure is a simple slide agglutination test. It is usual to test an isolate first against a polyvalent O serum covering groups A to I. If this is positive, then tests are conducted with the individual group sera. Further serologic characterization is carried out in reference laboratories. Some important serovars of *Salmonella* are listed in Table 17–6.

Some *Proteus* species react with the polyvalent salmonella sera. Many *Salmonella* serovars are diphasic with flagellar antigens in phase 1 (specific) and phase 2 (nonspecific). A culture of *Salmonella* may have organisms in just one phase or in both. In the former, the culture, although capable of developing the alternative phase, usually maintains a constant phase through several generations. To obtain the complete antigenic formula of the *Salmonella,* and hence to determine the serovar, both flagellar phases must be identified.

Table 17–6. Antigens of Important Salmonella *Serovars Recovered from Animals*

Serovars	Group	Somatic antigens	Flagella antigens Phase 1	Flagella antigens Phase 2	Chickens, Turkeys	Swine	Cattle	Equines	All other birds and animals	Reptiles	Feed and all other sources
S. typhimurium	B	1,4,[5],12	i	1,2	+	+	+	+	+	·	+
S. derby	B	1,4,[5],12	g,f	[1,2]	+	+	·	·	·	·	·
S. agona	B	4,12	f,g,s	–	·	+	+	·	+	·	·
S. saint paul	B	1,4,[5],12	e,h	1,2	+	·	·	·	·	+	·
S. heidelberg	B	1,4,[5],12	r	1,2	+	·	·	·	·	+	·
S. san diego	B	4,[5],12	e,h	e,n,z$_{15}$	+	·	·	·	·	·	·
S. typhisuis	C$_1$	6,7	c	1,5	·	·	·	·	·	·	·
S. choleraesuis	C$_1$	6,7	c	1,5	·	+	·	·	·	·	·
S. choleraesuis biovar *Kunzendorf*	C$_1$	6,7	[c]	1,5	·	+	·	·	·	·	·
S. infantis	C$_1$	6,7,14	r	1,5	+	·	·	·	·	·	·
S. oranienburg	C$_1$	6,7	m,t	–	·	·	·	·	·	·	·
S. montevideo	C$_1$	6,7,14	g,m,[p],s	–	+	·	·	·	·	·	·
S. newport	C$_2$	6,8	e,h	1,2	·	·	·	·	·	·	·
S. muenchen	C$_2$	6,8	d	1,2	·	·	·	·	·	·	·
S. manhattan	C$_2$	6,8	d	1,5	·	+	·	·	·	·	+
S. kentucky	C$_3$	8,20	i	z$_6$	·	·	+	·	·	·	·
S. panama	D$_1$	1,9,12	1,v	1,5	·	+	·	·	·	·	·
S. gallinarum	D$_1$	1,9,12	–	–	·	·	·	·	·	·	·
S. pullorum	D$_1$	9,12	–	–	+	·	·	·	·	·	·
S. enteritidis	D$_1$	1,9,12	g,m	[1,7]	·	·	+	·	·	·	·
S. dublin	D$_1$	1,9,12,[Vi]	g,p	–	·	·	+	·	·	+	·
S. anatum	E$_1$	3,10	e,h	1,6	+	·	·	·	·	·	·
S. london	E$_1$	3,10	1,v	1,6	·	+	·	·	·	·	·
S. meleagridis	E$_1$	3,10	e,h	1,w	·	·	·	·	·	·	·
S. give	E$_1$	3,10	1,v	1,7	·	·	·	·	·	·	·
S. muenster	E$_1$	3,10	e,h	1,5	·	·	+	·	·	·	·
S. newington	E$_2$	3,15	e,h	1,6	·	·	·	·	·	·	·
S. worthington	G$_2$	1,13,23	z	1,w	·	·	·	·	·	·	·
S. cubana	G$_2$	1,13,23	z$_{29}$	[z$_{37}$]	·	·	+	·	·	·	·
S. cerro	K	6,14,18	z$_4$z$_{23}$	[1,5]	·	+	·	·	·	·	·

In italics, O antigen whose presence is due to phage conversion; [ ], antigen present or absent; +, commonly isolated; ·, occasionally isolated.

Adapted from Carter, M.E. and Chengappa, M.M.: Enterobacteria. *In* Diagnostic Procedures in Veterinary Bacteriology and Mycology. 5th Ed. Edited by G.R. Carter and J.E. Cole. New York, Academic Press, 1990.

Table 17–7. Appearance of Important Enterobacteria on Selective Media

Enterobacteria	Brilliant Green Agar	MacConkey Agar	Hekton Enteric Agar
Coliforms: *Escherichia coli* *Enterobacter* *Klebsiella*	Inhibited. If present, are yellowish-green.	Grow and are red. *Enterobacter* and *Klebsiella* may be larger and mucoid.	Grow and are yellow-orange or yellow-green. *Enterobacter* and *Klebsiella* may be larger and mucoid.
Proteus	Grow; don't spread; yellowish-green. Sucrose-negative strains are colorless.	Grow and may spread. Colorless.	Grow; may spread, colorless; H_2S-positive strains are black.
Salmonella	Grow. Red because of peptone hydrolysis.	Grow; colorless.	Grow; H_2S-positive strains are black; H_2S-negative strains are colorless.

Lysogenization by certain converting phages may change the O-antigenic formulas of the salmonellae. In antigenic groups A, B, and D, the presence of O-antigen 1 (factor 1) is associated with lysogenization; however, the presence or absence of this factor in strains of these groups does not alter the name of the serovar. In group E, however, phage E15 alters the O-antigen 3,10 to 3,15, resulting in *S. anatum* becoming *S. newington*.

To prevent smooth-rough (S-R) dissociation, the freshly isolated strains are maintained on media with no added carbohydrate. Rough strains often autoagglutinate in saline and consequently are unsuitable for typing. Serovars with flagella may give rise to nonflagellated variants, and this change is usually irreversible. *S. pullorum* is permanently without flagella.

The antigenic schema for the salmonellae in subgroup III (*Arizona*) is based on O and H antigens. The antigenic formulas of most *Arizona* serovars have been converted to *Salmonella* formulas for inclusion in the Kauffmann-White scheme.

Salmonella biovars have the same antigenic formula, but they may differ in certain biochemical reactions and in their disease manifestations.

Klebsiella

At least 77 capsule types of *Klebsiella* have been described (K1 to K72, K74, K79 to K82). K1, K5, and K7 are the predominant types in metritis in mares. K1, K2, and K3 types are predominant in pneumonic cases in humans.

RESISTANCE

Like most vegetative forms of bacteria, enterobacteria are not especially resistant to physical and chemical influences. Sunlight and desiccation kill them readily; freezing does not.

ISOLATION AND CULTIVATION

The organisms grow well on ordinary unenriched culture media. Selective media are available that favor the growth of some genera (Tables 17–7 and 17–8). Tissues, feces, or intestinal material is usually submitted for culture.

Procedures for isolation and cultivation are outlined in Figure 17–1.

The colonies of the various enterobacteria on blood agar look much the same with few exceptions. Colonies on selective media, however, show considerable differences among genera (see Table 17–7).

IDENTIFICATION

After observing the kinds and numbers of colonies, several are inoculated in triple sugar iron agar (TSI). This medium is used for fermentation of lactose, sucrose, and glucose and production of H_2S and gas. It is inoculated first into the butt, then streaked on the slant and incubated for 18 hours at 37° C. The following reactions may be obtained:

1. Alkaline slope (red) and acid butt (yellow): glucose fermentation only.
2. Acid slope (yellow) and acid butt (yellow): lactose or sucrose fermentation or both; glucose fermentation.
3. Blackening along the stab line or butt: H_2S production.
4. Gas bubbles in agar: some fermentative enterobacteria produce gas, whereas many others do not.

The reactions on TSI are observed (Table 17–9). These, along with the so-called IMViC reactions (indole, methyl red, Voges-Proskauer [acetylmethyl carbinol], citrate [utilization]) and the other reactions listed in Table 17–10, identify the principal genera. The definitive identification of some

Table 17–8. Media for the Isolation and Identification of the Enterobacteriaceae

Medium	Key Nutrients	Indicators	Detected	Inhibitors	Bacteria Inhibited	Bacteria Favored
Selenite F broth	Lactose	None	–	Sodium selenite	Coliforms	*Salmonella, Shigella, Proteus*
Tetrathionate broth	None	None	–	Bile salts, iodine	Coliforms, gram-positives	*Salmonella, Shigella*
Triple sugar iron agar (TSI)	Glucose 0.1%, Lactose 1.0%, Sucrose 1.0%	Phenol red, ferrous ammonium sulfate	Carbohydrate fermentation, gas and H_2S production	None	None	Most
MacConkey agar	Lactose	Neutral red	Lactose fermentation	Bile salts, crystal violet	Gram-positives	Enteric bacteria and other gram-negatives
Brilliant green agar	Lactose, sucrose	Phenol red	Lactose or sucrose fermentation	Brilliant green	Coliforms, *Shigella*	*Salmonella, Proteus*
Hektoen enteric agar	Lactose, sucrose	Bromthymol blue and Andrade's indicator	Sugar fermentation, H_2S production	Bile salt	Gram-positives	Enteric bacteria
Salmonella-shigella agar	Lactose	Neutral red	Lactose fermentation, H_2S production	Bile salt, brilliant green	Gram-positives	Enteric bacteria
Simmons' citrate agar	Sodium citrate	Bromthymol blue	Growth from citrate as sole source of carbon	None	Bacteria unable to use citrate as sole C source	Citrate-positive organisms
MR-VP broth	Glucose	Add after incubation to two different culture tubes: methyl red, and VP1 (alpha naphtol) VP2 (KOH)	Acid from glucose =+ Acetyl-methyl carbinol from glucose = +	None	–	–
Tryptone broth (for indole)	Tryptophan	Add Kovac's reagent after incubation	Indole production from tryptophan	None	–	–

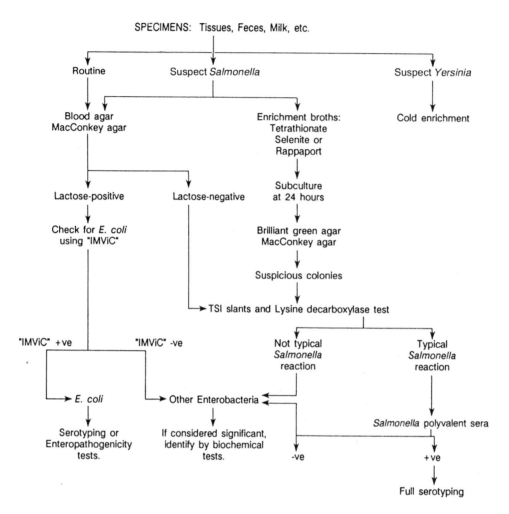

Figure 17–1. Sequence of procedures for the isolation and identification of enterobacteria. Adapted from Carter, M.E., and Chengappa, M.M.: Enterobacteria. *In* Diagnostic Procedures in Veterinary Bacteriology and Mycology. 5th Ed. Edited by G.R. Carter and J.E. Cole. New York, Academic Press, 1990.

species of enterobacteria can be determined from Table 17–11.

Some *Proteus* species may spread or swarm over the agar plate; swarming is inhibited if the agar is increased to 4%. The spreading edges of two different strains of *Proteus* on an agar plate are inhibited before union takes place (Dienes' phenomenon). In contrast, the spreading edges of the same strain fuse imperceptibly. This can be of epidemiologic significance in urinary tract infections.

Several serologic procedures have been developed in recent years for the rapid detection of *Escherichia coli* and *Salmonella* antigens in tissue specimens and fecal samples. They are the fluorescent antibody test, the passive hemagglutination

procedure, the ELISA, the radiometric assay, and the latex agglutination procedure. Species-specific DNA probes are being evaluated currently for the identification of many members of the family *Enterobacteriaceae*. Specific DNA probes are being used in some laboratories for the identification of adhesion (K99, K88, 987P, and K41), enterotoxin (ST and LT), and verotoxin (SLT-1, SLT-II, and SLT-IIv) genes of *Escherichia coli*.

TREATMENT

Tetracyclines, chloramphenicol (especially for *Salmonella typhi*), ampicillin, neomycin, penicillin, amoxicillin, apramycin, and sulfonamides have been used. There are multiple-drug-resistant

Table 17–9. Reactions of Some Important Enterobacteria on Triple Sugar Iron Agar

Slant	Butt	Gas	H₂S	Sugars Attacked (Acids)	Probable Identification
A	A	−	−	G,L,(S)	*Escherichia coli*
A	A	+	−		
A	A	+	−	G,L,S	*Klebsiella*
K	A	+	−	G	*Salmonella*
K	A	−	+	G	
K	A	+	+	G	
A	A	+	+	G,L,(S)	*Proteus*
K	A	−	−	G	
K	A	+	−	G	
K	A	+	+	G	
A	A	+	−	G,L,(S)	*Enterobacter*
K	A	+	+	G	*Edwardsiella*
K	A	+	−	G	*Morganella*
A	A	−	−	G,L,S	*Serratia*
A	A	+	−	G,L,S	
K	A	−	−	G	
A	A	+	−	G,L,(S)	*Citrobacter*
A	A	+	+	G,L,(S)	
K	A	−	−	G	
K	A	+	+	G	
K	A	−	−	G	*Providencia*
K	A	+	−	G	
K	A	−	−	G	*Yersinia*

K, alkaline; A, acid; L, lactose; S, sucrose; G, glucose; L, (S), lactose and/or sucrose.

Table 17–10. Differentiation of the Principal Genera of the Enterobacteriaceae.

Test	*Escherichia*	*Shigella*	*Salmonella*	*Citrobacter*	*Klebsiella*	*Enterobacter*	*Hafnia*	*Serratia*	*Proteus*	*Providencia*	*Yersinia*
Indole	+	(−)	−	−	(−)	−	−	−	(+)	+	(−)
Methyl red	+	+	+	+	−	−	(+)	(−)	+	+	(+)
Voges-Proskauer	−	−	−	−	+	+	(+)	+	(−)	−	−
Simmons' citrate	−	−	d	+	+	+	(+)	+	+	+	−
H₂S (TSI)	−	−	+	(+)	−	−	−	−	+	−	−
Urease	−	−	−	dw	+w	(+)	−	dw	+	−	(+)
Motility at 36° C	(+)	−	+	+	−	+	+	+	+	+	−
Lysine	d	−	+	−	+	−	+	+	−	−	−
Ornithine	d	d	+	d	−	+	+	+	(+)	−	(−)
Phenylalanine	−	−	−	−	−	−	−	−	+	+	−
Gas from glucose	+	−	+	+	+	+	+	(+)	(+)	−	−
Lactose	+	−	−	d	+	+	(−)	(−)	−	−	−
Sucrose	d	−	−	d	+	+	d	+	+	d	(−)

+, >90% of isolates positive; −, >90% of isolates negative; d, delayed positive (3 to 5 days); w, weak reaction; (+), majority positive but less than 90% positive; (−), majority negative, but less than 90% negative.
Adapted from Koneman, E.W., Allen, S.D., Dowell, V.R., Jr., and Sommers, H.M.: Diagnostic Microbiology. Philadelphia, J.B. Lippincott, 1979.

strains. The plasmids involved are transferred among enteric organisms primarily by conjugation. Included in the plasmid (R factor) is the resistance transfer factor (RTF) and genes for resistance to several drugs. They appear to diminish permeability to the corresponding drugs. There are complex interrelations among the enteric bacteria. Serologic type may be based on a small difference in a single macromolecule. There are many opportunities for genetic recombination. In salmonellosis there may be carriers after treatment.

IMMUNITY

Escherichia coli bacterins are used to immunize cows and sows to prevent disease in their young. Because of antigenic heterogeneity, however, they are considered of limited value. Mini-cell and pilus vaccines have been developed and appear to be of value. Sows have been vaccinated orally with field cultures of *E. coli*. Attenuated live *Salmonella typhimurium* and *S. dublin* vaccines are used in cattle in England and the United States. Various salmonellae, such as *S. choleraesuis* and *S. typhimurium*, are incorporated in bacterins, alone or with other bacteria. A vaccine containing live attenuated *S. choleraesuis* is being used currently. An *S. dublin* bacterin is used to prevent salmonellosis in calves. Because immunity to salmonellosis is probably predominantly cell-mediated, the value of bacterins is questionable. Synthetic *Escherichia coli* heat-stable enterotoxin has been used as an immunogen in cattle and swine; its value is questionable.

PUBLIC HEALTH SIGNIFICANCE

Salmonella

Reservoir and Sources of Infection. The carrier state may be considerable in domestic (including poultry) and wild animals; turtles and other pets may also shed salmonellae. Human patients, both sick and convalescent, and subclinical carriers may shed organisms.

Other sources are feces of humans and animals; whole eggs, especially duck eggs; egg products; meat and meat products; poultry; and fertilizers and animal feeds prepared from bones, fish meal, and meat.

Transmission. Infections and epidemics are usually traceable to various food products derived from meat, eggs, milk, and poultry. Other means of infection derive from food and water contaminated with rodent feces, from infected food handlers, and from contaminated equipment and utensils. Sporadic cases occur from direct contact with an infected animal or person.

Yersinia

The genus now contains 10 species. These species resemble the Enterobacteriaceae more closely than the classic pasteurellae. All species are facultative intracellular parasites. The genus was established and described by Kitasato and Yersin independently in 1894. *Y. enterocolitica*, *Y. pestis*, and *Y. pseudotuberculosis* are important animal and human pathogens. *Y. ruckeri* causes enteric redmouth of fish. Other yersiniae (see Table 17–1) are not known to cause infection in humans and animals.

Yersinia pestis

Synonym. *Pasteurella pestis.*

Pathogenesis and Pathogenicity. All virulent strains produce exotoxin, which is the likely cause of death from plague. The toxin is composed of two protein components, toxin A and toxin B, with molecular weights of 240,000 and 120,000, respectively. Other factors thought to have a role in the virulence of *Yersinia pestis* include production of bacteriocin, coagulase, and fibrolytic enzymes; encapsulation of strains; production of V-W antigens; calcium dependence in culture; ability to synthesize purines; and the formation of pigmented colonies on hemin media. Virulent strains resist phagocytosis and can grow within macrophages. Endotoxin undoubtedly contributes to tissue damage in plague.

Plague is fundamentally a disease of rats and wild rodents. Humans are considered accidental hosts.

Bubonic and pneumonic forms of plague in humans can be epidemic. The disease is transmitted by fleas. Fleas become infected from rats in which the disease is bubonic and similar to that seen in humans. Buboes is the term used for infected lymph nodes. The bubonic form can give rise to the pneumonic form, which is highly contagious and usually fatal if not treated.

Sylvatic plague occurs in wild rodents other than rats. At least 38 species of wild rodents, including marmots and squirrels, have been found to be susceptible. Fleas transmit it to humans and various rodents. Sylvatic plague has given rise to outbreaks of bubonic and pneumonic plague. Natural infections have been reported in dogs, cats, camels, elephants, buffaloes, and deer.

Between 1910 and 1951, 523 cases of bubonic plague in humans were reported in the United States, and the fatality rate was 65%. Outbreaks have occurred in California, Louisiana, Florida, Texas, and Washington. In addition, sporadic cases have been reported from Arizona, Idaho, New

Table 17-11. Differentiation of Some Enteric Bacteria by Biochemical Tests

	Indole production	Methyl red	Voges-Proskauer	Citrate	Hydrogen sulfide (TSI)	Urease	Phenylalanine	Lysine decarboxylase	Arginine dihydrolase	Ornithine decarboxylase	KCN (growth)	Motility at 36° C	Gelatin liquefaction	Malonate	Glucose (gas)	Lactose	Sucrose	Mannitol	Dulcitol	Salicin	Adonitol	Inositol	Sorbitol	Arabinose	Raffinose	Rhamnose	Esculin hydrolysis	ONPG (-galactosidase)
Citrobacter amalonaticus	+	+	-	(+)	-	(+)	-	-	(+)	+	+	+	-	(-)	+	d	(-)	+	-	d	-	-	+	+	-	+	-	+
C. diversus	+	+	-	+	-	(+)	-	-	d	+	+	+	-	+	+	d	d	+	d	(-)	+	-	+	+	d	+	-	+
C. freundii	-	+	-	+	(+)	d	-	-	d	(-)	+	+	-	(-)	+	d	d	+	d	-	+	-	+	+	d	+	-	+
Edwardsiella tarda	+	+	-	-	+	-	-	+	-	+	-	+	-	-	+	-	-	+	-	-	-	-	-	-	-	-	-	-
E. ictaluri	-	-	-	-	-	-	-	+	-	d	-	-	-	-	d	-	-	-	-	-	-	-	-	-	-	-	-	-
Enterobacter aerogenes	(-)	-	+	+	-	(-)	-	+	-	+	+	(+)	-	d	+	d	+	+	-	+	+	+	+	+	+	+	+	+
E. agglomerans	-	d	d	d	-	d	(-)	-	-	-	d	(+)	-	d	+	d	(+)	+	(-)	d	-	(-)	d	+	d	(+)	d	+
E. cloacae	-	-	+	+	-	+	-	-	+	+	+	+	-	(+)	+	+	+	+	(-)	(+)	(-)	(-)	+	+	+	+	d	+
E. gergoviae	-	d	+	+	-	+	-	+	-	+	-	+	-	+	+	d	+	+	-	+	(-)	-	-	+	+	+	+	+
Escherichia coli	+	+	-	-	-	-	-	(+)	(-)	d	-	d	-	-	+	+	d	+	d	d	-	-	+	+	d	(+)	d	+
Klebsiella oxytoca	+	d	+	+	-	+	-	+	-	-	-	-	-	+	+	+	+	+	d	+	+	+	+	+	+	+	+	+
K. pneumoniae	-	(-)	+	+	-	+	-	+	-	-	+	-	-	+	+	+	+	+	d	+	+	+	+	+	+	+	+	+
Morganella morganii	+	+	-	-	-	+	+	-	-	+	+	+	-	-	(+)	-	-	-	-	-	-	-	-	-	-	-	-	-
Proteus mirabilis	-	+	(-)	d	+	+	+	-	-	+	+	+	+	-	+	-	(-)	-	-	d	-	-	-	-	-	-	-	-
P. vulgaris	+	+	-	(-)	+	+	+	-	-	-	+	+	+	-	(+)	-	+	-	-	(+)	-	-	-	-	-	-	(+)	-
Providencia rettgeri	+	+	-	+	-	+	+	-	-	-	+	+	-	-	-	-	(-)	+	-	d	+	+	-	-	-	d	d	-
P. stuartii	+	+	-	+	-	d	+	-	-	+	+	(+)	-	+	-	-	d	(-)	-	-	+	+	-	-	-	-	-	-
Shigella boydii	d	+	-	-	-	-	-	-	-	-	-	-	-	-	-	-	-	+	-	-	-	-	d	d	d	-	-	-
S. sonnei	-	+	-	-	-	-	-	-	-	+	-	-	-	-	-	-	-	+	-	-	-	-	-	+	-	d	-	+
Salmonella subgroup 1	-	+	-	+	+	-	-	+	d	+	-	+	-	+	+	-	-	+	d	-	-	-	+	+	-	+	-	-
subgroup 3 (Arizona)	-	+	-	+	+	-	-	+	(+)	+	-	+	-	+	+	d	-	+	-	-	-	-	+	+	-	+	-	-
Serratia liquefaciens	-	(+)	(+)	+	-	-	-	+	-	+	+	+	+	-	d	-	+	+	-	+	-	d	+	+	+	(-)	+	+
S. marcescens	-	(-)	+	+	-	(-)	-	+	-	+	+	+	+	-	d	-	+	+	-	+	d	(+)	+	-	-	-	+	+
S. odorifera	d	(+)	(+)	+	-	-	-	+	-	d	d	+	+	+	-	+	d	+	-	d	d	+	+	+	d	+	d	+
Yersinia enterocolitica	d	+	-	-	-	(+)	-	-	-	+	-	-	-	-	-	-	+	+	-	d	d	d	-	+	-	-	-	+
Y. pestis	-	(+)	-	-	-	-	-	-	-	-	-	-	-	-	-	-	-	+	-	d	-	-	-	d	(-)	+	(+)	(+)
Y. pseudotuberculosis	-	(+)	-	-	-	+	-	-	-	-	-	-	-	+	-	-	-	+	-	(-)	-	-	-	d	-	+	(+)	d

-, 0–10% of strains positive; (–), 11–25% of strains positive; d, 26–75% of strains positive; +, 90–100% of strains positive; (+), 76–89% of strains positive.

Adapted from Carter, M.E., and Chengappa, M.M.: Enterobacteria. In Diagnostic Procedures in Veterinary Bacteriology and Mycology. 5th Ed. Edited by G.R. Carter and J.E. Cole. New York, Academic Press, 1990.

Mexico, Nevada, Oregon, and Utah. Fortunately, many of the foci of sylvatic plague are situated in sparsely populated and isolated rural districts where the fleas of wild rodents do not have the opportunity to bite humans.

Isolation, Cultivation, and Identification. The organism is not fastidious. Identification is made on the basis of the criteria presented in Table 17–11. It is closely related to *Y. pseudotuberculosis*, with which it shares many antigens. It differs from this organism in that it is nonmotile at 20 to 25° C.

Yersinia pseudotuberculosis

Synonym. *Pasteurella pseudotuberculosis.*

Pathogenicity. This organism produces pseudotuberculosis in various rodents, guinea pigs, cats, chinchilla, and turkeys; epididymo-orchitis of rams; abortion in goats; and occasional infections in swine, buffaloes, cattle, sheep, deer, and wild birds. The infection in small animals initially involves the mesenteric nodes, with spread from the caseous abscesses to the liver and spleen particularly.

In humans, infections simulating typhoid and appendicitis (mesenteric adenitis) occur.

Virulent strains of *Yersinia pseudotuberculosis* carry a 40 to 50 megadalton plasmid. Virulence factors associated with the plasmid are calcium dependency, expression of V-W antigens, autoagglutination, production of certain membrane proteins, and lethality in mice.

Antigens. Six serotypes are based on somatic and flagellar antigens.

Identification. *Y. pseudotuberculosis* is motile at 22° C; *Y. pestis* is not. See Table 17–11 for additional differential characteristics.

Yersinia enterocolitica

Pathogenicity. This organism, which resembles *Y. pseudotuberculosis*, causes gastroenteritis, mesenteric adenitis, and a wide variety of infrequent infections in humans. It seems likely that the reservoir of *Y. enterocolitica* is the intestine of wild and domestic animals. Many of the infections in animals resemble those caused by *Y. pseudotuberculosis*. Ileitis, gastroenteritis, and mesenteric adenitis are probably the most common disease processes. Most strains produce a heat-stable enterotoxin.

Isolation has been made from chinchilla, hares, deer, rabbits, dogs, pigs, horses, mink, various avian species, goats, cattle, sheep, water, and milk. The organism has been isolated from a considerable percentage (25%) of mesenteric nodes of swine and also from tongues (35%).

Identification. The organism can be cultivated without difficulty by a "cold enrichment" procedure like that used for *Listeria monocytogenes*. Growth is better at room temperature or lower than 37° C. Identification is made on the basis of morphologic, cultural, and biochemical characteristics (see Table 17–11).

Yersinia enterocolitica shares an antigen with the classic *Brucella* species and thus may give rise to false *Brucella* agglutination reactions. There are more than 50 serotypes and several biotypes, many of which do not appear to be pathogenic. New species *Yersinia intermedia*, *Y. frederiksenii*, and *Y. kristensenii* have been established for strains that differ biochemically from those of human origin.

Treatment. Both *Y. pseudotuberculosis* and *Y. enterocolitica* are susceptible to tetracyclines, trimethoprim-sulfamethoxazole, aminoglycosides, kanamycin, and chloramphenicol.

Because the *Yersinia* are facultative intracellular parasites and because the infections they cause may be acute, early and adequate treatment is particularly important.

FURTHER READING

D'Aoust, J.Y.: Pathogenicity of foodborne *Salmonella*. Int. J. Food Microbiol. *12*:17, 1991.

Donnenberg, M.S., and Kaper, J.B.: Enteropathogenic *Escherichia coli*. Infect. Immun. *60*:3953, 1992.

Edelman, R., and Levine, M.M.: Summary of a workshop on enteropathogenic *Escherichia coli*. J. Infect. Dis. *147*:1108, 1983.

Evans, M.G., Waxler, G.L., and Newman, J.P.: Prevalence of K88, K99, and 987P pili of *Escherichia coli* in neonatal pigs with enteric colibacillosis. Am. J. Vet. Res. *47*:2431, 1986.

Ewing, W.H.: Differentiation of Enterobacteriaceae by Biochemical Reactions. Atlanta, Centers for Disease Control, 1973.

Farmer, III, J.J., et al.: Biochemical identification of new species and biogroups of Enterobacteriaceae isolated from clinical specimens. J. Clin. Microbiol. *21*:46, 1985.

Farmer, J.J., III, and Kelly, M.T.: *Enterobacteriaceae*. In Manual of Clinical Microbiology. 5th Ed. Edited by A. Balows, et al. Washington, D.C., American Society for Microbiology, 1991.

Franz, J.C., et al.: Investigation of synthetic *Escherichia coli* heat-stable enterotoxin as an immunogen for swine and cattle. Infect. Immun. *55*:1077, 1987.

Holland, R.E.: Some infectious causes of diarrhea in young farm animals. Clin. Microbiol. Rev. *3*:345, 1990.

Holland, R.E., Sriranganathan, N., and DuPont, L.: Isolation of enterotoxigenic *Escherichia coli* from a foal with diarrhea. J. Am. Vet. Med. Assoc. *194*:389, 1989.

Janke, B.H., et al.: Attaching and effacing *Escherichia coli* infection as a cause of diarrhea in young calves. J. Am. Vet. Med. Assoc. *196*:897, 1990.

Kikuchi, N., Iguchi, I., and Hiramune, T.: Capsule types of *Klebsiella pneumoniae* isolated from the genital tract of mares with metritis, extragenital sites of healthy mares, and the genital tract of stallions. Vet. Microbiol. *15*:219, 1987.

Kramer, T.T., Roof, M.B., and Matheson, R.R.: Safety and efficacy of an attenuated strain of *Salmonella choleraesuis* for vaccination of swine. Am. J. Vet. Res. *53*:444, 1992.

McWhorter, A.C., et al.: *Trabulsiella guamensis,* a new genus and species of the family *Enterobacteriaceae* that resembles *Salmonella* subgroups 4 and 5. J. Clin. Microbiol. *29:*1480, 1991.

Moon, H.W.: Mechanisms in the pathogenesis of diarrhea: A review. J. Am. Vet. Med. Assoc. *172:*443, 1978.

Okerman, L.: Enteric infections caused by non-enterotoxigenic *Escherichia coli* in animals: occurrence and pathogenicity mechanisms. A review. Vet. Microbiol. *14:*33, 1987.

Pelzer, K.D.: Salmonellosis. J. Am. Vet. Med. Assoc. *195:*456, 1989.

Pospischil, A., et al.: Attaching and effacing bacteria in the intestines of calves and cats with diarrhea. Vet. Pathol. *24:*330, 1987.

Raybould, T.J.G., Crouch, C.F., and Acres, S.D.: Monoclonal antibody passive hemagglutination and capture enzyme-linked immunosorbent assays for direct detection and quantitation of F41 and K99 fibrial antigens in enterotoxigenic *Escherichia coli.* J. Clin. Microbiol. *25:*278, 1987.

Riet-Correa, F., et al.: *Yersinia pseudotuberculosis* infection of buffaloes (*Bubalus bubalis*). J. Vet. Diagn. Invest. *2:*78, 1990.

Rubin, R.H., and Weinstein, L.: Salmonellosis. New York, Stratton, 1977.

Scholl, D.R., et al.: Clinical application of novel sample processing technology for the identification of salmonellae by using DNA probes. J. Clin. Microbiol. *28:*237, 1990.

Shiozawa, K., et al.: Virulence of *Yersinia pseudotuberculosis* isolated from pork and from the throats of swine. Appl. Environ. Microbiol. *54:*818, 1988.

Soderlind, O., Thafvelin, B., and Mollby, R.: Virulence factors in *Escherichia coli* strains isolated from Swedish piglets with diarrhea. J. Clin. Microbiol. *26:*879, 1988.

Toma, S.: Human and nonhuman infections caused by *Yersina pseudotuberculosis* in Canada from 1962 to 1985. J. Clin. Microbiol. *24:*465, 1986.

Turk, J., et al.: Coliform septicemia and pulmonary disease associated with canine parvoviral enteritis: 88 cases (1987–1988). J. Am. Vet. Med. Assoc. *196:*771, 1990.

Wray, C., and Callow, R.J.: The detection of salmonella infection in calves by the fluorescent antibody test. Vet. Microbiol. *19:*85, 1989.

18

Pseudomonas, Aeromonas, Plesiomonas, and Vibrio

Principal Characteristics

The pseudomonads are gram-negative, aerobic (sugars split by oxidation), medium-size rods. They are motile by one or several polar flagella (except *Pseudomonas mallei*), catalase- and oxidase-positive, and some species produce water-soluble pigments.

More than 90 species of pseudomonads are listed in the current *Bergey's Manual of Systematic Bacteriology*, Vol. 1. They occur widely in nature and are classified in the family Pseudomonadaceae. Three species are of considerable pathogenic significance in animals: *P. aeruginosa* causes pyogenic infections, *P. pseudomallei* causes melioidosis, and *P. mallei* causes glanders. The natural habitat of the first two species is water, soil, and decaying vegetation; *P. mallei* is an obligate parasite. *P. aeruginosa* also may be found on the skin and mucous membranes, and in feces. *P. pseudomallei* only occurs naturally in tropical areas. *P. maltophilia, P. stutzeri, P. fluorescens, P. cepacia, P. putida*, and other pseudomonads rarely cause infections in animals.

The genera *Aeromonas, Plesiomonas*, and *Vibrio* are currently listed in the family Vibrionaceae. They occur widely in nature, including sea water and fresh water and in association with aquatic animals. Several species are pathogens or potential pathogens for humans, animals, and marine creatures.

Pseudomonas aeruginosa

Pathogenesis

P. aeruginosa possess pili, which facilitate adherence to epithelial cells with subsequent colonization. The failure to colonize on normal cells results from a protective coating of fibronectin protein present on epithelial cell surfaces. Colonization only takes place when the fibronectin coat is disrupted as the result of infection or mechanical trauma. Colonization by *P. aeruginosa* is not confined to the surface of the epithelial cells. The organism can colonize deep tissues as well, including tissues exposed to burns and trauma. As in other gram-negative bacteria the capsule and lipopolysaccharide of *P. aeruginosa* offer considerable protection to the organism against phagocytic destruction.

P. aeruginosa produces numerous extracellular toxins and enzymes. Those that may play a role in the production of disease are fibrinolysin, elastase, lecithinase, lipase, proteases, hemolysins (heat-stable and heat-labile), leukocidin, alginate, phospholipase C, esterase, enterotoxin, and exotoxin A. In addition, *P. aeruginosa* produces a deep-blue, chloroform-soluble pigment, pyocyanin, and a yellow-green, water-soluble pigment, fluorescein. These pigments exhibit antimicrobial activities against a wide range of bacteria and some fungi. The enterotoxin of *P. aeruginosa* is responsible for the diarrhea seen during intestinal infection.

166

Hemolysins of *P. aeruginosa* act synergistically with a phosphatase on lipids and lecithin to produce necrosis. These heat-stable and heat-labile hemolysins also break down pulmonary surfactant with resulting atelectasis. Among the extracellular products, exotoxin A is the most potent. This toxin kills cells in the same way that diphtheria toxin does. It catalyzes the transfer of ADP-ribose from nicotinamide-adenine dinucleotide (NAD) to elongation factor 2, thereby inhibiting protein synthesis in the host cell. Neither toxin A nor elastase can be detoxified efficiently by standard inactivating procedures. Exotoxin A is toxic for monocytes and for the bone marrow of humans and animals. It is lethal for mice and is considered important in virulence. Toxigenic strains are more virulent than nontoxigenic strains.

PATHOGENICITY

This species is a frequent contaminant in disease processes, and isolation alone is not necessarily significant. Its significance in mixed infections, particularly with streptococci and staphylococci, may be questionable. Repeated isolation in pure culture strongly indicates pathogenicity.

P. aeruginosa is an opportunist in weakened tissues (burns), wounds, debilitated patients, individuals with malignancies and immunodeficiencies, and young animals. It may replace bacteria that have been eliminated from infectious processes by antimicrobial treatment, and it sometimes causes a fatal septicemia. Infections are rare in healthy, normal individuals.

Some diseases or conditions with which *P. aeruginosa* has been associated are:

All animals: wound infections, abscess formation, diarrhea, and ear, urinary, and genital infections; nosocomial infections.

Horse: abortion, corneal and guttural pouch infections.

Cattle: mastitis, abortion, infertility, and granuloma of skin and subcutis.

Dogs and cats: prostatitis, cystitis, dermatitis, postoperative septicemia, ear infection, and endocarditis.

Fowl: septicemia and respiratory infections.
Mink: hemorrhagic pneumonia.
Sheep: "green wool" and dermatitis.

Humans: wound, urinary, corneal, and inner ear infections and fatal infections involving trachea, lungs, heart valves, meninges, and brain; septicemia, osteomyetitis, arthritis, cellulitis, and phlebitis; diarrhea caused by intestinal infection; and nosocomial infections.

Specimens

Urine, pus, affected tissues, and swabs from infected tissue surfaces.

ISOLATION AND CULTIVATION

All strains grow well on ordinary nutrient media. Colonies are irregular, spreading, translucent, and 3 to 5 mm in diameter, and may show a bluish-metallic sheen. Beta-hemolysis is usually observed around colonies growing on blood agar plates. A distinctive grape-like odor is usually apparent, regardless of the medium used.

P. aeruginosa does not grow anaerobically.

Medium-sized, gram-negative rods are seen in smears. They cannot be distinguished morphologically from the enteric bacteria.

IDENTIFICATION

Two pigments are commonly produced by these bacteria, both of which are water-soluble: pyocyanin (bluish-green), which is chloroform-soluble ("blue pus bacillus") and fluorescein or pyoverdin (yellowish-green), which is not chloroform-soluble. Both pigments may be found in media, but not always. Occasionally a strain produces a dark-red pigment (pyorubin) or a brown-black pigment (pyomelanin). Pyocyanin can be extracted from a slant culture by pouring chloroform over the pigment. All strains are oxidase-positive.

Fluorescein fluoresces under ultraviolet light, but *P. fluorescens*, an occasional contaminant, also produces fluorescein. *P. fluorescens* does not grow well at 37° C, however.

Other features of *P. aeruginosa* are motility by polar flagella and gelatin liquefaction. It is oxidase-positive, peptonizes litmus milk, utilizes citrate, is indole-negative, and reduces nitrate. The oxidation/fermentation (O/F) test is positive for oxidation. Differential features of the more important pseudomonads are listed in Table 18–1.

ANTIGENIC NATURE

The species is heterogeneous, with 17 serotypes based on differences in O antigens. Strains can be typed by bacteriophages and pyocins (bacteriocins), but serotyping is less cumbersome. Killed vaccines are used in burn patients and to prevent hemorrhagic septicemia in mink.

RESISTANCE

In general, these organisms resemble other vegetative bacteria except that they are more resistant to high dilutions of quaternary ammonium compounds and phenolic compounds. Pus is protective. They have been known to survive in quaternary ammonium disinfectants containing hard water or fragments of cork and plastic. With ade-

Table 18–1. *Differentiation of Important* Pseudomonas *Species*

	P. aeruginosa	P. maltophilia	P. fluorescens	P. pseudomallei	P. mallei
Glucose oxidation	+	+	+	+	+
Maltose oxidation	−	+	V	+	+
SS agar	+	−	+	−	−
Oxidase	+	−	+	+	−
Motility	+	+	+	+	−
Starch hydrolysis	−	−	−	+	V
Cetrimide agar	+	−	+	+	−
Growth at 42° C	+	V	−	−	−
Pigment	Pyocyanin: water- and chloroform-soluble; Fluorescein: water-soluble; Pyorubin: occasional strains	None, but a yellow to brown water-soluble tyrosine produced	Fluorescein: water-soluble	None	None

V, variable reactions.

quate moisture, *P. aeruginosa* can survive for long periods on water faucets, utensils, floors, instruments, baths, humidifiers, and respiratory care equipment. Pseudomonads are susceptible to ethylene oxide or heat (55° C for 1 hour).

TREATMENT

Infections caused by *P. aeruginosa* do not usually respond well to chemotherapy. Gentamicin and other aminoglycosides, such as amikacin, tobramycin, and colistin (polymyxin E), are used, but resistant forms develop during prolonged treatment. Carbenicillin, ticarcillin, and polymyxin are also employed. In severe infections, carbenicillin may be combined with gentamicin. Because of the high concentration of polymyxin in the urine, this drug is especially effective in *Pseudomonas* urinary infections. Third-generation cephalosporins, e.g., cefoperazone and cefotaxime, and quinolones, e.g., enrofloxacin, are quite effective. Neither streptomycin nor the tetracyclines are too active. Sulfonamides, especially sulfadiazine, sulfamerazine, and sulfamethazine, are sometimes of value. Combination therapy with two or even three antibiotics is occasionally chosen for serious infections. Multiple-type drug resistance caused by R factors is encountered frequently. The clinical efficacy of antimicrobial drugs against pseudomonads is difficult to predict based on in vitro data.

Multiple *P. aeruginosa* infections are uncommon in veterinary practice. When encountered, proper isolation procedures, strict sanitary measures, and effective disinfection are necessary for control.

Pseudomonas pseudomallei

This organism is found in tropical soils and water in Southeast Asia, Central Africa, and northern Australia.

MODE OF INFECTION

In both humans and animals, the organisms are thought to gain entry by inhalation or ingestion, or through wounds and abrasions.

PATHOGENICITY

The disease in humans and animals varies from a benign pulmonary form to a systemic form with visceral nodules (little pus unless secondary bacteria) and a terminal septicemia. The human disease is called melioidosis or pseudoglanders. Although melioidosis is frequently seen in immunodeficient patients, it can occur as a single independent disease without any predisposing condition.

Although the disease in animals can be septicemic, often it is chronic and characterized by nodules in the lungs, liver, spleen, lymph nodes, and subcutis. The acute disease occurs more often in young animals. In spite of extensive lesions, animals may appear normal. Among the animals infected are cattle, sheep, goats, pigs, horses, dogs, cats, primates, and rodents.

Endotoxin, exotoxin, proteases, and hemolysin are some of the biologically active substances. Their precise role in the pathogenesis of melioidosis is not known.

The most useful specimens for laboratory examination are pus and material from nodular lesions, urine, blood, and sputum (humans).

Criteria for identification are given in Table 18–1.

TREATMENT

Sulfonamides and broad-spectrum antibiotics are effective, but the treatment of choice appears to be trimethoprim-sulfamethoxazole. The response largely depends on the extent of the lesions.

Pseudomonas mallei

HABITAT AND OCCURRENCE

P. mallei is an obligate pathogen of horses, other solipeds, humans, and carnivores. Glanders (farcy), the disease it causes, has been eradicated from North America, and Central and Western Europe. It still occurs, however, in parts of Asia, the Middle East, and Africa.

MODE OF INFECTION

The organisms usually enter via the respiratory tract.

PATHOGENICITY

No exotoxin has been described; endotoxin is probably significant. Glanders is a contagious, usually chronic disease of horses characterized by the formation of tubercle-like nodules (granulomas) that frequently break down to form ulcers. Three forms of the disease are seen, depending on the principal location of the lesions, viz., nasal, pulmonary, or skin (farcy). Cattle, swine, rats, and birds are resistant to infection.

Humans, and particularly members of the cat family, may be infected. All infections usually terminate fatally if not treated.

SPECIMENS

Tissue containing early nodules or pus from ulcers.

ISOLATION AND IDENTIFICATION

P. mallei grows on blood and serum agar and is oxidative rather than fermentative. Colonies are shallow, round, convex, and opaque, and become yellowish green or brown on aging. On blood agar, colonies tend to be slimy. For identification, see Table 18–1.

TREATMENT, IMMUNITY, AND CONTROL

The most effective drugs are streptomycin and sulfadiazine. No vaccines or bacterins are used.

Control is by mallein testing (analogous to tuberculin testing), with the elimination of reactors. Mallein is injected intrapalpebrally. Immunity is predominantly cell-mediated.

Aeromonas

Members of *Aeromonas* are facultatively anaerobic, gram-negative rods. All are motile (except *A. salmonicida* and *A. media*) with a single polar flagellum. Peritrichous flagella are seen in young cultures grown on solid media. They occur widely in fresh water, sewage, and soil, and on fishes. They produce catalase and oxidase, and utilize glucose and other carbohydrates (Table 18–2). They grow well on most laboratory media at room temperature (optimum 22 to 28° C); however, most can be cultivated satisfactorily at 37° C. Some strains of *A. hydrophila* produce a brown pigment in 2 to 3 days on infusion agar. Most strains of *A. hydrophila* are beta-hemolytic.

A. hydrophila is a pathogen of reptiles, fish, and amphibians. Guinea pigs and mice can be experimentally infected. *A. hydrophila* has been recovered from a variety of animals and birds, including cattle, swine, dogs, horses, several avian species, and wild, zoo, and laboratory animals; however, it is only rarely pathogenic in these animals. It causes furunculosis in salmonid fishes. *Aeromonas* species have been implicated as the cause of cellulitis, diarrhea, septicemia, urinary tract infections, osteomyelitis, meningitis, peritonitis, otitis, and endocarditis in humans.

Known virulence factors of *A. hydrophila* are a heat-stable cytotonic toxin, a heat-labile cytotoxin, and surface adhesins.

Table 18–2. *Differentiation of Aeromonas, Plesiomonas, and Vibrio*

Tests	Aeromonas	Plesiomonas	Vibrio
Susceptible to 0/129*			
10 µg	−	V	V
150 µg	−	+	+
Lipase production	(+)	−	(+)
Na⁺ is required for growth	−	−	+[†]
Gelatin hydrolysis	+	−	+
Oxidase	+	+	+[‡]
Acid:			
Sucrose	+	−	(+)
Mannitol	+	−	(+)
Inositol	−	+	−

* Vibriostatic agent 2,4-diamino-6,7 diisopropylpteridine phosphate.
[†] Except *V. cholerae* and *V. mimicus.*
[‡] Except *V. metschnikovii.*
V, variable; (+), most positive.
Adapted from Finegold, S.M. and Baron, E.L.: Vibrionaceae family. *In* Bailey and Scott's Diagnostic Microbiology. 7th Ed. St. Louis, The C.V. Mosby Co., 1986.

170   *Bacteria*

Plesiomonas

Plesiomonas shigelloides (formerly *Aeromonas shigelloides*) is the only species in the genus *Plesiomonas*. It is a facultatively anaerobic, gram-negative rod with polar flagella. Nonmotile strains have been recognized occasionally from clinical specimens. This species occurs widely in water, fish, and other aquatic animals. Like *Aeromonas*, *P. shigelloides* produces oxidase and catalase and ferments glucose. The organism grows well on the common laboratory media at 37° C and is nonhemolytic on blood agar. The minimum and maximum growth temperatures are 8° and 42° C, respectively.

The organism has been recovered from the gut of fish and from a variety of animals, including cattle, goats, dogs, cats, monkeys, swine, snakes, and toads. It has been implicated only rarely in infection of domestic animals. *P. shigelloides* causes diarrhea in humans. Infection has been associated with travel to or residence in tropical and subtropical areas. Most infections are thought to result from drinking contaminated water or eating raw seafood. Cellulitis, septicemia, and meningitis also have been reported in humans.

P. shigelloides produces heat-labile and heat-stable enterotoxins. Their exact role in the pathogenesis is not known.

Vibrio

Members of the genus *Vibrio* are facultatively anaerobic, gram-negative, straight or curved rods; they are motile with polar flagella. Cultures grown on solid media possess numerous lateral flagella. All produce oxidase (except *V. metschnikovii* and *V. gazogenes*) and ferment glucose readily without gas. Most species grow well at 30 to 35° C on commonly used laboratory media, but only a few species can grow at 4 or 40° C.

Vibrio species are found in seawater and fresh water, where they can cause diseases in aquatic animals. Only one species, *V. metschnikovii*, has been reported to cause an infrequent fatal disease of young chickens and other avian species. The disease is characterized by the sudden onset of severe enteritis with diarrhea. At least five species of *Vibrio* are known to cause or be associated with diarrhea in humans. Among these is *V. cholerae*, the cause of human cholera. *V. parahaemolyticus* is a major cause of gastroenteritis in humans. The disease is associated with the consumption of inadequately cooked seafood. In addition, various vibrios have been isolated from the following human specimens: blood, wounds, eyes, ears, and gallbladder.

FURTHER READING

Ashdown, L.R., and Koehler, J.M.: Production of hemolysin and other extracellular enzymes by clinical isolates of *Pseudomonas pseudomallei*. J. Clin. Microbiol. *28*:2331, 1990.

Dance, D.A.B.: Melioidosis: the tip of the iceberg? Clin. Microbiol. Rev. 4:52, 1991.

Dogget, R.G. (ed.): *Pseudomonas aeruginosa:* Clinical Manifestations of Infection and Current Therapy. New York, Academic Press, Inc., 1979.

Donovan, G.A., and Gross, T.L.: Cutaneous botryomycosis (bacterial granulomas) in dairy cows caused by *Pseudomonas aeruginosa*. J. Am. Vet. Med. Assoc. *184*:197, 1984.

Durack, D.T.: *Pseudomonas aeruginosa:* A ubiquitous pathogen. *In* Mechanisms of Microbial Disease. Edited by M. Schaechter, et al. Baltimore, Williams & Wilkins. 1993.

Erskine, R.J., et al.: *Pseudomonas* mastitis: Difficulties in detection and elimination from contaminated wash-water systems. J. Am. Vet. Med. Assoc. *191*:811, 1987.

Herrington, D.A., et al.: In vitro and in vivo pathogenicity of *Plesiomonas shigelloides*. Infect. Immun. *55*:979, 1987.

Honda, T., et al.: The thermostable direct haemolysin of *Vibrio parahaemolyticus* is a pore-forming toxin. Can. J. Microbiol. *38*:1175, 1992.

Iglewski, B.: Probing *Pseudomonas aeruginosa*, an opportunistic pathogen. Am. Soc. Microbiol. News *55*:303, 1989.

Lausen, N.C.G., Richter A.G., and Large, A.L.: *Pseudomonas aeruginosa* infection in squirrel monkeys. J. Am. Vet. Med. Assoc. *189*:1216, 1986.

Palleroni, N.J.: The *Pseudomonas* Group. Durham, England, Meadowfield Press Ltd., 1978.

von Graevenitz, A., and Altwegg, M.: *Aeromonas* and *Plesiomonas*. *In* Manual of Clinical Microbiology. 5th Ed. Edited by A. Balows. Washington, D.C., American Society for Microbiology, 1991.

Woods, D.E., et al.: Role of pili in adherence of *Pseudomonas aeruginosa* to mammalian buccal epithelial cells. Infect. Immun. *29*:1146, 1980.

19

Pasteurella and Francisella

There is no justification for including *Francisella* with *Pasteurella* other than convenience and tradition. *Francisella tularensis* was once, with little justification, called *Pasteurella tularensis*.

PRINCIPAL CHARACTERISTICS OF PASTEURELLA

Species of *Pasteurella* are of small gram-negative rods or coccobacilli. They are non-motile, non-spore-forming, facultatively anaerobic, oxidase positive, and fermentative (except for *P. anatipestifer*).

Bergey's Manual of Systematic Bacteriology, Vol 1, recognizes the following species:

1. *P. multocida*: may occur as commensals in the upper respiratory and digestive tracts of several animal species.
2. *P. haemolytica*: may occur as commensals in the upper respiratory and digestive tracts of several animal species.
3. *P. pneumotropica*: may occur as commensals in the upper respiratory and digestive tracts of several animal species.
4. *P. ureae*: found in the upper respiratory tract of humans.
5. *P. gallinarum*: commensal in upper respiratory tract of chickens; occasionally causes low-grade respiratory infections in chickens.
6. *P. aerogenes*: commensal in the intestine of swine; rarely pathogenic.
7. *P. anatipestifer*: a nonfermenter that really does not belong in the genus *Pasteurella*.

The correct taxonomic position of some species of *Pasteurella* is still in doubt. A new classification has been proposed based mainly on DNA analysis.

It is particularly useful in that it gives names to organisms that were frequently referred to as *P. multocida*-like or *Pasteurella*-like because they differed in one or more characteristics from recognized species. Species included in the new classification and their differentiation are presented in Table 19–1. Their significance is summarized briefly as follows.

Three species of *P. multocida* have been proposed: *P. multocida* ssp. *multocida*; *P. multocida* ssp. *septica*; and *P. multocida* ssp. *gallicida*. The subspecies *multocida* contains most of the strains that cause significant disease in domestic animals. *P. multocida* ssp. *septica* is recovered from various sources, including dogs, cats, birds, and human beings. It is most important in wound infections that result when people are bitten by dogs and cats. *P. multocida* ssp. *gallicida* is recovered from avian species and may occasionally cause fowl cholera. The three subspecies are differentiated by minor differences in their fermentation of carbohydrates. The identification of these subspecies may be useful in epidemiologic studies, but their recognition is of little significance for practitioners. Most diagnostic laboratories will probably continue to use the name *P. multocida* without naming the subspecies.

The new names and brief comments on their significance are given below.

Pasteurella dagmatis. This is a commensal organism of the oro- and nasopharynx of dogs and cats. In human beings, it causes local and systemic infections resulting from animal bites. These strains are identical to the Henriksen biotype of *P. pneumotropica*.

171

Table 19–1. *Differential Characteristics of Species in the Proposed Reclassification of the Genus Pasteurella*

Taxon	NAD requirement	Ornithine	Indole	Urease	Acid produced within 24 to 48 hr from:						
					Trehalose	Maltose	D-Xylose	L-Arabinose	Mannitol	Sorbitol	Dulcitol
P. multocida ssp. multocida	−	+	+	−	d	−	d	−	+	+	−
P. multocida ssp. septica	−	+	+	−	+	−	+	−	+	−	−
P. multocida ssp. gallicida	−	+	+	−	−	−	+	d	+	+	+
P. dagmatis	−	−	+	+	+	+	−	−	−	−	−
P. gallinarum	−	−	d	−	+	+	−	−	−	−	−
P. canis	−	+	+	−	d	−	d	−	−	−	−
P. stomatis	−	−	+	−	+	−	−	−	−	−	−
P. anatis	−	+	−	−	+	−	+	−	+	−	−
Pasteurella species B	+	−	+	−	+	d	+	−	+	−	+
Pasteurella species A	+	−	−	−	+	d	d	+	d	−	−
P. langaa	−	−	−	−	−	−	−	−	+	−	−
P. avium	d	−	−	−	+	−	d	−	+	−	−
P. volantium	+	d	−	−	+	+	d	−	+	d	−

NAD, nicotinamide adenine dinucleotide; d, different results observed.
Adapted from Mutters, R. et al. Reclassification of the genus *Pasteurella* Trevisan 1887 on the basis of deoxyribonucleic acid homology, with proposals for the new species *Pasteurella dagmatis, Pasteurella canis, Pasteurella stomatis, Pasteurella anatis,* and *Pasteurella langaa.* Int. J. Syst. Bacteriol. 35:309-322, 1985.

Pasteurella gallinarum. Commensal in upper respiratory tract of chickens; occasionally causes low-grade respiratory infections in chickens.

Pasteurella canis. This new species includes many of the *P. multocida*-like strains from canine mouths and dog-bite infections.

Pasteurella stomatis. This species has been recovered from the respiratory tracts of dogs and cats. Many of the *Pasteurella* strains recovered from cats, and some recovered from dogs, are *P. multocida* (ssp. *multocida* or ssp. *septica*). *Pasteurella* species have a low capacity for causing disease in dogs and cats. They are usually secondary invaders and involved in mixed infections.

Pasteurella anatis. This species has been recovered from the intestinal tracts of ducks.

Little information is available on the significance of the varieties *Pasteurella* A and *Pasteurella* B listed in Table 19–1, because few strains have been studied.

Pasteurella langaa. This species has been isolated from the respiratory tracts of normal chickens.

Pasteurella avium and *P. volantium.* The former was known previously as *Haemophilus avium*. *Pasteurella avium* and *P. volantium* have been recovered from the respiratory tracts of normal chickens.

Additional species. *P. ureae*, which is only recovered from humans, has been renamed *Actinobacillus ureae*.

The authors of this new classification concluded that *Pasteurella haemolytica* biotypes A and T and *P. pneumotropica* biotypes Jawetz and Heyl do not belong in the genus *Pasteurella* and are more closely related to the *Actinobacillus* group. They found that *Pasteurella aerogenes* did not belong in the genus *Pasteurella* and that its correct taxonomic position is not yet known.

Several new species have been proposed in recent reports. An aerogenic species, *P. caballi*, was isolated from equine clinical specimens. It is a commensal of the upper respiratory tract of horses and was considered to have a causal role in upper respiratory infections, pneumonia, peritonitis, and a mesenteric abscess. The new species *P. granulomatis* is associated with a severe, progressive, fibrogranulomatous disease of cattle in southern Brazil. Lesions caused by *Dermatobia hominis* may initiate the disease process. An organism given the name *P. testudinis* occurs as a commensal in tortoises. Two new species of probably minor significance have been established recently. They are *P. lymphangitidis* from bovine lymphangitis and *P. mairi* from porcine abortions.

DISTRIBUTION AND HABITAT

Pasteurella organisms are distributed worldwide. The species previously listed (except for *P. ureae*) occur as commensals in the upper respiratory and digestive passages of animals, e.g., *P. multocida* is found in the mouth of cats and the tonsils and nasal passages of swine; *P. haemolytica* is found in the nasopharynx of some normal cattle and sheep.

Pasteurella multocida

HISTORICAL

The first significant report of an organism of this species was made by Bollinger in 1878.

MODE OF INFECTION

Infection may be acquired by contact, inhalation, or ingestion; rarely is it transmitted by biting arthropods.

PATHOGENESIS

As in other gram-negative infections, endotoxins no doubt play a role in pathogenesis. Various environmental stresses play an important role in predisposition to infection. Passage of the infecting agent from animal to animal results in enhancement of virulence. *P. multocida* is a frequent secondary invader in pneumonic disease; however, it may also be a primary cause of disease, as in fowl cholera and epizootic hemorrhagic septicemia. When it is primary, septicemia frequently occurs.

A thermolabile toxin is produced by some type A and D strains recovered from swine and other animals. Some investigators think that the toxigenic cultures alone, or together with *Bordetella bronchiseptica*, cause atrophic rhinitis of swine. It is thought that *B. bronchiseptica* infection of the turbinate mucosa facilitates colonization by toxigenic strains of *Pasteurella multocida*. Toxigenic strains of *P. multocida* have been isolated from disease in humans.

Among the properties of the *P. multocida* toxin are the following: mainly cell-associated and appears to be released when bacteria die; polypeptide with molecular weight 125,000 to 160,000; heatlabile; dermonecrotic (guinea pig skin); lethal for mice; and immunogenic. The gene encoding for the toxin has been cloned and expressed in *Escherichia coli*. The recombinant toxin has properties comparable to those of the original purified toxin.

PATHOGENICITY

The diseases with which *Pasteurella multocida* is associated are too numerous to review fully. It may be a primary agent but more frequently it is a secondary invader when resistance of the animal is reduced by various stresses. It may be secondary to a primary virus, mycoplasma, or other bacterium.

P. multocida is a primary or more frequently a secondary invader in pneumonia of cattle, swine, sheep, goats, and other species. As a secondary invader, it is frequently involved in the bovine pneumonic pasteurellosis and in enzootic pneumonia of pigs. As mentioned earlier, toxin-producing strains, alone or with *Bordetella bronchiseptica*, cause the important economic disease of swine called atrophic rhinitis. It is considered the primary cause of fowl cholera and epizootic hemorrhagic septicemia of cattle and water buffaloes. Epizootic hemorrhagic septicemia occurs in many tropical and subtropical countries but is rare in the United States and South America. *Pasteurella multocida* is one of the causes of the pleuro-pneumonia form of "snuffles" in rabbits; it is a cause of severe mastitis of cattle and sheep; and it is responsible for a variety of sporadic infections in animals, including encephalitis, meningitis, and abortion. Atrophic rhinitis in rabbits caused by *P. multocida* has been reported.

Because dogs and cats harbor these organisms in their mouths as commensals, humans and other animals are frequently infected by bites. A wide variety of infections have been reported in humans including sinusitis, pneumonia, peritonitis, urinary tract infection, endocarditis, otitis, meningitis, abscesses, cellulitis, tonsillitis, appendicitis, bacteremia, and septicemia. Human infections are frequently secondary to some primary disease process.

DIRECT EXAMINATION

Bipolar organisms can be demonstrated in blood smears in septicemias. This is of minor significance except as an aid in the diagnosis of epizootic hemorrhagic septicemia.

SPECIMENS

Specimens are selected according to the location of the infectious process. The organisms survive well in transport media and in refrigerated and frozen tissues.

ISOLATION AND CULTIVATION

Definitive diagnosis is based on isolation and identification of *P. multocida*. Good primary growth requires media enriched with serum or blood. Colonies appear after incubation for 24 hours at 37° C in air or in an atmosphere of 6 to 8% CO_2. They are usually of moderate size, round, and grayish. Some strains produce large mucoid colonies. Fresh cultures have a characteristic odor.

Smears reveal small, gram-negative rods and coccobacilli. Marked pleomorphism is not uncommon.

IDENTIFICATION

Of special significance are nonmotility, indole production, lack of hemolysis, and production of oxidase (Table 19–2). In contrast, *P. haemolytica* is beta-hemolytic, indole-negative, and grows poorly on MacConkey agar. Some strains are weak oxidase producers. Cultures of *P. multocida* that are aberrant in one or two biochemical characteristics are occasionally encountered.

EXPERIMENTAL ANIMALS

Mice and rabbits are susceptible to most strains. Lethal infections develop within one or several days. Mouse inoculation is occasionally used to recover *P. multocida* from heavily contaminated specimens, e.g., nasal swabs from pigs.

ANTIGENIC NATURE

The types identified on the basis of differences in capsular substances (polysaccharides) are types A, B, D, E, and F.
1. Type A: causes fowl cholera, pneumonia, and many other infections of various animals.
2. Type B: causes epizootic hemorrhagic septicemia in Asia, the Middle East, and southern Europe.
3. Type D: recovered relatively infrequently from various infections in many animals but frequently from pneumonia and atrophic rhinitis in swine.
4. Type E: causes epizootic hemorrhagic septicemia in Africa.
5. Type F: recovered from turkeys; its role in disease is not yet clear.

Capsular types may be subdivided further into somatic types (16 thus far) on the basis of serologic differences in lipopolysaccharides (somatic or O antigens). A serotype is designated by the capsular type, followed by the number representing the somatic type, e.g., serotype B:2 is the cause of epi-

Table 19–2. Differential Characteristics of Important Pasteurella spp.

| | Beta hemolysis | MacConkey Agar | Indole | Oxidase | Urease | Ornithine Decarboxylase | Fermentation: Acid/Gas | | | | |
							Glucose	Lactose	Sucrose	Maltose	Mannitol
P. multocida	–	–	+	+	–	(+)	A	(–)	A	(–)	(A)
P. haemolytica (Table 19–3)	+	+	–	+	–	(–)	A	(A)	A	A	A
P. pneumotropica	–	–	+	+	+	+	A	(A)	A	A	–
P. gallinarum	–	–	–	+	–	+/–	A	–	A	A	–
P. ureae	–	–	–	+	+	–	A	–	A	A	A
P. aerogenes	–	+	–	+	+	(+)	AG	–	AG	AG	–
P. anatipestifer	–	–	–	–	–	NA	–	–	–	–	–
P. caballi	–	–	–	+	–	+/–	AG	A	NA	A	A

(+), most positive; (–), most negative; +/–, positive and negative strains; NA, not available.

demic hemorrhagic septicemia. Different varieties within a serotype can be identified by DNA fingerprinting.

TREATMENT

The following antibacterial drugs have been widely used: penicillin and streptomycin; tetracyclines; sulfonamides, including sulfamerazine and sulfamethazine; and chloramphenicol if strains are resistant to the less toxic drugs. Sulfaquinoxaline is the drug of choice in fowl cholera. Ceftiofur (naxel), a third-generation cephalosporin, has been shown to be effective in the treatment of pneumonia in cattle caused by *P. multocida* and *P. haemolytica*. For many years, antibiotic resistance was uncommon, but currently some clinical isolates have displayed multiple resistance. Antibiotic resistance plasmids have been found in strains of *P. multocida* causing fowl cholera and pneumonia in cattle.

IMMUNITY

Immunity is predominantly humoral.

Pasteur's first vaccine was developed to prevent fowl cholera. It was an attenuated strain that was not altogether satisfactory. In recent years, vaccines consisting of live attenuated strains, administered in drinking water, have been employed to prevent fowl cholera. Several live attenuated vaccines are being employed to prevent pneumonic pasteurellosis in cattle with varying degrees of success.

Whole-broth killed cultures (bacterins) with a high concentration of organisms, some containing adjuvants, have been used widely to prevent the following *P. multocida* infections:

1. Fowl cholera: there is a problem of different serotypes resulting in bacterin "breaks," i.e., the causal serotype may not be in the bacterin.
2. Pneumonic pasteurellosis: with or without *P. haemolytica* and the viruses PI-3 and IBR.
3. Pneumonia in sheep: with *P. haemolytica*.
4. Hemorrhagic septicemia: type B or type E strains.

Pasteurella haemolytica

Two different biotypes of *P. haemolytica* have been identified, viz., biotype A and biotype T. They differ in several characteristics, including pathogenicity, antigenic nature, and biochemical activity (Table 19–3). The name *P. trehalosi* has been proposed for *P. haemolytica*, biotype T.

PATHOGENICITY

All strains of *P. haemolytica* elaborate a soluble cytotoxin (leukotoxin) that kills alveolar macro-

phages and other leukocytes of ruminants, thus breaching the lung's primary defense mechanism. Some properties of the cytotoxin are the following: produced by all serotypes of *P. haemolytica;* thermolabile; is protein of relatively large molecular weight; resembles the alpha-hemolysin of *Escherichia coli;* and is immunogenic. The DNA fragment responsible for leukotoxin has been successfully cloned in *E. coli*. There is considerable evidence that the cytotoxin plays an important role in the pathogenesis of pneumonia in ruminants.

Pasteurella haemolytica has a primary or secondary role in pneumonia of cattle, goats, and sheep and is frequently recovered from the bronchopneumonic lungs of cattle with shipping fever. Other important diseases in which this organism is involved are mastitis of ewes and septicemia of lambs.

Laboratory animals are refractory to experimental infection. Gastric mucin and hemoglobin have been used to enhance the virulence of *P. haemolytica* for mice.

A distinct variety of *P. haemolytica* can cause infrequent low-grade infections in poultry and swine. *P. haemolytica* of chicken, turkey, and swine origin differ in certain biochemical characteristics from the conventional ruminant strains, and in addition, the former strains cannot be typed. The taxonomic position of these "atypical" strains is not yet clear. They are referred to as *P. haemolytica*-like. Some produce leukotoxin.

ISOLATION AND CULTIVATION

Direct examination is of limited value.

Media containing serum or blood are required for good growth. Colonies are round, grayish, and usually somewhat smaller than those of *P. multocida*. They are usually surrounded by a zone of beta-hemolysis. This zone varies considerably and may be no larger than the colony, and thus it is not apparent unless the colony is removed. Bovine blood is more suitable than that of sheep or horses for the demonstration of hemolysis.

IDENTIFICATION

Smears from colonies disclose small gram-negative rods or coccobacilli. It is of special significance in identification that they are beta-hemolytic, indole-negative, nonmotile, and grow on MacConkey agar (see Table 19–2). A *P. haemolytica*-like organism frequently can be recovered from the upper respiratory tract of chickens and turkeys. It differs in hemolysis, which is stronger, and differs biochemically from typical cultures of *P. haemolytica*.

Table 19–3. Differential Characteristics of Biotypes of **Pasteurella haemolytica**

	Biotype A	Biotype T
Fermentation:		
arabinose	+	−
trehalose	−	+
salacin	−	+
xylose	+	−
lactose	+	−
Susceptibility to penicillin:	(except serotype 2) high	low
Serotypes:	1,2,5,6,7,8,9,11,12, 13,14,16	3,4,10,15
Principal location in normal host:	nasopharynx	tonsils
Principal disease association:	Pneumonia in cattle and sheep; septicemia in nursing lambs.	Septicemia in feeder lambs

Modified from Biberstein, E.L.: Biotyping and serotyping of *Pasteurella haemolytica*. Methods Microbiol. *10*:253, 1978.

TREATMENT

Treatment is essentially the same as that for *P. multocida*. Multiple drug resistance is encountered, and antibiotic resistance plasmids have been demonstrated.

ANTIGENIC NATURE AND IMMUNITY

P. haemolytica is heterogeneous and somewhat resembles *P. multocida* in that it has capsular and somatic varieties. The somatic antigens are so complex that serotypes are designated according to differences in capsular substances, e.g., type 1 is the most common type in bovine pneumonia. There are 16 serotypes of *P. haemolytica* based on capsular antigens. These antigens are recognized by an indirect hemagglutination procedure (Table 19–3).

Immunity is thought to be predominantly humoral.

Bacterins containing both *P. haemolytica* and *P. multocida* are widely used in cattle and sheep, although their value is questionable. Claims of efficacy in the prevention of bovine pneumonic pasteurellosis have been made for several live and subunit vaccines.

Pasteurella pneumotropica

This organism can be recovered from the nasopharynx of some guinea pigs, rats, hamsters, mice, dogs, and cats. It is usually a secondary invader in pneumonic disease in mice and rats, and has been implicated in enteritis of hamsters. It is not a significant pathogen in dogs and cats.

It resembles *P. multocida* culturally but can be distinguished biochemically (see Table 19–2). Some strains may split sugars with the production of gas.

Pasteurella anatipestifer

The name *Riemerella anatipestifer* has been proposed recently for this species. It was found to have a phylogenetic affiliation within the *Flavobacterium-Cytophaga* rRNA homology group.

Pasteurella anatipestifer causes infectious serositis, a highly acute disease of ducklings, various water fowl, chickens, turkeys, and pheasants. This disease has often had an adverse effect on the commercial duck industry. A widely distributed serofibrinous exudate is found in the acute form of the disease.

Francisella tularensis

This organism was first isolated in Tulare County, California, in 1912. *F. tularensis* is the only significant species in this genus. *F. novicida*, which was recovered from water, is not known to infect animals or humans; recent studies suggest that it belongs in a biogroup of *F. tularensis*. Two biovars of *F. tularensis* have been found in the United States. Type A (*F. tularensis* ssp. *tularensis*) biovars are highly virulent and are associated with rabbits. Type B (*F. tularensis* ssp. *paleartica*) biovars are less virulent and are associated with disease of muskrats and beavers. Type A biovars exhibit citruline ureidase activity but type B biovars do not. About 80% of human cases of tularemia in the United States are caused by type A biovars.

PRINCIPAL CHARACTERISTICS

F. tularensis is a small, pleomorphic, nonmotile, noncapsulated, aerobic, gram-negative rod or coccobacillus. It is a facultative intracellular parasite that is oxidase negative, nonfermentative, and requires cystine for isolation.

PATHOGENICITY

Tularemia is principally a disease of wild animals; however, humans, as well as some domestic animals and fowl, are susceptible. In nature, the disease is frequently transmitted from infected to susceptible hosts by insect vectors. These include wood ticks, dog and rabbit ticks, the deer fly, fleas, black flies, mites, mosquitoes, and lice. The organism can be transmitted transovarially in female ticks.

The prevalence of tularemia in wild rabbits in the United States has been estimated to be approximately 1%. In North America, the cottontail rabbit is the reservoir of infection for nearly 70% of the human cases. Other naturally susceptible animals are squirrel, opossum, beaver, woodchuck, muskrat, skunk, coyote, fox, cat, sheep, deer, bullsnake, game birds, and domestic fowl.

PATHOGENESIS

The most characteristic feature of the disease is focal, granulomatous lesions of a variety of organs and lymph nodes that may undergo necrosis and suppuration. After spread from the point of entry to dependent lymph nodes, a bacteremia results in small abscessing granulomas in visceral organs and lymph nodes. Small, necrotic, granulomatous foci in the liver, spleen, and lymph nodes are the characteristic gross lesions observed in wild rabbits.

The manner in which *F. tularensis* causes disease is not understood. Endotoxin is probably an important factor; an exotoxin has not been found. The organism, however, is highly toxic for macrophages. Immunity is primarily cell-mediated, and delayed hypersensitivity may contribute to tissue damage.

PUBLIC HEALTH SIGNIFICANCE

Humans may become infected as a result of contact with infected animals or their discharges; animal bites; ingestion of contaminated water and partially cooked meat; and inhalation of fecal droplets of ticks.

The human disease may assume several forms, but the most common is the ulceroglandular form, with the development of papule, ulcer, and lymph node enlargement, in that order. Depending on the portal of entry, the other forms are the oculoglandular, glandular, gastrointestinal, pneumonic, and typhoidal. All forms may give rise to the systemic form, but the pneumonic and typhoidal forms are considered the most dangerous.

ISOLATION AND CULTIVATION

Note: The organism is highly infectious for humans, and isolation should not be attempted without proper biocontainment facilities.

It grows well on cystine-blood agar; cystine is essential for growth. Minute and dewdrop-like colonies yield small, gram-negative rods and coccobacilli. There is a characteristic greenish discoloration surrounding the colonies.

Guinea pig inoculation is sometimes used to overcome contaminants. The organism can be recovered without difficulty from terminally ill guinea pigs.

IDENTIFICATION

Biochemical tests are difficult to perform and are not usually carried out. The fluorescent antibody (FA) procedure is widely used to identify the organisms. Identification of specific antibodies by enzyme-linked immunosorbent assay (ELISA) or agglutination in the sera of guinea pigs inoculated with infectious material is confirmatory.

A four-fold rise in titer in the agglutination test with paired sera is supportive of a diagnosis in humans.

TREATMENT

Streptomycin is the drug of choice. Early treatment usually eliminates organisms from lesions.

IMMUNITY

This is primarily cell-mediated. A live attenuated vaccine is used in people whose risk of infection is high.

FURTHER READING

Adlam, C., and Rutter, J.M. (eds.): Pasteurella and Pasteurellosis. London, Academic Press, 1989.

Bain, R.V.S., de Alwis, M.C.L., Carter, G.R., and Gupta, B.K.: Hemorrhagic septicemia. FAO Animal Production and Health Paper, No. 323. Rome, Food and Agricultural Organization of the United Nations, 1982.

Biberstein, E.L.: Biotyping and serotyping of *Pasteurella haemolytica.* Methods Microbiol. *10*:253, 1978.

Brennan, P.C., Fritz, T.E., and Flynn, R.J.: *Pasteurella pneumotropica:* Cultural and biochemical characteristics, and its association with disease in laboratory animals. Lab. Anim. Care *15*:307, 1965.

Carter, G.R.: Pasteurellosis: *Pasteurella multocida* and *Pasteurella haemolytica.* Adv. Vet. Sci. *11*:321, 1967.

Carter, G.R.: Serotyping *Pasteurella multocida*. Methods Microbiol. *16*:247, 1984.

Chengappa, M.M., Carter, G.R., and Chang, T.S.: Hemoglobin enhancement of experimental infection of mice with *Pasteurella haemolytica*. Am. J. Vet. Res. *44*:1545, 1983.

Collins, F.M.: Mechanisms of acquired resistance to *Pasteurella multocida* infection: A review. Cornell Vet. *67*:103, 1977.

Donnio, P.Y., et al.: Dermonecrotic toxin production by strains of *P. multocida* isolated from man. J. Med. Microbiol. *34*:333, 1991.

Fodor, L., et al.: Characterization of a new serotype of *Pasteurella haemolytica* isolated in Hungary. Res. Vet. Sci. *44*:399, 1988.

Frank, G.H., and Wessman, G.E.: Rapid plate agglutination procedure for serotyping *Pasteurella haemolytica*. J. Clin. Microbiol. *7*:142, 1978.

Heddleston, K.L., Gallagher, J.E., and Rebers, P.A.: Fowl cholera: Gel diffusion precipitin test for serotyping *Pasteurella multocida* from avian species. Avian Dis. *16*:925, 1972.

Kilian, M., Frederiksen, W., and Biberstein, E.L. (eds.): *Haemophilus, Pasteurella* and *Actinobacillus*. New York, Academic Press, 1981.

Long, G.W., et al.: Detection of *Francisella tularensis* in blood by polymerase chain reaction. J. Clin. Microbiol. *31*:152, 1993.

Markham, R.J.F., and Wilkie, B.N.: Interaction between *Pasteurella haemolytica* and bovine alveolar macrophages: Cytotoxic effect on macrophages and impaired phagocytosis. Am. J. Vet. Res. *41*:18, 1980.

Patten, B.E., et al. (eds.): Pasteurellosis in Production Animals. Proceedings, International Workshop, Bali, Indonesia, 1992.

Canberra, Agricultural Centre for International Research, 1993.

Petersen, S.K., and Foged, N.T.: Cloning and expression of the *Pasteurella* toxin gene, tox A, in *Escherichia coli*. Infect. Immun. *57*:3907, 1989.

Reilly, J.R.: Tularemia. *In* Infectious Diseases of Wild Mammals. Edited by J.W. Davis. Ames, Iowa State University Press, 1970.

Ribeiro, G.A., Carter, G.R., Frederiksen, W., and Riet-Correa, F.: A *Pasteurella haemolytica*-like bacterium from a progressive granuloma of cattle in Brazil. J. Clin. Microbiol. *27*:1401, 1989.

Rimler, R.B., and Rhoades, K.R.: Serogroup F, a new capsular serogroup of *Pasteurella multocida*. J. Clin. Microbiol. *25*:615, 1987.

Rutter, J.M., and Luther, P.D.: Cell culture assay for toxigenic *Pasteurella multocida* from atrophic rhinitis of pigs. Vet. Rec. *114*:393, 1984.

Sandhu, T.S., Rhoades, K.R., and Rimler, R.: *Pasteurella anatipestifer* infection. *In* Diseases of Poultry. 9th Ed. Edited by B.W. Calnek, et al. Ames, IA, Iowa State University Press, 1991.

Schlater, L.K., et al.: *Pasteurella caballi*, a new species from equine clinical specimens. J. Clin. Microbiol. *27*:2169, 1989.

Shewen, P.E., and Wilkie, B.N.: Cytotoxin of *Pasteurella haemolytica* acting on bovine leukocytes. Infect. Immun. *35*:91, 1982.

Sneath, P.H.A., and Stevens, M.: *Actinobacillus rossii* sp. nov., nom. rev., *Pasteurella bettii* sp. nov., *Pasteurella lymphangitidis* sp. nov., *Pasteurella mairi* sp. nov., and *Pasteurella trehalosi* sp. nov. Int. J. Syst. Bacteriol. *40*:148, 1990.

Yung-Fu C., Young, R.Y., Post, D., and Struck, D.K.: Identification and characterization of the *Pasteurella haemolytica* leukotoxin. Infect. Immun. *55*:2348, 1987.

20

Actinobacillus

Principal Characteristics of *Actinobacillus*

Species of the genus *Actinobacillus* are gram-negative, nonmotile, small rods. They are non-spore-forming, aerobic, facultatively anaerobic, and fermentative.

The following species are recognized by *Bergey's Manual of Systematic Bacteriology:* (1) *A. lignieresii;* (2) *A. equuli;* (3) *A. suis* (causes septicemia and other infectious processes in pigs); (4) *A. capsulatus* (causes arthritis in rabbits); and (5) *A. actinomycetemcomitans* has a role in periodontal disease and endocarditis in humans. Although it is infrequently recovered from animals it has been associated with epididymitis in rams. An organism named *A. rossi* has been recovered from the vaginas of postparturient sows. Its significance is not yet clear.

There are three species which probably do not belong in the genus *Actinobacillus:* (1) *A. actinoides,* which produces pneumonia in calves and seminal vesiculitis in bulls; it is probably the same as *Haemophilus sommus;* (2) *A. seminis,* which causes epididymitis in young rams—a disease resembling that caused by *Brucella ovis*—and purulent polyarthritis and gangrenous mastitis in sheep; and (3) *A. salpingitidis,* which is found in the oviduct and respiratory tract of chickens, and occasionally causes salpingitis and peritonitis.

All of these organisms probably occur as commensals, giving rise to exogenous and endogenous infections. *A. pleuropneumoniae,* formerly *Haemophilus pleuropneumoniae,* the cause of swine pleuropneumonia, is a recent addition to the genus.

Actinobacillus lignieresii

Historical

A. lignieresii was described by Lignieres and Spritz in 1902 as one of the causes of bovine actinomycosis.

Distribution and Habitat

It is worldwide in distribution and occurs as a commensal in the alimentary tract of cattle. Six serotypes (somatic antigens) have been identified. Their occurrence correlates with geographic and host species origin.

Mode of Infection

The organism usually produces a sporadic, endogenous disease, but on occasion several animals in a herd may be infected. It gains entrance to the oral mucosa through injuries to the tissue.

Pathogenicity

Actinobacillosis is seen most commonly in cattle, less commonly in sheep, and rarely in pigs, dogs, and humans. Lesions usually consist of multiple, granulomatous abscesses. In cattle and sheep, these occur most frequently around the head and neck region. The lesion commences as a firm nodule that eventually ulcerates and discharges a viscous, white to faintly green pus that contains small granules. The granules are greyish-white and usually less than 1 mm in diameter. By comparison, the sulfur granules of actinomycosis are several millimeters in diameter.

Unlike actinomycosis, the infection is spread via the lymphatics. Lesions may involve the tongue (wooden tongue), lungs, and less frequently other internal organs. Rarely, granulomatous abscesses occur in the udder of the sow.

Several cases of an acute, suppurative bronchopneumonia and infected horse- and sheep-bite wounds have been reported in humans.

DIRECT EXAMINATION

Small, gram-negative rods are demonstrable within granules. The granules are examined in the same manner as those from actinomycosis: wash, examine granule under a coverslip in 10% NaOH, prepare smear and stain. The granules in actinobacillosis are small (< 1 mm), grey, and white.

SPECIMENS

Pus and necrotic material from early, nondischarging lesions are submitted.

ISOLATION AND CULTIVATION

A. lignieresii can be recovered consistently if clinical material is seeded onto serum or blood agar and incubated at 37° C; 10% CO_2 stimulates growth.

Small, translucent, smooth, and glistening colonies resembling those of *P. multocida* are evident in 24 to 48 hours. Stained smears disclose small gram-negative rods or coccobacilli.

IDENTIFICATION

The organism can only be identified precisely by biochemical criteria (see Table 20–1).

IMMUNITY

Little is known about the immune response in this disease. The granulomatous nature of the lesions suggests a strong component of cellular immunity.

TREATMENT

Advanced cases are not usually treated. In others, surgical drainage along with a broad-spectrum antibiotic or a sulfonamide is employed. Potassium iodide given orally is useful in reducing the inflammation. Treatment must be prolonged.

Table 20–1. Differential Characteristics of Actinobacillus *Species*

	A. lignieresii	A. equuli	A. suis	A. capsulatus	A. actinomycetemcomitans	A. pleuropneumoniae	"A. seminis"
Hemolysis (sheep)	–*	V	+	–	–	+	–
CAMP reaction	–	–	–	–	–	+	–
Catalase	+	–	+	+	+	V	–
Hydrogen sulfide	+	V	–	–	–	+	–
Arabinose	–	–	+	+	–	–	+
Cellobiose	–	–	+	+	–	–	–
Esculin	–	–	+	(+)	–	–	–
Lactose	(+)	+	+	+	–	–	–
Mannitol	+	+	–	+	V	–	–
Melibiose	–	+	+	+	–	–	–
Salicin	–	–	+	+	–	–	–
Sorbitol	–	–	–	+	–	–	–
Sucrose	+	+	+	+	–	+	–
Trehalose	–	+	+	+	–	–	–

*Some strains of *A. ligniersii* from horses are hemolytic.
(+), late reaction; V, variable.
Adapted from Phillips, J.E.: *Actinobacillus*. In Diagnostic Procedures in Veterinary Bacteriology and Mycology. Edited by G.R. Carter and J.R. Cole, Jr., 5th Ed. New York, Academic Press, 1990.

Actinobacillus equuli

HABITAT

This organism is commonly found in the intestinal tract of normal horses.

MODE OF INFECTION

Mode of infection is probably by ingestion. Infrequently it may be via the umbilicus or across the placenta (prenatal). *Strongylus* larvae may carry the organism into arteries.

PATHOGENICITY

In foals the disease caused by *A. equuli* is called shigellosis or viscosum infection ("sleepy foal disease"). Many foals develop the disease within a few hours or days of birth. Those dying within 24 hours of life have a severe enteritis. Those living for several days develop a purulent nephritis, frequently with concomitant pneumonia and joint infections.

The following manifestations may be seen in older horses: lameness due to purulent arthritis; infected aneurysms leading to systemic involvement; and infrequent abortion in mares.

Septic arthritis, endocarditis, suppurative nephritis, septicemia, and mastitis are occasionally seen in swine.

SPECIMENS

Affected tissues, purulent material, feces, and blood are submitted.

ISOLATION AND CULTIVATION

The organism grows well on blood agar. The colonies of fresh isolates are rough in appearance but mucoid in character, probably due to a mucinous ("sticky") capsule. They may lose their mucoid character on transfer. Some strains are beta-hemolytic.

IDENTIFICATION

The principal differential features are given in Table 20–1.

CONTROL AND TREATMENT

Immunization is not practiced, and little is known about the immunology of the infection.

Strains are antigenically heterogeneous. Good sanitation at parturition, with disinfection of the umbilicus, is important. Prophylactic treatment of all foals shortly after birth with penicillin and streptomycin, or tetracyclines has been effective.

Actinobacillus pleuropneumoniae

Synonyms: *Haemophilus pleuropneumoniae, H. parahaemolyticus.*

This important pathogen of swine has been transferred from *Haemophilus* to the genus *Actinobacillus*. Like other *Actinobacillus* spp., it is a commensal of the upper respiratory tract of some pigs. The disease it causes, swine pleuropneumonia, is of great economic importance.

MODE OF INFECTION

The organism is transmitted by direct and indirect contact and infection is via the respiratory tract, most commonly by inhalation of infectious material.

PATHOGENICITY AND PATHOGENESIS

The morbidity and mortality of swine pleuropneumonia is usually very high in newly infected pigs of all age groups. Acute, subacute, and chronic respiratory infections are seen. The acute form is characterized by a severe fibrinous pleuropneumonia. The chronic form, which often occurs in feeder pigs, is characterized by pleuritis, pleural adhesions, and pulmonary sequestration and abscessation.

It has been hypothesized that antigen (endotoxin)-antibody complexes damage blood vessel endothelium and result in vasculitis, thrombosis with consequent edema, necrosis, infarction, and hemorrhage. In addition to lipopolysaccharide, the capsule, and cytotoxins have a role in virulence and pathogenesis. The cytotoxins belong to RTX (repeats in structural toxin) cytolysin family. These pore-forming toxins are hemolytic (resemble the alpha hemolysin of *E. coli*). They are heat-labile, immunogenic, and thought to be responsible for the severe lesions.

ANTIGENIC NATURE AND SEROLOGY

At least 12 serotypes have been identified based upon differences in capsular polysaccharide antigens. Serotypes 1, 5, and 7 are the most commonly isolated ones in North America. Serologic tests are not used for diagnosis, but may be useful in surveys, epidemiological studies, and efforts at elimination of the disease from herds.

ISOLATION AND CULTIVATION

A. pleuropneumoniae is usually isolated on blood agar. Most strains require the V factor (NAD), which can be supplied by yeast extract or a staphylococcus streak. Two colony types may be seen, a round "waxy" type and a flat, soft, glistening variety; both types are hemolytic. A positive CAMP reaction is seen with a β-toxin-producing staphylococcus.

IDENTIFICATION

The characteristic cellular and colonial morphology, along with the V factor requirement and a positive CAMP reaction, strongly suggests *A. pleuropneumoniae*. Definitive identification is based upon the characteristics listed in Table 20–1.

IMMUNITY

Immunity in swine pleuropneumonia is predominantly humoral. Maternal immunity protects neonates for 5 to 9 weeks. Capsular antigens elicit protective antibodies. Bacterins confer homologous protection and reduce mortality, but they do not completely prevent chronic pulmonary lesions. Polyvalent bacterins only protect against serotypes contained in the bacterin. In contrast, natural infection and aerosol exposure provide cross-serotype protection. Several mutant vaccines have shown promise.

TREATMENT

A. pleuropneumoniae is susceptible to many antimicrobial drugs including tetracyclines, chloramphenicol, spectinomycin, erythromycin, nitrofurazone, ampicillin, trimethoprim-sulfonamides, gentamycin, and penicillin G. Antimicrobial susceptibility tests should be carried out because multiple-drug-resistant strains have emerged. Resistance has been attributed to R-plasmids. Beta-lactamase resistance to penicillin and ampicillin has been reported.

Actinobacillus suis

This organism was first isolated from disease in swine in 1962. It is worldwide in distribution and probably occurs as a commensal in the tonsils and on mucous membranes of the respiratory and genital tracts of pigs. Route of infection is probably via the upper digestive or respiratory tract, and the umbilicus. The organisms are thought to gain access to the vascular system via the upper respiratory tract.

A. suis is most frequently associated with acute septicemia in young pigs (less than 6 months of age.) The organism has also been implicated in arthritis, pneumonia, pericarditis, nephritis, meningitis, and metritis in older pigs. A cytotoxin in the RTX family, similar to the cytotoxin or hemolysin of *A. pleuropneumoniae*, has been described. Its role in pathogenesis is not clear.

FURTHER READING

Allen, J.G.: Bronchopneumonia in calves in Western Australia associated with *Actinobacillus actinoides*. Aust. Vet. J. 52:100, 1976.

Bulgin, M.S., and Anderson, B.C.: Association of sexual experience with isolation of various bacteria in cases of ovine epididymitis. J. Am. Vet. Med. Assoc. *182*:372, 1983.

Burrows, L.L., and Lo. R.Y.C.: Molecular characterization of an RTX toxin determinant from *Actinobacillus suis*. Infect. Immun. 60:2166, 1992.

Campbell, S.G., Whitlock, R.H., Timoney, J.F., and Underwood, A.M.: An unusual epizootic of actinobacillosis in dairy heifers. J. Am. Vet. Med. Assoc., *166*:604, 1975.

Escande, F., et al.: Deoxyribonucleic acid relatedness among strains of *Actinobacillus* spp. and *Pasteurella ureae*. Int. J. Syst. Bact. 34:309, 1984.

Fales, W.H., et al.: Antimicrobial susceptibility and serotypes of actinobacillus (*Haemophilus*) pleuropneumonia recovered from Missouri swine. J. Vet. Diagn. Invest. 1:16, 1989.

Inzana, T.L.: Virulence properties of *Actinobacillus pleuropneumoniae*. Microb. Pathog. *11*:305, 1991.

Inzana, T.J., and Mathison, B.: Serotype specificity and immunogenicity of the capsular polymer of *Haemophilus pleuropneumoniae* serotype 5. Infect. Immun. 55:1580, 1987.

Inzana T.J., Todd, J., and Veit, H.P.: Safety, stability, and efficacy of noncapsulated mutants of *Actinobacillus pleuropneumoniae* for use in live vaccines. Infect. Immun. 61:1682, 1993.

Killian, M., Nicolet, J., and Biberstein, E.L.: Biochemical and serological characterization of *Haemophilus pleuropneumoniae* (Matthews and Pattison, 1961). Shope 1964 and proposal of a neotype strain. Int. J. Syst. Bacteriol. *28*:20, 1978.

Killian M., Frederiksen, W., and Biberstein, E.L. (eds.): *Haemophilus, Pasteurella and Actinobacillus*. New York, Academic Press, 1981.

Mair, N.S., et al.: *Actinobacillus suis* in pigs. J. Comp. Pathol. *84*:113, 1974.

Peel, M.M., et al.: *Actinobacillus* spp. and related bacteria in infected wounds of humans bitten by horses and sheep. J. Clin. Microbiol. 29:2535, 1991.

Phillips, J.E.: Antigenic structure and serological typing of *Actinobacillus lignieresii*. J. Pathol. Bacteriol. *93*:463, 1967.

Phillips, J.E.: *Actinobacillus*. In Bergey's Manual of Systematic Bacteriology. Vol. 1. Edited by N.R. Kreig. Baltimore, Williams & Wilkins, 1984.

Samitz, E.M., and Biberstein, E.L.: *Actinobacillus suis*-like organisms and evidence of hemolytic strains of *Actinobacillus lignieresii* in horses. Am. J. Vet. Res. 52:1245, 1991.

Sneath, P.H.A. and Stevens, M.: *Actinobacillus rossi* sp. nov., *Actinobacillus seminis* sp. nov., nom. rev., *Pasteurella bettii* sp. nov., *Pasteurella lymphangitidis* sp. nov., *Pasteurella mairi* sp. nov., and *Pasteurella trehalosi* sp. nov. Int. J. Syst. Bacteriol. *40*:148, 1990.

Watt, D.A., Banford, V., and Nairin, M.E.: *Actinobacillus seminis* as a cause of polyarthritis. Aust. Vet. J. *46*:515, 1971.

Windsor, R.S.: *Actinobacillus equuli* infection in a litter of pigs. Vet. Rec. *92*:178, 1983.

21

Campylobacter and Helicobacter

Principal Characteristics of *Campylobacter*

Campylobacter organisms are spirally curved (one or more spirals, gram-negative, pleomorphic rods; they are motile by a single polar flagellum, microaerophilic (3 to 15% O_2) to anaerobic, and oxidase-positive. They do not attack carbohydrates.

In contrast, *Vibrio* organisms are aerobic, facultatively anaerobic, and fermentative.

More than 13 species of *Campylobacter* have been described in the literature. Only some are considered pathogenic for animals. *Campylobacter* spp. are found on the mucous membrane of reproductive tracts, in the intestinal tract, and in the oral cavity of humans and animals.

Campylobacter fetus

Strains of *C. fetus* comprise two subspecies, *C. fetus* subsp. *fetus* and *C. fetus* subsp. *venerealis*. Subspecies *venerealis* can further be separated on the basis of H_2S production into two biotypes, *venerealis* and *intermedius*.

Historical

C. fetus was first recognized as a cause of abortion in cows by McFadean and Stockman in 1909.

Distribution and Mode of Infection

C. fetus is widespread. It is transmitted by ingestion or fomites. It is also present in semen and is spread venereally by the bull but not by the ram. Distribution of the two biotypes of subspecies *venerealis* is variable. Biotype *venerealis* is generally more widespread, whereas biotype *intermedius* is predominantly seen in some parts of the United States, Argentina, and the northern half of Australia.

Pathogenicity

Subspecies *venerealis* is found in the prepuce of the asymptomatic bull and the genital tract of the cow and heifer. It produces both infections and a carrier state in cattle. It also causes infertility (epizootic bovine infertility) and occasionally abortion in cattle. Subspecies *fetus* is found in the intestine of cattle, sheep, and humans. It causes abortion in cattle (sporadic) and sheep (multiple).

Subspecies *fetus* is also found in the genital tract of infected sheep and cattle, and in aborted fetal tissues; these serve as sources of this subspecies. Subspecies *fetus* has also been recovered from an aborted equine fetus and from aborted goat fetuses.

Subspecies *venerealis* has not been associated with human infection, whereas subspecies *fetus* has been recognized as an infrequent cause of systemic infections and meningitis, pericarditis, peritonitis, salpingitis, septic arthritis, abortions, and abscesses.

Effects are considered to result in part from endotoxins. The uterine mucosa is infected with

184

subsp. *venerealis,* resulting in a metritis. As a consequence, the embryo may die and be resorbed. The organism may be shed from the uterus for a long period.

During the course of infection with subsp. *fetus,* the organisms invade the uterus and multiply in the fetus. The infected fetuses are usually aborted. If birth occurs, the newborn may only live for a few hours.

SPECIMENS

Special methods are employed for the collection of cervical mucus and preputial secretions for culture. Fetal stomach contents or fetal tissues are also suitable for culture. Filtration may be used to aid recovery; *Campylobacter* can pass through a 0.65 μm membrane filter.

DIRECT EXAMINATION

C. fetus can be demonstrated in the fetal stomach contents by negative staining and by phase microscopy. A specific fluorescent antibody reagent can be used to identify *C. fetus* in preputial washings, cervical mucus, and fetal stomach contents, but it does not distinguish between subspecies.

ISOLATION AND CULTIVATION

In order to recover and grow the organism, the material submitted must be fresh.

Special media (e.g.; Clark and Dufty medium) containing antibiotics are available to reduce growth of contaminants. An atmosphere containing 10% CO_2 should be used. Air should be reduced to one third and replaced with nitrogen for subsp. *venerealis.*

Isolation media are available commercially; they are nutritively rich and selective. Plates are incubated at 37°C in an atmosphere of 10% CO_2. The oxygen content of the atmosphere should be reduced to 6%.

Fine pin-point colonies are seen after 3 to 6 days of incubation. Smears reveal small, gram-negative rods that assume various forms—short and long, both curved and S-shaped. Long wavy filaments may be seen in some cultures.

IDENTIFICATION

Most nonpathogenic strains of *Campylobacter* are catalase-negative. One of these is *C. sputorum* subsp. *bubulus,* which is found in the genital tract of male and female cattle and sheep. Differential characteristics are listed in Table 21–1.

SEROLOGIC DIAGNOSIS

The serum agglutination test may be of value if interpreted carefully. Sera should be taken from several aborting cows 3 weeks to 4 months after abortion. The cervical mucus agglutination test is more reliable.

ANTIGENIC NATURE AND SEROLOGY

There are considerable antigenic differences among subspecies, although they are composed of strains that are closely related serologically and immunologically. Serotyping of the two subspecies has not been widely employed in the characterization of field isolates.

RESISTANCE

Campylobacter spp. do not survive outside the host for more than several hours unless protected from drying and sunshine.

TREATMENT

Campylobacter spp. are susceptible to a number of antibiotics, but treatment is not usually feasible. Losses caused by the bovine disease may be reduced with penicillin and streptomycin. Irrigation of the uterus and prepuce with streptomycin is sometimes carried out. Tetracycline administered in feed or by injection may reduce the incidence of ovine abortion.

IMMUNITY

Bacterins composed of killed *C. fetus* subsp. *venerealis* combined with adjuvants such as oil, alum, or related compounds are of some value in cattle, but immunity is of short duration. Vaccination has been used in an effort to eliminate the carrier state in bulls. Bacterins are also used to prevent the ovine disease. The relative importance of humoral and cell-mediated immunity is not known, but it seems likely that the former is most important in protective immunity.

CONTROL OF EPIZOOTIC BOVINE INFERTILITY

Semen is routinely treated with streptomycin and penicillin. Breeding by artificial insemination will result in eventual elimination of *C. fetus* subsp. *venerealis.* Infected bulls should be removed. *C. fetus* subsp. *venerealis* can be eliminated from a herd but subsp. *fetus* cannot.

*Table 21–1. Differentiation of Important **Campylobacter** Species and Subspecies*

Species and Subspecies	Principal Hosts	Catalase	Nitrate Reduction	H₂S TSI	H₂S Lead Acetate Strips	Growth in		Growth at	
						1% Glycine	3.5% NaCl	25° C	42° C
C. fetus ss. venerealis	Cattle	+	–	–	–	–	–	+	–
ss. fetus	Cattle, sheep	+	–	–	+	+	–	+	–
C. jejuni	Cattle, sheep, dog, cats, human, avian	+	–	–	+	+	–	–	+
C. sputorum ss. sputorum	Humans	–	+	+	+	+	–	+	+
ss. bubulus	Cattle, sheep	–	+	+	+	+	+	(+)	+
C. mucosalis	Swine	–	+	+	+	–	–	+	+
C. fecalis	Cattle, sheep	+	+	+	+	+	(+)	–	+
C. coli	Swine, chickens, humans	+	–	–	+	+	–	–	+
C. hyointestinalis	Swine, humans	+	+	+	+	+	–	+	(–)

(+), most grow at this temperature; (–), poor growth at this temperature.

Campylobacter mucosalis

C. mucosalis (formerly C. sputorum subsp. mucosalis) is oxidase positive and catalase negative (Table 21–1).

This bacterium can be recovered in large numbers from the mucosa of pigs with swine proliferative enteritis but not from the mucosa of healthy pigs.

There is considerable evidence now that this organism may not be involved in the etiology of swine proliferative enteritis. This is a disease complex that includes intestinal adenomatosis, necrotic enteritis, regional ileitis, and proliferative hemorrhagic enteropathy. These are diseases of postweaned and adult pigs characterized by an enteritis varying in severity from chronic to peracute and involving mainly the ileum.

C. mucosalis can also be recovered from the oral cavity and intestinal contents of clinically healthy pigs.

Because of difficulty in its isolation, diagnosis of the disease is best made by macroscopic and microscopic examination of the ileum, by the use of special staining procedures, or by direct examination of mucosal scrapings. An indirect fluorescent antibody test can be used to demonstrate intracellular organisms in epithelial cells in feces.

Colonies on blood agar are about 1.5 mm at 48 hours. Older cultures yield organisms that tend to be more coccoid and filamentous. A slide agglutination procedure is routinely used in many diagnostic laboratories for rapid identification.

Three serovars of C. mucosalis (A, B, and C) have been identified in pigs.

Campylobacter hyointestinalis

This relatively new species of Campylobacter has also been recovered from lesions of swine prolifer-

ative enteritis. It has not been established clearly that this organism is the cause of the disease. It has also been recovered from the intestine of cattle, hamsters, and humans. In humans, C. hyointestinalis has been associated with gastrointestinal disease.

In addition to the procedures described above for C. mucosalis, C. hyointestinalis can be identified with DNA probes in fecal and mucosal specimens.

Campylobacter jejuni

At one time this organism was thought to be the cause of a disease called "winter dysentery" of cattle.

C. jejuni occurs frequently as a commensal in the intestinal tract of many species of domestic and wild animals, including birds and poultry. Dogs and cats frequently shed this organism in their feces, and there are several claims that it can cause a febrile enteritis with diarrhea in these animals. In addition, C. jejuni is known to cause diarrheic illness in cattle, goats, pigs, lambs, mink, and ferrets. The organism also causes abortion in bitches, does, and heifers, and mastitis in cows. C. jejuni is an important cause of enteritis in human beings. Among the signs are fever, abdominal pain, nausea, vomiting, blood in the stool, and diarrhea. Infections have been traced to animal and human carriers and food and water contaminated by feces. A case of bursitis caused by C. jejuni in a human has been reported recently.

C. jejuni is the cause of avian infectious hepatitis (vibrionic hepatitis) of chickens. This is a widespread disease characterized by a low mortality, high morbidity, chronic course, and hemorrhagic and necrotic changes in the liver.

Some strains of C. jejuni produce a heat-labile enterotoxin, which is thought to be responsible for diarrheic disease. Little information is available on the antigenic structure of this species. Certain strains of *C. jejuni* also produce a toxic factor for mouse hepatocytes; it is different from enterotoxins.

Campylobacter coli

This organism was mistakenly thought to be the cause of swine dysentery. It occurs as a commensal in the intestinal tract of poultry, swine, and human beings and is not known to be a significant pathogen. However, it occasionally causes enteritis in humans and pigs. *C. coli* also produces a heat-labile enterotoxin.

It is difficult to distinguish from *C. jejuni*.

ISOLATION AND IDENTIFICATION

Those species just discussed are isolated using essentially the same procedures as described for *C. fetus*. Special measures such as filtration, the use of antibiotics, and below surface sampling (*C. mucosalis*) are used to reduce contaminants. Growth is slow and colonies of the various species resemble those of *C. fetus*, except that those of *C. mucosalis* have a dirty yellow appearance.

In avian hepatitis *C. jejuni* can be demonstrated in bile by phase microscopy. This organism grows readily in a candle jar.

Identification is based on growth characteristics and biochemical reactions (see Table 21–1). Species specific DNA probes are being used in some diagnostic laboratories for the identification of *C. jejuni*, *C. coli*, and *C. hyointestinalis* in feces.

A commercial latex agglutination test is available for the identification of *C. jejuni*, *C. coli* and other *Campylobacter* spp. An ELISA is available for the serodiagnosis of *C. jejuni* infection.

TREATMENT

Among the drugs that have been used to treat human, canine, and feline infections caused by *C. jejuni* are erythromycin, the aminoglycosides, chloramphenicol, and the tetracyclines.

Other *Campylobacter* spp.

C. upsaliensis has been recovered from feces of both healthy and diarrheic dogs and cats and from feces of healthy children. The exact role of this organism in diarrheic illnesses has not been established.

C. sputorum subsp. *bubulus* is a commensal found in healthy cattle and sheep. It is not known to cause disease in cattle or sheep. *C. fecalis* has been recovered from ovine feces and from bovine semen and vaginas. Clinical significance of this organism is not known. Suggestions have been made to reclassify *C. fecalis* and *C. sputorum* subsp. *bubulus* as biovars of *C. sputorum*.

Intracellular *Campylobacter*-like organisms have been described recently from cases of porcine proliferative enteritis. They are antigenically unrelated to the other campylobacters isolated from pigs. These organisms have not been grown in conventional bacteriologic media. Although their relationship to the pathogenesis of the disease is not known, their consistent presence during the disease suggests they are significant.

PUBLIC HEALTH SIGNIFICANCE

Veterinarians, farmers, packing house workers, and others associated with cattle and sheep occasionally sustain infections due to *C. fetus*. Diseases attributed to these infections are abortions, enteritis, endocarditis, and fever with bacteremia. Human infections with *C. jejuni*, *C. hyointestinalis*, *C. coli*, and other *Campylobacter* spp. were discussed earlier.

Helicobacter

These spiral-shaped organisms resemble campylobacteria and were previously classified in the genus *Campylobacter*. *Helicobacter pylori* has been isolated from humans with chronic gastritis including gastric ulcers and is thought to be etiologically significant. *H. felis*, a possible veterinary pathogen, was first recovered from a domestic cat. Inoculation of this organism into gnotobiotic mice and Beagle dogs resulted in gastritis similar to that caused by *H. pylori* in humans. Helicobacteria are prolific producers of urease. This enzyme contributes to the ability of the organism to colonize the stomach by providing an alkaline environment. *H. mustelae* has been recovered from the normal and inflamed mucosa of ferrets.

FURTHER READING

Blaser, M.J., LaForce, F.M., Wilson, N.A., and Wang, W.L.L.: Reservoirs of human campylobacteriosis. J. Infect. Dis., *141*:665, 1980.

Burnens, A.P., and Nicolet, J.: Detection of *Campylobacter upsaliensis* in diarrheic dogs and cats, using a selective medium with cefoperazone. Am. J. Vet. Res., *53*:48, 1992.

Butzler, J.P. (ed.): Campylobacter Infection of Man and Animals. Boca Raton, Florida, CRC Press Inc., 1984.

Eaton, K.A., et al.: Essential role of urease in pathogenesis of gastritis induced by *Helicobacter pylori* in gnotobiotic piglets. Infect. Immun., *59*:2470, 1991.

Fox, J.G., Moore, R., and Ackerman, J.I.: *Campylobacter jejuni*-associated diarrhea in dogs. J. Am. Vet. Med. Assoc., *183*:1430, 1983.

Fox, J.G., et al.: "*Campylobacter upsaliensis*" isolated from cats as identified by DNA relatedness and biochemical features. J. Clin. Microbiol., *27*:2376, 1989.

Gebhart, C.J., Ward, G.E., and Murtaugh, M.P.: Species-specific cloned DNA probes for the identification of *Campylobacter hyointestinalis*. J. Clin. Microbiol., *27*:2717, 1989.

Gebhart, C.J., et al.: Cloned DNA probes specific for the intracellular *Campylobacter*-like organism of porcine proliferative enteritis. J. Clin. Microbiol., *29*:1011, 1991.

Kita, E., et al.: Hepatotoxic activity of *Campylobacter jejuni*. J. Med. Microbiol., *33*:171, 1990.

Lee, A., et al.: Role of *Helicobacter pylori* in chronic gastritis. Vet. Pathol., *29*:487, 1992.

Lindblom, G., Kaijser, B., and Sjogren, E.: Enterotoxin production and serogroups of *Campylobacter jejuni* and *Campylobacter coli* from patients with diarrhea and from healthy laying hens. J. Clin. Microbiol., *27*:1272, 1989.

Minet, J., Grosbois, B., and Megraud, F.: *Campylobacter hyointestinalis*: an opportunistic enteropathogen. J. Clin. Microbiol., *26*:2659, 1988.

Penner, J.L.: The genus *Campylobacter*: a decade of progress. Clin. Microbiol. Rev., *1*:157, 1988.

Prescott, J.F., and Brein-Mosch, C.W.: Carriage of *Campylobacter jejuni* in healthy and diarrheic animals. Am. J. Vet. Res., *42*:164, 1981.

Smibert, R.M.: The genus *Campylobacter*. Ann. Rev. Microbiol., *32*:673, 1978.

Smibert, R.M.: Genus *Campylobacter*. *In* Bergey's Manual of Systematic Bacteriology. Vol. 1. Edited by N.R. Krieg. Baltimore, Williams & Wilkins, 1984.

Thompson, L.M., et al.: Phylogenetic study of the genus *Campylobacter*. Int. J. Syst. Bacteriol., *38*:190, 1988.

Williams, L.P.: Campylobacteriosis. J. Am. Vet. Med. Assoc., *193*:52, 1988.

22

Haemophilus and Taylorella

PRINCIPAL CHARACTERISTICS OF *Haemophilus*

Species of the genus *Haemophilus* are small, gram-negative rods and filaments. They are nonmotile, facultatively anaerobic, and require X or V factor or both.

More than a dozen species are listed in *Bergey's Manual of Systematic Bacteriology* (Vol. 1). Most are associated with humans and animals as commensals on mucous membranes of the upper digestive, respiratory, and genital tracts. Some are potential pathogens. Except for *H. somnus*, they require one or both of the following factors for growth: (1) X factor: requirement for the iron porphyrin, hemin; supplied by blood agar or chocolate agar; (2) V factor: nicotinamide adenine dinucleotide (NAD) or one of its riboside precursors; supplied by fresh yeast extract, staphylococcal growth, or chocolate agar.

Nucleic acid hybridization studies have shown that members of the genus *Haemophilus* are genetically heterogeneous. The two species *H. avium* and *H. pleuropneumoniae* have been transferred to the genera *Pasteurella* and *Actinobacillus*, respectively. Some other species may be reclassified eventually. *Haemophilus equigenitalis*, which clearly did not belong in the genus *Haemophilus* for genetic and biochemical reasons, has been placed in a newly created genus, *Taylorella*.

The hosts and X and V factor requirements of some important species are given in Table 22–1.

MODE OF INFECTION

This is most frequently by inhalation. Fomites may be involved. Infections may be endogenous or exogenous.

PATHOGENESIS

Virulence is associated with capsule (polysaccharide) formation, and it is likely that endotoxin has an important role. Young or previously unexposed animals are most susceptible. Stresses and crowding may be contributory.

H. influenzae gains entrance to human tissues via the respiratory tract, usually with an initial nasopharyngitis. If this infection is not checked, it may lead to sinusitis, otitis media, and pneumonia. If a bacteremia develops, joint infections and meningitis may follow. A somewhat similar pathogenesis is seen with some of the varieties of *Haemophilus* that infect animals, e.g., *H. parasuis* and *H. paragallinarum*. Disease caused by *H. somnus* probably has a somewhat similar development.

Haemophilus somnus

Because this organism does not require either the X or V factor, it cannot be classed as a true *Haemophilus*.

H. somnus infection of cattle is manifested by four principal syndromes: (1) respiratory involvement, with pneumonia and bacteremia; (2) localization in the central nervous system, with thromboembolic meningoencephalitis ("sleepers"); (3) joint infec-

189

Table 22–1. *Hosts and X and V Factor Requirements of Important Species of* **Haemophilus**

Species	Hosts	Requirement for X	Requirement for V
H. influenzae	Humans	+	+
H. parainfluenzae	Humans and cats; probably cattle, sheep, fowl	–	+
H. parasuis	Swine	–	+
H. haemoglobinophilus	Dogs (preputial sac)	+	–
H. paragallinarum	Chickens	–	+
H. aphrophilus	Humans, dogs (infrequent)	+	–
H. paracuniculus	Rabbit	–	+
H. somnus	Cattle	–	–
H. influenzaemurium	Mice	+	–
H. ovis	Sheep	+	–

tion accompanied by arthritis; and (4) reproductive failure. More than one syndrome may be seen in the same animal. The neural manifestation of the disease is frequently fatal. Outbreaks are often associated with stress and are frequently seen in feedlot cattle. Asymptomatic carriers are also common. It is not clear whether the absence of clinical signs in carriers is due to a difference in the host response or to a difference in the virulence of isolates. In some cases, the carrier isolates appear to be less virulent than those from diseased animals. Other infections are tracheitis, laryngitis, mastitis, conjunctivitis, otitis, and septicemia.

Organisms can be demonstrated in brain lesions. They can be recovered from semen samples and preputial washings of healthy bulls. Isolation can be made on media supplemented with blood and yeast in 10% CO_2 (mandatory). Definitive identification requires several biochemical tests.

According to DNA studies *Histophilus ovis* and *Haemophilus agni* are indistinguishable from *H. somnus*. *Histophilus ovis* and *H. agni* are commensals of the genital tract of sheep and have been reported as causes of epididymitis and orchitis in rams, and pneumonia, mastitis, myositis, polyarthritis, meningitis, and septicemia in sheep.

Haemophilus parasuis

H. parasuis is a secondary invader in swine influenza, other pneumonias, and the primary agent of Glässer's disease, a disease of young pigs characterized by a polyserositis and occasionally by meningitis. The signs and lesions resemble those of polyserositis caused by *Mycoplasma hyorhinis*. Arthritis and pneumonia are seen mainly in older pigs. Acute myositis in SPF sows associated with *H. parasuis*, has been reported.

Haemophilus paragallinarum

H. paragallinarum is the cause of infectious coryza of chickens. This disease has both acute and chronic forms and is characterized by nasal discharge, sneezing, and edema of the face. There are high morbidity and low mortality rates sometimes with significant economic losses because of the reduction in growth and egg production. Recovered chickens may carry and shed the organism for long periods.

PATHOGENICITY OF SOME SPECIES OF LESSER IMPORTANCE

H. haemoglobinophilus (H. canis) has been recovered from the genital tract of dogs. It has been implicated in cystitis in dogs and is thought to have a role in canine neonatal and genital infections.

H. influenzaemurium causes respiratory infections and conjunctivitis in mice.

H. aphrophilus has been shown to cause endocarditis in humans. It has been recovered from the pharynx of dogs.

H. avium has been transferred to the genus *Pasteurella*. It is a nonpathogenic commensal that can be confused with *H. paragallinarum*; in contrast to this organism, it is catalase-positive.

H. ovis has been reported twice in sheep, as a commensal and as a cause of bronchopneumonia.

H. paracuniculus has been isolated from rabbits. Its significance is not known.

The name *H. felis* has been proposed for a commensal organism recovered from the nasopharynx of apparently normal cats. It requires CO_2 and V factor for growth.

SPECIMENS

Haemophilus spp. are fragile and do not survive long when removed from the host. Clinical material is best frozen (dry ice preferred) and delivered to the laboratory within 24 hours. Refrigeration and transport media may not be sufficient to assure viability.

ISOLATION AND IDENTIFICATION

The most important species of *Haemophilus* that cause animal disease will grow on blood agar, with a *Staphylococcus* streak (growth) providing the V factor. Blood agar supplies sufficient hemin; chocolate agar supplies both X and V factors. If *Haemophilus* is suspected, blood plates with a *Staphylococcus* streak should be incubated in air containing 10% CO_2. *H. somnus* does not grow initially without CO_2.

Plates are incubated for 24 to 48 hours. Small dewdrop colonies appear after 24 hours of incubation. If the V factor is required, the small colonies will appear near the *Staphylococcus* streak (satellite growth).

For practical purposes identification is based on morphologic and colonial characteristics, X or V factor requirement or both, and host, lesions, and clinical signs. Species can be identified using a number of biochemical tests; however, because of the fastidious growth requirements of these organisms, such tests are not carried out routinely in the diagnostic laboratory. For precise identification, refer to *Bergey's Manual of Systematic Bacteriology*, Vol. 1, 1984. Some differential characteristics of the more important species are given in Table 22–2.

RESISTANCE

Haemophilus species are fragile. They are sensitive to sunlight and drying and are readily killed by common disinfectants.

IMMUNITY

Immunity to *Haemophilus* species is thought to be predominantly humoral. Most species are antigenically heterogeneous. A number of serotypes of *H. somnus*, *H. parasuis*, and *H. paragallinarum* have been identified. Based on an immunodiffusion test using heat-stable antigens, 15 serovars of *H. parasuis* have been recognized. Nine serotypes of *H. paragallinarum* and 15 serotypes of *H. somnus* have been identified. Specific capsular antibodies are considered important in protection. Bacterins are used to prevent infectious coryza and *H. somnus* infection in cattle.

Serological tests, including agglutination, ELISA, and agar gel precipitation tests, are used to detect birds carrying *H. paragallinarum*. Agglutination, ELISA, and complement-fixation tests are used in serological surveys for *H. somnus* exposure and infection.

TREATMENT

Haemophilus spp. are susceptible to penicillin, gentamycin, spectinomycin, tetracyclines, sulfonamides, chloramphenicol, neomycin, and erythromycin. Susceptibility tests should be carried out because resistant strains may be encountered. Drugs are usually administered in food or water.

Taylorella equigenitalis

This organism causes contagious equine metritis (CEM), an acute, highly contagious venereal disease of mares and female ponies characterized by a metritis, cervicitis, and copious, purulent vaginal discharge. Abortions may occur within the first 60 days. Stallions are infected and spread the disease during coitus but show no clinical signs. Spread may also be by contaminated equipment and attendants.

The disease has been reported from the United Kingdom, France, many other European countries, Australia, and Japan. The disease appeared in Kentucky in 1978 and Missouri in 1979.

PATHOGENESIS

The infection is mainly transmitted to the mare at coitus from infected stallions. The organism is found on the surface of the penis, in the preputial smegma, and in the urethral fossa. The infection can also be spread between mares and stallions by attendants, fomites, and especially by instruments.

Table 22–2. Some Differential Characteristics of Important Haemophilus spp. and Taylorella equigenitalis

Species	Required X	Required V	Indole	Urease	Hemolysis	CAMP Reaction	Catalase	Oxidase	Acid: Glucose	CO_2 Enhances Growth
H. parasuis	–	+	–	–	–	–	+	–	+	+
H. paragallinarum	–	+	–	–	–	–	–	–	+	+
H. somnus	–	–	+	–	–	–	–	+	+	+
T. equigenitalis	–	–	–	–	–	–	+	–	–	+

The infectious process appears to be confined to the mucous membrane of the uterus, cervix, and vagina, with accompanying endometritis, cervicitis, and vaginitis. There has been no evidence of spread to other tissues and organs. The organism may reside for long periods in the clitoral sinuses and fossa of mares. No lesions are seen in the stallion.

The discharge from the vulva contains large numbers of neutrophils, many of which harbor *T. equigenitalis*. The edematous uterine mucosa initially contains many neutrophils and mononuclear cells with later a predominance of plasmocytic cells.

DIAGNOSIS

Clinical: The copious mucopurulent discharge occurring after breeding or during the breeding season should be highly suspicious.

Laboratory: The disease can only be diagnosed definitively by the isolation and identification of the causal agent. The following tests have been used: complement fixation, agglutination (plate and tube) and passive hemagglutination. Infected stallions are serologically negative, as are some carrier mares.

LABORATORY SPECIMENS

Swabs from the cervix, urethra, and clitoral fossa, including the clitoral sinuses of the mare and the prepuce, urethral fossa and penile sheath of the stallion, should be refrigerated and sent to the laboratory in a transport medium (preferably Amies) as soon after being collected as possible.

ISOLATION AND IDENTIFICATION

The organism can be isolated on eugonagar or chocolate agar that has been incubated for several days in air containing 5 to 10% CO_2. Small colonies similar in appearance to those of *Haemophilus* spp. appear after 24 hours of incubation. Although fastidious and rather unreactive biochemically, *T. equigenitalis* can be shown to be oxidase, catalase, and phosphatase-positive. Some stimulation of growth is obtained with the X factor but not the V factor. Strains both sensitive and resistant to streptomycin have been isolated. Some differential characteristics are listed in Table 22–2.

TREATMENT

Intrauterine irrigation with nitrofurazone, ampicillin, or penicillin daily for 5 to 10 days is effective. Ampicillin or penicillin are given parenterally for the same period. The penis should be cleaned and the prepuce irrigated on at least five occasions with chlorhexidine and nitrofurazone. One week after treatment, mares and stallions must be checked to determine if they are negative for the organism. Three successive cultures at weekly intervals should be negative.

Conception rates for mares and breeding rates for stallions return to normal the following breeding season.

IMMUNITY

Immunity would seem to be of a low order and mainly antibody-mediated. There is evidence that previously infected mares can be reinfected several weeks after being culturally negative. Both local and systemic antibodies can be demonstrated by various procedures in mares but not in stallions. Bacterins do not prevent the disease but the severity is lessened.

CONTROL AND PROPHYLAXIS

If the disease is suspected, state and federal veterinary officials should be notified. The suspected infected stallion should not be used for further breeding until shown to be culturally negative. All animals suspected or known to be infected should be kept under strict isolation until shown to be negative by culture.

The organism is fragile, and evidence indicates that it will not survive in discharge material outside the host for more than several days.

FURTHER READING

Acland, H.M., Allen, P.Z., and Kenney, R.M.: Contagious equine metritis: distribution of organisms in experimental infection of mares. Am. J. Vet. Res., 44:1197, 1983.

Albritton, W.L., et al.: Heterospecific transformation in the genus *Haemophilus*. Mol. Gen. Genet., 193:358, 1984.

Biberstein, E.L.: *Haemophilus*. In Diagnostic Procedures in Veterinary Bacteriology and Mycology. Edited by G.R. Carter and J.R. Cole, Jr. 5th Ed. New York, Academic Press, 1990.

Blackall, P.J.: The avian haemophili. Clin. Microbiol. Rev., 2:270, 1989.

Dierkes, R.E., and Hanna, S.A.: Epizootiology and pathogenesis of *Haemophilus somnus* infection. J. Am. Vet. Med. Assoc., 163:866, 1975.

Humphrey, J.D., et al.: Occurrence of "*Haemophilus somnus*" in bovine semen and in the prepuce of bulls and steers. Can. J. Comp. Med., 46:215, 1982.

Inzana, T.J., et al.: Isolation and characterization of a newly defined *Haemophilus* species from cats: "*Haemophilus felis*". J. Clin. Microbiol., 30:2108, 1992.

Kielstein, P., and Ropp-Gabuelson, V.J.: Designation of 15 serovars of *Haemophilus parasuis* on the basis of immunodiffusion using heat-stable antigen extracts. J. Clin. Microbiol., 30:862, 1992.

Kilian, M., Nicolet, J., and Biberstein, E.L.: Biochemical and serological characterization of *Haemophilus pleuropneumoniae* (Matthews and Pattison, 1961). Shope 1964 and proposal of a neotype strain. Int. J. Syst. Bacteriol., 28:20, 1978.

Kilian, M., Frederiksen, W., and Biberstein, E.L. (eds.): *Haemophilus, Pasteurella* and *Actinobacillus*. New York, Academic Press, 1981.

Kilian, M., and Biberstein, E.L.: Genus 11 *Haemophilus. In Bergey's Manual of Systematic Bacteriology.* Vol. 1. Edited by N.R. Krieg. Baltimore, Williams & Wilkins, 1984.

Morozumi, T., and Nicolet, J.: Some antigenic properties of *Haemophilus parasuis* and a proposal for serological classification. J. Clin. Microbiol., 23:1022, 1986.

Myers, L.E., et al.: Genomic fingerprinting of "*Haemophilus somnus*" isolates by using a random-amplified polymorphic DNA assay. J. Clin. Microbiol., 31:512, 1993.

Nielsen, R., and Danielsen, V.: An outbreak of Glässer's disease. Nord. Vet. Med. 27:20, 1975.

Panciera, R.J., Dahlgren, R.R., and Rinker, H.B.: Observations on septicemia of cattle caused by a *Haemophilus*-like organism. Pathol. Vet., 5:212, 1968.

Patrick, J., et al.: Proposal of a new serovar and altered nomenclature of *Haemophilus paragallinarum* in the Kume hemagglutinin scheme. J. Clin. Microbiol., 28:1185, 1990.

Sugimoto, C., Isayama, Y., Sakazaki, R., and Kuramochi, S.: Transfer of *Haemophilus equigenitalis* Taylor, et al. 1978 to the genus *Taylorella* gen. nov. as *Taylorella equigenitalis* comb. nov. J. Clin. Microbiol., 9:155, 1983.

Taylor, C.E.D., et al.: The causative organism of contagious equine metritis. 1977. Proposal for a new species to be known as *Haemophilus equigenitalis*. Equine Vet. J., 10:136, 1978.

Walker, R.L., Biberstein, E.L., Pritchett, R.F., and Kirkham, C.: Deoxyribonucleic acid relatedness among "*Haemophilus somnus,*" "*Haemophilus agni,*" "*Histophilus ovis,*" "*Actinobacillus seminis,*" and *Haemophilus influenzae*. Int. J. Syst. Bact., 35:46, 1985.

23

Bordetella and Moraxella

PRINCIPAL CHARACTERISTICS OF *Bordetella*

Species of the genus *Bordetella* are small, gram-negative rods and coccobacilli. They are aerobic, catalase and oxidase-positive, and do not ferment carbohydrates (metabolism respiratory). There are both motile and nonmotile species.

Only four species are recognized:
1. *Bordetella bronchiseptica:* natural hosts are animals; causes respiratory disease.
2. *B. avium:* causes rhinotracheitis (coryza) of turkey poults.
3. *B. pertussis:* natural host is humans; causes whooping cough (pertussis).
4. *B. parapertussis:* natural host is humans; causes parapertussis, a mild form of whooping cough.

Bordetella bronchiseptica

HABITAT

B. bronchiseptica is a commensal in the upper respiratory tract of dogs, cats, swine, rabbits, horses, guinea pigs, rats, and possibly other animals.

MODE OF INFECTION AND TRANSMISSION

Infections may be endogenous or exogenous. Inhalation is the principal mode of infection. Spread is by direct and indirect contact and fomites.

PATHOGENESIS

Considerable variation exists among *B. bronchiseptica* strains in their ability to colonize and produce disease in pigs and other animals. Most *B. bronchiseptica* strains possess pili and flagella. These structures appear to correlate with growth phase and colonial morphology. Adherence of *B. bronchiseptica* to epithelial cells of the respiratory tract is facilitated by the presence of pili. *B. bronchiseptica* seems to have a strong affinity for respiratory mucin. This affinity for mucin receptor appears to help the organism to adhere and colonize the nasal mucosa of young pigs. Virulent strains of *B. bronchiseptica* produce an extracellular enzyme, adenylate cyclase, which is capable of altering cellular functions of the host including phagocytosis and intracellular killing. In addition, the enzyme has the ability to immobilize the respiratory tract cilia (ciliostasis).

B. bronchiseptica possesses an intracellular, heat-labile toxin with a molecular weight of approximately 145 kilodaltons. The toxin, a single-chain polypeptide, is inactivated by trypsin, formalin, and glutaraldehyde. It is lethal when injected intraperitoneally into mice and produces necrosis when injected intradermally into the guinea pig. The toxin, also known as dermonecrotic toxin, is at least partially responsible for the production of nasal turbinate atrophy (atrophic rhinitis) in piglets, and experimentally in rabbits, rats, and mice. The toxin impairs the ability of osteoblasts to differentiate, which leads to turbinate atrophy. It appears that the severe turbinate atrophy sometimes seen in pigs is due to mixed infection with *B. bronchiseptica* and toxigenic *Pasteurella multocida.*

Other factors that may have a role in the pathogenesis of the disease are: production of acid and alkaline phosphatases, hemolysin, adhesin, endotoxin, and cytotoxin. The exact role of these enzymes and toxic products is not clearly understood.

PATHOGENICITY

Infection results in respiratory disease that is usually subacute to chronic in nature. Diseases or conditions with which *B. bronchiseptica* has been associated are:

Swine—atrophic rhinitis and severe bronchopneumonia in young pigs.

Dogs—infectious tracheobronchitis (kennel cough), bronchopneumonia following distemper viral infection.

Rabbits, guinea pigs, rats—bronchopneumonia, upper respiratory infections, and septicemia.

Cats and horses—respiratory infections.

B. bronchiseptica is seldom infectious for humans; however, the organism has been implicated as the cause of bronchitis, pneumonia, septicemia, bacteremia, sinusitis, endocarditis, peritonitis, meningitis, wound infections, and terminal sepsis.

Fatal infections can be produced in guinea pigs by injection of fresh cultures intraperitoneally. A case of pneumonia in a koala has been reported recently.

ISOLATION AND CULTIVATION

The organism is aerobic, can be cultured on blood or serum agar, and may be beta-hemolytic. Small, circular, dewdrop colonies appear in 48 hours. On further incubation, colonies enlarge, becoming flat and glistening. Stained smears disclose small gram-negative rods or coccobacilli.

Special media are available for culturing material from nasal swabs in the testing of swine herds for *B. bronchiseptica* and thus infectious atrophic rhinitis. These media greatly reduce the number of extraneous bacteria. *B. bronchiseptica* forms distinctive colonies on Bordet-Gengou agar, a blood-based medium used routinely for *B. pertussis.* The colonies of *B. bronchiseptica* on this medium are smooth, dome-shaped, and have a "mercury droplet" appearance.

IDENTIFICATION

B. bronchiseptica is motile, indole-negative, and does not produce H_2S. Urease is produced, and the tests for oxidase and catalase are positive. Litmus milk: alkaline, turning from blue to black in 5 to 10 days. Because drug resistance has been encountered in *B. bronchiseptica,* it is advisable to carry out susceptibility tests on isolates. Carbohydrates are not fermented. For additional criteria, see Table 23–1.

ANTIGENS

The following types of antigens from *B. bronchiseptica* have been described: flagellar H antigens, heat-labile surface K antigens, heat-stable surface O antigens and fimbrial antigens. Based primarily on heat-stable surface antigens, *B. bronchiseptica* cell types have been divided into three smooth phases and one rough phase. It is antigenically related to other members of the *Bordetella* genus. A 68 kilodalton outer membrane protein of *B. bronchiseptica* has been shown to be an important protective antigen against disease in piglets.

IMMUNITY

Immunity to *B. bronchiseptica* appears to be mainly humoral. It is included in mixed and other bacterins to aid in the prevention of respiratory disease and infectious atrophic rhinitis in swine. It is combined with *Pasteurella multocida* in bacterins to prevent snuffles in rabbits. It is sometimes used with other agents to produce antisera to aid in the prevention and treatment of the pneumonia encountered in distemper. Bacterins and live vaccines are used currently to prevent "kennel cough" in dogs. A live avirulent vaccine has been licensed for use in sows (intramuscular) and piglets (intranasal) to prevent atrophic rhinitis.

TREATMENT AND CONTROL

B. bronchiseptica is susceptible to tetracycline, chloramphenicol, carbenicillin, erythromycin, polymyxin B, gentamycin, streptomycin, kanamycin, and sulfonamides. It is usually resistant to penicillin. Long-acting oxytetracycline injected at 9-day intervals seems to help reduce atrophic rhinitis in pigs.

Sulfonamides are administered to swine in their feed or water for several weeks; the drug is present on nasal mucous membranes. A tylosin-sulfonamide combination in feed and water is an alternative treatment. Before an animal is considered free

Table 23–1. *Differential Characteristics of Some Nonfermentative Gram-Negative Bacteria*

TSI and Kligler's: alkaline slant, alkaline or neutral butt, no gas, and no H₂S production	Principal Host	Beta-Hemolysis	Growth on MacConkey Agar	Growth on Salmonella, Shigella Medium	Oxidase	Motility	Pigment	Gelatinase	Nitrate Reduction	Urease	Citrate	Oxidation Maltose	Oxidation Xylose	Oxidation Glucose
Acinetobacter calcoaceticus	Animals and humans	–	+	(+)	–	–	–	–	–	V	+	(–)	+	+
Acinetobacter lwoffii	Animals and humans	–	+	–	–	–	–	–	–	–	+	–	–	–
Alcaligenes faecalis	Animals and humans	–	+	(+)	+	+	–	–	–	–	+	–	–	–
Bordetella avium	Turkeys, chickens	–	+	+	+	+	–	–	–	–	–	–	–	–
Bordetella bronchiseptica	Animals	+	+	–	+	+	–	–	+	+	+	–	–	–
Moraxella bovis	Cattle	+	–	–	+	–	–	+	(–)	–	–	–	–	–
Moraxella species	Animals	–	(–)	–	+	–	–	V	V	V	–	–	–	(–)

(+), most strains positive; (–), most strains negative; V, variable.

of the infection, at least three successive nasal swabs should be negative for *B. bronchiseptica*.

Bordetella avium

Synonym: *Alcaligenes faecalis*.

There was some doubt as to whether this organism belonged to the *Alcaligenes* or *Bordetella* genus, but a recent comprehensive study that included DNA hybridization has placed it in the latter group.

This organism is the cause of the economically important disease of turkeys, rhinotracheitis (turkey coryza). The disease is highly contagious and is characterized by oculonasal discharge, sneezing, dyspnea, decreased weight gain, and tracheal collapse. Under field conditions, the disease is often particularly severe due to increased stress and secondary infection. It has also been isolated from the respiratory tracts of other avian species. The organism appears to have a primary or secondary role in respiratory disease in chickens. It colonizes ciliated tracheal epithelium leading to inflammation and destruction of the epithelium and tracheal rings.

B. avium produces a dermonecrotic toxin which is a heat-labile protein with a molecular weight of approximately 155 kilodaltons. It is lethal to mice, guinea pigs, young chickens, and turkey poults and produces dermonecrosis when injected intradermally into guinea pigs, chickens, and turkey poults. Other virulence factors include pili, tracheal cytotoxin, and hemagglutinin.

B. avium resembles *B. bronchiseptica* in its growth and cultural characteristics, but it differs from it in that it does not produce urease. Additional differential characteristics are provided in Table 23–1. Analysis of fatty acids is helpful in differentiating *B. avium* from other gram-negative bacteria.

Live attenuated vaccines of *B. avium* appear to offer significant protection against the disease.

Principal Characteristics of *Moraxella*

Moraxella are small, gram-negative aerobic, nonmotile rods. They are catalase- and oxidase-positive, do not utilize carbohydrates, and do not require X and V factors.

Of the 10 species described in *Bergey's Manual of Systematic Bacteriology (Vol. 1)* only one, *M. bovis*, is significant in animal disease. *M. lacunata* has been recovered infrequently from infections in animals.

Moraxella bovis

Habitat

The organism may be found as a commensal on the conjunctiva or in the nasopharynx of cattle.

Transmission

M. bovis is spread most commonly by flies (*Musca autumnalis*, *M. domestica* and *Stomoxys calcitrans*) but it can also be spread by direct contact, aerosol, and fomites.

PATHOGENESIS AND PATHOGENICITY

M. bovis is considered the cause of pinkeye, infectious bovine keratoconjunctivitis or infectious ophthalmia of cattle. Both young and adult cattle are susceptible. It is seen more commonly in the beef breeds and is aggravated by grazing in tall grass, by a dry dusty environment, and by insects. Other predisposing factors include prolonged exposure to sunlight (ultraviolet light), breed susceptibility, and concurrent viral (bovine herpesvirus), mycoplasmal, or ureaplasmal infections. Vitamin A deficiency is known to be a contributing factor in some outbreaks. Carrier animals are one of the sources of infection. Pinkeye is a highly contagious worldwide disease of cattle which occurs frequently during the summer.

Some *M. bovis* strains possess pili that aid in adherence and colonization. Virulent strains are piliated and produce rough colonies which are beta-hemolytic. In addition, certain strains of *M. bovis* produce a cytotoxin that is toxic to bovine neutrophils. It is produced only by hemolytic strains and is thought to play an important role in the pathogenesis of the disease.

ISOLATION AND CULTIVATION

Good growth is obtained on standard media; it is enhanced by the addition of blood or serum. Colonies are usually round, translucent, grayish-white, 1 mm to 2 mm in diameter, and surrounded by a narrow zone of beta hemolysis. After 48 to 72 hours, colonies enlarge and become somewhat flattened, with raised centers.

Stained smears reveal gram-negative or gram-variable coccobacilli, usually occurring in pairs (diplobacilli) and less frequently in short chains. *M. bovis* is nonmotile, nonsporeforming, and encapsulated.

IDENTIFICATION

No acid is produced in the usual fermentation media. Litmus milk becomes alkaline; it does not reduce nitrates, does not form indole, liquefies gelatin slowly, does not grow on MacConkey agar, and catalase production is variable. (see Table 23–1). A fluorescent antibody test is also used frequently for rapid identification of *M. bovis* in tears or from cultures.

IMMUNITY

Immunity to the disease is of short duration and relapses are common.

Although a number of vaccines and bacterins have been developed and used in recent years, their efficacy in field trials has been variable, ranging from no effect to a reduced morbidity. However, vaccines prepared to contain pili appear to provide significant protection against infectious bovine keratoconjunctivitis.

TREATMENT

Cattle are confined to shady areas, and adequate vitamin A is provided. Chloramphenicol, gentamicin, triple antibiotic (neomycin, bacitracin, and polymyxin B), penicillin, nitrofurazone, erythromycin, sulfonamides, or tetracyclines are administered locally (topically), systemically, or by subconjunctival injection. Repeated applications are required. Measures should be taken to control flies. If feasible clinically affected animals should be segregated. Reduction in the number of carrier animals may be accomplished by the use of systemic antibiotics.

Other *Moraxella* spp.

M. lacunata has been isolated from guinea pigs, aborted equine fetuses, septicemia in a goat, and from various clinical specimens from dogs and pigs. This organism has also been isolated from goats with viral pneumonia and encephalitis. *M. phenylpyruvica* has been recovered from the genitourinary tract and brain of sheep and cattle, the genitourinary tract of pigs, and the intestine of a goat.

FURTHER READING

Baptista, P.J.H.P.: Infectious bovine keratoconjunctivitis: A review. Br. Vet. J., *135*:255, 1979.

Bemis, D.A., Carmichal, L.E., and Appel, M.F.G.: Naturally occurring respiratory disease in a kennel caused by *Bordetella bronchiseptica*. Cornell Vet., *67*:282, 1977.

Bemis, D.A., and Wilson, S.A.: Influence of potential virulence determinants on *Bordetella bronchiseptica*-induced ciliostasis. Inf. and Immunity, *50*:35, 1985.

Daniel, M.G., et al.: An up-to-date review of atrophic rhinitis. Vet. Med., *81*:735, 1986.

Gentry-Weeks, C.R., Cookson, B.T., Goldman, W.E., et al.: Dermonecrotic toxin and tracheal cytotoxin, putative virulence factors of *Bordetella avium*. Inf. and Immunity, *56*:1698, 1988.

Goodnow, R.A.: Biology of *Bordetella bronchiseptica*. Microbiol. Rev., *44*:722, 1980.

Hellwig, D.H., Arp, L.H., and Fingerland, J.A.: A comparison of outer membrane proteins and surface characteristics of adhesive and non-adhesive phenotypes of *Bordetella avium*. Avian Dis., *32*:787, 1988.

Horiguchi, Y., et al.: *Bordetella bronchiseptica* dermonecrotizing toxin suppresses in vivo antibody responses in mice. FEMS Microbiol. Letters, *90*:229, 1992.

Horiguchi, Y., Nakai, T., and Kume, K.: Effects of *Bordetella bronchiseptica* dermonecrotic toxin on the structure and function of osteoblastic clone MC3-E1 cells. Infect. Immun., *59*:1112, 1991.

Ishikawa, H., and Isayama, Y.: Evidence for sialyl glycoconjugates as receptors for *Bordetella bronchiseptica* on swine nasal mucosa. Inf. and Immunity, *55*:1607, 1987.

Kagonyera, G.M., George, L., and Miller, M.: Effects of *Moraxella bovis* and culture filtrates on ^{51}Cr-labeled bovine neutrophils. Am. J. Vet. Res., *50*:18, 1989.

Kersters, K., et al.: *Bordetella avium* sp. nov., isolated from the respiratory tracts of turkeys and other birds. Int. J. Syst. Bacteriol., *34*:56, 1984.

Kobisch, M., and Novotny, P.: Identification of a 68-kilodalton outer membrane protein as the major protective antigen of *Bordetella bronchiseptica* by using specific-pathogen-free piglets. Infect. Immun., *58*:352, 1990.

Lee, S.W., Way, A.W., and Osen, E.G.: Purification and subunit heterogeneity of pili of *Bordetella bronchiseptica*. Inf. and Immunity, *51*:586, 1986.

Letcher, J., Weisenberg, E., and Jonas, A.: *Bordetella bronchiseptica* pneumonia in a Koala. J. Am. Vet. Med. Assoc., *202*:985, 1993.

Leyh, R., and Griffith, R.W.: Characterization of the outer membrane proteins of *Bordetella avium*. Inf. and Immunity, *60*:958, 1992.

Magyar, T., et al.: The pathogenesis of turbinate atrophy in pigs caused by *Bordetella bronchiseptica*. Vet. Microbiol., *18*:135, 1988.

Mobely, D.M., et al.: Effect of pH, temperature and media on acid and alkaline phosphatase activity in "clinical" and "nonclinical" isolates of *Bordetella bronchiseptica*. Can. J. Comp. Med., *48*:175, 1984.

Moore, C.J., Mawhinney, H., and Blackall, P.J.: Differentiation of *Bordetella avium* and related species by cellular fatty acid analysis. J. Clin. Microbiol., *25*:1059, 1987.

Moore, L.J., and Rutter, J.M.: Antigenic analysis of fimbrial proteins from *Moraxella bovis*. J. Clin. Microbiol., *25*:2063, 1987.

Moore, C.P., and Miller, R.B.: Infectious and Parasitic Eye Diseases of Cattle. *In* Current Veterinary Therapy. 3: Food Animal Practice. Editor-in-Chief, J. Howard. Philadelphia, W.B. Saunders Co., 1993.

Oliveira, A.S., and Gil-Turnes, C.: Studies on the antigenic relationships of six adherent isolates of *Bordetella bronchiseptica*. Vet. Microbiol., *18*:325, 1988.

Papasian, C.J., et al.: *Bordetella bronchiseptica* bronchitis. J. Clin. Microbiol., *25*:575, 1987.

Rosenbusch, R.F. and Ostle, A.G.: *Mycoplasma bovoculi* infection increases ocular colonization by *Moraxella bovis* in calves. Am. J. Vet. Res., *47*:1214, 1986.

Smith, I.M., and Baskerville, A.J.: A selective medium facilitating the isolation and recognition of *Bordetella bronchiseptica*. Res. Vet. Sci., *27*:187, 1979.

Wilt, G.R., et al.: Plasmid content of piliated and nonpiliated forms of *Moraxella bovis*. Am. J. Vet. Res., *51*:171, 1990.

Woolfrey, B.F., and Moody, J.A.: Human infections associated with *Bordetella bronchiseptica*. J. Clin. Microbiol., *4*:243, 1991.

24

Brucella

Principal Characteristics of *Brucella*

Brucella are small, gram-negative, nonmotile, nonspore-forming rods. They are aerobic and carboxyphilic, catalase- and urease-positive, and produce no acid from carbohydrates in conventional peptone media.

They are not found living apart from animals and all are pathogenic, facultative intracellular parasites with a predilection for the reticuloendothelial system and the reproductive tract. The following species are recognized:

B. abortus

B. melitensis

B. suis

B. ovis

B. canis

B. neotomae: recovered from sand rats

Historical

Brucella melitensis was identified by Bruce in Malta in 1887. *B. abortus* was first recognized by Bang in 1897, and *B. suis* was discovered by Traum in 1914. In 1918, Alice Evans showed the taxonomic relationship between *B. abortus* and *B. melitensis* and identified the first *Brucella* of human origin in the United States.

Mode of Infection

The common routes of infection in humans and animals are via the mucous membranes of the digestive tract, genital tract (cow or sow from bull and boar), and skin.

Pathogenesis of Brucellosis

The organism passes from the point of entry via the lymphatics to the regional lymph nodes, and after multiplication to the thoracic duct and then via the bloodstream to the parenchymatous organs and other tissues. The brucellae are principally intracellular in polymorphonuclear leukocytes (PMNLs) and macrophages. Granulomatous foci develop in lymphatic tissues, liver, spleen, bone marrow, and other locations. On occasion these granulomatous foci or nodules may abscess. Hypersensitivity to elements of brucella organisms, including endotoxin, may play a role in pathogenesis.

The predilection that brucellae have for the ungulate placenta, fetal fluids, and testes of the bull, ram, and boar is attributed to erythritol. This polyhydric alcohol has been shown to stimulate the growth of *Brucella*. It is not present in the human placenta. The growth of the vaccine strain, *B. abortus* 19, is not stimulated by erythritol. Virulent strains of *B. abortus* can survive and multiply within PMNLs and macrophages better than avirulent strains. *B. abortus* releases 5' guanosine monophosphate and adenine which inhibit the degranulation of peroxidase-positive granules of PMNLs. This contributes to intracellular survival. Rough strains bind to IgG and other serum proteins nonspecifically; smooth strains do not. It appears that the outer membrane proteins are exposed in rough organisms. There is evidence that the virulence factor for *Brucella* is a surface cell-wall carbohydrate that is responsible for binding to B lymphocytes.

IMMUNITY

The immunity acquired from natural infection is not always sufficient to prevent reactivation of infection or reinfection. This low level of immunity in some humans results in the chronic and relapsing nature of the disease. Bactericidal serum antibodies and neutrophils can destroy organisms that are not within phagocytic cells. There is no correlation between levels of antibodies and acquired immunity. Acquired immunity is mainly cell-mediated; however, maximal immunity would seem to depend upon the interrelationship of cellular and humoral responses.

ANTIGENIC NATURE

Like many other gram-negative bacteria, *Brucella* exhibit smooth-to-rough colonial dissociation. The change from S to R is associated with loss of virulence, a tendency to autoagglutination, and loss of antigens that elicit agglutinins specific for smooth strains. The S and R colonial variants are detected by examining colonies in oblique light. The vaccine strain *B. abortus* 19 is an intermediate mutant that, although low in virulence, is antigenic (elicits agglutinins).

All *Brucella* spp. are closely related and some share a number of antigens. *B. abortus, B. melitensis,* and *B. suis* possess two important surface antigens designated A and M, which are present on the LPS protein complex. *B. abortus* contains more A antigen than M; *B. melitensis* has more M than A; and *B. suis* has an intermediate pattern but, like *B. abortus,* has more A than M. *B. canis* and *B. ovis* are antigenically rough and do not possess the A and M antigens. Both possess an R surface antigen.

Brucella abortus, B. melitensis, B. suis, and *B. canis*

Cattle. Brucellosis is one of the most important diseases of cattle. It has great public health and economic significance. The disease in cattle is almost always caused by *B. abortus.*

The organism is highly infectious and usually gains entrance to the body as a result of (1) ingestion of food, water, and milk contaminated with uterine discharges, urine, or feces of an infected animal; (2) penetration of the skin; or (3) service by an infected bull.

The incubation period is usually from 30 to 60 days. In the cow the infection localizes, usually after a bacteremia, in the placenta of the gravid uterus (placentitis). If the animal is not pregnant, there is usually localization in the udder (interstitial mastitis) and adjacent lymph nodes. Organisms are shed in the milk. It may also localize in the liver, lungs, lymph nodes, or spleen, where it produces granulomatous foci. Cows may remain infected for years.

In the bull, infection may localize in the testicle, epididymis, or seminal vesicle, and abscessation is a common sequela. *Brucella* organisms may be discharged in the semen. Noninfected bulls usually do not become infected as a result of serving an infected cow, but infected bulls infect cows.

The consequences of the bovine disease are loss of calves as a result of abortion at 6 months or later (about one third of infected animals usually abort), and sterility or infertility of either the male or female.

Control. Bovine brucellosis has been eliminated from several countries and from many states in the United States. The procedure that has been followed involves blood testing (agglutination test) of all cattle, and the removal of reactors (titer 1:100 or higher). So that cattle will be less susceptible to reinfection, calfhood vaccination is recommended, and in some circumstances is mandatory. The attenuated live vaccine (strain 19 *B. abortus* biotype 1) is used in female calves 4 to 12 months of age. They develop an agglutination reaction, which usually decreases or disappears soon. If the reaction at 1:200 or higher persists past 30 months of age, the animal is considered a reactor. Because strain 19 may cause infertility in some male calves, its use is restricted to females.

The card test, which uses only one serum dilution and stained antigen, is rapid, sensitive, and useful as a field screening test. The agglutination, ELISA and complement-fixation tests have been adapted to the rapid microtiter system. A number of other tests are performed when the specificity of the reaction is in doubt or in the case of persisting vaccinal reactions. Complement-fixation, rivanol precipitation, and mercaptoethanol agglutination detect primarily IgG antibodies. Rivanol and mercaptoethanol break down IgM. A drop in titer with the rivanol and mercaptoethanol tests may indicate a vaccinal titer as opposed to one caused by chronic natural infection.

The brucellosis ring test for agglutinins shed from the udder is performed three times each year on milk from herds whose milk is sold. If there are reactors to this very sensitive test, or if there is any evidence of brucellosis in a herd, a blood test is carried out.

The Particle Concentration Fluorescence Immunoassay (PCFIA) is another sensitive test that utilizes submicron polystyrene beads to which soluble antigens and a fluorescence marker are attached. The test is available commercially.

Regulations and procedures relating to the brucellosis eradication program are involved, and students are referred to publications of the U.S. Department of Agriculture for further details.

Swine. Although low in the United States, the incidence in swine is difficult to estimate, because testing is not compulsory. *B. abortus* and *B. melitensis* rarely infect swine.

Swine of all ages are susceptible. Nursing pigs may become infected as a result of ingesting milk from infected sows. Older animals usually become infected by ingesting contaminated food, water, or soil. Infected boars transmit the disease by coitus. Swine brucellosis is characterized by abortion, sterility, birth of stillborn or weak pigs, focal abscessation in various organs, spondylitis and lameness. If given sufficient time, many animals will fully recover and free their tissues of the organism. Abortion may occur at any time during gestation; gilts and sows usually abort only once. Unlike cattle, infected sows may eliminate the infection but remain susceptible to reinfection.

Brucellosis is a more generalized infection in hogs than in cattle. Following bacteremia, the organism may localize in lymph nodes, spleen, liver, kidneys, uterus, mammary glands, urinary bladder, seminal vesicles, testicles, accessory sex glands, and bones. Unlike *B. abortus* in the cow, *B. suis* may persist for some time in the sow's uterus, causing metritis and sterility. In some instances, it has been isolated from uterine discharges after 30 months.

Control. Three plans are used to eradicate swine brucellosis: (1) Elimination of the infected herd and restocking with brucellosis-free swine. (2) Infected animals are separated from the noninfected ones and eventually slaughtered. The noninfected gilts, boars, and weanling pigs serve as the nucleus for a clean herd. Testing is carried out frequently and all infected animals are removed. (3) If the incidence of infection is low, reactors are removed and the herd is retested at 30-day intervals. Reactors are removed until the entire herd is negative on retest.

Swine do not react immunologically (humoral) to the same degree that cattle do, and consequently the agglutination test is less reliable. The card test is considered more accurate than the agglutination test. The other serological tests used for cattle may also be used for swine.

Following two consecutive negative herd tests not less than 90 days apart, the herd is eligible for Validated Brucellosis-Free Herd status. Vaccination is not employed.

Dog. *B. abortus* and *B. suis* have been isolated occasionally from sporadic infections in dogs. Canine brucellosis caused by *B. canis* was first recognized as a problem in beagle breeding kennels. The disease is known to be widely distributed throughout the general dog population, although the incidence is low. The mode of infection, transmission, and pathogenesis of the canine disease resembles that of brucellosis in cattle, swine, or goats. Expelled tissues and vaginal discharges of aborted bitches and the urine of infected males are primary sources of the infectious agent. Other means of transmission are copulation and nursing.

The incubation period after oral infection is 6 to 21 days. The bacteremic phase of the disease may last as long as 2 years, and other than a lymphadenopathy, dogs show little evidence of infection. Infected bitches usually abort in the last trimester. Those puppies that are not dead when aborted soon die. Following abortion there is a yellow-brown to dark brown discharge that persists for 1 to 6 weeks. Another possible result of infection of the bitch is resorption of the fetuses. Infections of bones may give rise to chronic osteomyelitis and diskospondylitis.

Prostatitis, epididymitis, and testicular atrophy with decreased spermatogenesis are common in the male and may result in irreversible sterility.

Diagnosis. This is usually accomplished by the agglutination test and by isolation of the organism from blood, urine (male), fetal organs, and vaginal swabs. A positive agglutination reaction of 1:200 or higher with the mercaptoethanol test indicates infection. The slide screening agglutination test is reliable when negative, but positive samples should be retested by the tube test. An agar gel precipitin test has been found to be sensitive and accurate in detecting infection.

Control. Treatment is not practiced. The disease is eliminated from kennels by blood testing, followed by elimination of reacting dogs. Only dogs free of brucellosis, i.e., those that are negative to at least two tests, are added to brucellosis-free breeding kennels. A satisfactory vaccine has not yet been developed.

Humans. Infections are caused by the three classic species and *B. canis*. In heavy swine-raising areas, *B. suis* infections are more prevalent; *B. melitensis* infections are seen in goat-raising areas, and *B. abortus* infections in areas with infected cattle. Pasteurization has greatly reduced the incidence of brucellosis in humans.

Organisms are thought to penetrate the unbroken skin and mucous membranes. Important sources are microbiology laboratories, infected cows (obstetric work), and unpasteurized milk and other dairy products. Multiple infections in laboratory workers due to *B. melitensis* have been reported recently. Slaughterhouse workers and veterinarians frequently contract the disease.

The disease can vary from quite mild to very severe. The incubation period ranges from 8 to 90 days. Those under 14 years of age are less susceptible. There is usually a bacteremia resulting in a variety of symptoms, including undulating fever, profuse perspiration, and rheumatic and neuralgic pains. The course is variable and relapses are frequent. Most patients totally recover within a year or two, even without treatment. The organism may localize in the liver, lymph nodes, or bones. The chronic disease may last as long as 20 years with intermittent relapses of varying intensity. Abortion is rare in women, perhaps resulting from the absence of erythritol in the human placenta. Symptoms in the chronic form are thought to be caused by hypersensitivity to *Brucella* protein. Infections due to *B. suis* and *B. melitensis* may be more serious than those caused by *B. abortus*. Infections due to strain 19 have been reported.

Diagnosis. The agglutination test although useful in the early and acute disease may be negative in chronic infections. The Coombs test, which detects incomplete antibody, is usually positive in cases of chronic disease. The complement-fixation test is superior to the agglutination test for chronic infections. Reagents for ELISAs are available commercially. These procedures measure total IgG and IgM anti-*Brucella* antibodies. They are highly sensitive and eliminate the troublesome prozones of agglutination procedures.

Treatment. Treatment is effective in humans if begun early. Oral doxycycline with rifampin administered for 30 days is preferred to prolonged treatment with a tetracycline and streptomycin. With the former, there are fewer side effects and infrequent relapses. Treatment of the chronic disease is not always satisfactory because organisms are intracellular and there are inaccessible foci (or focus), often in bone.

Goats. Although accurate data are not available, tests indicate that the incidence of brucellosis in goats in the United States is approximately 1%. The majority of infections in goats are caused by *B. melitensis*. Essentially the means of diagnosis and control are the same as those used for cattle.

Horse. *B. abortus* and *B. suis* have been recovered, along with other organisms, from cases of suppurative bursitis (fistulous withers and poll evil). Brucellae have also been recovered from muscles, tendons, and osteoarthritic lesions in various locations in the horse. There is little information on the relationship between serological titers and infection.

Sheep. *B. abortus* causes occasional infections, resulting in abortions.

DIRECT EXAMINATION

Modified Ziehl-Neelsen and Koster's stains are useful in demonstrating brucellae in smears from the placenta (cotyledons) in bovine abortion. Cells of the chorion are packed with organisms which stain red against a blue background. Organisms can also be demonstrated directly in smears from vaginal mucus, semen, and various tissues. Direct and indirect fluorescent antibody staining can also be used.

ISOLATION AND CULTIVATION

Good growth is obtained on tryptose, potato, liver infusion, and blood agar. Colonies are round, entire, smooth, glistening, and translucent. Young colonies are 1 mm to 2 mm in diameter; they may become 5 mm to 8 mm on continued incubation. *B. abortus* requires 10% CO_2 for initial isolation. Plates should be incubated for as long as 30 days.

Small rods, single, or in pairs or short chains, are seen in smears from colonies.

IDENTIFICATION

The different species can be identified by the characteristics listed in Table 24–1. With additional tests, a number of biotypes (biovars) of each of the classic species can be identified. For growth in the presence of dyes, the latter are incorporated in tryptose agar. A number of bacteriophages are available to aid in the identification of *Brucella* spp.

Monospecific sera prepared to react with A, M, and R antigen, are used to aid identification (see Table 24–1). They are prepared by adsorption of the sera with the appropriate *Brucella* species (see "Antigenic Nature" above). Fluorescent antibody staining is used for generic identification. Organisms from colonies can be presumptively identified as brucellae by a slide agglutination test using *B. abortus* antiserum.

EXPERIMENTAL ANIMALS

Guinea pigs can be readily infected with infectious material. They are useful if material is badly contaminated or the numbers of organisms are very small. Infected guinea pigs will yield pure

Table 24–1.　Differentiation of **Brucella** *Species and their Biotypes (Biovars)*

Species	Biotype	Urease	CO₂ Requirement	H₂S Production	Growth on Dyes		Agglutination in Sera		
					Thionin (20 μg/ml)	Basic Fuchsin (20 μg/ml)	A	M	R
B. melitensis	1	V	–	–	–	+	–	+	–
	2	V	–	–	–	+	+	–	–
	3	V	–	–	–	+	+	+	–
B. abortus	1	+	(+)	+	–	+	+	–	–
	2	+	(+)	+	–	–	+	–	–
	3	+	(+)	+	+	+	+	–	–
	4	+	(+)	+	–	(+)	–	+	–
	5	+	–	–	–	+	–	+	–
	6	+	–	(+)	–	+	+	–	–
	7	+	–	(+)	–	+	+	+	–
	9	+	(–)	+	–	+	–	+	–
B. suis	1	+	–	+	+	–	+	–	–
	2	+	–	–	–	–	+	–	–
	3	+	–	–	+	+	+	–	–
	4	+	–	–	+	(–)	+	+	–
B. canis		+	–	–	+	–	–	–	+
B. ovis		–	+	–	+	(–)	–	–	+
B. neotomae		+	–	+	–	–	+	–	–

V, variable; (+), most are positive; (–), most are negative.

cultures and develop a significant agglutination titer.

RESISTANCE

All species are readily killed by commonly used chemical disinfectants and pasteurization. Organisms are fairly resistant to some environmental conditions, e.g., *B. abortus* will survive for 4½ hours when exposed to direct sunlight; 4 days in urine; 5 days on cloth at room temperature; and 75 days in an aborted fetus during cool weather.

IMMUNIZATION

Strain 19 vaccine, a live attenuated (*B. abortus* biotype 1) strain, was developed by Buck in 1930. It is not considered transmissible. In vaccinated calves, agglutination titers usually fall to negative levels in 4 to 6 weeks. As mentioned above, there is the problem of persisting reactors. If an animal is positive (1:200) after 30 months, it is considered a reactor. Adjuvant bacterins, e.g., vaccine 45/20, are used in some countries; 45/20 has been used live or dead to reduce losses in adult cattle. Strain 19 has also been used in adult cattle. Because 45/20 is a rough strain, the immune response to it can be distinguished from that caused by infection. When used as a killed vaccine, two doses provide protection for about a year.

Immunity in brucellosis is predominantly cell-mediated.

Brucella ovis

This organism causes a widespread, sexually transmitted disease of sheep characterized in the ram by orchitis, epididymitis, and impaired fertility, and in some ewes by placentitis and abortion. The ram is more susceptible than the ewe and more rams develop lesions than ewes. Infection of ewes originates almost exclusively from infected rams, and the disease is effectively controlled by the elimination of the rams. Various vaccination procedures have been used successfully to prevent rams from becoming infected. *Brucella melitensis* Rev. 1 live, attenuated vaccine has been used with success to immunize rams against *B. ovis* infection. This vaccine and the *B. melitensis* H 38 killed vaccine result in rams being positive in *B. melitensis* serologic tests.

Control and elimination of the disease are accomplished by complement fixation testing, semen examination (staining, including FA and Koster's method, and culture), and culling of rams with palpable lesions. ELISA, hemagglutination, and immunodiffusion tests have also been used successfully to detect infections. Two consecutive negative tests of flocks indicate absence of the infection.

FURTHER READING

Anaj, D.F., et al.: Evaluation of ELISA in the diagnosis of acute and chronic brucellosis in human beings. J. Hyg., (Camb.) *97:*457, 1986.

Biberstein, E.L., McGowan, B., Olander, H., and Kennedy, P.C.: Epididymitis in rams: Studies on pathogenesis. Cornell Vet. 54:27, 1964.

Brown, G.M., et al.: Characterization of *Brucella abortus* strain 19. Am. J. Vet. Res., 33:759, 1972.

Buchanan, T.M., Baber, L.C., and Feldman, R.A.: Brucellosis in the United States, 1960-1972. An abattoir-associated disease. Part. 1. Clinical features and therapy. Medicine, 53:403, 1974.

Busch, L.A., and Parker, R.L.: Brucellosis in the United States. J. Infect. Dis., 125:289, 1972.

Canning, P.C., Roth, J.A., and Dejoe, B.L.: Release of 5' guanosine monophosphate and adenine by *Brucella abortus* and their role in the intracellular survival of the bacteria. J. Infect. Dis., 154:464, 1986.

Carmichael, L.E., and Bruner, D.W.: Characteristics of a newly recognized species of *Brucella* responsible for infectious canine abortion. Cornell Vet., 58:579, 1968.

Carmichael, L.E., and Greene, C.E.: Canine Brucellosis. *In* Infectious Diseases of the Dog and Cat. Edited by C.E. Greene. Philadelphia, W.B. Saunders Company, 1990.

Cornell, W.D. et al.: *Brucella suis* biovar 3 infection in a Kentucky swine herd. J. Vet. Diagn. Invest., 1:20, 1989.

Crawford, R.P., Williams, J.D., Huber, J.D., and Childers, A.B.: Biotypes of *Brucella abortus* and their value in epidemiologic studies of infected cattle herds. J. Am. Vet. Med. Assoc., 175:1274, 1979.

Denny, H.R.: A review of brucellosis in the horse. Equine Vet. J., 5:121, 1973.

Deyoe, B.L.: Brucellosis. *In* Disease of swine. 6th Ed. Edited by A.D. Leman, et al. Ames, Iowa, Iowa State University Press, 1986.

Forbes, L.B.: *Brucella abortus* infection in 14 farm dogs. J. Am. Vet. Med. Assoc., 196:911, 1990.

Hall, W.A., Ludford, C.G., and Ward, W. H.: Infection and serological responses in cattle given 45/20 vaccine and later challenged with *Brucella abortus*. Aust. Vet. J., 52:409, 1976.

Harrington, Jr., R., and Brown, G.M.: Laboratory summary of brucella isolations and typing. Am. J. Vet. Res., 37:1241, 1976.

Hubbert, N.L., Bech-Nielsen, S., and Barta, O.: Canine brucellosis: Comparison of clinical manifestations with serologic test results. J. Am. Vet. Med. Assoc., 177:168, 1980.

Hughes, K.L., and Claxton, P.D.: *Brucella ovis* infection. I. An evaluation of microbiological, serological, and clinical methods of diagnosis in the ram. Aust. Vet. J., 44:41, 1968.

Luchsinger, D.W., and Anderson, R.K.: Longitudinal studies of naturally acquired *Brucella abortus* infection in sheep. Am. J. Vet. Res., 40:1307, 1979.

McDevitt, D.G.: Brucellosis and the veterinary surgeon. Vet. Rec., 88:537, 1971.

Moore, J.A., Gupta, B.M., and Conner, G.H.: Eradication of *Brucella canis* infection from a dog colony. J. Am. Vet. Med. Assoc., 153:523, 1968.

Nicoletti, P.: Prevalence and persistence of *Brucella abortus* strain 19 infections and prevalence of other biotypes in vaccinated adult dairy cattle. J. Am. Vet. Med. Assoc., 178:143, 1981.

Nicoletti, P.: The epidemiology of bovine brucellosis. Adv. Vet. Sci. Comp. Med., 24:69, 1981.

Rahaley, R.S., Denis, S.M. and Smeltzer, M.S.: Comparison of the enzyme-linked immunosorbent assay and complement fixation for detecting *Brucella ovis* antibodies in sheep. Vet. Rec., 113:467, 1983.

Schurig, G.G., Hammerberg, C., and Fenkler, B.R.: Monoclonal antibodies to *Brucella* surface antigens associated with the smooth lipopolysaccharide complex. Am. J. Vet. Res., 45:967, 1984.

Slaszkiewica, J., et al.: Outbreak of *Brucella melitensis* among microbiology laboratory workers in a community hospital. J. Clin. Microbiol., 29:287, 1991.

Smith, H., et al.: Erythritol: A constituent of bovine foetal fluids which stimulates the growth of *B. abortus* in bovine phagocytes. Br. J. Exp. Pathol., 43:31, 1962.

Thoen, C.O., and Enright, F.: *Brucella. In* C.L. Gyles and C.O. Thoen (eds.) Pathogenesis of Bacterial Infections in Animals. Ames, Iowa State University Press, 1986.

Walker, R.L., Leamaster, B.R., Stellflug, J.N., and Biberstein, E.L.: Association of age of ram with distribution of epididymal lesions and etiological agent. J. Am. Vet. Med. Assoc., 188:393, 1986.

Wilfert, C.M.: *Brucella. In* Zinser Microbiology. Edited by W.K. Joklik, et al. 20th Ed. Norwalk, Connecticut, Appleton & Lange, 1992.

Young, E.J., and Corbel, M.J. (eds.): Brucellosis: Clinical and Laboratory Aspects. Boca Raton, Florida, CRC Press, Inc., 1989.

25

Mycobacteria

PRINCIPAL CHARACTERISTICS OF MYCOBACTERIA

Mycobacteria are gram-positive, nonbranching, acid-fast, small rods. They are nonmotile, non-spore-forming, aerobic, and do not have aerial hyphae. They split sugars oxidatively.

Members of this genus may be grouped as follows:

1. The classic species have been recognized for many years as causes of disease in humans and animals:

> Mycobacterium bovis
> M. avium
> M. tuberculosis
> M. paratuberculosis
> M. leprae

M. avium and M. intracellulare are indistinguishable phenotypically; thus they are frequently referred to as M. avium-intracellulare complex.

2. A number of other mycobacteria, called "anonymous," "unclassified," or "atypical," were first placed in categories by Runyon (1959). He established four groups based on rate of growth, colony morphology, and pigment production.

Group I. Photochromogenic, producing pigmented (yellow) colonies only after exposure to light; slow-growing in that it requires 7 days or more for visible growth; e.g., M. kansasii, M. marinum, M. asiaticum, M. simiae.

Group II. Scotochromogenic, i.e., producing yellow or orange pigment in the absence of light;

slow-growing; e.g., M. gordonae, M. scrofulaceum, M. szulgai, M. xenopi.

Group III. Nonphotochromogenic, producing no or slight pigment with exposure to light; slow-growing; e.g., M. avium, M. intracellulare, M. terrae, M. ulcerans.

Group IV. Variable pigmentation; grows rapidly in that there is visible growth in less than seven days; e.g., M. phlei, M. smegmatis, M. fortuitum, M. chelonei.

Many of the organisms within each of these groups have now been speciated on the basis of cultural and biochemical characteristics, and thus the groups introduced by Runyon have been expanded and more precisely defined. The groups and some of the important species are listed in Table 25–1. A number of species of these groups are recovered not infrequently from animals and are considered significant pathogens. Many species of these groups can sensitize animals to tuberculin.

TUBERCULOSIS CAUSED BY M. bovis, M. avium, AND M. tuberculosis

HISTORICAL

M. tuberculosis was probably first seen in tissues by Baumgarten and Koch in 1882. Koch cultivated M. tuberculosis and reproduced the disease in the period from 1882 to 1884.

MYCOBACTERIAL CELL CONSTITUENTS

None of the mycobacteria has yet been shown to produce exotoxins. The way in which they produce

Table 25–1.   Pathogenicity and Source of Some "Atypical" Mycobacteria

Group I	
M. kansasii	Has been isolated from the lymph nodes of cattle, swine, and other animals. Causes pulmonary infections in humans.
M. marinum	Isolation from cold-blooded animals. Causes swimming pool granuloma in humans.
M. asiaticum	Pulmonary infections in humans; pathogenic to mice.
M. simiae	Pulmonary infections in humans.
M. genaveuse*	Has been isolated from AIDS patients and pet birds.
Group II	
M. scrofulaceum	Cervical lymph nodes of animals and children.
M. xenopi	Several reports of isolation from animals.
Group III	
M. avium† (M. avium-intra-cellulare complex)	28 serotypes recognized; 1, 2, and 3 are usually pathogenic for birds. Serotypes 4 to 20 have been isolated from humans and animals but do not produce progressive disease in chickens. A number of serotypes produce tuberculosis in swine, horses, dogs and cats. Strains formerly called the Battey bacilli cause serious human infections.
M. ulcerans	Skin ulcers in humans; Rats, mice, rabbits, and guinea pigs are susceptible.
Group IV	
M. fortuitum	Pulmonary infections in humans; skin infections in cats; lymph node infections and mastitis in cattle; joint and respiratory infections in pigs; pneumonia in dogs.
M. phlei	Soil; nonpathogenic.
M. smegmatis	Soil and smegma; mastitis in cattle.
M. chelonei	Several reports of human infections.

*This organism is similar to *M. simiae*, group affiliation not clear.

† Although traditionally one of the classic species, it is listed here because it contains various serotypes that do not produce progressive disease in chickens and because *M. avium* and *M. intracellulare* are virtually indistinguishable phenotypically and biochemically.

disease is not understood clearly. The chemistry of the tubercle bacilli is quite complex. They have a high concentration of lipids, 20 to 40% dry weight, which is thought to be in part responsible for their resistance to humoral defense mechanisms and to disinfectants, acids, and alkalis.

The thick cell wall of mycobacteria is rich in mycolic acid and other complex lipids, making it hydrophobic and impermeable to aqueous stains without heat. Heat is applied in the Ziehl-Neelsen stain. The cell wall of mycobacteria contains N-glycolyl-muramic acid rather than N-acetyl-muramic acid.

Some of the specific lipids are the following:

Mycolic Acids. They are β-hydroxy fatty acids that vary in size with species and are responsible for acid-fastness, the property of retaining carbol fuchsin after application of the decolorizer, acid alcohol.

Mycosides. They are responsible for control of cellular permeability (resistance to water-soluble enzymes, antibiotics, and disinfectants). They are associated with cord factor and wax D, a mycoside that enhances the immune response. Wax D and various proteins induce delayed hypersensitivity. Recent evidence supports the hypothesis that factors responsible for virulence reside in mycosides, certain sulfolipids and sulfatides.

Glycolipids. They result in toxicity, a granulomatous response, and enhanced survival of phagocytosed mycobacteria. Cord factor, a glycolipid, is responsible for the characteristic colonial growth (long palisade-like growth resembling serpentine cords) of virulent mycobacteria. Chemically, the cord factor is made up of trehalose-6-6'-dimycolate.

SOME FACTORS CONTRIBUTING TO TUBERCULOSIS

1. Crowding is important because the number of organisms from carriers is higher under crowded conditions, e.g., among stabled cattle as opposed to range cattle.
2. Genetic factors play a role in susceptibility; some races are more susceptible, e.g., American Indian and Eskimo.
3. There is both natural and acquired resistance to tuberculosis, the latter as a result of previous exposure.

PATHOGENESIS

The local manifestations depend upon the route of invasion. In inhalation, the route is via the lungs and tracheobronchial lymph nodes. In ingestion, it is usually through the mesenteric nodes and intestinal wall and to the liver via the portal system. Organisms from lymph nodes may reach the thoracic duct with general dissemination. Animals develop delayed hypersensitivity and cell-mediated immunity, usually with a lessening of multiplication and dissemination. It is thought that delayed hypersensitivity of an exaggerated level attributable to large amounts of tubercular antigen may have a destructive effect on tissues. Most foci are microscopic and most disappear. Some, however, may persist for years and in some instances may progress to form the characteristic tubercle.

Miliary tuberculosis is an acute form of the disease, with general dissemination and production of large numbers of small tubercles.

MODE OF INFECTION

M. bovis. Organisms leave the host in respiratory discharges, feces, milk, urine, semen, and genital discharges. Infection is by inhalation. Localized lesions of lymph nodes of head and nodes of lungs and parenchyma of lungs are produced. In calves, mode of infection may be by ingestion. Lesions are seen in intestinal wall, mesenteric nodes, liver and spleen, and secondarily in lungs.

M. avium. Shed in feces; acquired mainly by ingestion of contaminated food, water, and soil. Lesions may be found anywhere but usually involve intestines, liver, spleen, and bone marrow. Lung lesions are infrequent.

M. tuberculosis. Shed in the sputum and respiratory discharges. Direct spread by droplet infection and by fomites. Lesions are found in lungs and lymph nodes principally.

PATHOGENICITY

M. bovis. Cattle are a natural host; swine are readily and severely infected. Cases have also been found in dogs, horses, and sheep (rare). Cats are susceptible and may perpetuate the bovine disease. In cattle, there is pulmonary tuberculosis with involvement of associated lymph nodes. Infection of viscera and bones occurs in humans, especially from milk. Chickens are resistant but rabbits, mice, and guinea pigs are very susceptible (generalized infections).

M. avium. (See Table 25–1) Chickens are most susceptible; other birds can be infected; not all infected chickens have gross lesions. Crowding is an important factor. Water fowl are quite resistant but house birds are susceptible. In swine, disease usually occurs in lymph nodes of the head. Cattle are refractory but sensitized. Mink fed infected chickens will become infected. Infections in humans are of little consequence. Guinea pigs are slightly susceptible; rabbits are quite susceptible. Sporadic cases have been reported in horses, dogs, and cats.

M. tuberculosis. Occurs in humans and primates, the latter acquired from humans. Cattle are sensitized by the human organism. In swine, disease usually occurs in lymph nodes of the head and organisms are acquired by eating uncooked garbage. Parrots are susceptible. Chickens are rarely infected. Dogs can be infected. Cats are very resistant. Guinea pigs and mice are very susceptible and rabbits are slightly susceptible. In elephants the pulmonary form occurs.

DIRECT EXAMINATION

Great care should be exercised in handling suspicious clinical materials.

The organism can be demonstrated in smears from lesions by employing acid-fast stains. The organisms are small, straight, or slightly curved, and they occur singly or in clumps. They stain red by the Ziehl-Neelsen acid-fast stain.

An alternative staining procedure uses fluorescein dyes. Acid-fast organisms tested by this procedure stain yellow. A negative smear does not mean that the specimen is negative for acid-fast organisms.

ISOLATION AND CULTIVATION

Frequently, a preliminary diagnosis of tuberculosis is made on the basis of the demonstration of typical acid-fast organisms in characteristic lesions. Definitive diagnosis of tuberculosis requires isolation and identification. Isolation should be attempted only if the laboratory is equipped with proper biocontainment facilities.

One procedure for isolation and cultivation from clinical material, e.g., nodules, is as follows:
1. Trim fat off tissues.
2. Add 10 ml of 4% NaOH containing phenol red indicator.
3. Grind tissue in a sterile mortar with sterile sand.
4. Neutralize sediment with 2N HCl for a maximum of 30 minutes.
5. Centrifuge at low speed for 20 minutes.
6. Decant supernatant fluid.
7. Inoculate sediment onto Löwenstein-Jensen slants and egg yolk agar slants, and incubate at 37°C for up to eight weeks. The glycerol in the slants has an inhibitory effect on *M. bovis*, which grows better on egg-base media without glycerol.
8. Stain and identify growth.

Cultural characteristics of classic species of *Mycobacteria* are presented in Table 25–2.

IDENTIFICATION

This is now based principally on cultural, morphologic, growth, and biochemical characteristics. Definitive identification is usually carried out in a reference laboratory. Some of the characteristics

Table 25–2.   Cultural Characteristics of Classic Species of Mycobacteria

M. bovis	M. avium	M. tuberculosis
Dry, sparse, delicate, nonluxuriant. Growth on solid media incubated at 37° C usually appears within 3–6 weeks.	Moist, slimy, glistening, luxuriant, frequently yellow or gray. Growth on solid media incubated at 40°–42° C usually appears within 2–3 weeks.	Dry, crumbly, luxuriant; colonies are usually yellowish with roughened surfaces. Growth on solid media incubated at 37° C usually appears within 2 weeks.

used to differentiate important mycobacteria are listed in Table 25–3. Identification based on cultural characteristics can take several days to several weeks. To identify mycobacteria from clinical specimens in a relatively shorter period of time, commercially available, species-specific isotopic and nonisotopic DNA probes have been used in some laboratories.

ANTIGENIC NATURE AND SEROLOGY

M. bovis and *M. tuberculosis* are antigenically closely related. Monoclonal antibodies appear to be helpful in recognizing the antigenic variations between these two species. DNA homology between *M. bovis* and *M. tuberculosis* is nearly 100%. *M. avium* can be readily differentiated serologically from *M. bovis* and *M. tuberculosis*.

M. avium antigenically resembles the so-called Battey bacilli, *M. intracellulare*. Both are sometimes referred to as the *M. avium-intracellulare* complex or *M. avium* complex, and both belong in Runyon's group III. The trend now is to refer to the complex as *M. avium*. Serotypes of this species are referred to in Table 25–1. Species-specific DNA probes have been constructed and used for the rapid identification of *M. avium* and *M. intracellulare*.

The serological diagnosis of mycobacterial infections (except for paratuberculosis) in animals and humans is not reliable. Sufficiently sensitive, specific, and standardized testing procedures are not available.

RESISTANCE

In general, mycobacteria are rather resistant to various physical influences and chemical disinfectants. Their considerable resistance is partly due to the presence of lipid in the cell wall. Species causing tuberculosis retain their viability in putrefying carcasses and in moist soil for 1 to 4 years and survive for at least 150 days in dry bovine feces. Freezing temperatures have little if any effect. Drying is only effective when the organisms are also exposed to direct sunlight. They are fairly resistant to acids and alkalis; however, phenols (5%), Lysol (3%), cresols, formaldehyde (3 to 8%), alkaline glutaraldehyde (2%), and cresylic acids are fairly effective. In addition, sodium hypochlorite

at 1:200 or 1:1000 concentration and phenol-soap mixtures or other phenol derivates are suitable for laboratory use.

TREATMENT

Treatment may not be feasible or desirable in animals. One of the most useful drugs in the treatment of tuberculosis is isoniazid. It is used in humans with para-aminosalicylic acid or ethambutol and occasionally with streptomycin, constituting "triple therapy." The results are usually excellent and the first three drugs may be given for up to 3 years; streptomycin is usually discontinued after several months. Other drugs used mainly in humans are thioacetazone, pyrazinamide, viomycin, cycloserine, ethionamide, pyrazinamide kanamycin and capremycin. Strains may develop resistance to streptomycin, and toxicity to vestibular and auditory nerves may be encountered. Strains are also found that are resistant to isoniazid. Rifampin is also a useful drug that may be used with isoniazid. Rifabutin, a derivative of rifampin, appears to be effective against rifampin-resistant mycobacteria. Isoniazid has been employed prophylactically to control tuberculosis in zoos and animal parks.

IMMUNITY

Although antibodies are produced in tuberculosis, immunity is primarily cell-mediated. The only vaccine used to any extent is the BCG vaccine (bacille Calmette Guérin). It is a live bovine strain that was attenuated by growth in potato-glycerin bile medium through several hundred transfers. It is used for the prevention of tuberculosis in children and calves, in whom the disease is prevalent. It has not been used in the United States because it has no place in an eradication program; it sensitizes animals to tuberculin.

Hypersensitivity to tuberculin indicates some resistance to tuberculosis. The tuberculin reaction is sometimes negative (anergy) if the infection is overwhelming or if there is a deficiency in cell-mediated immunity.

Field Diagnosis and Control

In the field, diagnosis is carried out by means of the tuberculin test, which depends upon a reaction of the delayed hypersensitivity type. Several tuberculins are used; all contain mycobacterial proteins, to which infected animals may be hypersensitive. Koch's "Old Tuberculin," which has been used widely in the standardization of tuberculins, is a filtrate of an 8-week-old culture of *M. tuberculosis*. The tuberculin used for the routine testing of cattle in the United States is prepared from strains of *M. bovis*. Avian tuberculin is used in the comparative test (double intradermal) in cattle as well as in swine and poultry. PPD (purified protein derivative) is a relatively pure tuberculin.

The tuberculin tests commonly used are

1. Intradermal: dose 0.1 ml tuberculin; read at 72 hours; firm swelling indicates a positive reaction. This is the most widely used test. The sites of inoculation in cattle are the caudal fold, the vulvar lips, or the sides of the neck. The neck skin is the most sensitive site.
2. Comparative cervical: intradermal inoculation of regular and avian tuberculin at two different sites in the neck. Read at 72 hours by measuring swelling.
3. Ophthalmic: mostly used on primates; 0.1 ml of a 1:10 dilution of regular "bovine" tuberculin is inoculated intradermally into the upper eyelid. Some require three negative tests at 30-day intervals before animals are moved out of quarantine.

The tuberculosis eradication program is based upon the detection and slaughter of infected animals as determined by the tuberculin test. Prior to an organized control program, the infection rate of bovine tuberculosis in the United States was approximately 5%. In 1917, the test and slaughter eradication program was initiated by the Bureau of Animal Industry. By 1940, when the country was accredited, the infection rate had dropped to 0.46%, and by 1957 to 0.156%. At least 85% of the current reactors do not have gross lesions, and it was for this reason that the comparative cervical test was introduced. During this 40-year period, over 400 million dollars was spent to control and eradicate the disease.

The absence of infected cattle and the pasteurization of milk have all but eliminated human infection with *M. bovis*.

General Steps in the Control of Bovine Tuberculosis

The system of surveillance followed by the USDA is briefly as follows:

1. When suspected tuberculosis lesions are found in cattle during routine postmortem examination, the veterinary meat inspector submits specimens to the Veterinary Services Diagnostic Laboratory (USDA, Ames, Iowa). If mycobacterial infection is confirmed, the federal veterinarian in charge of the state involved is informed.
2. The regular tuberculin test is then applied to the herd or herds of origin.
3. If the original infection was caused by *M. bovis* (based upon pathologic examination or cultivation or both), the procedure of choice is

Table 25–3. In Vitro Tests for Identifying Some Clinically Significant Mycobacteria

Mycobacterium	Growth Rate 43°C	Growth Rate 37°C	Growth Rate 31°C	Niacin	Nitrate Reduction	Cord Formation	Thiophen-2-carboxylic acid-hydrazide	NaCl Tolerance	Tween Hydrolysis	Chromogenicity	Arylsulfatase at 3 Days	Glycerol Inhibition
M. tuberculosis		M		+	+	+	+	–	–	–	–	+
M. bovis		M		–	–	+	–	–	–	–	–	–
*M. avium**	M	M	M	–	–	–	+	–	–	–	–	+
M. kansasii		M	S	–	+	V	+	–	+	+	–	+
M. marinum			S	–	–	–	+	–	+	+	–	+
M. scrofulaceum		M	S	–	–	–	+	–	–	+	–	+
M. xenopi	S	S		–	–	–	+	–	–	+	V	+
M. fortuitum		R	R	–	+	V	+	+	–	–	+	+
M. chelonei		R	R	V	–	–	–	–	–	–	+	+

–, negative—absence or inhibition; +, positive—production or growth; V, variable; R, rapid (1 to 6 days); M, moderate (6 to 14 days); S, slow (more than 14 days).

* Includes strains previously identified as *M. intracellulare*. *M. avium* serotypes 1 and 2 grow best at 43°C; some strains of serotypes 3 through 28 grow best at 22° to 30° C.

From Thoen, C.O.: *Mycobacterium. In* Diagnostic Procedures in Veterinary Bacteriology and Mycology. 5th Ed. Edited by G.R. Carter and J.R. Cole, Jr. New York, Academic Press, 1990. Reprinted with permission.

liquidation of the herd. If it is not completely depopulated, the herd is quarantined for 10 months and a series of retests are carried out. Reactors are removed and slaughtered. If infection is extensive, depopulation is always recommended.

4. The comparative test is used mainly after the regular test has revealed questionable responses in routine testing. The action taken on the reactors and those animals classed as suspicious (based upon comparative responses) depends upon their number and the size of the herd. The so-called "scattergram" is used as the guide. Many suspicious and responding animals may have no gross lesions (NGL).

DECONTAMINATION OF INFECTED PREMISES

After depopulation, manure, litter, hay, straw, and other accumulated extraneous material are removed from the stables and barnyard and burned. The stables, building, and barnyard (if structural) are brushed, scraped, and washed down with water under pressure. Within several days, a disinfectant is applied under pressure to saturate the same structures. When depopulation is carried out because of tuberculosis, the premises are not repopulated for at least 30 days. The two disinfectants preferred in tuberculosis eradication are a cresylic compound or sodium orthophenylphenate. Different disinfectants are used for different diseases.

Mycobacterium leprae

M. leprae causes leprosy (Hansen's disease), a chronic disease affecting the skin and peripheral nerve trunks of humans. The incubation period may be up to 20 years. It occurs worldwide but is most prevalent in tropical countries and is infrequent in countries in temperate regions. It has not been cultivated in vitro, but experimental infections have been produced in the armadillo, mice, hamsters, rats, ground squirrels, hedgehogs, and monkeys. Mice and the 9-banded armadillo are the most susceptible.

Nonclassic Mycobacteria

This includes a large number of species, only a small number of which are pathogenic and clinically significant (see Table 25–1). Some were initially placed in the Runyon groups discussed earlier. They are worldwide in distribution, occurring and living in soil. The species distribution varies with the kind of soil and various climatic and environmental factors. They can sometimes be isolated from animal feces. Generally severe infections caused by some species of these mycobacteria occur in humans and animals only after impairment of the body's defense mechanisms.

ISOLATION AND IDENTIFICATION

These mycobacteria grow well on Löwenstein-Jensen medium and other culture media used for the growth of mycobacteria. The procedures used for isolation are the same as those referred to earlier for the classic species. Some of the characteristics used for the identification of both classic and nonclassic species are listed in Table 25–3.

SKIN TUBERCULOSIS OF CATTLE

Mycobacteria have been demonstrated from skin lesions consisting of cold, firm, rounded swellings and fluctuant thick-walled abscesses. They occur most commonly in the skin of the lower parts of the leg, and they may soften and ulcerate. Because of the lymphatic distribution of lesions, the term ulcerative lymphangitis has been used. The organisms, which have not been cultivated, may sensitize cattle to tuberculin.

A leprosy of cattle and water buffaloes has been described in the Far East. It is not clear whether this condition is distinct from the skin tuberculosis of cattle just described. The distribution of the lesions is similar, and the organisms have not been cultivated in vitro.

FELINE LEPROSY

Cat leprosy is presumed to be an infectious disease caused by an as yet uncultivated *Mycobacterium*. The disease is characterized by the formation of single and multiple granulomas or nodules of the skin 1 to 3 cm in diameter. They are painless and move freely. Some may be ulcerous and discharge a slight, serosanguineous exudate. Affected cats are usually in good health and only in rare cases does the disease become generalized.

There is some experimental evidence that the causal agent is identical to *M. lepraemurium*, the cause of rat leprosy, and it has been suggested that cats acquire the infection via rat bites.

Long, slender, acid-fast rods can be demonstrated in smears from the nodules.

Treatment involves the surgical removal of nodules, which do not usually recur. Variable results have been obtained with the anti-leprosy (human) drug dapsone. Streptomycin and isoniazid are toxic for the cat.

Mycobacterium paratuberculosis

HISTORICAL

This organism was first observed by Johne and Frothingham in 1895. In 1906 Bang demonstrated that the disease was distinct from tuberculosis and caused by a different organism. Twort first isolated the organism from infected tissue in 1910.

DISTRIBUTION

M. paratuberculosis is found worldwide, and cattle, sheep, and goats are the principal ruminants affected. Because there is no national eradication plan for this disease in the United States, it is difficult to determine its precise incidence. It may be sufficiently prevalent in some dairy herds to constitute a real problem. Annual death losses within an infected herd may reach 10%.

MODE OF INFECTION

Animals are infected by ingestion of food and water contaminated by feces. The incidence of subclinical cases shedding organisms intermittently may be as high as 15%. Vertical transmission has been suggested but is as yet unsubstantiated.

PATHOGENICITY

Little is known regarding the pathogenesis of the disease. Iron appears to play an important role in the pathogenesis. Presence of a large quantity of intracellular iron correlates well with the severity of lesions. High levels of iron and iron-containing compounds are also positively correlated with fecal shedding of organisms from infected cattle. Experimental infections can be established orally or intravenously. Dosage of organisms is probably important in establishing infections. Toxic substances have not been demonstrated.

In cattle there is a chronic enteritis, often with severe diarrhea. The diarrhea in sheep, goats, and other ruminants is usually less severe or absent. The incubation period may be a year or more. Calves are susceptible but do not show signs until adulthood. The disease is usually progressive, leading to emaciation and death. Mortality is caused in large part by the malabsorption of amino acids and the loss of protein into the intestine (protein-losing enteropathy). The ileum and colon are usually involved, and the infection may extend to the rectum in advanced cases. The mucous membrane becomes corrugated and thickened because of epithelioid and giant cells, both of which contain many organisms. Large numbers of organisms may be shed in the feces.

M. paratuberculosis has been isolated from the udder and reproductive tracts of both male and female cattle. Disseminated paratuberculosis of both kidneys of a cow has been reported. Bovine fetal infection with the organism has also been reported. Mice, hamsters, pigs, and horses have been infected experimentally.

M. paratuberculosis has been isolated from the tissues of several human patients with Crohn's disease. Micro- and macroscopically, Crohn's disease (Crohn's eleitis) is very similar to Johne's disease. Whether or not *M. paratuberculosis* has a role in the cause of Crohn's disease remains to be determined.

DIRECT EXAMINATION

The organisms are often difficult to demonstrate in smears, and failure to demonstrate organisms does not exclude Johne's disease. A number of smears may have to be examined. Thin smears are made from feces, intestinal mucosa (terminal ileum preferred) in the dead animal, and rectal mucosa in the live animal. The rectal smears may only be positive in advanced cases. On the average, the rectal smear will only detect about 25% of infected animals. A small piece of the rectum is pinched out, washed, and then squeezed between two slides. The resulting smear and other smears are stained by the Ziehl-Neelsen method. Johne's bacilli occur singly and in characteristic clumps and stain a pinkish red. Bovine feces frequently yield saprophytic acid-fast organisms that can be mistaken for Johne's bacilli.

A reliable but complicated procedure (laparotomy) is to examine smears of biopsies of mesenteric lymph nodes in the region of the terminal ileum for acid-fast organisms.

ISOLATION AND CULTIVATION

The organism grows very slowly, and cultivation and identification may take months. The feces or tissue is treated for contaminants. A medium containing mycobactin (extract of *M. phlei*) is used. Colonies appear in 4 to 12 weeks.

IDENTIFICATION

In smears organisms appear as short, thick, small, acid-fast rods similar to the avian tubercle bacillus. Identification is based on cultural (including growth rate and mycobactin dependency), morphologic and staining characteristics and sero-agglutination.

ANTIGENIC NATURE AND SEROLOGY

The antigenic relationship between this organism and the avian tubercle bacillus is indicated by the fact that animals with Johne's disease often react to avian tuberculin.

Serologic tests that are available for the diagnosis of paratuberculosis in animals include the ELISA, complement fixation test, agar gel immunodiffusion test, fluorescent antibody test, radioimmunoassay, and hemagglutination test. Species-specific DNA probes have been used for rapid identification of *M. paratuberculosis* in bovine feces.

RESISTANCE

M. paratuberculosis resembles other mycobacteria in its resistance to physical and chemical influences; it will survive in contaminated stables for months.

CONTROL

The intravenous johnin test will detect about 80% of cases found to be infected by cultural methods. A positive reaction is indicated by a temperature rise of 1.5° F or greater. The complement-fixation test is used as a screening procedure, but it is not as reliable as culture of the feces.

Recent work indicates that an agar gel immunodiffusion test may be as reliable or possibly more reliable than culture for the diagnosis of clinical paratuberculosis.

The following steps are recommended for controlling paratuberculosis:*

1. Animals with persistent diarrhea or chronic weight loss should be isolated or sent to slaughter.
2. Culture the feces from all animals 2 years old or older every 6 months and remove and slaughter animals (and their offspring) whose cultures are positive.
3. Adults from the herd should be sold only for slaughter or to quarantine feedlots. Calves of culturally negative dams may be sold on the open market if they are separated from the dams at birth, raised apart, and have a negative reaction to johnin not more than 30 days before sale.
4. Clean and disinfect the premises after the removal of infected animals. The cresylic disinfectants and sodium orthophenylphenate (when used in the same dilutions that are recommended for disinfecting premises contaminated with *M. bovis*) are suitable for use

on premises contaminated with *M. paratuberculosis*.

5. Calf-rearing quarters should have separate cleaning and feeding equipment, which should never be exchanged with the equipment used for the mature animals because calves are easily infected.
6. Continue surveillance (at intervals of not less than 5 or more than 7 months) until there have been four consecutive negative fecal cultures of all animals 2 years of age or older.
7. Purchase only animals with johnin-negative tests from herds with no history of the disease.
8. If artificial insemination is used, semen should come from culturally negative bulls.

IMMUNITY

Recovery from the disease is rare. Bacterins have been used in sheep and calves with some success, but immunization has not been widely practiced and is not permitted in cattle in some countries. Vaccinated animals may be johnin- and tuberculin-positive.

As in tuberculosis, immunity in Johne's disease is considered to be predominantly cell-mediated.

FURTHER READING

Anonymous: Laboratory methods in veterinary mycobacteriology. Ames, Iowa, Veterinary Services Laboratories, APHIS, 1974.
Chengappa, M.M., Kadel, W.L., Maddux, R.L., and Greer, S.C.: An unusual isolation of *Mycobacterium fortuitum* from pig joints. Vet. Med./Sm. Anim. Clin., *78*:1273, 1983.
Drolet, R.: Disseminated tuberculosis caused by *Mycobacterium avium* in a cat. J. Am. Vet. Med. Assoc., *189*:1336, 1986.
Dubina, J., Sula, L., Kubin, M., and Varekova, J.: Incidence of *Mycobacterium avium* and *M. intracellulare* in cattle and pigs. J. Hyg. Epidemiol. Microbiol. Immunol., *18*:15, 1974.
Gilmour, N.J.L.: The pathogenesis, diagnosis and control of Johne's disease. Vet. Rec., *99*:433, 1976.
Hines, S.A., Buergelt, C.D., Wilson, J.H., and Bliss, E.L.: Disseminated *Mycobacterium paratuberculosis* infection in a cow. J. Am. Vet. Med. Assoc., *190*:681, 1987.
Hoop, R.K., et al.: Mycobacteriosis due to *Mycobacterium genavense* in six pet birds. J. Clin. Microbiol., *31*:990, 1993.
Hurley, S.S., Splitter, G.A., and Welch, R.A.: Development of a diagnostic test for Johne's disease using a DNA hybridization probe. J. Clin. Microbiol., *27*:1582, 1989.
Kreeger, J.M.: Ruminant paratuberculosis—a century of progress and frustration. J. Vet. Diagn. Invest., *3*:373, 1991.
Lofstedt, J., and Jakowski, R.M.: Diagnosis of avian tuberculosis in a horse by use of liver biopsy. J. Am. Vet. Med. Assoc., *194*:260, 1989.
McFadden, J., et al.: Mycobacteria in Crohn's disease: DNA probes identify the wood pigeon strain of *Mycobacterium avium* and *Mycobacterium paratuberculosis* from human tissue. J. Clin. Microbiol., *30*:3070, 1992.
Merkal, R.S.: Laboratory diagnosis of bovine paratuberculosis. J. Am. Vet. Med. Assoc., *163*:1100, 1973.

*Based on Larsen, A.B.: Paratuberculosis: the status of our knowledge. J. Am. Vet. Med. Assoc., *161*:1539, 1972.

Merkal, R.S.: Paratuberculosis: Advances in cultural, serologic, and vaccination methods. J. Am. Vet. Med. Assoc., *184*:939, 1984.

Morfitt, D.C., Matthews, J.A., Thoen, C.O., and Kluge, J.P.: Disseminated *Mycobacterium avium* serotype 1 infection in a seven-month-old cat. J. Vet. Diagn. Invest., *1*:354, 1989.

Murray, A., Moriarty, K.M., and Scott, D.B.: A cloned DNA probe for the detection of *Mycobacterium paratuberculosis.* New Zealand Vet. J., *37*:47, 1989.

Patterson, C.J., et al.: Accidental self-inoculation with *Mycobacterium paratuberculosis* bacterin (Johne's bacterin) by veterinarians in Wisconsin. J. Am. Vet. Med. Assoc., *192*:1197, 1988.

Righter, J., Hart, G.D., and Howes, M.: *Mycobacterium chelonei:* Report of a case of septicemia and review of the literature. Diagn. Microbiol. Infect. Dis., *1*:323, 1983.

Rohde, R.F., and Shulaw, W.P.: Isolation of *Mycobacterium paratuberculosis* from the uterine flush fluids of cows with clinical paratuberculosis. J. Am. Vet. Med. Assoc., *197*:1482, 1990.

Saito, H., et al.: Identification and partial characterization of *Mycobacterium avium* and *Mycobacterium intracellulare* by using DNA probes. J. Clin. Microbiol., *27*:994, 1989.

Schaefer, W.B.: Incidence of serotypes of *Mycobacterium avium* and atypical mycobacteria in human and animal disease. Am. Rev. Resp. Dis., *97*:18, 1968.

Schultze, W.D., and Brasso, W.B.: Characterization and identification of *Mycobacterium smegmatis* in bovine mastitis. Am. J. Vet. Res., *48*:739, 1987.

Seitz, S.E., et al.: Bovine fetal infection with *Mycobacterium paratuberculosis.* J. Am. Vet. Med. Assoc., *194*:1423, 1989.

Shackelford, C.C., and Reed, W.M.: Disseminated *Mycobacterium avium* infection in a dog. J. Vet. Diagn. Invest., *1*:273, 1989.

Sherman, D.M., Markham, J.F., and Bates, F.: Agar gel immunodiffusion test for diagnosis of clinical paratuberculosis in cattle. J. Am. Vet. Med. Assoc., *185*:179, 1984.

Snider, W.R.: Tuberculosis in canine and feline populations. Am. Rev. Resp. Dis., *104*:877, 1971.

Sweeny, R.W., Whitlock, R.H., and Rosenberger, A.E.: *Mycobacterium paratuberculosis* cultured from milk and supramammary lymph nodes of infected asymptomatic cows. J. Clin. Microbiol., *30*:166, 1992.

Thoen, C.O.: Mycobacterium. *In* Diagnostic Procedures in Veterinary Bacteriology and Mycology. Edited by G.R. Carter and J.R. Cole, Jr. 5th Ed. New York, Academic Press, 1990.

Turnwald, G.H., et al.: Survival of a dog with pneumonia caused by *Mycobacterium fortuitum.* J. Am. Vet. Med. Assoc., *192*:64, 1988.

Whipple, D.L., Kapke, P.A., and Anderson, P.R.: Comparison of a commercial DNA probe test and three cultivation procedures for detection of *Mycobacterium paratuberculosis* in bovine feces. J. Vet. Diag. Invest., *4*:23, 1992.

Wilkinson, G.T.: Cat leprosy. *In* The Veterinary Annual. Edited by G.S.G. Grunsell and F.W.G. Hill. Bristol, England, Scientechnica, 1978.

26

Actinomyces, Nocardia, and Dermatophilus

The gram-positive organisms discussed in this chapter are referred to generally as the actinomycetes. Included are the genera, *Actinomyces, Nocardia, Streptomyces, Actinomadura,* and *Dermatophilus.* They are sometimes called "higher bacteria" because they have some of the cultural and morphologic characteristics of the fungi. These include extensive filamentation, branching, usually the production of some aerial hyphae with asexual spores or conidia, and rather tenacious colonies. Some produce club-shaped cells and acid-fast elements that bear a resemblance to the corynebacteria and mycobacteria.

Nocardia are closely related to *Corynebacterium* and *Mycobacterium* but differ from *Actinomyces* in the chemical composition of their cell walls and their guanine-cytosine content.

Actinomyces

PRINCIPAL CHARACTERISTICS

Actinomyces are gram-positive, nonacid-fast rods that may show branching. They are nonmotile and nonspore-forming; microaerophilic or anaerobic (except for *A. viscosus* and *A. naeslundii*); and catalase-negative (except for *A. viscosus*) and fermentative.

All of the actinomyces causing disease in animals and humans occur as commensals in the oral cavity.

Significant species are *Actinomyces bovis, A. israelii* (causes actinomycosis in humans), *A. naeslundii* (causes infrequent infections in humans), and *A. viscosus.*

Actinomyces bovis

HISTORICAL

Bollinger described the disease (actinomycosis) and the organism in 1877.

HABITAT

A. bovis is a commensal in the oral cavity of cattle and probably of some other animals.

MODE OF INFECTION

Infections are initiated in wounds of the mucous membrane of the upper digestive tract.

PATHOGENESIS

Exotoxins have not been demonstrated. Organisms grow in the "anaerobic" damaged tissue, causing abscesses. Infectious material may be aspirated into the lungs, producing pulmonary actinomycosis, or swallowed, producing visceral or abdominal actinomycosis.

PATHOGENICITY

A. bovis causes a subacute or chronic progressive disease principally of cattle characterized by the

214

development of indurated, granulomatous, suppurative lesions involving bone and soft tissue. Abscesses discharge through fistulas; tortuous sinuses result from the burrowing process.

Cattle. The disease involves the mandible or other bony tissue of the head ("lumpy jaw"). Seen less often are orchitis, mastitis, and lesions of the liver and other internal organs. Actinomycosis is rare in sheep.

Pigs. In pigs the disease results in abscesses of the liver and other internal organs; in sows it causes chronic granulomatous suppurative mastitis (see *Actinomyces suis* below).

Dogs and Cats. Infection is rare in these animals. *A. bovis* and *Actinobacillus lignieresii* are occasionally found together.

Humans. Lesions involve the face, neck, lung, breast, and lymph nodes.

DIRECT EXAMINATION

A small amount of pus is placed in a Petri dish and washed to expose the small 1 to 3 mm sulfur granules associated with the disease. The actinomycotic granules are larger than the grey-white granules seen in actinobacillosis. A granule is transferred to a slide, and a drop of 10% sodium hydroxide is added. A coverslip is placed on the granule, and it is crushed by gentle pressure. In actinomycosis the characteristic "ray fungi" with club-shaped margins can be seen under low power microscopy. The "clubs" are caused by a gelatinous sheath and the deposition of calcium phosphate around the terminal filaments. The granule is held together by a polysaccharide-protein complex.

The coverslip is removed and the material spread to make a smear. This is dried, fixed, and stained by the Gram method. If the granules are from an actinomycotic lesion, delicate, intertwined, branching, gram-positive filaments are seen.

ISOLATION AND CULTIVATION

The organism grows well on blood agar, brain heart infusion agar, and in thioglycolate broth. An anaerobic atmosphere containing 5 to 10% CO_2 is preferred. Colonies are white, rough, nodular, and difficult to remove. The radiating mycelia can be seen under a dissecting microscope. Small cottony colonies may be seen suspended discretely in thioglycolate broth.

MORPHOLOGY AND STAINING

Gram-stained smears from growth on solid or fluid media reveal masses of gram-positive rods and slightly branched filaments.

IDENTIFICATION

A strongly presumptive identification is usually made on the basis of the gross pathology, characteristic sulfur granules, and demonstration of the gram-positive branching filaments. Cultivation of an organism from characteristic lesions and granules in animals possessing the morphologic characteristics of *A. bovis* is usually considered sufficient for identification.

Definitive differentiation of *A. bovis* from other *Actinomyces* and from anaerobic diphtheroids can be accomplished by various biochemical tests (Table 26–1).

TREATMENT

Establish and maintain drainage of abscesses. Penicillin is the preferred antibiotic; tetracyclines, chloramphenicol, and streptomycin have also been used. Iodides given orally or intravenously are also effective.

Actinomyces viscosus

This organism differs from other *Actinomyces* in that it grows aerobically and is catalase-positive. It has been isolated from the human and canine oral cavity, from periodontal disease in humans and hamsters, and most frequently from actinomycosis in dogs. Several isolates have been recovered from other animals.

In the past some of the diagnoses of nocardiosis in the dog may actually have been actinomycosis due to *A. viscosus*. Actinomycosis in the dog is characterized by the presence of actinomycotic granules containing gram-positive, nonacid-fast, filamentous organisms that resemble *A. bovis* morphologically.

Two forms of actinomycosis have been seen in the dog. The more common is the localized granulomatous abscess involving mainly the skin and subcutis. This form responds well to treatment. The other form principally involves the thorax, with or without extension to the abdominal cavity. Pyothorax with granulomatous lesions of thoracic tissues and accumulation of pleural and pericardial fluid containing soft grey-white granules are characteristic of this deep form.

Table 26–1. **Differentiation of Actinomyces *species***

Test	A. bovis	A. israelii	A. naeslundii	A. viscosus	A. pyogenes
Aerotolerance	M or An	M or An	F	F	F
Catalase	–	–	–	+	–
Nitrate red	–	+	+	+	–
Gelatinase	–	–	–	–	+
Fermentation:					
Mannitol	–	+	–	–	–
Lactose	–	(–)	–	–	(+)
Sucrose	+	+	+	+	V
Salicin	–	(+)	V	(+)	–
Glycerol	–	–	–	V	V
Xylose	–	(+)	–	–	V
Arabinose	–	(–)	–	–	V
Raffinose	–	(+)	+	+	–

M, microaerophilic; An, anaerobic; F, facultative; V, variable; ( ), most strains.

Skin pustules and nodules in a horse, caused by *A. viscosus*, have been reported.

A. viscosus may be cultivated at 37°C on blood and brain heart infusion agar (and broth) but not on Sabouraud agar. Colonies are readily apparent in 3 to 7 days. See Table 26–1 for differential characteristics.

Prolonged antimicrobial therapy, e.g., with penicillin and tetracycline, and surgical drainage are effective in the treatment of canine actinomycosis.

Actinomyces pyogenes

Synonym: *Corynebacterium pyogenes*

PATHOGENESIS AND PATHOGENICITY

This species is a common commensal on the mucous membranes of the nasopharynx of cattle, sheep, and swine. It may be shed from apparently normal udders and is frequently recovered from tonsils and retropharyngeal lymph nodes.

Infections arise when the organisms gain entrance to tissue as a result of various injuries and other infections, including those caused by viruses, mycoplasmas, and other bacteria. Dissemination to lungs and other tissues may be hematogenous. It is frequently found in mixed infections, e.g., with *Fusobacterium necrophorum* in bovine liver abscesses.

A. pyogenes produces a relatively weak hemolytic protein exotoxin which kills mice intravenously and produces skin necrosis. Antitoxin can be demonstrated in naturally infected animals but its correlation with protection is questionable. A protease, which may be identical to the gelatinase produced by the organism, has been suggested as a possible virulence factor. Abscesses are variable in size with a usually substantial fibrous capsule. The character and odor of the pus depends upon whether the infection is pure or mixed. *Fusobacte-*

rium necrophorum, *Bacteroides* spp., and other anaerobes may be responsible for a foul odor.

A. pyogenes is a very important pyogenic organism of cattle, sheep, and swine. Among the infections it causes mainly in these species are: chronic abscessing mastitis particularly in cows; chronic suppurative pneumonia, frequently with mycoplasmas and *Pasteurella* spp.; septic arthritis; vegetative endocarditis (cattle); endometritis and pyometra; umbilical infections; infections of wounds and surgical incisions; and seminal vesiculitis (bulls and boars). Infections may affect single or multiple animals.

ISOLATION AND IDENTIFICATION

Gram-stained smears of pus disclose small, slender gram-positive pleomorphic rods which may be somewhat curved and clubbed at the ends. The organism grows readily on blood agar producing pinpoint, glistening strep-like beta-hemolytic colonies in 48 hours. With age, colonies become opaque and dry. *A. pyogenes* is the only one of the potentially pathogenic actinomyces that produces gelatinase. Important characteristics used in identification of this species are listed in Table 26–1.

TREATMENT

A. pyogenes is susceptible to penicillin, ampicillin, erythromycin, chloramphenicol, tetracyclines, and sulfonamides. Resistant strains have been reported, but are uncommon. Because of the nature of infections—abscesses with thick fibrous capsules—the response to antimicrobial treatment is poor.

IMMUNITY

The immune response to *A. pyogenes* has received little attention. Serum antibodies, including those against toxin, are detectable, but their significance is not clear. They are not necessarily correlated with protection. The organism and its products have been included in vaccines and bacterins, but the value of such products remains doubtful.

Other *Actinomyces* Species

Actinomyces hordeovulnaris. This species has been isolated from dogs with localized abscesses and systemic infections characterized by one or more of the following: pleuritis, peritonitis, pyothorax, and septic arthritis. The infections were initially reported from California and were associated with grass of *Hordeum* spp.

The organism, which is pleomorphic with branching filaments, grows well on blood agar in an anaerobic atmosphere; a candle jar is satisfactory. White colonies somewhat adherent, achieve a diameter of 2mm in 72 hours. Characteristics used in identification are listed in Table 26–1.

Actinomyces suis. This name has been proposed for strains of *Actinomyces* recovered from actinomycosis of the mammary gland of sows. Although these strains resemble *A. bovis* and *A. israelii* they have minor biochemical and antigenic differences.

Actinomyces **spp.** Unspeciated *Actinomyces* are occasionally associated with supra-atlantal bursitis (poll evil) and supraspinous bursitis (fistulous withers) in horses and various infections of other animals including the dog. These infections are usually initiated by various injuries.

Nocardia

PRINCIPAL CHARACTERISTICS

Nocardia are nonmotile, nonspore-forming, gram-positive rods that usually show branching and aerial hyphae. They are aerobic, split sugars by oxidation, and may be partially acid-fast.

There is considerable confusion in the taxonomy of *Nocardia.* Several species, all soil-borne, have been described. Three are considered important pathogens: *N. asteroides* in domestic animals and humans; *N. caviae (N. otitidiscaviarum)* in the guinea pig and humans, and as a cause of bovine mastitis; and *N. brasiliensis,* one of the causes of nocardiosis in humans.

The disease bovine farcy, originally thought to be caused by *N. farcinica,* is now claimed to be caused by one of two species of mycobacteria; however, some still consider *N. farcinica* to be the cause. Some workers give the name *N. farcinica* to strains, others consider them to be *N. asteroides.*

Nocardia asteroides

HISTORICAL

Nocard (a French veterinarian) was probably the discoverer of this organism or a closely related one (*N. farcinica*) from a disease of cattle—bovine farcy—in 1888.

HABITAT

N. asteroides is found widely distributed in the soil as a saprophyte.

MODE OF INFECTION

Infection is by inhalation or wounds (hands and feet of agricultural laborers). It is not considered contagious and is exogenous.

PATHOGENESIS

The pathogenesis of nocardiosis is somewhat like that of actinomycosis. Infection begins as a nodule or pustule, with subsequent induration. There is usually rupture, with suppuration and regression, followed by exacerbation and spread, with additional abscess formation and production of interlocking sinuses. Toxins have not been demonstrated. Like *Rhodococcus, Mycobacterium,* and *Corynebacterium,* the cell walls of *Nocardia* possess mycolic acids. Fractions of the cell walls of *Nocardia* like those of *Mycobacterium* increase the antitumor and antimicrobial activities of macrophages.

Experimentally virulent *N. asteroides* can grow within and destroy macrophages. The resistance of this species to oxidative killing by human neutrophils and monocytes has been attributed to noncardial catalase and superoxide dismutase. Some human strains of *N. asteroides* display an as yet unexplained neurotropism.

PATHOGENICITY

Nocardiosis is usually a chronic progressive disease characterized by suppurating, granulomatous lesions. Sporadic infections may be seen in many animal species.

Cattle. It occurs as an acute or chronic mastitis with granulomatous lesions and draining fistulous tracts.

Dogs and Cats. There is a localized form of the disease, with subcutaneous lesions (mycetomas) or lymph node involvement or both. In the dog, there is a thoracic form with occasional extension to the abdominal cavity. Like actinomycosis in the dog caused by *A. viscosus,* there is a suppurative pleuritis or peritonitis or both, with the accumulation of pleural, pericardial, and peritoneal fluid. Abscesses may be found in the heart, brain, liver, and kidneys as well. Severe halitosis, gingivitis, and ulceration of the oral cavity are common in dogs with nocardial stomatitis.

Horses. Nocardiosis is infrequent in the horse; however, respiratory and disseminated nocardiosis have been reported in immunosuppressed horses.

Unlike actinomycosis, granules are not found in infections due to *N. asteroides.* Because the treatments of nocardiosis and actinomycosis is different, it is very important that a correct diagnosis be made.

Humans. The most common forms are pulmonary nocardiosis and a subcutaneous form. The systemic disease with CNS involvement is usually fatal.

DIRECT EXAMINATION

Gram-stained smears of pus reveal gram-positive branching filaments with or without clubs. The acid-fast stain of most strains shows retention of some of the carbolfuchsin.

EXPERIMENTAL ANIMALS

Guinea pigs are susceptible to experimental infection if the organisms are administered in gastric mucin.

ISOLATION AND CULTIVATION

The organism grows on unenriched media and on blood agar and Sabouraud agar, at 25°C or 37°C. Growth is evident in 4 or 5 days, and colonies are irregularly folded, raised and smooth, or granular. The color varies from white through yellow to deep orange. Gram-positive partially acid-fast branching mycelial filaments, which break up into bacillary and coccoid forms, are evident under oil immersion. The presence of mycelial elements distinguishes *Nocardia* from saprophytic and atypical mycobacteria. The mycelial forms of *Nocardia* can be readily seen in slide cultures on Sabouraud dextrose agar. The mycelial elements may give regular cultures a powdery appearance.

IDENTIFICATION

A presumptive identification is based on pathology, demonstration of typical organisms in clinical material, and on colonial, cultural, morphologic, and staining characteristics. Although pathogenic nocardiae are usually partially acid-fast some strains are not. Nocardiae reduce nitrate and are catalase positive. See Table 26–2 for differentiation of important species.

Streptomyces spp. and *Actinomadura* spp. have aerial hyphae, are not acid-fast, and are not pathogenic for mice and guinea pigs. They are occasionally isolated from mycetomas in animals in the tropics. Rapidly growing *Mycobacterium* spp., which occur widely, can be distinguished by their occurrence as rods rather than as fragmenting hyphae and by their strong acid-fastness.

N. caviae and *N. brasiliensis* are differentiated from *N. asteroides* on the basis of several biochemical reactions (see Table 26–2).

ANTIGENIC NATURE AND SEROLOGY

N. asteroides and *N. brasiliensis* have some antigens in common, and they share antigens with mycobacteria. Little is known regarding the antigenic makeup of *N. asteroides.*

TREATMENT

Treatment consists of surgical debridement and drainage of lesions. Antimicrobial susceptibility tests should be performed as some resistant strains have been encountered. Some drugs that have been effective are sulfamethoxazole-trimethoprim, sulfonamides, especially sulfadiazine, novobiocin, ampicillin, and tetracyclines. In some cases antibiotic administration must be continued for periods as long as 12 weeks. Penicillin is not effective.

There is no effective treatment for nocardial mastitis.

Streptomyces and *Actinomadura*

These nonacid-fast actinomycetes are rarely causes of infections in animals. *Streptomyces griseous* and *Actinomadura madurae* have been isolated infrequently from mycetomas in cats and goats, respectively.

Dermatophilus congolensis

Dermatophilus congolensis is a gram-positive, branching, filamentous rod. It is aerobic, nonsporeforming, and not acid-fast; zoospores are motile.

It is generally agreed that there is only one species. The earlier literature refers to several different species. The disease produced is called streptothricosis or dermatophilosis. It is worldwide in distribution, and although it may affect many animal

Table 26–2. *Differentiation of Important* **Nocardia** *species*

Species	Decomposition of			
	Casein	Tyrosine	Xanthine	Urea
N. asteroides	–	–	–	+
N. brasiliensis	+	+	–	+
N. caviae (*N. otitidiscaviarum*)	–	–	+	+

species, it is seen most frequently in cattle, sheep, goats, and horses.

HISTORICAL

Streptothricosis of cattle was first described by Van Saceghem in 1915 in the Belgian Congo.

HABITAT

As far as is known, *Dermatophilus congolensis* is an obligate parasite living only on animals.

MODE OF INFECTION

Infection is spread by contact, fomites, and biting insects. Moist conditions probably promote its dissemination.

PATHOGENICITY

Streptothricosis or dermatophilosis has been encountered in horses, cattle, sheep, goats, dogs, cats, deer, squirrels, and humans. Recent studies indicate that the disease is widely prevalent, especially in cattle. It is an infection involving the superficial layers of the skin and is characterized by the formation of crusts or scabs varying in size from quite small to about 2.5 cm. In advanced cases, large areas of the skin may be involved as a result of coalescence of smaller lesions. Removal of the scab leaves a moist depressed area.

A severe form of the disease has been responsible on occasions for deaths of calves, sheep, and goats.

In sheep, the disease is referred to as mycotic dermatitis and is seen in three forms: (1) dermatitis of the wool-covered areas or "lumpy wool;" (2) dermatitis of the face and scrotum; and (3) dermatitis of the lower leg and foot, which may result in a severe ulcerative dermatitis referred to as "strawberry foot rot."

Several cases, acquired from animals, have been described in humans. Infections can be produced experimentally in the rabbit. The disease in cats is probably initiated by puncture wounds. Abscesses develop involving the subcutis, muscles, and lymph nodes; chronic draining fistulas may result.

DIRECT EXAMINATION

Smears are made from scabs softened with distilled water and then stained by the Giemsa or Gram method. Segmenting (longitudinal and transverse) filaments and coccoid spores stain deep purple. The spores are seen in packets.

ISOLATION AND CULTIVATION

The organism grows well on blood agar, tryptose agar, and other media. Small, rough, greyish-white colonies appear in 24 to 48 hours; they have fimbriated lace-like borders, enlarge to 4 mm in diameter on further incubation, and become yellowish to yellow-orange. The organism can usually be recovered in the conventional manner on blood agar.

MORPHOLOGY AND STAINING

Motile zoospores approximately 1 μm in diameter are formed as a result of the septation of hyphal elements; they possess polar flagella and can be seen in wet mounts from colonies. Gram-positive, branching hyphal elements in various stages of segmentation are seen in stained smears. The hyphal elements are larger and more irregular in shape than the filaments of *Streptomyces* and *Nocardia*.

IDENTIFICATION

This is usually based upon the findings of the characteristic morphologic elements in the Giemsa-stained crusts and scabs, and growth of organisms with the cultural features of *D. congolensis*. Immunofluorescent staining has been used to identify the organism in clinical specimens.

IMMUNITY

Animals can remain infected for long periods; however, when they are cleared of infection, reinfection does not occur. Vaccines have not proved effective in field trials.

TREATMENT

The disease has been effectively treated in some animals by a single large dose of combined penicillin and streptomycin. It is important that both drugs be used. Tetracyclines and chloramphenicol are also effective. Removal of scabs with a brush and mild soap is recommended before topical application of iodine compounds, copper sulfate, or other solutions. Mild cases usually respond to regular grooming and isolation in dry quarters.

FURTHER READING

Albrecht, R., et al.: *Dermatophilus congolensis* chronic nodular disease in man. Pediatrics, 53:907, 1974.

Arroyo, J.C., Nichols, S., and Carrol, G.F.: Disseminated *Nocardia caviae* infection. Am. J. Med., 62:409, 1977.

Buchanan, A.M., et al.: *Actinomyces hordeovulnaris* sp. nov., an agent of canine actinomycosis. J. Syst. Bact., 34:439, 1984.

Carakostas, M.C., Miller, R.T., and Woodward, M.G.: Subcutaneous dermatophilosis in a cat. J. Am. Vet. Med. Assoc., 185:675, 1984.

Davenport, A.A., Carter, G.R., and Schermer, R.G.: Canine actinomycosis due to *Actinomyces viscosus:* Report of six cases. Vet. Med. Sm. An. Clin., 69:1442, 1974.

Davenport, A.A., Carter, G.R., and Beneke, E.S.: *Actinomyces viscosus* in relation to other actinomycetes and actinomycosis. Vet Bull., 45:313, 1975.

Franke, F.: Aetiology of actinomycosis of the mammary gland of the pig. Zentrabl. Bakteriol., 223:111, 1973.

Hardie, E.M., and Barsanti, J.A.: Treatment of canine actinomycosis. J. Am. Vet. Med. Assoc., 180:537, 1982.

How, S.J., and Lloyd, D.H.: Use of monoclonal antibody in the diagnosis of infection by *Dermatophilus congolensis*. Res. Vet. Sci., 45:416, 1988.

Jones, R.T.: Subcutaneous infection with *Dermatophilus congolensis* in a cat. J. Comp. Path., 86:415, 1976.

Kirpensteijn, J., and Fingland, R.B.: Cutaneous actinomycosis and nocardiosis in dogs: 48 cases (1980–1990). J. Am. Vet. Med. Assoc., 201:917, 1992.

Kurup, P.V., et al.: Nocardiosis: A review. Mycopathology, 40:194, 1970.

Lechtenberg, K.F., Nagaraja, T.G., Leipold, H.W., and Chengappa, M.M.: Bacteriologic and histologic studies of hepatic abscesses in cattle. Am. J. Vet. Res., 49:58, 1988.

Lloyd, D.H., and Sellers, K.C.: Dermatophilus Infection in Animals and Man. New York, Academic Press, 1976.

Mostafa, I.E.: Bovine nocardiosis (cattle farcy): A review. Vet. Bull., 36:189, 1966.

Pier, A.C., Richard, J.L., and Farrell, E.F.: Fluorescent antibody and cultural technics in cutaneous streptothricosis. Am. J. Vet. Res., 235:1014, 1964.

Rhoades, H.E., Reynolds, H.A., Jr., Rahn, D.P., and Small, E.: Nocardiosis in a dog with multiple lesions of the central nervous system. J. Am. Vet. Med. Assoc., 142:278, 1963.

Reinke, S.I., et al.: Actinomycotic mycetoma in a cat. J. Am. Vet. Med. Assoc., 189:446, 1986.

Rippon, J.W.: Actinomycosis, Nocardiosis. In Medical Mycology. 3rd Ed. Philadelphia, W.B. Saunders, 1988.

Schaal, K.P.: Genus *Actinomyces*. In Bergey's Manual of Systematic Bacteriology, Vol. 2. Edited by P.H.A. Sneath, et al. Baltimore, William & Wilkins Co., 1986.

Specht, T.E., et al.: Skin pustules and nodules caused by *Actinomyces viscosus* in a horse. J. Am. Vet. Med. Assoc., 198:457, 1991.

Stewart, G.H.: Dermatophilosis: A skin disease of animals and man. Part I. Vet. Rec., 91:537, 1972.

Stewart, G.H.: Dermatophilosis: A skin disease of animals and man. Part II. Vet. Rec., 91:555, 1972.

Swerczek, T.W., Schiefer, B., and Nielsen, S.W.: Canine actinomycosis. Zbt. Vet. Med. Bull., 15:955, 1968.

Watts, T.C., Olsen, S.M., and Rhoades, C.S.: Treatment of bovine actinomycosis with isoniazid. Can. Vet. J., 14:223, 1973.

27

Spirochetes

The spirochetes are classified in the families Spirochaetaceae and Leptospiraceae of the order *Spirochaetales*. There are five genera in the family Spirochaetaceae. However, only the genera *Borrelia* and *Serpulina* (formerly under *Treponema*) have species that cause disease in animals. Two species in the genus *Treponema*, *T. pallidum* and *T. partenae*, cause syphilis and yaws, respectively, in humans. The genus *Leptospira* is currently in the family Leptospiraceae. Differentiation of the genera is based mainly on morphology. Spirochetes of the three significant genera are slender, spiral, actively motile, flexible organisms that divide by transverse fission. The spirochetes are 3 to 20 μm long and 0.09 to 0.5 μm wide.

In nature these organisms are found in water, soil, decaying organic materials, and in or upon the bodies of plants, animals, and humans. The majority are saprophytes, a few are commensals, and some are pathogenic, causing diseases in both animals and humans.

Morphologically, spirochetes are relatively slender, helically coiled, round on cross-section, and have a varying number of spirals. The three basic cellular elements are the outer sheath, which encompasses the cell, the axial filament or fibril, and the protoplasmic cylinder, which includes the cell wall and cell membrane. The outer sheath, whose function is not known, appears to act as a unit membrane.

All these spirochetes have axial filaments that resemble flagella. The axial filaments wind around the protoplasmic cylinder under the outer sheath. It is thought that they may be responsible for motility. Insertion of the axial filament is by a proximal hook and insertion discs. The hook is an extension of the axial filament shaft and bends toward the protoplasmic cylinder. The insertion discs are plate-like and are inserted into a depression at the end of the cell. The number of insertion discs varies with the genus. *Borrelia* have two; *Treponema* and *Serpulina* have one; and *Leptospira* have three to five.

Motility involves rapid rotation around the long axis, flexation of cells, and locomotion along a helical path. Spirochetes may be anaerobic, aerobic, or microaerophilic.

All spirochetes are relatively inactive biochemically, and differentiation by this means is difficult. Identification is usually based on morphologic and antigenic properties.

Although spirochetes are gram-negative, they stain poorly. They may be demonstrated by the following special procedures: Giemsa or Wright stain (the larger ones); India ink or nigrosin (negative stain); silver impregnation (coating increases their size); darkfield microscopy; and immunofluorescence.

Some distinguishing characteristics of the three genera are summarized in Table 27–1.

Borrelia anserina

This species of *Borrelia* causes a significant disease in domestic fowls, fowl spirochetosis. For the most part speciation of *Borrelia* is based on the arthropod vector involved.

221

Table 27–1. Distinguishing Features of **Borrelia**, **Treponema/Serpulina**, *and* **Leptospira**

Characteristic	Borrelia	Treponema/Serpulina	Leptospira
Length	3 to 20 μm	5 to 20 μm	6 to 20 μm
Width	0.25 to 0.5 μm	0.09 to 0.5 μm	0.1 to 0.2 μm
Ends	Taper terminally to fine filaments	Pointed, may have terminal filaments	One or both ends have a semicircular hook
Spirals:			
number	4 to 8, loose	6 to 14, regular, angular	Many, fine, tight
amplitude	3 μm	1 μm	0.4 to 0.5 μm
Motility	Lashing, cork-screw-like	Rotating, undulating, stiffly flexible	Spinning, undulating
Cultivation	Readily, anaerobic	Some difficult; anaerobic	Readily, aerobic
Staining:			
Gram	Yes	No	Faint
Giemsa	Yes	Poor	Poor
silver impregnation	Not necessary	Yes	Yes

PATHOGENICITY

B. anserina is the cause of fowl spirochetosis (avian borreliosis), a disease of chickens, ducks, turkeys, geese, pheasants, pigeons, canaries, and some wild birds. Although an uncommon disease in the United States, it is of considerable economic importance in many countries. The disease is characterized by an acute septicemia with accompanying fever, diarrhea, drowsiness, and emaciation. It is transmitted by the bites of ticks; *Argas persicus* is the principal vector. The organism may be passed in eggs to the next generation of ticks. Other arthropods may also transmit this spirochete.

The spleen may be enlarged and mottled, and anemia is usually present. Surviving birds recover after about 2 weeks and have long-lasting immunity.

DIRECT EXAMINATION

Diagnosis is easily made by demonstration of the organism in carbol fuchsin or Giemsa-stained blood, spleen, and liver smears. It can also be readily demonstrated by darkfield microscopy and immunofluorescence.

ISOLATION AND IDENTIFICATION

B. anserina can be readily cultivated in the turkey or chicken embryo and in enriched media containing rabbit tissue. Diagnosis is based upon demonstration of typical *Borrelia* from poultry with characteristic lesions and clinical signs.

TREATMENT, PREVENTION, AND CONTROL

Penicillin, chloramphenicol, streptomycin, kanamycin, tylosin, and tetracyclines are effective in treatment.

A bacterin made from chicken embryo cultures is used for prevention. Attempts should be made to eliminate ticks.

Relapsing Fever

This disease, caused by a number (more than 10) of *Borrelia* species including *B. recurrentis*, occurs sporadically in the United States and is distributed worldwide. It is characterized by recurrent febrile attacks, during which the organism can be recovered from the blood. It is transmitted from human to human by lice; from animal to animal, especially rodents, by ticks; and from animal to human by ticks. The developmental cycle takes place in ticks. Rodents are probably a natural reservoir.

Borrelia burgdorferi

HISTORICAL

B. burgdorferi causes Lyme disease in humans and animals. It is an arthropod-borne disease which occurs in North America, Europe, the former USSR, Japan, and possibly elsewhere. The disease was first recognized in 1975 in children from Lyme, Connecticut. The organism was first cultured in 1981 from a tick, *Ixodes dammini* in New York.

PATHOGENICITY

The disease has been reported from both domestic and wild animals. Several cases of naturally occurring Lyme disease in dogs have been reported with transient or recurrent arthritis being the most common clinical sign. Some infected dogs develop renal disorders. Arthritis, encephalitis, uveitis, and laminitis have been recognized in infected horses and cows. *B. burgdorferi* has been recovered from the liver of a passerine bird; the significance of this isolation was not apparent.

B. burgdorferi is transmitted primarily by *Ixodes dammini*. However the spirochete has been isolated from other ticks including *I. pacificus, I. ricinus, I. persulcatus,* and *Dermacentor variabilis*. White-footed mice, meadow voles, and Eastern chipmunks are also known to carry this spirochete. Intrauterine transmission of spirochetes in bitches has been reported recently. Antibodies to *B. burgdorferi* have been detected in cottontail rabbits. This finding could be epidemiologically important.

Three stages of Lyme disease have been recognized in humans. First: skin rashes, stiffness of joints and neck, headaches, and lymphadenopathy; second: multiple skin patches, arthritis, and central and peripheral nervous systems disorders; and third: chronic arthritis, chronic neurologic symptoms, and cardiac signs caused by occlusion of arteries to the heart.

EXPERIMENTAL INFECTION

Although characteristic skin lesions have been produced experimentally in rabbits, hamsters, rats, and guinea pigs, a laboratory model for arthritis has not been developed. Experimentally infected white-footed mice develop long lasting spirochetemia.

LABORATORY DIAGNOSIS

Culture of the spirochete in laboratory media is difficult; modified Kelly medium has been successfully used. Serologic procedures are the most reliable methods for rapid diagnosis of the disease. Established tests include the indirect fluorescent antibody procedure, enzyme-linked immunosorbent assay and fluorescence immunoassay. An ear punch biopsy method has been introduced for the detection of *B. burgdorferi* in rodents. Reagents for the serodiagnosis are available commercially.

Serpulina hyodysenteriae

This gram-negative, oxygen-tolerant, anaerobic spirochete produces a dysentery in SPF pigs (not germ-free pigs) that is indistinguishable from what in the past has been called vibrionic or swine dysentery. There is evidence that *Bacteroides fragilis* and *Fusobacterium necrophorum* are important secondary agents in the etiology of swine dysentery. Asymptomatic carriers of *S. hyodysenteriae* are encountered.

Pigs of any age may be affected. The disease is manifested by a bloody diarrhea that may terminate in death or a chronic form characterized by a diphtheritic inflammatory process involving the mucosa of the cecum, large intestine, and rectum. Dehydration and emaciation are common in chronically affected pigs. There is also a less acute form that involves loss of weight and condition, and mild diarrhea.

Virulence factors of this organism have not been fully characterized; however, endotoxin and hemolysin are thought to be important in pathogenesis.

Nine serotypes of *S. hyodysenteriae* have been described based on differences in LPS antigens in an agar gel double immunodiffusion test.

DIRECT EXAMINATION

The demonstration of this organism in material taken from lesions provides a strong presumptive diagnosis of swine dysentery.

The methods used for the demonstration of *S. hyodysenteriae* in mucosa and feces involve the examination of wet mounts with the phase or darkfield microscope and of Giemsa, crystal violet or Victoria blue-stained smears with the light microscope. It is a large flexible spirochete that moves rapidly in a snake-like or eel-like fashion. Considerable experience is necessary in order to distinguish *Serpulina* from other spirochetes.

ISOLATION AND IDENTIFICATION

Isolation is not usually practiced. Diagnosis is usually made on the basis of clinical signs and a positive direct examination.

S. hyodysenteriae can be isolated from filtered feces or ground colonic mucosa on serum-enriched blood agar containing spectinomycin (400 μg/ml) to prevent the growth of undesirable bacteria. Plates are incubated anaerobically at 42°C for 48 hours. The small, white translucent colonies have a zone of clear hemolysis. In contrast, *S. innocens* is weakly beta-hemolytic. Stained smears of *S. hyodysenteriae* disclose a loosely coiled organism. *S. hyodysenteriae* will grow at 37°C, but growth is better and more selective at 42°C.

Several selective media have been described and used with varying degrees of success for the isolation of *S. hyodysenteriae*. BJ and CVS media have been highly recommended for the isolation of this spirochete. The BJ medium contains an extract of pig feces to promote growth of *S. hyodysenteriae* and 5 antimicrobials to inhibit other fecal bacteria; whereas, the CVS blood agar base medium contains three antimicrobial agents. It is oxidase- and catalase-negative.

Both direct and indirect fluorescent antibody procedures have been used effectively for identification. Species-specific DNA probes have been employed experimentally for detection of animals infected with this spirochete. Other methods of identification include a rapid slide agglutination procedure, growth inhibition by discs containing specific antiserum, and biochemical and enzyme tests. Several serological procedures have been used for the serodiagnosis of swine dysentery. An enzyme-linked immunoassay appears to be the most sensitive test. It is useful as a herd test but not as an individual animal test as it produces false positive and false negative results.

TREATMENT

Among the compounds used to treat swine dysentery are lincomycin, tylosin, erythromycin, bacitracin, carbadox, dimetridazole, gentamicin, sodium arsanilate, tiamulin, virginiamycin, and spiramycin. Some of these drugs and others are administered in feed or water for prophylaxis as well as treatment.

In vitro susceptibility tests may be indicated because antimicrobial resistance to some of these drugs has been encountered.

IMMUNITY

Immunity is predominantly humoral in that hyperimmune serum is protective.

CONTROL

This is particularly difficult because of asymptomatic carriers. Serologic tests such as the ELISA may be useful in detecting these carriers. Bacterins appear to provide considerable protection against *S. hyodysenteriae* infection. Rodent control is an important part of control programs.

Serpulina innocens

S. innocens is a nonpathogenic spirochete present in the intestine of pigs. It is weakly beta-hemolytic and sometimes confuses the diagnosis of swine dysentery as it resembles *S. hyodysenteriae*.

Treponema paraluis-cuniculi

This organism is the cause of a widespread disease, rabbit syphilis or vent disease. It is a true venereal disease in which lesions consisting of vesicles and scabs are seen mainly involving the prepuce, vagina, and perineal region. Thick scaly crusts persist in the female for months. Penicillin is an effective treatment.

Diagnosis is by the demonstration of organisms from lesions using stains or darkfield microscopy. *T. paraluis-cuniculi* has not been cultivated in vitro.

Leptospira

Leptospirosis is primarily a disease of animals. It is transmitted from animals to humans infrequently.

The basic taxon of the genus *Leptospira* is the serovar (formerly serotype). There are more than 180 parasitic serovars and 19 serogroups. Two species, *L. interrogans* and *L. biflexa*, have been proposed for the "pathogenic or parasitic" and the "saprophytic" leptospires, respectively. As mentioned, the pathogenic leptospires are included in the species *L. interrogans*. In the new classification the former species name, now serovar, is added to *L. interrogans*, e.g., *L. canicola* becomes *L. interrogans* serovar *canicola* and *L. hardjo* becomes *L. interrogans* serovar *hardjo*. We will use the older more widely used names, each of which represents a serovar. The microscopic agglutination test, which is widely used to detect antibodies, is highly serovar-specific. There are both group- and serovar-specific antigens. Serologic procedures are used in the identification of serovars after isolation and cultivation.

Because of insufficient taxonomic data, the various *Leptospira* species are not listed and described in Bergey's Manual of Systematic Bacteriology. There are free-living serovars as well as serovars that are parasitic and pathogenic for humans and domestic animals. Each serovar appears to have certain animal species as natural hosts. Some important serovars, their natural hosts (principally in the United States), and their occurrence in domestic animals are given in Table 27–2. Humans and animals may be infected with a wide variety of serovars, although most infections in domestic animals are caused by only a few serovars of *Leptospira*.

MODE OF INFECTION AND TRANSMISSION

The source of the organism is urine from infected or carrier animals. Water, litter, and food may serve as fomites. The organisms can live in alkaline water for days. Direct or indirect infection may be via nasal, oral, or conjunctival mucous membranes and abraded skin. Leptospiras are destroyed in the stomach.

PATHOGENESIS

After epithelial penetration, there is hematogenous dissemination with localization and proliferation in parenchymatous organs, particularly the liver, for up to 16 days. This causes fever, anemia, subserous and submucosal hemorrhages, conjunctivitis, icterus, and often meningitis and agalactia. The kidney is also infected, frequently resulting in nephrosis and uremia, with shedding of organisms in the urine possibly for months. The lesions, signs, and severity vary with different serovars. Death may occur during the febrile stage or later caused by toxemia resulting from liver and kidney damage. Although the pathogenic mechanisms are not

Table 27–2. **Important Leptospira** *Species or Serovars and Their Hosts**

Serovars	Known Host (Natural)	Occurrence in			
		Humans	Dogs	Cattle	Swine
icterohemorrhagiae	Rat, mouse, raccoon, opossum	Common	Occasional	Reported	Reported
canicola	Dog, cattle, swine, skunk, jackal	Common	Common	Rare	Occasional
pomona	Cattle, swine, skunk, raccoon, wildcat, opossum, horse	Occasional	Rare	Common	Common
autumnalis	Opossum, raccoon, mouse	Rare	?	?	?
ballum	Mice, grey fox, rat, opossum, raccoon, wildcat, skunk, rabbit, grey squirrel	?	?	?	?
grippotyphosa	Raccoon, mouse, fox, squirrel, rabbit, bobcat	Rare	Occasional	Occasional	Occasional
bataviae	Rat, mouse	Rare	?	?	?
hardjo	Cattle	Rare	?	Common	?
sejroe	Opossum, raccoon, mouse	?	?	Sporadic	?
hebdomadis	Opossum, raccoon	?	?	?	?
australis	Opossum, raccoon, fox	?	?	?	?
bratislava	Swine	?	Reported	?	Reported

*Data principally applicable to the United States.
?, Not known.

known, there is considerable damage to vascular endothelium.

Virulent strains produce more cytotoxic protein than avirulent strains. The exact role of this protein in the disease is not clear. The hemolysin of *Leptospira* appears to be responsible for intravascular hemolysis.

CANINE LEPTOSPIROSIS

This disease is primarily caused by serovar *canicola* and less frequently by serovar *icterohemorrhagiae*. The dog is considered an incidental host for serovars *grippotyphosa, autumnalis, australis, pomona,* and *bratislava.* Although the exact incidence is unknown, surveys have shown that up to 38% of dogs in various parts of the United States show serologic evidence of exposure or disease.

Infected dogs and rats sporadically shed *Leptospira* in their urine and serve as sources of *canicola* and *icterohemorrhagiae* infections. Dogs may shed *Leptospira* in their urine for 2 to 6 months; rats usually shed for longer periods of time. Organisms may survive in nature for approximately 3 weeks if environmental conditions are favorable. The viability of organisms is influenced by the pH of the urine of dogs and rats, and alkaline pH favors viability.

Clinical. Infections may be latent to severe. A chronic progressive nephritis may follow acute *canicola* infection, with death occurring long after

the initial infection; however, some dogs recover and renal function is regained. These animals may shed organisms in the urine for long periods. Four principal forms are recognized: (1) the hemorrhagic form, (2) the icteric form, (3) the uremic or subacute form, and (4) the inapparent form. The first two forms are primarily caused by serovar *icterohaemorrhagiae,* whereas the latter two forms are usually caused by serovar *canicola.* In the initial stages of the disease, the first three forms are characterized by depression, anorexia, vomiting, and diarrhea or constipation. Serovar *grippotyphosa* occasionally causes severe leptospirosis in dogs.

Diagnosis. There are several methods:
1. Examination of urine by darkfield microscopy. Experience is required to recognize *Leptospira.* They autolyse rapidly and formalin should be added to preserve them.
2. Serologic tests:
   a. paired sera; look for a fourfold rise in titer;
   b. plate screening test: if positive, do plate dilution test;
   c. plate dilution test: if positive at 1:60 or greater (classed as positive or current infection), then do the microscopic agglutination test (agglutination lysis); this is the preferred serologic procedure. If the titer is 1:100 or higher, it is considered of diagnostic significance. It is preferable to have

a fourfold increase in paired sera. However, not all cases of leptospirosis produce significant serologic titers.

3. Isolation, cultivation, and identification: isolation from urine or blood is not usually feasible. Filtration or the addition of 5-fluorouracil may be used to reduce contaminants. *Leptospira* are aerobic and may be cultivated in special media at 30° C.
4. Guinea pig or hamster inoculation: blood, urine, or tissue is used; when bacteremic the experimental animal's blood is used for isolation and cultivation.
5. Histopathology: organisms may be demonstrated in kidney sections with special stains.
6. A fluorescent antibody technique can be used to identify *Leptospira* in tissues and urine sediment.

BOVINE LEPTOSPIROSIS

This disease is principally caused by serovar *pomona*. Serovar *hardjo* causes fewer abortions but results in infertility. Occasionally serovar *grippotyphosa*, *canicola*, or *icterohemorrhagiae* is involved. Three to 11% of cattle show serologic evidence of infection; 2 to 4% are estimated to be actively infected.

Sources. Sources of the organisms are cattle and swine with leptospiruria and wild animals. Cattle may shed for 3 months, but not in large numbers and irregularly. Outbreaks of leptospirosis are often associated with heavy rainfall. Leptospirosis is infrequent under dry conditions.

Clinical. The infection may be latent in a herd and may be precipitated by stress. Infections are characterized by a variety of clinical signs including fever, diarrhea, anemia, icterus, and hemoglobinuria. Acute infections sometimes result in abortion.

Diagnosis. Diagnosis of bovine leptospirosis is similar in principle to that of the canine disease; serologic tests are used almost exclusively. An enzyme-linked immunosorbent assay has been used to detect antibodies (IgM and IgG) against serovars *pomona* and *hardjo* in cattle.

PORCINE LEPTOSPIROSIS

Serovar *pomona* is the principal cause of leptospirosis in pigs.

Other serovars including *canicola*, *grippotyphosa*, *icterohaemorrhagiae*, and *bratislava* are also involved in porcine leptospirosis. Serovar *bratislava*, a relatively new serovar, has been one of the predominant serovars in swine in England and Ireland. Serologic studies conducted in recent years showed that *bratislava* is also widespread in swine in the United States. Serovar *bratislava* is extremely difficult to culture in the laboratory media. However, rare isolations have been made in the United States from sows following abortion.

Serologic evidence indicates a 3 to 22% level of infection; probably 2 to 4% are actively infected.

Sources. The organisms may be found in swine or cattle, and skunks, raccoons, opossums, wildcats, or deer. Organisms may be shed for 3 months; shedding is irregular and not in large numbers.

Clinical. Infections are mostly subclinical or latent. Unthriftiness, abortion, fever, icterus, and anemia are among the signs observed. Metritis and meningoencephalitis are observed occasionally.

Diagnosis. Diagnosis follows that of canine infections; serologic tests are used almost exclusively. *Leptospira* can be recovered from and demonstrated in aborted fetuses.

EQUINE LEPTOSPIROSIS

Leptospirosis appears to be an important disease of horses. Most infections are caused by serovar *pomona*. Rare infection caused by serovar *Kennewicki* has also been reported. There is usually a transient febrile illness, with icterus and occasionally abortions. Recurrent iridocyclitis (moon blindness or periodic ophthalmia) may be a sequela.

IMMUNITY

Immunity appears to be mainly humoral in that the organisms are not intracellular and bacterins (killed organisms) elicit considerable protection, although of short duration (less than a year). The levels of antibody resulting from vaccination are low and do not affect serologic testing. There is little cross-immunity between serovars.

Dogs. Bacterins usually contain serovars *canicola* and *icterohemorrhagiae*.

Cattle. Bacterins contain serovar *pomona*; some bacterins contain serovars *hardjo*, *grippotyphosa*, *canicola*, and *icterohemorrhagiae* as well. *Leptospira* may be combined with other antigens, including viruses.

Swine. Bacterins contain serovar *pomona*. Some bacterins contain other serovars including *bratislava*.

Treatment and Control. Combined penicillin and streptomycin are recommended for treatment; early administration is important. Treatment may be of no avail if renal damage is extensive. Heavy doses of streptomycin may eliminate the carrier state. The tetracycline and macrolide antibiotics are also effective.

If leptospirosis is a recurring problem, preventive measures such as effective rat control, fencing off of potentially contaminated ponds and streams, and the careful screening of replacement stock should be implemented. Although *Leptospira* will survive for days in alkaline water, they will only live for about 12 hours in sewage, and they are very susceptible to drying and heat.

Public Health Significance

Human beings acquire leptospirosis from infected domestic animals, rodents, and contaminated water. The disease is referred to by several names, including Weil's disease, Fort Bragg fever, and swineherd's disease. Various serovars of *Leptospira*, including *canicola*, *icterohemorrhagiae*, and *pomona*, can infect humans. Veterinarians, slaughterhouse workers, and farmers are at particular risk. The acute form of the human disease is similar to that seen in some animals and is characterized by febrile jaundice and nephritis.

The laboratory diagnosis of the human disease is essentially the same as that described earlier for the dog.

It is thought that treatment will only affect the course of the disease if it is initiated within 4 days of onset. The same antibiotics are used as recommended for animals.

FURTHER READING

Anderson, J.F., et al.: Involvement of birds in the epidemiology of the Lyme disease agent *Borrelia burgdorferi*. Infect. Immun., *51*:394, 1986.

Barbour, A.G.: Laboratory aspects of Lyme borreliosis. Clin. Microbiol. Rev., *1*:399, 1988.

Bernard, W.V., et al.: Leptospiral abortion and leptospiruria in horses from the same farm. J. Am. Vet. Med. Assoc., *202*:1285, 1993.

Bernard, W.V., et al.: Serologic survey for *Borrelia burgdorferi* antibody in horses referred to a mid-Atlantic veterinary teaching hospital. J. Am. Vet. Med. Assoc., *196*:1255, 1990.

Bolin, C.A., and Cassells, J.A.: Isolation of *Leptospira interrogans* serovar *bratislava* from stillborn and weak pigs in Iowa. J. Am. Vet. Med. Assoc., *196*:1601, 1990.

Burgess, E.C., et al.: Arthritis and systemic disease caused by *Borrelia burgdorferi* infection in a cow. J. Am. Vet. Med. Assoc., *191*:1468, 1987.

Chengappa, M.M., et al.: Laboratory procedures for diagnosis of swine dysentery. Report of the Committee on Swine Dysentery. Published by Am. Assoc. Vet. Lab. Diagnosticians, 1989, p. 1–14.

Donahue, J.M., et al.: Diagnosis and prevalence of leptospira infection in aborted and stillborn horses. J. Vet. Diagn. Invest., *3*:148, 1991.

Ellinghausen, H.C., Jr.: Virulence, nutrition and antigenicity of *Leptospira interrogans* serotype *pomona* in supplemented and nutrient depleted bovine albumin medium. Ann. Microbiol. (Inst. Pasteur), *124*:477, 1973.

Ellinghausen, H.C., Jr.: Variable factors influencing the isolation of leptospires involving culture ingredients and testing. Proc. 79th Meeting U.S. Animal Health Assoc., 1975.

Ellis, W.A., et al.: Bovine leptospirosis: Microbiological and serological findings in aborted fetuses. Vet. Rec., *110*:147, 1982.

Ellis, W.A., et al.: Isolation of leptospires from the genital tract and kidneys of aborted sows. Vet. Rec., *118*:294, 1986.

Ellis, W.A., et al.: Prevalence of *Leptospira interrogans* serovar *hardjo* in the genital and urinary tracts of non-pregnant cattle. Vet. Rec., *118*:11, 1986.

Gustafson, J.M., et al.: Intrauterine transmission of *Borrelia burgdorferi* in dogs. Am. J. Vet. Res., *54*:882, 1993.

Hansen, L.E.: Immunology of bacterial diseases with special reference to leptospirosis. J. Am. Vet. Med. Assoc., *170*:991, 1977.

Li, Z., Belanger, M., and Jacques, M.: Serotyping of Canadian isolates of *Treponema hyodysenteriae* and description of two new serotypes. J. Clin. Microbiol., *29*:2794, 1991.

Lysons, R.J., et al.: A cytotoxin haemolysin from *Treponema hyodysenteria*—a probable virulence determinant in swine dysentery. J. Med. Microbiol., *34*:97, 1991.

Nielsen, J.N., et al.: Relationship among selected *Leptospira interrogans* serogroups as determined by nucleic acid hybridization. J. Clin. Microbiol., *27*:2724, 1989.

Nielsen, J.N., et al.: *Leptospira interrogans* serovar *bratislava* infection in two dogs. J. Am. Vet. Med. Assoc., *199*:351, 1991.

Pennell, D.R., et al.: Evaluation of a quantitative fluorescence immunoassay (FIAX) for detection of serum antibody to *Borrelia burgdorferi*. J. Clin. Microbiol., *25*:2218, 1987.

Rentko, V.T., et al.: Canine leptospirosis: A retrospective study of 17 cases. J. Vet. Internal Med., *6*:235, 1992.

Roush, J.K., et al.: Rheumatoid arthritis subsequent to *Borrelia burgdorferi* infection in two dogs. J. Am. Vet. Med. Assoc., *195*:951, 1989.

Sinsky, R.J., and Piesman, J.: Ear punch biopsy method for detection and isolation of *Borrelia burgdorferi* from rodents. J. Clin. Microbiol., *27*:1723, 1989.

Stanton, T.B.: Proposal to change the genus designation *Serpula* to *Serpulina* gen. nov. containing the species *Serpulina hyodysenteriae* comb. nov. and *Serpulina innocens* comb. nov. Int. J. Syst. Bacteriol., *42*:189, 1992.

Stringfellow, D.A., et al.: Can antibody responses in cattle vaccinated with a multivalent leptospiral bacterin interfere with serologic diagnosis of disease? J. Am. Vet. Med. Assoc., *182*:165, 1983.

Wright, J.C., et al.: Use of an enzyme-linked immunosorbent assay for detection of *Treponema hyodysenteriae* infection in swine. J. Clin. Microbiol., *27*:411, 1989.

28

Miscellaneous Potential Pathogens, and Nonpathogens

There are a number of bacteria associated with animals, some as commensals and some as transients from the environment, which either do not cause disease or do so only infrequently. Because these organisms may be reported by the clinical microbiology laboratory as occurring in clinical materials, the practicing veterinarian should at least be acquainted with their names and probable origin. Culture purity, condition of the specimen, number of colonies, and repeated isolation must be considered in estimating the significance of these and other ordinarily nonpathogenic organisms. Some of these organisms, such as the *Acinetobacter* species, may replace other organisms in infectious processes that are more susceptible to antimicrobial drugs.

Several genera and groups of bacteria of the kind mentioned above are discussed briefly below. Some of their principal characteristics are listed in Table 28–1. Those readers interested in the definitive identification of these bacteria should consult the references at the end of this chapter.

Two species that do not belong in other chapters and do cause significant infections are *Streptobacillus moniliformis* and *Bacillus piliformis*. The algae *Prototheca*, and the *Legionella* bacteria are also discussed in this chapter.

Neisseria

They occur as commensals most commonly on the mucous membranes of the nasopharynx and conjunctiva of animals. Isolations are made occasionally from the intestines and genitourinary tracts of dogs. Some characteristics of *Neisseria* are given in Table 28–1.

In smears from cultures, these gram-negative cocci occur singly or in clumps. Cells taken from body fluids appear as diplococci with adjacent sides flattened.

The *Neisseria* spp. most frequently associated with animals are listed below. They have only infrequently been reported as causing disease in animals. Potentially pathogenic species grow best on media enriched with blood and serum.

N. animalis: isolated from the throats of guinea pigs.

N. denitrificans: isolated from the nasopharynx of guinea pigs.

N. canis: isolated from the nasopharynx of cats and dogs.

N. flavescens and *N. sicca:* recovered from the oropharynx of normal dogs.

N. lactamica: isolated from the conjunctival sacs of healthy dogs.

N. meningitidis: causes meningococcal meningitis of humans.

Table 28–1. Some Characteristics of Gram-negative Bacteria from Infrequent Infections and Clinical Specimens*

	Morphology	Oxidation/ Fermentation	MacConkey Agar	Motility	Oxidase	Other
Neisseria	Cocci	0 or neg.	−	−	+	
Branhamella	Cocci	0 or neg.	−	−	+	
Acinetobacter	Diplococci, rods	0 or neg.	+	−	−	
Flavobacterium	Rods	0	−	−	+	Yellow to orange colonies.
Weeksella	Rods	neg.	−	−	+	Urease positive.
CDC Group EF-4	Short rods or coccobacilli	0 or F	V	−	+	Urease negative. Two varieties: EF-4a and EF-4b
Chromobacterium	Rods	0 or F	+	+	V	Violet to purple colonies
Capnocytophaga	Rods (long, thin)	F	−	−	+	Urease negative. Candle jar or CO_2
Gardnerella	Rods coccobacilli	F	−	−	−	Beta-hemolytic, gram-variable

* All are catalase positive except *N. elongata.*
V, variable

N. gonorrhoeae: causative agent of gonorrhea.
N. parelongata (formerly CDC Group M-5): this organism has been recovered from dog-bite wounds in humans.

The species *N. ovis, N. caviae,* and *N. cuniculi* are now considered "false neisseria" and have been transferred to genus *Branhamella.*

Branhamella

Members of this gram-negative genus, which were previously included in the genus *Neisseria,* are closely related to *Moraxella.* In *Bergey's Manual of Systematic Bacteriology* (Vol. 1), *Branhamella* is considered one of the subgenera of *Moraxella.* The principal differences between *Neisseria* and *Branhamella* are genetic makeup and pathogenic potential. Some of their characteristics are given in Table 28–1. The following species are of veterinary significance:

B. ovis. It has been recovered from the conjunctiva of sheep and cattle, the upper respiratory tract of sheep, and in cultures from keratoconjunctivitis of goats, sheep, and cattle. It is considered a commensal with low pathogenic potential.

B. caviae. This species has been isolated from the conjunctiva of dogs and the throats of guinea pigs.

B. cuniculi. It has been recovered from the nasopharynx of marine pinnipeds and the oral cavity of rabbits.

B. catarrhalis (formerly *Neisseria catarrhalis*). It is part of the normal nasopharyngeal flora of humans in which it may cause bronchitis, pneumonia, otitis media, and sinusitis. It has been isolated from the pneumonic lungs of calves, the upper respiratory tract, the mouth, and the conjunctiva of dogs. Its pathogenic significance is unclear.

Branhamella species, although smaller than *Moraxella,* are similar morphologically. They are relatively inactive biochemically and thus are difficult to speciate.

Acinetobacter

Only one species, *Acinetobacter calcoaceticus,* is recognized in *Bergey's Manual of Systematic Bacteriology* (Vol. 1). However, recent taxonomic studies have identified 17 hybridization groups (genospecies). The two varieties of greatest veterinary significance are usually given the species names *A. calcoaceticus* and *A. lwoffii.*

Acinetobacter spp. occur frequently in soil, water and sewage, and as part of the normal flora of animals and humans. They are isolated frequently from clinical specimens. Occasionally they cause opportunistic infections in animals and they have been recovered from aborted fetuses, blood of sick dogs, and bronchopneumonia in mink.

Some characteristics that aid in their identification are: gram-negative, rods or diplococci, nonmotile, nonfermentative, negative in the O/F test, grow on MacConkey agar, catalase and oxidase negative. (see Table 28–1).

An *Acinetobacter*-like organism (CDC Control Group NO-1) associated with dog and cat bites has been reported recently.

Flavobacterium

Members of this genus occur widely in soil and water. Although they are not part of the normal flora of animals, their occurrence in soil and water results in their being isolated occasionally from animals and clinical specimens. Opportunistic infections occur in humans due to flavobacteria, and it would seem reasonable to expect similar infections in animals.

Flavobacteria are medium to long, narrow, nonmotile, gram-negative rods. Colonies are usually yellow to orange in appearance. A number of species have been described; *F. meningosepticum* is responsible for most human infections. These include meningitis, pneumonia, and septicemia, particularly in immune-compromised adults. Flavobacteria are occasionally recovered from dogs and other animals although infections appear to be rare.

Weeksella

Bacteria that were earlier called *Flavobacterium* sp. group IIj have now been named *Weeksella zoohelcum*. They are of interest because they are part of the normal flora of the mouth and paws of dogs and cats, and may cause bite or scratch infections in humans. They do not appear to cause significant infections in dogs and cats. Colonies on blood agar are large, mucoid, and sticky, and are difficult to remove from the agar surface. All strains hydrolyze urea rapidly (less than 5 min). They are gram-negative rods.

CDC Group EF-4

These are short, gram-negative rods or coccobacilli that give rise to small convex, mucoid, yellow to tan colonies. It has been proposed that this organism be included in the genus *Neisseria*. They are commensals in the mouth and nasopharynx of dogs and cats and are occasionally isolated from bite wounds in humans. They do not appear to cause infections in dogs or cats. However, pneumonia in a domestic cat and an African lion have been attributed to this organism.

Chromobacterium

Chromobacteria are short to medium, gram-negative, motile rods that occur in soil and water. They give rise to characteristic violet to purple colonies on media. Two species are recognized by *Bergey's Manual of Systematic Bacteriology* (Vol. 1), viz., *Chromobacterium violaceum* and *C. fluviatile*. Only the former has been incriminated in disease. Most infections, mainly suppurative pneumonia in swine and cattle, occur in tropical and subtropical countries, including the southern United States.

Capnocytophaga

Bacteria that were called DF-2 and DF-2-like strains are now called *Capnocytophaga canimorsus* and *C. cynodegmi*, respectively. These organisms are small, gram-negative, long, slender rods that are commensals in the mouth and nasopharynx of dogs and possibly cats. These two species are fastidious, slow-growing organisms believed to be the primary cause of several cases of septicemia, meningitis, endocarditis, cellulitis, diarrhea, lymphadenitis, wound infection, and keratitis in humans.

Gardnerella

This genus contains only one species, *Gardnerella vaginalis*. According to DNA and taxonomic studies, it is not related to any other known taxon. It is a gram-negative to gram-variable, small, nonmotile, pleomorphic, nonencapsulated rod. Some important characteristics are: facultatively anaerobic, fastidious in growth requirements, fermentative, catalase and oxidase negative, beta-hemolytic on rabbit and human blood agar but not on sheep blood agar.

G. vaginalis is associated with bacterial vaginosis in women. Recently *G. vaginalis* and *G. vaginalis*-like organisms have been recovered from the genital tracts of a large number of mares. Whether or not these organisms cause disease in the equine reproductive tract has not yet been determined.

Bacillus piliformis

This interesting gram-negative, intracellular organism, which is not a member of the *Bacillus* genus, is the cause of Tyzzer's disease.

PATHOGENICITY

The organism probably occurs frequently in the intestine of rodents. Under circumstances of stress such as experimentation, cortisone treatment, or thymectomy, it causes enteritis, colitis, and hepatitis. The latter is evidenced by livers with diffusely distributed pale grey necrotic foci. Organisms are probably carried to the liver from intestinal infection. The disease may occur sporadically or as a serious epizootic in mice, rats, gerbils, hamsters, rabbits, and monkeys. Sporadic infections have been reported in the cat, dog, foal, fox, coyote, and calf.

DIAGNOSIS

Smears are made from the necrotic foci in the liver and stained with Giemsa. Long, slender organisms are seen in the cytoplasm of hepatic cells. Very long, thin, tortuous filaments are sometimes seen as well as short bacillary forms and occasionally filaments with moniliform swellings. Tapering and beading of the filaments are characteristic features. The organisms are motile by peritrichous flagella and have subterminal spores which are difficult to see in tissue sections.

What presumably are subclinical infections can be detected with a complement-fixation test. A fluorescent antibody has been used to identify organisms in smears.

ISOLATION AND CULTIVATION

The organism has not been cultivated on artificial media. It can be cultivated in the yolk sac of embryonated chicken eggs and cell cultures.

TREATMENT AND CONTROL

Broad-spectrum antibiotics in the drinking water are effective against *Bacillus piliformis*. While cleaning and disinfecting, it should be kept in mind that the spores of *B. piliformis* are somewhat resistant. A temperature of 80°C will kill them in 30 minutes. Tyzzer's disease can be prevented by establishing colonies free of *B. piliformis*. It is also susceptible to penicillin, ampicillin and erythromycin. Treatment of clinical cases is ordinarily not successful.

Streptobacillus moniliformis

S. moniliformis is a facultatively anaerobic, gram-negative, highly pleomorphic rod that forms filaments with moniliform swellings and L forms under certain conditions. Pioneering studies on L forms were carried out with this species. Its precise taxonomic position has not been determined. *S. moniliformis* is a normal inhabitant of the upper respiratory tract of wild and laboratory rats and some other rodents.

PATHOGENICITY

The organism is a secondary invader in chronic murine pneumonia of rats and a primary cause of a disease of mice characterized by septicemia, septic arthritis, hepatitis, and lymphadenitis. Serious infections in turkeys have been attributed to rat bites.

Infections in humans initiated by rat bites (rat-bite fever) are characterized by septicemia and polyarthritis.

Outbreaks of infection in humans due to ingestion of contaminated food, including milk, are termed Haverhill fever. Respiratory and gastrointestinal symptoms are more common in these infections.

Spirillum minus or *S. minor* (most likely belongs in the genus *Aquaspirillum*) is another cause of rat-bite fever in humans. The organism is carried by rats and mice, and the disease it causes in humans is clinically similar to that caused by *S. moniliformis*.

ISOLATION, CULTIVATION, AND IDENTIFICATION

The organism can be grown in blood or serum-enriched media incubated for at least 8 days. Isolation from humans is most readily accomplished with blood cultures. Identification is usually based upon the characteristic cultural and morphologic features of the organism. Confirmation is obtained by a number of biochemical tests.

S. minor has not been cultivated in vitro. It is demonstrable in wet mounts and stained smears.

Legionella pneumophila

This fastidious, gram-negative, small rod is the cause of Legionnaires' disease. The first cases involved members of the American Legion attending a convention in Philadelphia in 1976. The organism was first propagated in guinea pigs and embryonated eggs, but specially formulated media are now available for its cultivation. Since the discovery of *L. pneumophila*, other closely related potentially pathogenic bacteria have been identified, and all have been placed in the family Legionella-ceae. They are free-living organisms that are widely distributed in many water-associated environments. Although infections in animals would appear to be rare, antibodies to this species have been reported in cattle, sheep, horses, antelope, and buffalo.

Diseases caused by this group of organisms may take several forms, of which a multisystem illness with pneumonia is the best known. Only a small number of persons exposed develop clinical disease, and symptoms may include all gradations from asymptomatic or mild to acute. The direct fluorescent antibody procedure can be used for the rapid identification of the organism. Special culture and serologic procedures are available.

Cat-Scratch Disease (CSD)

This well-known non-contagious disease of humans is also known as cat-scratch fever and benign lymphoreticulosis. CSD is of veterinary interest because it usually results from contact with a cat. The cause was unknown for many years, but recently it has been claimed that the causal agent is the rickettsia *Rochalimaea henselae*. This organism, which has been associated with fever and angiomatosis in humans, can infect cats for long periods without causing disease. It is a small, pleomorphic, gram-negative rod which, unlike most rickettsiae, can grow extracellularly and on lifeless media.

Pathogenicity and Pathogenesis

CSD affects children predominantly and there is almost always a history of contact with a cat. Most cases occur in the late summer and autumn. The cats involved are normal and usually less than a year of age. It is suggested that the bacterium may be a commensal of the mouth and skin.

Infection may result from a cat scratch, a puncture wound, or entrance via the conjunctiva (Parinaud's oculoglandular syndrome). A red or pink macule develops at the site of entrance, followed by a vesicle which ruptures and encrusts. A papule less than 1 cm in diameter persists for a number of weeks. Unilateral regional lymphadenopathy (axillary, cervical or trochlear) develops with enlargement and occasional suppuration. This regional lymphadenopathy is the predominant sign of CSD.

Diagnosis

This is usually accomplished by staining smears of material collected from the early lesion. When stained by the Warthin-Starry silver stain, the bacteria are pleomorphic, coccoid and small (less than 1 μm in diameter). They are usually extracellular and may appear as microcolonies.

Although isolation and identification are not necessary for diagnosis, cultivation is accomplished in brain-heart infusion media and blood agar. Five weeks incubation may be required for the appearance of colonies. The latter are whitish, invaginated, tenacious, and may be imbedded in the medium.

A highly specific skin test using an antigen heat-treated pus from lymph nodes has been used effectively in diagnosis. Serologic test systems (e.g., indirect FA) for antibodies to *R. henselae* in humans and cats are available commercially. A polymerase chain reaction procedure has been used to identify the causal agent in biopsies.

Treatment/Prevention

The disease is usually self-limiting; most infections are resolved spontaneously. Tetracyclines and ciprofloxacin have been effective. Disposal of cats thought to be involved is not indicated. Transmission to humans is prevented by avoiding bites and scratches by cats.

Lactobacillus

These long, slender, pleomorphic, gram-positive rods, which are part of the normal flora of the mouth, vagina, and intestinal tract of animals are rarely pathogenic. The presence of large numbers of lactobacilli in vaginal secretions indicates a healthy vagina. They are oxidase negative and may be facultative or strictly anaerobic.

Among the several species most frequently isolated from human clinical specimens is *Lactobacillus acidophilus*. Cultures of *L. acidophilus*, sometimes in milk (sweet acidophilus milk), have been administered to animals and humans to treat intestinal disorders. The idea is to replace the "undesirable" intestinal bacteria.

Kurthia

These large, gram-positive, motile rods resemble *Bacillus* spp. but do not produce spores. They are soil saprophytes and rarely result in infections.

Oerskovia

These soil saprophytes are actinomycetes that are seen as branching gram-positive filamentous forms. Most strains produce a yellow pigment, and they are rarely involved in infections.

Prototheca

Members of this genus are microscopic, colorless achlorophyllic algae of the family Chlorellaceae. They are ubiquitous in nature and are occasionally recovered from clinical specimens in which they are not usually significant. However, there have been several reports of human and animal infections. The agents are infrequent opportunists that would appear to produce disease only if the host's resistance is impaired. *Prototheca* have been reported to cause bovine mastitis, localized infection in a cat, and disseminated protothecosis in the dog.

Treatment with amphotericin B and ketoconazole has shown promise in human infections.

Small colonies that resemble those of *Cryptococcus* spp. appear on Sabouraud agar (25° C) and blood agar (37° C) in 24 hours. They are hyaline and globose in form, without a capsule. They are larger than bacteria with width and length as great as 13 to 16 μm. Eight or more characteristic endospores are produced by internal segmentation. Five species have been identified using the fluorescent antibody technique.

FURTHER READING

Boulder, I., Cohen, A., Tamarin-Landau, R., and Sompolinsky, D.: Isolation of *Legionella pneumophila* from calves and the prevalence of antibodies in cattle, sheep, horses, antelopes, buffaloes, and rabbits. Vet. Microbiol., *13*:313, 1987.

Brenner, D.J., Hollis, D.G., Fanning, G.R., and Weaver, R.E.: *Capnocytophaga canimorsus* sp. nov. (Formerly CDC Group DF-2), a cause of septicemia following dog bite, and *C. cynodegmi* sp. nov., a cause of localized wound infection following dog bite. J. Clin. Microbiol., *27*:231, 1989.

Carithers, H.A.: Cat-scratch disease: An overview based on a study of 1200 patients. Am. J. Dis. Child., *139*:1124, 1985.

Craigie, J.: *Bacillus piliformis* (Tyzzer) and Tyzzer's disease of the laboratory mouse. 1. Propagation of the organism in the embryonated eggs. Proc. R. Soc. Lond. (Biol.), *165*:35, 1966.

Drolet, R., Kenefick, K.B., Hakomaki, M.R., and Ward, G.E.: Isolation of group eugonic fermenter-4 from a cat with multifocal suppurative pneumonia. J. Am. Vet. Med. Assoc., *189*:311, 1986.

Fenwick, B.W., Jang, S.S., and Gillespie, D.S.: Pneumonia caused by a eugonic fermenting bacterium in an African lion. J. Am. Vet. Med. Assoc., *183*:1315, 1983.

Ganaway, J.R.: Effect of heat and selected chemical disinfectants upon activity of spores of *Bacillus piliformis* (Tyzzer's disease). Lab. Anim. Sci., *30*:192, 1980.

Groves, M.G., and Harrington, K.S.: *Rochalimaea henselae* infections: Newly recognized zoonoses transmitted by domestic cats. J. Am. Vet. Med Assoc., *204*:267, 1994.

Guibourdenche, M., Lambert, T., and Riou, J.Y.: Isolation of *Neisseria canis* in mixed cultures from a patient after a cat bite. J. Clin. Microbiol., *27*:1673, 1989.

Hanner, T.L., et al.: Characterization of eugonic fermenters group EF-4 by polyacrylamide gel electrophoresis and protein immuno-blot analysis. Am. J. Vet. Res., *52*:1065, 1991.

Harrington, D.D.: *Bacillus piliformis* infection (Tyzzer's disease) in two foals. J. Am. Vet. Med. Assoc., *168*:58, 1976.

Hollis, D.G., et al.: Characterization of Centers for Disease Control Group NO-1, a fastidious, nonoxidative, gram-negative organism associated with dog and cat bites. J. Clin. Microbiol., *31*:746, 1993.

Inzana, T.J.: Miscellaneous glucose-nonfermenting gram-negative bacteria. *In* Diagnostic Procedures in Veterinary Bacteriology and Mycology. 5th Ed. Edited by G.R. Carter and J.R. Cole, Jr. New York, Academic Press, 1990.

Joseph, P.G., Sivendar, R., Anwar, M., and Fong, S.F.: *Chromobacterium violaceum* infection in animals. Kajian Vet. (Malaysia-Singapore), *3*:55, 1971.

Lyons, R.W.: *Acinetobacter calcoaceticus*. Clin. Microbiol. Newsletter, *5*:87, 1981.

Migaki, G., et al.: Canine protothecosis: Review of the literature and report of an additional case. J. Am. Vet. Med. Assoc., *181*:794, 1982.

Pickett, M.J., Hollis, D.G., and Bottone, E.J.: Miscellaneous Gram-Negative Bacteria. *In* Manual of Clinical Microbiology. 5th Ed. Edited by A. Balows, et al. Washington, D.C. American Society for Microbiology, 1991.

Piot, P.: *Gardnerella, Streptobacillus, Spirillum*, and *Calymmatobacterium*. Ibid.

Qureshi, S.R., Carlton, W., and Olander, H.J.: Tyzzer's disease in a dog. J. Am. Vet. Med. Assoc., *168*:602, 1976.

Rakich, P.M., and Latimer, K.S.: Altered immune function in a dog with disseminated protothecosis. J. Am. Vet. Med. Assoc., *185*:681, 1984.

Regnery, R., Martin, M., and Olson, J.: Naturally occurring *Rochalimaea henselae* infection in the domestic cat. Lancet *340*:557, 1992.

Salmon, S.A., et al.: Characterization of *Gardnerella vaginalis* and *G. vaginalis*-like organisms from the reproductive tract of the mare. J. Clin. Microbiol., *29*:1157, 1991.

Sippel, W.L., Medina, G., and Atwood, M.B.: Outbreaks of disease in animals associated with *Chromobacterium violaceum*. 1. The disease in swine. J. Am. Vet. Med. Assoc., *124*:467, 1954.

Spencer, T.H., Gannaway, J.R., and Waggie, K.S.: Cultivation of *Bacillus piliformis* (Tyzzer) in mouse fibroblasts (3T3 cells). Vet. Microbiol., *22*:291, 1990.

Wear, D.J., et al.: Cat-scratch disease: A bacterial infection. Science, *221*:1403, 1983.

Welch, D.F., et al.: *Rochalimaea* sp. nov., a cause of septicemia, bacillary angiomatosis, and parenchymal bacillary peliosis. J. Clin. Microbiol., *30*:275, 1992.

Wilkie, J.S.N., and Barker, I.K.: Colitis due to *Bacillus piliformis* in two kittens. Vet. Path., *22*:649, 1985.

29

Rickettsia and Chlamydia

The rickettsiae and chlamydiae are obligate intracellular organisms that are now classed as bacteria. At present they are classified in the orders Rickettsiales and Chlamydiales. They contain the families listed below.

ORDER RICKETTSIALES

Family Rickettsiaceae. These are usually parasites of the gut cells of arthropods; transmission is from arthropod to animal. Capillary endothelium is attacked, producing thrombi that result in hemorrhagic skin rashes. This family is sub-divided into tribe I, Rickettsiae, tribe II, Ehrlichieae, and tribe III, Wolbachieae (invertebrates). Important genera are: *Rickettsia, Cowdria, Ehrlichia, Neorickettsia,* and *Coxiella.*

Family Bartonellaceae. These bacteria parasitize mammalian erythrocytes; there is an intermediate arthropod host. They are rod-shaped and multiply by division inside or outside the host cell. None of the genera is of veterinary significance.

Family Anaplasmataceae. These organisms also parasitize mammalian erythrocytes; there is an intermediate arthropod host. They are spherical, multiply intracellularly, and have sac-like appendages. No organelles are seen, as in protozoa. Important genera are: *Anaplasma, Aegyptianella, Haemobartonella,* and *Eperythrozoon.*

ORDER CHLAMYDIALES

Family Chlamydiaceae. Transmission is by inhalation and ingestion, and there is considerable evidence of vector-borne infection. Epithelial cells of the lung and mucosal membranes as well as vascular endothelium and mobile phagocytes are parasitized. The important genus is *Chlamydia.*

SOME FEATURES OF RICKETTSIAE AND CHLAMYDIAE

Only rickettsiae and chlamydiae of the families Rickettsiaceae and Chlamydiaceae are discussed here. There is a lack of basic information on members of the families Bartonellaceae and Anaplasmataceae.

There are fundamental differences between the chlamydiae and the rickettsiae. The latter have cytochromes and their metabolic reactions are aerobic, whereas the former have not been shown to have cytochromes, and their metabolic reactions are essentially anaerobic. The chlamydiae also have a singular developmental cycle, while the rickettsiae multiply by simple binary fission.

Both are now classed as bacteria. They can be seen with the light microscope. All contain DNA and RNA and are susceptible to various antibiotics. They have cell walls, including two membrane systems, that resemble those of gram-negative bacteria. They stain reasonably well with Giemsa, Castaneda, Gimenez, and Macchiavello stains but poorly with Gram's stain. They are small, pleomorphic coccobacillary forms existing as obligate intracellular parasites. They possess many of the metabolic functions of bacteria but require exogenous cofactors from animal cells. Rickettsiae can generate their own energy, but they also depend on their host for some energy; whereas, Chlamydiae are more dependent on energy from their host cells. Rickettsiae can exchange their internal ADP for

ATP from the host cells. Rickettsiae can lose their viability in storage due to the loss of their intracellular ATP pool and several coenzymes.

Most rickettsiae and chlamydiae grow readily in the yolk sac of embryonated eggs and in cell cultures. Several species have been grown on artificial media.

FAMILY RICKETTSIACEAE

Morphology

These are minute coccobacilli, visible with the light microscope. They are usually about 0.3 to 0.6 μm in width and about 0.8 to 2.0 μm in length.

Mode of Infection

1. In mammals by direct penetration of skin as a result of feeding by an infected arthropod (tick, louse, flea, or mite). The organisms parasitize gut cells of arthropods.
2. In arthropods as the result of ingestion of blood of infected animals.
3. From arthropod to progeny by infected ova.
4. By inhalation and ingestion, as in Q fever.
5. By ingestion of infected flukes, as in salmon poisoning.

Pathogenesis

Noninfectious (ultraviolet irradiated) rickettsiae are toxic for mice and rats when administered intravenously. Death is caused by damage to capillary endothelial cells, producing loss of plasma, decrease in blood volume, and shock. The toxins have not been isolated and identified. Hemolysins are produced by some typhus rickettsiae. Rickettsiae contain endotoxin-like lipopolysaccharides. They are different from true endotoxins of gramnegative bacteria in that they act strongly to stimulate production of protective antibodies.

Infections begin in the vascular system; organisms proliferate in endothelial and phagocytic cells and are disseminated via the bloodstream. There is obstruction of small blood vessels because of hyperplasia of infected endothelial cells and resulting small thrombi. Fever, hemorrhagic rash, stupor, shock, and patchy gangrene of subcutis and skin are among the signs and lesions noted.

These clinical signs are thought to be due in part to endotoxin-like substances of rickettsiae. Steps involved in parasitization include: adherence, endocytosis, and phagosome destruction. The adherence is facilitated by the surface receptors of the host cell. After engulfment rickettsiae destroy the phagosomal membrane by phospholipase and then multiply within the cytoplasm or in certain cases (spotted fever) in the nucleus as well.

Pathogenicity

Diseases caused by the members of the *Rickettsiaceae* are listed in Table 29–1. Cat-scratch disease, whose rickettsial etiology has only recently been elucidated, is discussed in Chapter 28.

Diagnosis

The rickettsiae can be cultivated in the yolk sac of embryonated eggs and in cell cultures. Serologic procedures consist of agglutination and complement fixation tests that are available for some of the diseases (Q fever, typhus, and "spotted" fevers).

Heartwater. Giemsa-stained or immunofluorescently-stained smears from brain tissue; inoculation of susceptible cattle or mice.

Tropical Canine Pancytopenia. Giemsa-stained blood smears; characteristic inclusions in monocytes and neutrophils. Serologic: indirect fluorescent antibody test.

Equine Ehrlichiosis. Essentially the same as for canine ehrlichiosis (tropical canine pancytopenia).

Potomac horse fever. Giemsa- or fluorescent antibody-stained blood smears; culture in human histiocytes or canine monocytes; indirect fluorescent antibody test on paired serum samples; enzyme-linked immunosorbent assay on serum samples.

Salmon poisoning. Observation of characteristic fluke (*Nanophyetus salmincola*) eggs in feces. Giemsa-, Gimenez-, or Macchiavello-stained smears of fluid aspirated from lymph nodes.

Q Fever. Inoculation of chicken embryos, guinea pigs, and hamsters; detection of organisms in stained smears. Agglutination or complement fixation tests.

Immunity

Immunity is both cellular and humoral. Vaccines consisting of killed organisms are used to prevent epidemic typhus and Rocky Mountain spotted fever. Vaccines are not available for the prevention of the rickettsial diseases of animals; a vaccine in use for Potomac horse fever is being field tested.

Treatment

Tetracyclines and chloramphenicol in combination with a normal immune response are curative.

FAMILY ANAPLASMATACEAE

Genera of this family include *Anaplasma, Aegyptianella, Haemobartonella,* and *Eperythrozoon.* In Giemsa-stained blood smears, these organisms appear as pleomorphic bodies measuring 0.2 to 0.4 μm in diameter. They may be present on erythro-

Table 29–1.   Family Rickettsiaceae

Agent	Disease	Host	Transmission
Rickettsia rickettsii	Rocky Mountain spotted fever: mild to serious acute, febrile disease. Infections in animals usually mild.	Humans (mainly South Atlantic states), dogs.	Endemic in wood, rabbit, and dog ticks. In feces and all tissues of ticks (*Dermacentor, Amblyomma, Rhipicephalus*).
Cowdria ruminantium	Acute septicemia: "heartwater." High mortality.	Cattle, sheep, goats, wild ruminants in Africa, Caribbean.	*Amblyomma* ticks.
Ehrlichia bovis	Bovine ehrlichiosis.	Cattle.	*Ixodus* ticks.
Ehrlichia ovina	Ovine ehrlichiosis.	Sheep.	Tick transmission suspected.
Ehrlichia canis	Tropical canine pancytopenia or canine ehrlichiosis. Parasites of leukocytes. Long course; recurrent fever, weight loss, bleeding.	Dog.	Brown dog tick (*Rhipicephalus sanguineus*).
Ehrlichia platys	Canine infectious cyclic thrombocytopenia. Found only in platelets.	Dog.	Vector not known.
Ehrlichia phagocytophilia	"Grazing fever" in cattle; tick-borne fever in sheep.	Cattle, sheep.	*Ixodes* ticks.
Ehrlichia ondiri	Bovine petechial fever.	Cattle.	Vector not known.
Ehrlichia equi	Sporadic disease; fever, ataxia, leg edema, thrombocytopenia, anemia. Low mortality.	Horse.	Vector not known.
Ehrlichia risticii	Potomac horse fever: fever, anorexia, leukopenia, usually diarrhea; mortality as high as 30%. Also known as equine monocytic ehrlichiosis.	Horse.	Vector not known.
Neorickettsia helminthoeca	Salmon poisoning; 90% fatal. Acute, febrile, conjunctivitis, diarrhea.	Dogs, foxes, coyotes, bears, raccoons, ferrets.	Fish contain the infected helminth fluke, which encysts in muscles. Dogs and other hosts eat infested salmon. Flukes mature and release invasive rickettsiae; passed → snail → salmon.
Elokomin fluke fever agent	Similar agent occurring with *N. helminthoeca* or separately.		
Coxiella burnetti	Q fever: febrile pneumonitis. Rarely fatal. Endemic: some dairy cattle, sheep, goats, rats, and many other domestic and wild animals, which serve as reservoir. Occasional abortions.	Humans, some animals.	Ticks: infected for long periods. Agent in cow's milk, various discharges. Inhalation of contaminated dust; fomites. Differs from other rickettsiae in being relatively resistant to drying and heat.

cytes or free in the plasma of infected animals, and may occur in short chains or irregular groups.

Transmission is via arthropod vectors or parenteral inoculation of blood-containing tissue from an infected animal. Infections have been known to spread through a group of animals following improper disinfection of surgical instruments or syringes. The primary clinical feature is chronic anemia.

Anaplasma

The principal rickettsia in this genus is *Anaplasma marginale*. It causes anaplasmosis, an ar-

thropod-borne (at least 20 species of ticks) disease of cattle and other ruminants, which is manifested in acute, subacute, and chronic forms, with fever and varying degrees of anemia and icterus. If untreated the acute disease is frequently fatal. Asymptomatic carriers are common.

Anaplasmosis occurs widely in tropical and subtropical countries, principally in cattle and water buffaloes. Calves under 6 months are relatively resistant to the clinical disease but may become carriers.

A. ovis is a relatively avirulent rickettsia that sometimes occurs with *A. marginale* in Central Africa and the midwestern United States. Under some circumstances it can cause clinical anaplasmosis in sheep and goats.

A. centrale causes a milder form of anaplasmosis. It produces central bodies in erythrocytes that are almost identical to the marginal bodies seen with *A. marginale,* but located in the center of the cells.

Diagnosis

Anaplasmosis is diagnosed by the demonstration of the organisms as marginal bodies in erythrocytes of Giemsa-stained smears. Severe, prolonged infections with much red cell destruction may show few anaplasmas.

Indirect and direct immunofluorescence assays and the card agglutination, capillary agglutination, complement fixation, enzyme-linked immunosorbent assay, radioimmunoassay, and latex agglutination tests are used to detect animals that have been exposed or infected. More recently, genusspecific DNA probes are being used for the diagnosis of anaplasmosis by recognition of antigen.

Treatment

Tetracyclines are effective if given early. They are also effective in eliminating the carrier state when administered for prolonged periods.

Control and Prevention

Vectors should be reduced. Eradication can be accomplished by the removal of infected animals, although this is not usually feasible. Veterinarians working in endemic areas should be careful to disinfect instruments between animals when performing procedures such as dehorning, castration, vaccination, and blood collection.

Premunition of young animals, i.e., deliberate infection with virulent or attenuated *A. marginale,* is widely practiced in tropical and subtropical countries. In adult animals premunition should include concomitant tetracycline administration.

A vaccine consisting of killed organisms is available.

Aegyptianella

Aegyptianella infection of domestic and wild fowl is caused by *Aegyptianella pullorum,* and is seen in South Africa, Indochina, and the Balkans. Disease is spread by ticks and is frequently associated with fowl spirochetosis. Acute disease is characterized by high fever, diarrhea, anorexia, and paralysis. Giemsa-stained blood smears reveal multiple inclusions in erythrocytes, and the organisms may be present in phagocytes or free in the plasma. Aegyptianellae are susceptible to tetracyclines and dithiosemicarbazones.

Haemobartonella

Haemobartonella felis causes the widespread disease of cats, feline infectious anemia. It is characterized by acute, subacute, and chronic forms, all of which lead to anemia. In the acute disease clinical signs include variable fever (103° to 105° C), anorexia, jaundice, and splenomegaly. In the chronic form the clinical signs are less severe and temperatures may be normal or subnormal.

Transmission is via ingestion; an arthropod vector has not been identified. The disease occurs in a latent form in many cats and becomes clinical as a result of stress or concurrent disease.

Diagnosis

H. felis is a small, coccoid, rod-like or ring-shaped organism. Diagnosis is based upon the demonstration of numbers of characteristic organisms on the surfaces of erythrocytes of peripheral blood or bone marrow in Giemsa-stained smears or by the fluorescent antibody technique. A number of smears may have to be examined because *H. felis* may only appear in the blood periodically.

Treatment

Blood transfusions should be given if indicated. Tetracyclines are administered for 2 to 3 weeks.

Control and Prevention

External parasites should be controlled and blood donor cats should be screened to prevent the spread of the disease.

Other species of the genus, *H. canis, H. muris, H. bovis,* and *H. tyzzeri,* are infectious but usually do not cause disease in their respective hosts.

Eperythrozoon

Species of the genera *Eperythrozoon* and *Haemobartonella* are difficult to differentiate morphologically. Unlike *Haemobartonella,* the eperythrozoa often occur as ring forms and are present on erythrocytes and free in the plasma with equal frequency. As with most other members of the family Anaplasmataceae, *Eperythrozoon* have not been cultured in cell-free media, are transmitted by arthropods or parental inoculation of infected blood, and are susceptible to tetracyclines.

E. suis can cause a clinical disease in pigs characterized by icterus, anemia, inappetence, and weakness. The severity of the disease appears to be doserelated, and most infected pigs display no clinical signs, but carry the organism in a latent state. Diagnosis is based on the presence of ring-shaped bodies on erythrocytes in Giemsa- and fluorescent antibody-stained blood smears. Complement-fixation, indirect immunofluorescence, enzyme-linked immunosorbent assay and indirect hemagglutination have been employed. Another species, *E. parvum,* is a nonpathogenic parasite of swine and may be confused with *E. suis.* Both organisms appear to be widespread in the United States, particularly in the Midwest.

E. ovis has been associated with splenomegaly, hepatomegaly, anemia, and excessive pericardial fluid in lambs. Transmission is by mosquitoes and sand flies. Affected lambs are generally unthrifty and pastured lambs may show retarded growth. Demonstration of the organism in blood smears, complement fixation, and the indirect fluorescent antibody test are useful diagnostic aids.

Tetracyclines or sodium arsanilate in feed or water are effective in treating the disease.

Other members of this genus include *E. coccoides, E. wenyoni,* and *E. felis* which have been found in mice, cattle, and cats, respectively. Although they are sometimes associated with disease, they are most frequently observed in mixed infection with other blood parasites.

ORDER CHLAMYDIALES

Family Chlamydiaceae

Taxonomists now recognize four species of *Chlamydia,* viz., *C. trachomatis, C. psittaci, C. pneumoniae,* and *C. pecorum.* Strains of *C. trachomatis* are now considered to cause trachoma, lymphogranuloma venereum, and inclusion conjunctivitis in humans. Various strains of *C. psittaci* that may only differ serologically are considered to be the cause of the chlamydioses of animals. *C. pneumoniae* causes a variety of respiratory tract infections in humans worldwide. There is no known animal reservoir. *C. pecorum* is the most recently described species. It has been recovered from cattle and sheep with various diseases including sporadic encephalitis, infectious polyarthritis, pneumonia, and diarrhea.

All chlamydiae share a group (genus)-specific antigen. This antigen, also known as complement fixation antigen, is lipopolysaccharide in nature with a ketodeoxyoctanoic acid as the reactive moiety. In addition, chlamydiae possess species-specific and serovar (serotype)-specific antigens. Based on outer membrane protein antigens, using a microimmunofluorescence assay, more than 10 serovars of *C. psittaci* have been described.

Morphology and Multiplication

The highly infectious elementary bodies released from cells are spherical, with a diameter of approximately 0.25 μm.

They reproduce as follows. The mature parasites are spherical and from 0.2 μm to 1.0 μm in size. Elementary bodies (0.2 to 0.3 μm) invade host epithelial or mucosal cells, thereby yielding intracytoplasmic inclusions (up to 12 μm) filled with amorphous forms (0.1 μm diameter) that develop after various sequential changes. Then there is division and reduction in size with the production of highly infectious elementary bodies in approximately 30 hours.

Toxin Production

Toxins have not been demonstrated from *Chlamydia.*

Mode of Infection

Animals and humans are infected by the inhalation of infectious dust and droplets. In some chlamydioses, e.g., enzootic abortion of ewes, or enteritis, infection may take place by ingestion. There is evidence suggesting that arthropod-borne infections may occur.

Pathogenesis

The chlamydiae have a predilection for epithelial cells of the mucous membranes, although other tissues in a variety of locations are regularly infected. Pneumonia may develop from the inhalation of infectious dust and droplets. In enzootic abortion of ewes the mode of infection is ingestion, and organisms localize in cells of the placenta. Latency is a common feature of chlamydial infections. Latent infections are often activated by various stresses. Persistent antigenic stimulation provokes chronic inflammation in host tissues.

Ovine and bovine isolates can be classified by plaque reduction assay as Type I or Type II. Type I organisms are more frequently associated with abortion, genital infections, and enteritis, whereas conjunctivitis, pneumonia, encephalomyelitis, and polyarthritis are associated with Type II organisms.

Pathogenicity (Table 29–2)

Psittacosis or Avian Chlamydiosis. *C. psittaci* causes psittacosis, a disease of humans and psittacine birds (parakeets, parrots). It is commonly carried in the spleen and kidney of normal-appearing birds. As a result of certain influences or "stresses,"

Table 29–2. Principal Chlamydioses of Animals Caused by **Chlamydia psittaci**

Disease Syndrome	Species Affected	Characteristics
Abortion, infertility, and/or fetal infection:		
Enzootic ovine abortion	Sheep.	A wide-spread disease of sheep and other domestic animals. Typically manifested as abortion or stillbirth in mid-to-late gestation, but may result in the birth of weak offspring.
Bovine abortion and infertility	Cattle.	
Abortion and infertility in other domestic animals	Goats, pigs, horses, rabbits, mice.	
Orchitis/seminal vesiculitis	Cattle, sheep, guinea pigs.	Chlamydial elementary bodies shed in the semen. Has been observed in sheep herds with a high incidence of abortion. More commonly associated with infertility or repeated breeding. In rams, epididymitis is the most common form.
Pneumonia/pneumonitis Feline pneumonitis	Cats.	A frequent infection of cats. May begin with conjunctivitis and nasal discharge followed by interstitial bronchopneumonia.
Respiratory infection in other domestic animals	Calves, lambs, goats, foals, pigs, rabbits, dogs, mice.	
Conjunctivitis/rhinitis	Calves, lambs, pigs, cats, guinea pigs.	Associated with mucopurulent ocular discharge and keratoconjunctivitis.
Enteritis/diarrhea	Calves, sheep, goats, pigs, dogs, hares.	Primarily affects young animals and probably plays a role in transmitting chlamydial infections. Organisms may be shed in the feces of clinically normal or carrier animals.
Encephalomyelitis In cattle: Buss disease (sporadic bovine encephalomyelitis)	Calves, buffaloes, dogs.	May follow chlamydemia, although initial infection may be inapparent. Organisms localize in the synovial tissues, leading to polyarthritis. There is evidence for placental transmission.
Polyarthritis	Calves, lambs, pigs, foals.	A sporadic disease primarily of calves. Can be transmitted through the milk of the dam. May occur with or be preceded by rhinitis, arthritis or diarrhea. Affected animals walk with a staggering gait or in circles. Accompanied by profound depression, fever, anorexia, and weakness.

the organisms multiply and are shed in the feces in large numbers. The feces dry, producing a dust that is infectious to susceptible avian or mammalian hosts by inhalation or ingestion.

The human disease resulting from the inhalation of fecal dust is initially a pneumonitis. The organisms may spread via the blood, producing very serious systemic disease. Mortality may be as high as 20% in untreated individuals. In humans, 70% of the confirmed cases of *C. psittaci* infections are caused by exposure to caged pet birds.

Ornithosis is the name that was given to the chlamydiosis seen in nonpsittacine birds, e.g., pigeons, sparrows, and domestic poultry. Like psittacosis, this disease is also transmissible to humans. Some texts use the terms psittacosis and ornithosis synonymously. In turkeys the disease may be economically important.

C. psittaci causes infertility, conjunctivitis, and urogenital and cloacal infections in koalas.

Psittacosis or ornithosis is controlled by the isolation of imported psittacine birds and administration of chloromycetin or tetracycline in the feed or water for 45 days.

Laboratory Diagnosis

1. Demonstration of organisms or elementary bodies in stained smears and sections of lesions, e.g., smears of conjunctival scrapings in feline pneumonitis. Gimenez's stain is preferred for smears. Fluorescein labeled antibody may be used for the specific staining of smears.

2. Isolation and cultivation of organisms are usually done in the yolk sac of the chicken embryo, in mice, and also in irradiated cell cultures. Organisms are detected by staining

with fluorescein labeled antibody. Species identification requires serologic procedures to detect specific antigens. A direct immunofluorescence test kit is available commercially for confirmation of *C. psittaci* in culture.

3. Paired serum samples for (rising titers): complement fixation (group antigen); immunofluorescence (inhibition test); latex agglutination; and enzyme-linked immunoassay.

Immunity

Immunity is both cell-mediated and humoral. The serotype-specific antigen stimulates production of protective antibody. Vaccines consisting of suspensions of killed organisms are available for the prevention of feline pneumonitis and enzootic abortion of ewes, but their success is variable.

Treatment

Sulfonamides are effective for *C. trachomatis* subgroup A because these organisms synthesize their own folic acid. Subgroup B organisms *C. psittaci* (animal pathogens), require preformed folic acid and thus are not inhibited by sulfonamides. Penicillin results in the production of intracellular spheroplasts and is therefore not recommended. Tetracyclines and chloramphenicol are useful.

FURTHER READING

Anderson, A.A.: Serotyping of *chlamydia psittaci* isolates using serovar-specific monoclonal antibodies with the microimmunofluorescence test. J. Clin. Microbiol., 29:707, 1991.

Davidson, D.E., Jr., et al.: Prophylactic and therapeutic use of tetracycline during an epizootic of ehrlichiosis among military dogs. J. Am. Vet. Med. Assoc., 172:697, 1978.

Flammer, K.: Treatment of chlamydiosis in exotic birds in the United States. J. Am. Vet. Med. Assoc., 195:1537, 1989.

Foggie, A.: Chlamydial infections in mammals. Vet. Rec., 100:315, 1977.

Fukushi, H., and Hirai, K.: Proposal of *Chlamydia pecorum* sp. nov. for chlamydia strains derived from ruminants. Int. J. Syst. Bacteriol., 42:306, 1992.

Girjes, A.A., et al.: Two distinct forms of *Chlamydia psittaci* associated with disease and infertility in *Phascolactos cinereus* (Koala). Inf. Immun., 56:1897, 1988.

Grimes, J.E.: Serodiagnosis of avian *Chlamydia* infections. J. Am. Vet. Med. Assoc., 195:1561, 1989.

Hibler, S.C., Greene, C.E.: Rickettsial infections in dogs. Part I. Rocky mountain spotted fever and *Coxiella* infections. Compend. Contin. Educ. Pract. Vet., 7:856, 1985.

Hibler, S.C., Greene, C.E.: Rickettsial infections in dogs. Part II. Ehrlichiosis and infectious cyclic thrombocytopenia. Compend. Contin. Educ. Pract. Vet., 8:106, 1986.

Hibler, S.C., Greene, C.E.: Rickettsial infections in dogs. Part III. Salmon disease complex and Haemobartonellosis. Compend. Contin. Educ. Pract. Vet., 8:251, 1986.

Keefe, T.J., Holland, C.J., Salyer, P.E., and Ristic, M.: Distribution of *Ehrlichia canis* among military working dogs in the world and selected civilian dogs in the United States. J. Am. Vet. Med. Assoc., 181:236, 1982.

Meinkoth, J.H., et al.: Ehrlichiosis in a dog with seizures and nonregenerative anemia. J. Am. Vet. Med. Assoc., 195:1754, 1989.

Mohan, R.: Epidemiologic and laboratory observations of *Chlamydia psittaci* infection in pet birds. J. Am. Vet. Med. Assoc., 184:1372, 1984.

Moore, F.M., McMillan, M.C., and Petrak, M.L.: Comparison of culture, peroxidase-antiperoxidase reaction, and serum latex agglutination methods for diagnosis of chlamydiosis in pet birds. J. Am. Vet. Med. Assoc., 199:71, 1991.

Page, L.A., and Grimes, J.E.: Avian chlamydiosis (ornithosis). *In* Diseases of Poultry. 8th Ed. Edited by M.S. Hofstad. Ames, Iowa State University Press, 1984.

Palmer, J.E.: Prevention of Potomac horse fever. Cornell Vet., 79:210, 1989.

Schachter, J.: Chlamydial infections_past, present, future. J. Am. Vet. Med. Assoc., 195:1501, 1989.

Schachter, J.: Chlamydiae. *In* Manual of Clinical Microbiology. 5th Ed. Edited by A. Balows, et al. Washington, D.C. American Society for Microbiology, 1991.

Schnorr, K.L.: Chlamydial vaccines. J. Am. Vet. Med. Assoc., 195:1548, 1989.

Seamer, J., and Snape, T.: *Ehrlichia canis* and tropical canine pancytopaenia. Res. Vet. Sci., 13:307, 1972.

Smith, R.D., Hungerford, L.L., Armstrong, C.T.: Epidemiologic investigation and control of an epizootic of anaplasmosis in cattle in winter. J. Am. Vet. Med. Assoc., 195:476, 1989.

Storz, J.: Rickettsiae and Chlamydiae. *In* Diagnostic Procedures in Veterinary Bacteriology and Mycology. 5th Ed. Edited by G.R. Carter and J.R. Cole, Jr. New York, Academic Press, 1990.

Woldhalm, D.G., Stoenner, H.G., Simmons, R.E., and Thomas, L.A.: Abortion associated with *Coxiella burnettii* infection in dairy goats. J. Am. Vet. Med. Assoc., 173:1580, 1978.

Wyrick, P.B., Richmond, S.J.: Biology of chlamydiae. J. Am. Vet. Med. Assoc., 195:1507, 1989.

30

Mycoplasmas

HISTORICAL

The first mycoplasmal species, the cause of contagious bovine pleuropneumonia, was discovered by Nocard and Roux in 1898. The species discovered later were called pleuropneumonia-like organisms (PPLO).

GENERAL

The mycoplasmas are the smallest and simplest procaryotic cells capable of self-replication. They belong to the class Mollicutes and are classified in families and genera, as shown in Table 30–1. The mycoplasmas that are parasitic and pathogenic for animals are in the families Mycoplasmataceae and Acholeplasmataceae. The ureaplasmas are distinctive in that they hydrolyze urea. The genus *Acholeplasma* is separated from the genera *Mycoplasma* and *Ureaplasma* because the latter two require cholesterol.

These procaryotic organisms have no rigid cell wall and consequently are plastic and highly pleomorphic. They are bound by a limiting lipoprotein plasma membrane and occur in a variety of forms including spherical or pear-shaped cells and filamentous structures. Some divide by binary fission, while others have a reproductive cycle, unlike conventional bacteria. In the latter case, elongated forms break up into round forms or beads that may pass through a 0.15 μm filter. Most species of *Mycoplasma* use either glucose or arginine as their major source of energy.

Some occur as commensals on mucous membranes of the upper respiratory and digestive tracts, the genital tract, and the bovine udder.

MORPHOLOGY AND PHYSIOLOGY

Mycoplasmas in smears are seen as coccobacilli, coccal forms, ring forms, spirals, and filaments. They stain poorly (gram-negative), although Giemsa is useful. They are difficult to demonstrate in and from tissues. They range in size from 0.2 to 0.3 μm in diameter with variable length depending upon the form. They can readily pass a 0.45 μm membrane filter. Dark-field and phase contrast microscopy are recommended for studying the morphology of mycoplasmas in liquid media. Shapes of cells are distorted when examinations involve smears and conventional staining.

The genome of mycoplasmas and ureaplasmas is a circular, double-stranded DNA molecule 5×10^8 to 1×10^9 daltons. This is the smallest for any self-replicating procaryotic cell. That it has less genetic information than the genome of bacteria is indicated by its low guanine plus cytosine content. DNA studies do not support the theory that the L forms of bacteria are related to mycoplasmas (see Table 30–2).

CULTIVATION AND CULTURAL FEATURES

Most mycoplasmas require cholesterol or related sterols for growth and they are unable to synthesize purines and pyrimidines, thus the requirement for complex media.

They are usually grown on media consisting of beef infusion, peptone, NaCl, 20% horse serum and 10% yeast extract; agar is added to make a solid medium. Inhibitors of bacterial growth, which may be included, are penicillin (gram-positives) and

Table 30–1. Families and Genera of Mycoplasmas

Families and Genera	Approximate Number of Species	Sterol Requirement	Habitat	Other
Mycoplasmataceae:				
Mycoplasma	>60	+	Animals	
Ureaplasma	5	+	Animals	Produce urease
Acholeplasmataceae:				
Acholeplasma	8	–	Animals, soil, sewage, etc.	
Spiroplasmataceae:				
Spiroplasma	4	+	Plants and insects	Helical and motile, filaments
Unclassified genera:				
Anaeroplasma	2	Variable	Rumen of cattle and sheep	Anaerobic

Adapted from Joklik, W.K., Willet, H.P., Amos, D.B. and Wilfert, C.M. (eds.): Zinsser Microbiology. 19th Ed. Norwalk, Conn., Appleton & Lange, 1988.

thallium acetate (gram-negatives). Some additives may be required for the growth of some species.

Parasitic mycoplasmas contain 10% to 20% lipid and possess a relatively low content of nucleic acids as compared with bacteria. Most grow aerobically but some require nitrogen with 5% to 10% CO_2; they may be grown in chicken embryos and cell cultures.

T-mycoplasmas or ureaplasmas produce smaller colonies (T = tiny) than the conventional mycoplasmas. Unlike the other mycoplasmas, they can split urea. Special procedures are required for the cultivation and maintenance of these organisms.

COLONY MORPHOLOGY

After 2 to 6 days of aerobic incubation at 37° C, colonies on solid media are 10 to 600 μm in diameter. Under low power magnification colonies appear transparent, flat, and often resemble a fried egg. Colonies grow into the medium and are difficult to remove from the agar surface. Stained colony preparations can be made from culture plates using Dienes' stain. It distinguishes mycoplasmas from dwarf bacterial colonies but not from L forms of bacteria.

Agar cultures are transferred by pushing a block of agar, colony side down, over another plate with a glass rod. Blocks with colonies are dropped into broth. Care must be taken to obtain pure cultures.

PATHOGENESIS

Many of the mycoplasmas are commensals in the upper digestive, respiratory, and genital tracts. It is known that some species attach to cells by specific receptors; for a number of species the host cell attachment is mediated by sialic acid moieties. Intimate contact with host cells is necessary for assimilation of vital nutrients and growth factors, e.g., nucleic acid precursors, which mycoplasmas cannot synthesize. The small size and plastic nature of these organisms enable them to adapt to the

shape and contours of host cell surfaces. A high molecular weight protein has been identified as an important adhesin of *M. pneumoniae*. Some have a predilection for infecting mesenchymal cells lining serous cavities and joints; others parasitize tissues of the respiratory tract, including the lungs. Their attachment to cells of the respiratory tract may result in destruction of cilia predisposing to secondary bacterial infection. Species show considerable host specificity. They are extracellular parasites and one, *M. neurolyticum*, produces a membrane-associated toxin. The fibrinous exudate frequently present in infections protects them from antibody and antimicrobial drugs and contributes to chronicity. Bacterial secondary invaders are not uncommon.

Aside from the neurotoxin of *M. neurolyticum*, the mechanisms by which mycoplasmas cause disease are poorly understood. It is thought that a galactan capsule produced by *M. mycoides* has a pathogenic role. Cytotoxic glycoproteins and proteins have been isolated from the membranes of several species. Amongst the products produced during growth by some species, are capsular carbohydrate, hemolysins, proteolytic enzymes, ammonia, and endonucleases. It is suggested that accumulation of mycoplasmal metabolites may contribute to cytopathic effects and tissue damage.

Infections are frequently chronic and low grade. Various stresses predispose to these infections. Experimental disease is often difficult to produce.

MODE OF INFECTION

This is most frequently by inhalation. Infection may be endogenous or exogenous.

IMMUNE RESPONSE

The immune response is predominantly humoral. As in bacterial infections, the first antibodies to appear are IgM and IgA, followed by IgG. The CF antibodies—being mostly IgM—are found

Table 30–2. A Comparison of Characteristics of Mycoplasmas and L Forms

Mycoplasma	L-Phase Variants (L Forms) of Bacteria*
Elements of colonies smaller	Elements of colonies larger
Contain less DNA	Contain more DNA
GC ratio lower	GC ratio higher
Do not revert to bacteria	May revert
No antigenic relation to bacteria	Antigenic relations to parent bacterium
Require sterols (except *Acholeplasma*)	Do not require sterols
Usually pathogenic or parasitic	Not known to be pathogenic
DNA does not relate to bacteria	DNA shows kinship to bacteria

* L-phase variants occur spontaneously or as a result of the action on bacteria of antisera, antibiotics, salts of heavy metals, phage, and so forth.

early. IgG antibodies are mycoplasmacidal and may persist for many months. IgA antibodies are temporary; they block the adherence of mycoplasmas to host cells. Autoimmune phenomena have been reported in some *Mycoplasma* infections.

Various procedures are used to detect and measure antibodies, e.g., agglutination, agar gel precipitation, complement fixation, ELISA, and counter-immunoelectrophoresis.

PATHOGENICITY

There are a large number of *Mycoplasma* spp., associated with animals. They are listed along with their disease status in Table 30–3. The most important species of domestic animals are discussed briefly below.

AVIAN MYCOPLASMAS

The significant avian species are: *M. gallisepticum*, *M. meleagridis*, *M. synoviae*, and *M. iowae*. These and the other species are listed below.

M. gallisepticum (MG). This is the primary cause of chronic respiratory disease and air sac disease of chickens, turkeys, and other fowl; infectious sinusitis of turkeys; and synovitis. This disease of major economic importance results in reduced egg production, poor growth, and embryo death. Egg transmission is of major importance. Spread is also by direct and indirect (mainly droplets) contact.

Properties. It is beta-hemolytic, ferments a number of carbohydrates, and agglutinates chicken red cells.

M. synoviae (MS). This species is considered the cause of infectious synovitis of chickens and turkeys. Although all synovial membranes may be affected, the lesions involving the hock and wing joints are most apparent. *M. synoviae* has been isolated from the respiratory tracts of chickens and turkeys. Transmission is by eggs, aerosol, and direct contact.

Properties. It is pathogenic for chicken embryos and ferments glucose and maltose but not lactose, sucrose, or mannitol.

M. meleagridis (MM). MM causes airsacculitis of turkeys. Transmission is by eggs and then laterally to poults. Fomites may also contribute to spread. It is isolated from semen, vagina, bursa of Fabricius, air sacs, lungs, trachea, and sinuses.

Properties. It is nonhemolytic and does not ferment glucose.

M. iowae. This species is recovered from turkeys and chickens, in which it is considered a potential pathogen. It can cause exudative airsacculitis, and toe and leg deformities in young poults.

The following avian species are not considered pathogenic: *M. gallinarum, M. pullorum, M. gallinaceum, M. columbinasale, M. iners,* and *Acholeplasma laidlawii. M. anatis* has been associated with sinusitis in ducks.

MYCOPLASMAS OF SWINE

M. hyorhinis causes polyserositis and arthritis in young pigs and is a secondary invader in rhinitis and pneumonia. It is frequently found in the upper respiratory tract.

M. hyosynoviae causes arthritis in young and feeder pigs; it is frequently found in the upper respiratory tract.

M. hyopneumoniae is the primary cause of enzootic pneumonia of swine, the most widespread pneumonic disease of swine. Ordinarily it is a mild chronic disease whose effects are mainly reflected in delayed weight gains. As a result of various stresses the pneumonia, usually complicated by *Pasteurella multocida,* can become severe.

M. flocculare is a commensal of the upper respiratory tract which is sometimes isolated with *M. hyopneumoniae.* It is of low or questionable pathogenicity.

Several additional species of questionable disease significance are listed in Table 30–3.

Table 30–3.   *Mycoplasmas, Ureaplasmas, and Acholeplasmas Associated with Diseases of Animals*[a]

Animal Species Affected	Disease	Organisms
Cattle	Pneumonia	*Mycoplasma mycoides* ss. *mycoides* *M. bovis* *M. dispar* Ureaplasmas
	Arthritis	*M. bovis* *M. bovigenitalium*
	Mastitis	*M. bovis* *M. californicum* *M. canadense*
	Abortion	*M. bovis*
	Vaginitis	Ureaplasmas, *U. diversum* *M. bovigenitalium*
	Seminal vesiculitis	*M. bovis* *M. bovigenitalium*
	Uncertain	*M. bovirhinis* *M. alkalescens* *M. arginini* *M. bovoculi* *M. verecundum* *M. canadense* *M. alvi* *Acholeplasma modicum* *A. laidlawii*
Swine	Pneumonia	*M. hyopneumoniae*
	Arthritis	*M. hyorhinis* *M. hyosynoviae*
	Uncertain	*M. flocculare* *M. sualvi* *A. axanthum* *A. granularum* *M. hyopharyngis*
Sheep and Goats	Pneumonia Pneumonia, arthritis, mastitis	*M. ovipneumoniae* *M. mycoides* ss. *capri* *M. mycoides* ss. *mycoides* *M. agalactiae* *M. putrefaciens* *M. arginini* *M. capricolum*
	Conjunctivitis	*M. conjunctivae*
	Uncertain	*A. oculi*
Horses	Uncertain	*M. equigenitalium* *M. equirhinis* *M. subdolum* *M. felis* *M. arginini* *M. salivarium* *A. equifetale* *A. hippikon* *A. laidlawii*
Rats and Mice	Pneumonia	*M. pulmonis*
	Arthritis	*M. arthritidis*
	Rolling disease	*M. neurolyticum*

Table 30–3.   Mycoplasmas, Ureaplasmas, and Acholeplasmas Associated with Diseases of Animals[a] (Continued)

Animal Species Affected	Disease	Organisms
Guinea pigs	Uncertain	*M. caviae*
Dogs	Pneumonia	*M. cynos*
	Uncertain	*M. spumans*
		M. maculosum
		M. edwardii
		M. molare
		M. canis
		M. opalescens
Cats	Pneumonia	*M. felis*
		M. feliminutum
		M. gateae

[a] Adapted from Stalheim, O.H.V.: Mycoplasmas of animals. *In* Diagnostic Procedures in Veterinary Bacteriology and Mycology. Edited by G.R. Carter and J.R. Cole, Jr., 5th Ed. New York, Academic Press, 1990.

MYCOPLASMAS OF CATTLE

M. mycoides ss. *mycoides* (small colony type) causes contagious bovine pleuropneumonia (CBPP), a major plague of cattle that is enzootic in parts of Africa and Asia. CBPP is a highly contagious disease characterized by septicemia, frequently followed by localization in the thorax with extensive suppurative lesions involving the lungs, pleura, and pericardium.

Like many other mycoplasmas *M. bovis* can be found as a commensal in the respiratory and genital tracts. It is a frequent cause of mastitis, arthritis, and less frequently of genital infections. Diseases caused by other mycoplasmas (see Table 30–3) are pneumonia, arthritis, mastitis, abortion, vaginitis, and seminal vesiculitis.

Ureaplasmas have frequently been isolated from the genital tract, pneumonic lungs, semen, and milk of cows. They are not uncommon commensals and have a probable pathogenic potential. Recent reports suggest an etiologic role in bovine granular vaginitis and infertility.

The other mycoplasmas recovered from cattle are listed in Table 30–3.

MYCOPLASMAS OF SHEEP AND GOATS

Several *Mycoplasma* species cause important diseases of sheep and goats. These infections are referred to briefly.

Contagious caprine pleuropneumonia is an acute serofibrinous pleurisy and pneumonia that may involve an entire lobe. It is characterized by red and grey hepatization with characteristic hemorrhagic infarction. A severe arthritis may be a sequela of the bacteremia. This disease has been attributed to *Mycoplasma mycoides* subspecies *capri*, *M. capripneumoniae*, and *M. mycoides* ss. *mycoides*

(large colony). It occurs in Europe, Asia, and Africa, and there is evidence that it exists in the United States.

The "small colony" form of *M. mycoides* ss. *mycoides* is the causative agent of contagious bovine pleuropneumonia.

Contagious agalactia is an acute, subacute, or chronic disease of sheep and goats caused by *M. agalactiae* (other mycoplasmas, viz., *M. mycoides* ss. *mycoides*—large colony—and *M. capricolum* are claimed to cause similar syndromes). It is characterized by bacteremia (after ingestion), with localization and inflammatory activity in the udder, uterus, joints (arthritis), and eyes (conjunctivitis). There is interstitial mastitis, which without treatment may lead to extensive fibrosis. Contagious agalactia occurs in Mediterranean countries and some regions of Europe, Africa, and Asia.

Polyarthritis in sheep and goats is probably the most common and geographically widespread mycoplasmosis in these species. It is most often caused by *M. capricolum*.

M. ovipneumoniae is found as a commensal of the respiratory and genital tracts of sheep and goats. It is considered to produce primary infection in the lung which may become complicated by secondary invaders such as *Pasteurella haemolytica*.

Keratoconjunctivitis in sheep and goats is a worldwide disease caused by *M. conjunctivae*.

M. mycoides ss. *mycoides* (large colony) has been reported to cause epizootics in kids characterized by septicemia, polyarthritis, and pneumonia, with high morbidity and mortality rates. The organism is usually acquired from the milk of shedding females.

Other disease manifestations with which mycoplasmas have been associated are enzootic pneumonia, arthritis, conjunctivitis, vulvovaginitis, infertility, and central nervous system disorders. See also Table 30–3.

MYCOPLASMAS OF HORSES

A number of species have been isolated from various specimens from horses. Their pathogenic significance for the horse has yet to be established. There is evidence that *M. felis* causes pleuritis. See Table 30-3.

MYCOPLASMAS OF DOGS

Mycoplasma cynos is considered a cause of a rapidly spreading respiratory infection involving the lungs. By itself it may have little significance, but in combination with other bacteria and viruses it may cause a severe pneumonia. *M. canis* and *M. spumans* are reported to cause canine urinary tract infections.

Other species that have been recovered from the dog and whose significance is uncertain are *M. maculosum*, *M. edwardii*, *M. molare*, and *M. opalescens*.

MYCOPLASMAS OF CATS

M. felis has been occasionally associated with feline conjunctivitis and pleuritis in horses. *M. gateae*, *M. feliminutum*, and *M. felis* have been implicated in feline pneumonia.

MYCOPLASMAS OF OTHER SPECIES

Most of the mycoplasmas that have been recovered from domestic animals, rats, mice, and guinea pigs are listed in Table 30–3.

SPECIMENS AND DIAGNOSIS

The particular fragility of these organisms must be considered in the submission of specimens. They should be refrigerated and delivered to the laboratory within 48 hours. Mycoplasmas in tissues can be preserved for longer periods by freezing, preferably on dry ice.

Definitive diagnosis is usually based upon isolation and identification or detection of the mycoplasmas in tissues by a fluorescent antibody procedure. A number of serologic procedures including complement-fixation, agar gel immunodiffusion, enzyme-linked immunosorbent assay (ELISA) are used to detect affected animals.

IDENTIFICATION OF MYCOPLASMAS

The association of a culture with a lesion is suggestive of a particular organism, e.g., a *Mycoplasma* recovered from polyserositis in a young pig would probably be *M. hyorhinis*. Precise identification is sometimes difficult and may require the help of a reference laboratory. Obtaining a pure culture may be time consuming. Various procedures are used for different species.

1. An agglutination procedure is used to identify avian mycoplasmas. It is sometimes used for the identification of other species. Other serological procedures such as complement-fixation and enzyme-linked immunosorbent assays (ELISAs) have been used in antigen recognition.
2. Direct and indirect fluorescent antibody staining is used to identify organisms in smears and colonies on plates.
3. Growth inhibition tests: specific antisera inhibit growth of homologous immunotypes on agar. This is a particularly useful procedure, but antisera are not always available. Monoclonal antibodies are available for some species.
4. Other criteria: fermentation of sugars, colony characteristics, pathogenicity, hemagglutination, tetrazolium reduction, hemolysis; species specific DNA probes have been developed for identification of some mycoplasmas.

RESISTANCE

Mycoplasma are more fragile than bacteria because of the absence of a cell wall. They are readily killed by drying, sunshine, and the usual means of chemical disinfection.

TREATMENT

Mycoplasma are resistant to sulfonamides and penicillin. Tetracyclines, gentamicin, kanamycin, tylosin, spectinomycin, spiramycin, and erythromycin are effective in some infections. No standardized procedure is available for performing in vitro antimicrobial susceptibility tests.

CONTROL

Flocks have been established that are free of avian *Mycoplasma*. Chickens supplying eggs in such flocks must be negative to cultural and serologic procedures. Chicks and eggs are screened so that the flocks are maintained free of *Mycoplasma*. Dipping hatching eggs in an antibiotic solution has been effective in producing chicks free of *M. gallisepticum*.

Herds of pigs free of swine mycoplasmas and other important viral and bacterial pathogens (specific pathogen-free or SPF pigs) have been established from caesarian-delivered pigs raised in isolation.

IMMUNIZATION

Cattle are vaccinated with a live attenuated *M. mycoides* ss. *mycoides* strain to prevent contagious bovine pleuropneumonia.

Live, attenuated, and inactivated vaccines give partial protection against losses in egg production and infections due to *M. gallisepticum*. An inactivated, oil-adjuvant vaccine containing the latter organism has been approved for use in the United States. A vaccine against enzootic pneumonia of pigs is now available commercially.

FURTHER READING

Afshar, A.: Diseases of bovine reproduction associated with *Mycoplasma* infections. Vet. Bull., *45*:211, 1975.

Allam, N.M., Powell, D.G., Andrews, B.E., and Lemcke, R.M.: Isolation of *Mycoplasma* species from horses. Vet. Rec., *93*:402, 1973.

Amanfu, W., Weng, C.N., Ross, R.F., and Barne, H.J.: Diagnosis of mycoplasmal pneumonia of swine: Sequential study by direct immunofluorescence. Am. J. Vet. Res., *45*:1349, 1984.

Ball, H.J., and Mackie, D.P.: Experimental production of bovine and ovine mastitis with a *Mycoplasma canadense* isolate. Vet. Rec., *118*:72, 1986.

Bayoumi, F.A., Farver, T.B., Bushnell, B., and Oliveira, M.: Enzootic mycoplasmal mastitis in a large dairy during an eight year period. J. Am. Vet. Med. Assoc., *192*:905, 1988.

Bencina, D., and Bradbury, J.M.: Combination of immunofluorescence and immunoperoxidase techniques for serotyping mixtures of mycoplasma species. J. Clin. Microbiol., *30*:407, 1992.

Blikslager, A.T., and Anderson, K.L.: *Mycoplasma mycoides* subspecies *mycoides* as the cause of a subauricular abscess and mastitis in a goat. J. Am. Vet. Med. Assoc., *201*:1404, 1992.

Doig, P.A., Ruknke, H.L., and Palmer, N.C.: Experimental bovine ureaplasmosis. 1. Granular vulvitis following vulvar inoculation. Can. J. Comp. Med., *44*:252, 1974.

DaMassa, A.J., Waknell, P.S., and Brooks, D.L.: Mycoplasmas of sheep and goats. J. Vet. Diagn. Invest., *4*:101, 1992.

East, N.E., et al.: Milkborne outbreak of *Mycoplasma mycoides* subspecies *mycoides* infection in a commercial goat dairy. J. Am. Vet. Med. Assoc., *182*:1138, 1983.

Jang, S.S., Ling, G.V., Yamamoto, R., and Wolf, A.M.: Mycoplasma as a cause of urinary tract infection. J. Am. Vet. Med. Assoc., *185*:45, 1984.

Jasper, D.E.: *Mycoplasma* and mycoplasma mastitis. J. Am. Vet. Med. Assoc., *170*:1167, 1977.

Jones, G.E.: Mycoplasmas of sheep and goats: A synopsis. Vet. Rec., *113*:619, 1983.

Losos, J.L.: Contagious bovine and caprine pleuropneumonia. *In Infectious Tropical Diseases of Domestic Animals.* Essex, England, Longman Scientific and Technical, 1986.

Maniloff, J. (Editor-in-chief): Mycoplasmas: Molecular Biology and Pathogenesis. Washington, D.C., American Society for Microbiology, 1992.

Razin, S., and Freundt, E.A.: The Mycoplasmas. *In Bergey's Manual of Systematic Bacteriology,* Vol. 1. Edited by N.R. Krieg, et al. Baltimore, Williams & Wilkins, 1984.

Rosendahl, S.: Canine mycoplasmas: Their ecologic niche and role in disease. J. Am. Vet. Med. Assoc., *180*:1212, 1982.

Rosendahl, S.: Mycoplasmal Infections. *In* Infectious Diseases of the Dog and Cat. Edited by C.E. Greene. Philadelphia, W.B. Saunders Company, 1990.

Rosendahl, S., et al.: Detection of antibodies to *Mycoplasma felis* in horses. J. Am. Vet. Med. Assoc., *188*:292, 1986.

Stalheim, O.H.V.: Mycoplasmal respiratory disease of ruminants: A review and update. J. Am. Vet. Med. Assoc., *182*:403, 1983.

Stalheim, O.H.V.: Mycoplasmas of animals. In *Diagnostic Procedures in Veterinary Bacteriology and Mycology.* 5th Ed. Edited by G.R. Carter and J.R. Cole, Jr. New York, Academic Press, 1990.

Timoney, J.F., et al.: The genera of *Mycoplasma* and *Ureaplasma. In* Hagan and Bruner's Infectious Diseases of Domestic Animals; 8th Ed. Ithaca, N.Y., Comstock Publishing Associates, 1988.

Tully, J.G., and Whitcomb, R.G. (eds.): The Mycoplasmas. Vol. 2. Human and Animal Mycoplasmas. New York, Academic Press, Inc., 1979.

Whittlestone, P.: Enzootic pneumonia of pigs (EPP). Adv. Vet. Sci. Comp. Med., *17*:1, 1973.

Wilkinson, G.T.: Mycoplasmas of the cat. *In* The Veterinary Annual. Edited by C.S.G. Grunsell and F.W.G. Hill. Bristol, England, Scientechnica, 1980.

Yoder, H.W., Jr.: Avian mycoplasmas. *In* Diagnostic Procedures in Veterinary Bacteriology and Mycology. 5th Ed. Edited by G.R. Carter and J.R. Cole, Jr. New York, Academic Press, 1990.

Part III

FUNGI

31

Introduction to the Fungi and Fungous Infections

What follows in this chapter and chapters 32, 33, 34, and 35 is a very brief introduction to the fungi and the diseases they cause.

GENERAL CHARACTERISTICS OF THE FUNGI

For the most part the fungi are heterotrophic, aerobic, nonmotile and possess cell walls that somewhat resemble those of plants in chemical composition and structure. Some of their basic characteristics, including subcellular structure are described in Chapter 1. Fungi grow as single cells—the yeasts—or as multicellular filamentous colonies—the molds and mushrooms. The fungi are not photosynthetic, and consequently they are restricted to a saprophytic or parasitic existence. They are abundant and widespread in the soil, on vegetation, and in water, where they subsist on decaying vegetation and wood. Digestion of these materials is accomplished by the production of specific proteolytic, lipolytic, and glycolytic enzymes. The cell wall prevents osmotic lysis and protects against mechanical injury and entrance by harmful macromolecules.

The two principal kinds of fungi are the molds and the yeasts. The main element of the vegetative or growing form of the mold is the hypha, a branching tubular structure 2 to 10 μm in diameter. As growth begins, hyphae become intertwined to form a mycelium. The vegetative mycelium consists of the surface hyphae, while the hyphae that

arise above the surface are referred to as the aerial mycelium. Under certain conditions the hyphae of the aerial mycelium produce reproductive cells or spores. These are collectively referred to as fruiting bodies. The hyphae of many fungi are divided by cross-walls called septa. Some hyphae grow into the culture medium while others grow upward as "aerial hyphae." Some of the latter produce stalk-like structures referred to as conidiophores or sporangiophores which give rise to asexual spores called conidia. They are referred to by a variety of names (see Glossary below). The asexual spores or conidia are more resistant to physical and chemical agents than hyphae. Free conidia promote the aerial dissemination of fungi.

The yeasts are oval or spherical cells ranging in diameter from 3 to 5 μm. Some varieties of yeasts or yeast-like fungi produce chains of irregular yeast cells that are referred to as pseudohyphae. Some fungi that exist in the mycelial form at room temperature will convert to a yeast form at 37°C or when in the tissues of animals. These fungi are called dimorphic. Many of the properties of the fungi that distinguish them from bacteria are summarized in Table 1–1.

There are two independent classification systems for the fungi. One is based on anamorphs (asexual structures) and the other on teleomorphs (sexual structures). Sexual reproduction takes place by fusion of two haploid nuclei (karyogamy) followed by meiotic division of the diploid nucleus. Two hyphal protoplasts may unite (plasmogamy) and be followed immediately by karyogamy. The sexual state of many of the medically important fungi has not been demonstrated. Asexual reproduction which involves the division of nuclei by mitosis, would appear to be so efficient that sexual elements rarely occur with these fungi. The formal classification of the fungi is discussed in Chapter 1.

For this reason only asexual reproduction will be considered. The three mechanisms of asexual reproduction are (1) sporulation followed by germination of the spores (e.g., *Aspergillus* and *Penicillium*); (2) fragmentation of hyphae (e.g., *Coccidioides immitis*, *Geotrichum candidum*); and (3) budding of yeast cells (e.g., *Candida*, *Cryptococcus*).

The various reproductive structures are defined below and referred to later under specific disease-producing fungi.

The sexual stage of a number of the dermatophytic (ringworm) fungi has been observed, e.g., the sexual or perfect stage of *Microsporum nanum* is called *Nannizzia obtusa* (ascomycetes). Only the asexual stage is found in infected skin. The sexual stage of *Cryptococcus neoformans* is called *Filobasidiella neoformans*.

COMMONLY USED MYCOLOGIC TERMS

Arthrospore: An asexual spore formed by the disarticulation of the mycelium, as can be seen in *Geotrichum candidum*.

Ascospore: A sexual spore characteristic of the true yeasts or ascomycetes. It is produced in a sac-like structure called an ascus. This ascospore results from the fusion of two nuclei and is seen in *Saccharomyces* spp.

Ascus: The specialized sac-like structure characteristic of the true yeasts in which ascospores are produced. This is found in *Saccharomyces* spp.

Blastospore: A spore produced as a result of a budding process along the mycelium or from a single spore, as in *Saccharomyces* spp.

Chlamydospores: Thick-walled, resistant spores formed by the direct differentiation of hyphae, as seen in *Candida albicans* and *Histoplasma capsulatum*.

Clavate: Club-shaped such as the microconidia of *Microsporum nanum*.

Columella: The persisting dome-shaped upper portion of the sporangiophore, which can be seen in *Mucor* spp.

Conidium: An asexual spore formed from hyphae by abstriction, budding, or septal division, as in *Penicillium* spp.

Conidiophore: A stalk-like branch of the mycelium on which conidia develop either singly or in numbers as found in *Penicillium* spp.

Dematiaceous: A term used to denote the dark brown or black fungi such as *Phialophora* spp., and *Hormodendrum* spp.

Dimorphic: Having two forms or phases, referred to as the yeast form and mycelial form. *Blastomyces dermatitidis* is dimorphic.

Echinulate: Spiny, for example the macroconidia of *Microsporum*.

Ectothrix: Occurring outside the hair shaft, as do *Microsporum* spp.

Endogenous: Originating or produced from within. *Candida albicans* infections are usually considered endogenous.

Endothrix: Occurring inside the hair shaft as do *Trichophyton* spp., on occasion.

Exogenous: Originating from without, such as *Histoplasma capsulatum* infection.

Geophilic: Denotes fungi whose natural habitat is the soil, such as *Coccidioides immitis*.

Germ Tube: Tube-like structures produced by germinating spores. They develop into hyphae, as in *Candida albicans*.

Glabrous: The smooth form, for example, the glabrous form of *Geotrichum candidum*.

Hyphae: The filaments that compose the body or thallus of a fungus.

Macroconidia: Large, multinucleate conidia; they may be fusiform (spindle-shaped) or clavate (club-shaped). If divided by transverse and longitudinal septations, they are termed muriform (having walls). *Microsporum canis* produces them.

Microconidia: Small, single-celled conidia borne laterally on hyphae. They may be spherical, elliptical, oval, pyriform (pear-shaped) or clavate. *Microsporum canis* produces them.

Mycelium: A mat made up of intertwining, thread-like hyphae.

Nodes: The points on the stolons from which the rhizoids arise, as in *Rhizopus* spp.

Obovoid. Egg-shaped and having the larger portion at the distal end.

Pseudohyphae: Filaments composed of elongated budding cells that have failed to detach, as seen in *Candida albicans*.

Rhizoid: Root-like, branched hyphae extending into the medium, as in *Absidia* spp.

Septate: Has cross-walls or septa in the hyphae, as found in the hyphae of *Aspergillus*.

Sessile: Denotes attachment directly to a hypha without a stalk.

Sporangiophore: A specialized hypha bearing a sporangium, for example in *Rhizopus* spp.

Sporangium: A closed, often spherical structure in which asexual spores are produced by cleavage (e.g., *Rhizopus*).

Sterigmata: Specialized structures, short or elongated, borne on a vesicle and producing conidia, as seen in *Aspergillus*.

Stolon: A horizontal hypha or runner that sprouts where it touches the substrate. It forms rhizoids in the substrate, as observed in *Absidia* spp.

Vesicle: The terminal swollen portion of a conidiophore, which is seen in *Aspergillus*.

Yeasts: An ill-defined group of unicellular fungi lacking mycelium and reproducing asexually by blastospores and occasionally by sexually produced ascospores. The latter are the true yeasts (e.g., *Saccharomyces* spp.).

Zygospore: A thick-walled, sexual spore of the true fungi that results from the fusion of two similar gametangia, as in *Phycomycetes*.

FUNGOUS INFECTIONS: GENERAL CONSIDERATIONS

Fungi (excepting the dermatophytes) rarely cause disease in healthy immunocompetent animals. Disease usually results when there are debilitating conditions that favor the growth of fungi or when fungi accidentally penetrate host barriers. The fungi causing disease in animals and humans are broadly classified as follows:

1. *Frankly pathogenic fungi:* those that cause ringworm and the more common mycoses such as blastomycosis and histoplasmosis.
2. *Opportunistic fungi:* those that seldom cause disease. They are widespread in nature, constituting species of a number of genera, e.g., *Penicillium, Aspergillus, Mucor, Absidia,* and *Rhizopus*.

A number of circumstances may give rise to systemic fungous infections:

1. Prolonged administration of antibiotics. Mode of action:
   a. Lowered host resistance; mechanisms not known for certain; effect may be on phagocytosis or antibody production.
   b. Interfere with synthesis of vitamins by effect on normal microflora, e.g., vitamin K, vitamin B complex components.
   c. Upsets the microfloral balance, supressing bacteria and favoring fungi, as in intestinal candidiasis.
2. Radiation, steroid therapy, urethane, mustard gas, and folic acid antagonists may activate latent fungous and bacterial infections. Steroids inhibit inflammatory as well as antibody response.
3. Cancer: fungous infections occur in patients with leukemia or lymphoma, particularly if they are being treated with antibiotics or anticancer drugs. Some of the latter are strongly immunosuppressive. Fungous infections are not uncommon in debilitated patients with terminal malignancies.
4. Immunosuppressive therapy, for example with azathioprine; patients are more susceptible to aspergillosis, cryptococcosis, and various opportunistic fungi.
5. Cytotoxic drugs: ablation of the bone marrow in the treatment of leukemia.
6. Immune deficiencies: T-cell deficiency, thymic hypoplasia, and anergy.
7. Humans with diabetes or other endocrine disorders are more susceptible to opportunistic fungi.

SOME GENERAL FEATURES OF FUNGOUS INFECTIONS

1. Most fungi capable of causing disease in animals and humans are classified among the Fungi Imperfecti (see Chapter 1).
2. Diseases caused by fungi do not usually assume epidemic proportions. Some exceptions are the dermatophytoses and infrequently aspergillosis, histoplasmosis, and cryptococcosis. Only the dermatophytoses are communicable.
3. Conclusive proof that fungi produce classic exotoxins or endotoxins is as yet lacking.
4. Some features of most fungous diseases are:
   a. Low invasiveness and low virulence of the organism.
   b. Certain predisposing factors contributing to the establishment of infection.
      i. Production of a necrotic focus by trauma, infection, or ischemia.
      ii. Lowered general resistance.
      iii. Moist environment, e.g., *Candida* infections in humans.
      iv. Exposure to a large number of organisms, e.g., brooder pneumonia.
   c. Chronicity of infection leads to a granulomatous process that resembles the reaction to a foreign body.
   d. Immunity is considered to be more cell-mediated than antibody-mediated.
5. Infected and exposed animals may develop a sensitivity to the fungus in question. This

hypersensitivity is responsible in part for the pathologic effects produced. Hypersensitivity may contribute to dissemination of the infection within the host.

6. Many pathogenic fungi exhibit a significant tissue tropism. For example, *Histoplasma capsulatum* lives within macrophages and dermatophytes thrive on keratin.

7. Fungi are identified principally by the study of cultural characteristics and the microscopic morphology of the so-called "fruiting bodies" or reproductive elements.

IMMUNITY TO FUNGOUS INFECTIONS

IMMUNE RESPONSE

Most of the fungi produce diseases that are characterized by granulomatous lesions resembling those produced by mycobacteria and other bacterial facultative intracellular parasites. Most fungal infections are asymptomatic, limited, and readily eliminated by the animal. Such exposed animals will usually manifest a positive delayed-type hypersensitivity skin reaction.

Antibodies to the various fungi are found in all the mycotic diseases except the dermatophytoses. In these superficial infections the antibody-producing cells are not stimulated. Antibody titers may be negative or low in asymptomatic or mild infections. Immunity to fungous infections is more cell-mediated than humoral. Serum antibodies from infected animals do not protect normal animals from experimental infections.

Most animals exposed to or infected by fungi develop a hypersensitivity of the delayed type that is detectable by inoculation of fungi or their products into the skin. Hypersensitivity to products of fungi spread hematogenously is responsible for the skin eruptions accompanying the dermatophytoses ("id" eruption), candidiasis, and coccidioidomycosis. Hypersensitivity and resistance are closely related in the animal's response to infection. There is a correlation between recovery and the development and persistence of delayed hypersensitivity. When a state of anergy (absence of delayed hypersensitivity reaction) develops in a serious systemic infection, the prognosis is usually poor.

Skin tests analogous to the tuberculin test are used in blastomycosis, histoplasmosis, coccidioidomycosis, and sporotrichosis. Various elements of the fungus are inoculated intradermally. A reaction of the delayed hypersensitivity type constitutes a positive test. A positive test indicates either past or current infection, and the result is considered along with other information in arriving at a diagnosis. The test result may be negative if the animal is anergic.

SEROLOGY OF MYCOTIC INFECTIONS

The serologic diagnosis of mycotic infections of animals has received little attention. Some of the serologic procedures that are employed in important mycoses of humans are mentioned under specific diseases. Not all veterinary diagnostic microbiology laboratories are prepared to carry out these procedures. Assistance is sometimes available through the courtesy of some hospital and public health laboratories.

It should be kept in mind that many of the skin tests and serologic procedures referred to under specific diseases were developed for use in human beings and that animals may respond somewhat differently.

TREATMENT OF MYCOTIC INFECTION: GENERAL

Treatment in general is discussed below. Treatment of particular fungous diseases is discussed with the disease in subsequent chapters.

The polyene antibiotics produced by various *Streptomyces* spp. have revolutionized the treatment of mycotic diseases. The principal drugs in the polyene group are amphotericin B, nystatin, and pimaricin (natamycin). They combine with sterols in the cytoplasmic membrane of fungi and adversely affect its permeability. However, they may also bind to sterols in mammalian cell membranes resulting in toxicity. Sterols are not present in bacteria with the exception of mycoplasmas. They are present in red blood cells, however, and hemolytic anemia can be a side effect. Renal toxicity is the most serious side effect seen with amphotericin B. Because of its potential toxicity this drug is reserved for serious infections. Nystatin is used topically or orally for candida infections. Pimaricin is used to treat mycotic keratitis.

The drug 5-fluorocytosine (flucytosine) is useful in the treatment of candidiasis and cryptococcosis. Flucytosine is transported into fungal cells and hydrolyzed to 5-fluorouracil. The latter is incorporated into fungal RNA resulting in errors in the production of RNA. It is relatively nontoxic when given orally. Resistance of *Candida albicans* has been encountered.

The synthetic benzimidazole derivatives, called imidazoles, (two nitrogen molecules) and triazoles (three nitrogen molecules) have considerable antifungal activity. They affect the fungal cell wall and cell membrane, resulting in interference with nutri-

Table 31–1. Common Laboratory Procedures Used in the Diagnosis of Fungal Infections

Procedure	Purpose
Wet mount of tissue or mucus-containing specimens in 10% KOH	Strong alkali degrades tissue and mucus and permits visualization of fungi
Wet mount of portions teased from fungal colonies and mounted in lactophenol cotton blue	Permits observation of fungal morphology and presence of spores. Kills fungi and provides good contrast.
Tissue sections and clinical material stained with periodic-acid-Schiff (PAS) or methenamine silver stains	Both PAS and silver stain fungal cell walls to give good contrast with background in tissue sections and clinical materials
Sabouraud glucose agar for culture; incubation at room temperature (RT) for up to 6 weeks	Low pH of the medium and RT incubation favor growth of fungi over bacteria. Antibiotics, e.g., chloramphenicol and cycloheximide, may also be added to discourage bacterial and fungal growth.
Blood agar or brain heart infusion agar at 37° C for a week or more	Various fungi grow at 37° C. The yeast phase of dimorphic fungi grow on these media at 37° C.
Slide cultures, with inoculated blocks of Sabouraud's glucose agar (about 1 cm square and 2 or 3 mm deep) on a glass slide covered with a coverslip and incubated in a moist chamber at room temperature; when spores form, the coverslip is carefully removed and examined in a lactophenol cotton blue wet mount	Permits observation of relatively undisturbed fungal growth. Particularly useful for identification of fruiting bodies.

Adapted from: G.N. Myrvik and R.S. Weiser: Introduction to Medical Mycology. *In*: Fundamentals of Medical Bacteriology and Mycology, 2nd Ed. Philadelphia, Lea & Febiger, 1988.

ent utilization. Among the imidazoles miconazole, clotrimazole, econazole, and ketoconazole appear to be the most useful. Two important triazoles are fluconazole and itraconazole. Although side-effects are seen, they are not as serious as those that can accompany amphotericin B therapy. These drugs are being used to treat blastomycosis, histoplasmosis, dermatophytosis and candidiasis.

Griseofulvin is produced by *Penicillium griseofulvum*. It is a selectively toxic antibiotic that is specific for fungi whose walls contain chitin. It accumulates in the keratin layer where it inhibits the nucleic acid synthesis of dermatophytes.

The aromatic diamidine 2-hydroxy-stilbamidine was the first effective treatment for blastomycosis. It is still used in humans who tolerate it better than amphotericin B.

Iodides, usually given orally, are effective in the treatment of sporotrichosis. These compounds do not affect in vitro growth of *Sporothrix schenckii*. Their mechanism of action is not clear.

GROUPING OF FUNGOUS DISEASES

The fungous diseases are grouped in subsequent chapters as follows:
1. Dermatophytosis
2. Mycoses Caused by Yeasts and Yeast-like Fungi:
   Candidiasis
   Cryptococcosis
   Geotrichosis
   Malassezia
   Trichosporonosis
3. Subcutaneous Mycoses:
   Sporotrichosis
   Phaeohypomycosis
   Pythiosis
   Eumycotic Mycetoma
   Chromoblastomycosis
   Hyphomycosis
   Epizootic Lymphangitis
   Rhinosporidiosis
4. Systemic Mycoses:
   Zygomycosis
   Entomophthoromycosis
   Aspergillosis
   Blastomycosis
   Histoplasmosis
   Coccidioidomycosis
   Adiaspiromycosis

This is an arbitrary grouping, and occasionally the subcutaneous mycoses may produce systemic disease; conversely, some of the agents causing systemic disease may be confined to the subcutis.

Laboratory Procedures

Laboratory procedures commonly used in the diagnosis of fungous infections are summarized in Table 31–1.

Most fungi grow well on simple media at room temperature (22° to 25° C). The most commonly used media are variations of Sabouraud dextrose agar. The latter contains peptone, dextrose, and agar and has a pH of 5.6. The low pH inhibits the growth of bacteria. All fungi grow aerobically.

A number of fungi will grow in the yeast phase at 37° C. The media most commonly used at this temperature are blood agar and brain heart infusion agar.

Inocula should be large, and incubation periods exceeding a month may be required.

Cycloheximide (Actidione) may be added to Sabouraud agar to inhibit the growth of many saprophytic fungi. It should be remembered that it also inhibits some important fungi, e.g., *Pseudoallescheria boydii, Aspergillus fumigatus,* and *Cryptococcus neoformans*. Chloramphenicol is added to Sabouraud agar to inhibit bacteria.

Indication for culture may come from the detection of fungi in tissue sections particularly after special fungal stains are used.

A variety of media are used in mycology laboratories for special purposes, such as demonstration of chlamydospores, growth of some dermatophytes, and the presumptive identification of certain yeasts. Slide cultures (see Table 31–1) are particularly helpful in identifying many fungi.

Various probe-based methods, including the polymerase chain reaction (PCR) are being developed for the identification of pathogenic fungi in cultures and clinical materials. They are not yet widely used.

FURTHER READING

Ainsworth, G.C., and Austwick, K.C.: Fungal Diseases of Animals. 2nd Ed. Farnham Royal, England, Commonwealth Agricultural Bureaux, 1973.

Balows, A., Ausherman, R.J., and Hopper, J.M.: Practical diagnosis and therapy of canine histoplasmosis and blastomycosis. J. Am. Vet. Med. Assoc., 148:678, 1966.

Beneke, E.S. and Rogers, A.L.: Medical Mycology Manual. 4th Ed. Minneapolis, Burgess Publishing Co., 1980.

Campbell, M.C. and Stewart, J.L.: The Medical Mycology Handbook. New York, John Wiley & Sons, 1980.

Coleman, R.M. and Kaufman, L.: Use of the immunodiffusion test in the serodiagnosis of aspergillosis. Appl. Microbiol., 23:301, 1972.

Conant, N.F., Smith, D.T., Baker, R.D., and Calloway, J.L.: Manual of Clinical Mycology. 3rd Ed. Philadelphia, W.B. Saunders Co., 1971.

Ellner, P.D. and H.C. Neu: Understanding Infectious Disease. Chicago. Mosby-Year Book, Inc., 1992.

Fromtling, R.A.: Fungi. In Manual of Clinical Microbiology. 5th Ed. Editor-in-Chief. A. Balows. Washington, D.C. American Society for Microbiology, 1991.

Greene, C.E.: Clinical Microbiology and Infectious Diseases of the Dog and Cat. Philadelphia, W.B. Saunders Co., 1984.

Greene, C.E. (Editor): Infectious Diseases of the Dog and Cat. Philadelphia, W.B. Saunders Co., 1990.

Jackson, J.A.: Immunodiagnosis of systemic mycoses of animals: A review. J. Am. Vet. Med. Assoc., 188:702, 1986.

Jungerman, P.F. and Schwartzman, R.M.: Veterinary Medical Mycology. Philadelphia, Lea & Febiger, 1972.

Kaufman, L. and Reiss, E.: Serodiagnosis of fungal diseases. In Manual of Clinical Microbiology. 4th Ed. Edited by E.H. Lennette et al. Washington, D.C., American Society for Microbiology, 1985.

Kirk, R.W. (ed.): Current Veterinary Therapy VIII, Philadelphia, W.B. Saunders, 1983.

Lane, J.G. and Warnock, D.W.: The Diagnosis of *Aspergillus fumigatus* infection of the nasal chambers of the dog with particular reference to the value of the double diffusion test. J. Sm. Anim. Pract., 18:169, 1977.

Medoff, G. and Kobayashi, G.S. Strategies in the treatment of systemic fungal infections. N. Engl. J. Med., 302:145, 1980.

Moriello, K.A.: Ketoconazole: Clinical pharmacology and therapeutic recommendations. J. Am. Vet. Med. Assoc., 188:303, 1986.

Palmer, D.F., Kaufman, L., Kaplan, W., and Cavallaro, J.J.: Serodiagnosis of Mycotic Diseases. Springfield, Ill., Charles C Thomas, 1977.

Persing, D.H., et al. (Editors): Diagnostic Molecular Biology. Washington. American Society for Microbiology, 1993.

Pratt, W.B.: Chemotherapy of Infection. New York, Oxford University Press, 1977.

Rippon, J.W.: Medical Mycology. 3rd Ed. Philadelphia, W.B. Saunders Company, 1988.

Smith, J.M.B.: Opportunistic Mycoses of Man and Other Animals. Wallingford, England. CAB International Mycological Institute, 1989.

Weir, E.C., Schwartz, A., and Buergelt, C.D.: Short-term combination chemotherapy for treatment of feline cryptococcosis. J. Am. Vet. Med. Assoc., 174:507, 1979.

Ytturraspe, D.J.: Clinical evaluation of a latex particle agglutination test and a gel diffusion precipitin test in the diagnosis of canine coccidioidomycosis. J. Am. Vet. Med. Assoc., 158:1249, 1971.

32

Dermatophytosis

General

The dermatophytes that cause infections in animals and humans, and whose sexual stages have been characterized, belong to the phylum Deuteromycota. Before their sexual stage was known they were called Fungi Imperfecti. All dermatophytes of veterinary importance are in the genera of *Trichophyton* and *Microsporum*. Several species of dermatophytes in the subdivision *Deuteromycotina* are known to have sexual life cycles (perfect states or teleomorphs) and produce ascospores. These species are now classified in the family Gymnoascaceae of the subdivision *Ascomycotina*. The species that have perfect states in the genera *Trichophyton* and *Microsporum* are placed in the genera *Arthroderma* and *Nannizzia,* respectively. The perfect state is useful in the identification of certain species; its demonstration requires special technique. For purposes of identification diagnostic microbiologists are primarily concerned with the conidial state of isolates.

The term "ringworm" denotes a clinical entity rather than an infection caused by a specific dermatophyte. Dermatophytes are able to penetrate all layers of the skin, but are generally restricted to the cornified nonliving keratin layer of the skin and its appendages (hairs, nails, horns, and feathers). These fungi do not penetrate beyond the stratum corneum because of antifungal activity of serum and body fluids and possibly because of a lack of tolerance for temperature above 35° C.

Most dermatophytes are not fastidious in their nutritional needs. They are aerobic and require a moist milieu for growth. The formation of arthrospores which are responsible for infectivity is stimulated by carbon dioxide.

Origin and Distribution

The dermatophytes occur in all parts of the world. All ringworm fungi may have originated from soil forms, but a significant number of them appear to have abandoned their saprophytic existence to become parasites. This adaptive process appears to entail loss of their perfect state (sexual life cycle). Increasing adaptability to the human and animal host is thought to result in the gradual loss of both the perfect state and the ability to produce asexual spores.

Dermatophytes are highly host-adapted parasites although several, e.g., *Microsporum gypseum* and *M. nanum,* can survive for long periods in soil. Ringworm fungi are categorized as geophilic, zoophilic, and anthropophilic depending on their habitat and host preference. Geophilic fungi inhabit the soil, whereas zoophilic and anthropophilic fungi are primarily found as parasites of animals and humans, respectively. Some have a broad host range, while others infect only a few animal species (Table 32–1).

Transmission

Dermatophytes may be transmitted from animal to animal, from animals to humans, from one human to another, and from soil to either animals or humans by direct or indirect contact.

Extracellular Products

Very little is known about the extracellular products of the dermatophytes that may be important in

Table 32–1. **Summary of Principal Characteristics of Important Veterinary Dermatophytes***

Species	Principal Hosts	Fluores-cence	Arthro-spores	Cultural Features	Macroconidia	Microconidia	Other
M. canis	Dog and cat (most cases), humans, monkey, horse	+	Ectothrix, small, mosaic	White to buff; reverse: yellow to orange; rapid grower	Spindle-shaped, frequent	Few, sessile	Accessory structures similar to those of *T. gallinae*
M. gypseum	Dog, horse, cat	−	Ectothrix, large, chains	Buff; reverse: orange brown to yellow; moderately rapid	Ellipsoidal, septa 2–6, frequent	Sessile or on short sterigmata; clavate	Persists in soil; accessory structures similar to those of *T. gallinae*
M. nanum	Swine	−	Ectothrix, large, chains	White to buff; reverse: red; moderately rapid	Obovoid to ellipsoidal ovate; frequent	Clavate	Persists in soil
T. mentagrophytes†	Many animal species, including all domestic animals	−	Ectothrix, large, chains	Granular, light buff to tan; reverse: variable red, yellow, etc.; fairly rapid	Occurrence variable; spindle or clavate; 5–6 septa	Abundant, pyriform or clavate, sessile	*T. equinum* resembles *T. mentagrophytes* (see below)
T. verrucosum	Cattle, sheep	−	Ectothrix, large, chains	Deeply folded, white to brilliant yellow; slow	Requires thiamine; long and thin-walled. Rare	Abundant with thiamine; singly ovoid; pyriform or clavate	Chlamydospores; grows better at 37° than at 25° C
T. gallinae	Fowl	−	Ectothrix, large, chains	Radial folds, white to pale rose; reverse: red; moderately rapid	Infrequent; club-shaped and clavate	Singly on hyphae, pyriform to clavate	Chlamydospores, nodular bodies, pectinate bodies, racquet hyphae
T. equinum	Horse	−	Ectothrix, long chains	White, cottony, yellow edge; old colony velvety to cream-tan; reverse: yellow to red-brown	Rare; clavate Requires nicotinic acid	Many, spherical to pyriform	

*Other dermatophytes are encountered less frequently in the domestic animals. Among these are *T. rubrum*, reported from the dog; *M. audouinii*, reported from the dog and monkey; and *T. schoenleinii*, reported from horses and cats in Europe.

† Consists of three varieties, *erinacei*, *mentagrophytes*, and *quinckaenum*.

pathogenesis. They produce keratinases and some elaborate elastase and collagenase. These enzymes help provide nutrients by digesting host tissues. The extracellular products of certain dermatophytes may induce severe inflammation at the sites of infection in animals and humans.

PATHOGENESIS AND PATHOGENICITY

Infections caused by dermatophytes or keratinophilic fungi are referred to as dermatophytoses. The term formerly used, dermatomycosis, includes all fungal infections involving the skin. The fungi belonging to the genera *Microsporum* and *Trichophyton*, that do not cause ringworm in animals or humans, are not referred to as dermatophytes. Many species of *Microsporum* and *Trichophyton* cause ringworm in animals. The principal differential characteristics of important veterinary dermatophytes are listed in Table 32–1.

Infection by a dermatophyte may result in a state of hypersensitivity to the dermatophyte. The nature of the lesion depends to some extent on the immunologic response. The inflammation is most severe if there is a hypersensitivity reaction; however, this response may contribute to the resolution of the infection. The local inflammatory response

and the delayed-type hypersensitivity are attributed to galactomannan glycopeptides. It has been suggested that chronic dermatophytosis may be related to a modification of cell-mediated immunity. Vesicular lesions may appear on various parts of the body as part of a general allergic reaction. They result from the hematogenous spread of the fungi or its products. These lesions, which do not contain the organism, are called dermatophytids or "id" lesions or reactions. They are well known in humans and occasionally occur in animals.

Secondary bacterial invaders such as *Staphylococcus aureus* and *Staphylococcus intermedius* are common and they may cause pustules in hair follicles.

Dermatophytes can hydrolyze keratin. The infection is localized in the keratinized epidermis. This is thought to be due to the lack of sufficient concentration of available iron elsewhere. The epidermis and hair are the principal structures attacked in lower animals. Dermatophytosis is almost always superficial and most infections are self-limiting and rarely lead to death. However, long-lasting infection can cause severe lesions with concomitant discomfort for the animals and economic loss.

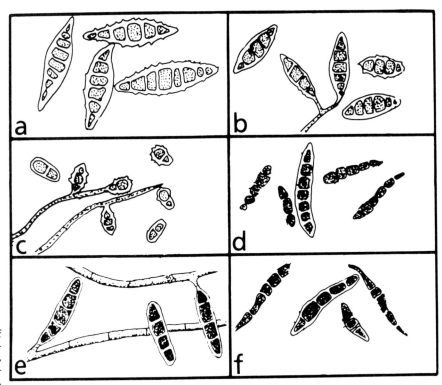

Figure 32–1. Macroconidia of important dermatophytes: a, *Microsporum canis*; b, *M. gypseum*; c, *M. nanum*; d, *Trichophyton mentagrophytes*; e, *T. equinum*; and f, *T. verrucosum*.

Characteristically, dermatophytosis is more frequently observed in stabled farm animals than in pastured animals. The incidence is usually higher during winter months, and the disease may clear up spontaneously in the spring and summer.

In domestic animals there are no apparent differences in the clinical appearances of infections produced by the different dermatophytes. The lesions in domestic animals are usually characterized by circular, scaly areas of alopecia with or without crust formation. In dogs and cats, lesions occur most frequently on the head and extremities. The head and tail are the most frequent locations in horses and cattle. Remissions are seen frequently in animals treated previously for clinical dermatophytosis.

PROCEDURE FOR THE LABORATORY DIAGNOSIS OF DERMATOPHYTOSIS

1. If feasible, examine patient in the dark with a Wood's lamp (filtered ultraviolet light, 3650 Å) to determine if fluorescence is present. If present, remove some fluorescing hairs with forceps for microscopic examination. Also remove hairs at edge of lesions for examination.

2. Hairs, nails, and skin scrapings are examined in 10% or 20% KOH under a coverslip for the presence of arthrospores or hyphae. The preparation should be gently warmed for about 10 minutes, or allowed to stand for about 30 minutes at room temperature to digest proteinaceous debris. The penetration and clarity can be enhanced by the addition of DMSO (36%) to the KOH (20%). Special staining procedures such as lactophenol cotton blue are used for better visualization before examining.

3. Regardless of whether arthrospores are found, material is inoculated onto Sabouraud agar containing cycloheximide and chloramphenicol. The former inhibit contaminating fungi and the latter contaminating bacteria. Do not discard plates until they have been incubated at room temperature (25 to 30° C) for at least a month. If *T. verrucosm* is suspected, the culture plate should also be incubated at 37° C as this temperature enhances growth of this fungus. For production of macroconidia, *T. verrucosum* (cattle) requires a medium supplemented with inositol and thiamine; *T. equinum* requires nicotinic acid. Yeast extract is a satisfactory source of these growth supplements.

4. If fungi grow, examine colonies grossly for morphology, texture, and pigment as seen under the colonies. Then examine the mycelium or other material microscopically in a

lactophenol cotton blue wet mount. The tape mount is a convenient procedure. The principal morphologic and cultural characteristics of the important dermatophytes of animals are summarized in Table 32–1. The morphology of the macroconidia of the major animal dermatophytes is shown in Figure 32–1. Their demonstration in cultures is significant in identification.

IDENTIFICATION OF DERMATOPHYTES

Knowledge of colony characteristics, microscopic morphology, and nutritional requirements are essential for identification of dermatophytes (Table 31–1). The size and shape of macro- and microconidia and the thickness of their cell walls are important microscopic characteristics for speciation. Detection of arthrospores outside (ectothrix) or inside (endothrix) the hairshaft may make possible the rapid diagnosis of ringworm. Speciation of *Trichophyton* may require the expertise of a reference laboratory. Commercial growth media (Trichophyton agars, Nos. 1 to 7) containing various growth factors are available to aid in the identification of species. Initial studies with monoclonal antibodies appear to provide a means for rapid identification of species of dermatophytes.

A medium called Dermatophyte Test Medium (DTM) is available commercially under a number of trade names. When dermatophytes grow on this modified Sabouraud agar (which contains phenol red), they change the yellow medium to red (alkaline), usually within two weeks. This is a useful screening medium. It is advisable to submit positive cultures to a microbiology laboratory for confirmatory examination as false-positive reactions occur.

TREATMENT

The affected animal or animals, if part of a group, should preferably be isolated. All affected animals should be treated topically with an antifungal solution. Clipping is indicated in animals with medium-to-long hair. Among the solutions used are lime-sulfur, chlorhexidine, captan, and povidone-iodine. If topical treatment alone is not effective, systemic therapy is indicated. Griseofulvin, which is given orally for at least a month, is widely used. Although dermatophytes are susceptible to ketoconazole and other related products, their use in large animals is costly; they are primarily used in small animals. The

"spot" treatment of lesions is not recommended as inapparent areas of infection may be missed. Cages, pens, rubbing posts, saddles, grooming tools, tack, etc., should be disinfected. Precautions should be taken to prevent human infections.

Dogs, and cats particularly, can be reinfected from an asymptomatic carrier. To determine if an animal is a carrier the entire body should be combed thoroughly with a new tooth brush. Collected hairs are cultured. Topical treatment is carried out pending the results of culture. Systemic treatment may also be necessary.

Cattle ringworm is often a problem in stabled animals; it usually clears up when cattle leave the stable. The topical antifungal solutions referred to above are effective.

Clorox and other antifungal preparations, including natamycin, are applied as sprays.

A live attenuated *T. verrucosum* vaccine, widely used in Europe, appears to be protective in cattle.

FURTHER READING

(Note: See also "Further Reading" for Chapter 31.)

Angarano, D.W., and Scott, D.W.: Use of ketoconazole in treatment of dermatophytosis in a dog. J. Am. Vet. Med. Assoc., *190*:1433, 1987.

Beneke, E.S., and Rogers, A.L.: Medical Mycology Manual, 4th Ed. Minneapolis, Burgess, 1980.

Carter, G.R.: Dermatophytes and dermatophytoses. *In*, Diagnostic Procedures, Veterinary Bacteriology and Mycology. 5th Ed. Edited by G.R. Carter and J.R. Cole, Jr. New York, Academic Press, 1990.

Dawson, C.O.: Ringworm in animals. Rev. Med. Vet. Mycol., *6*:223, 1968.

Ginther, O.J.: Clinical aspects of *Microsporum nanum* infection in swine. J. Am. Vet. Med. Assoc., *146*:945, 1965.

Grappel, S.F., Bishop, C.T., and Blank, F.: Immunology of dermatophytes and dermatophytosis. Bacteriol. Rev., *38*:222, 1974.

Kane, J., Padhye, A.A., and Ajello, L.: *Microsporum equinum* in North America. J. Clin. Microbiol., *16*:943, 1982.

Medleau, L., and Chalmers, S.A.: Ketoconazole for treatment of dermatophytosis in cats. J. Am. Vet. Med. Assoc. *200*:77, 1992.

Oldenkamp, E.P., and Spanoghe, L.: Natamycin treatment of ringworm in cattle. Netherlands J. Vet. Sci., *102*:124, 1977.

Oldenkamp, E.P.: Treatment of ringworm of the horse with natamycin. Vet. Rec., *11*:36, 1979.

Pratt, W.B.: Chemotherapy of Infection. New York, Oxford University Press, 1977.

Reppon, J.W.: Medical Mycology. 3rd Ed. Philadelphia, W.B. Saunders Company, 1988.

Tilton, R.C., and McGinnis, M.R.: Dermatophytes. *In*, Clinical and Pathogenic Microbiology. Edited by B.J. Howard. Washington, The C.V. Mosby Co., 1987.

Weitzman, I., and Kane, J.: Dermatophytes and agents of superficial mycoses. *In*: Manual of Clinical Microbiology. 5th Ed. Edited by E.H. Lennette, et al. Washington, American Society for Microbiology, 1991.

33

Mycoses Caused by Yeasts or Yeast-like Fungi

CANDIDIASIS (MONILIASIS, THRUSH)

A number of species of *Candida* can be differentiated by biochemical tests. All *Candida* occur saprophytically. The important species from the standpoint of disease is *C. albicans*. It is a normal inhabitant of the digestive tract, oral cavity, and vagina. Infections are usually endogenous.

The following *Candida* species have been implicated as causes of bovine mastitis: *C. albicans, C. parapsilosis, C. guilliermondii, C. krusei, C. pseudotropicalis, C. rugosa,* and *C. tropicalis. C. parapsilosis* has caused bovine abortion and *C. rugosa* has been implicated in pyometra in a mare.

PATHOGENICITY

Infections by *C. albicans* occur most frequently on mucous membranes of the digestive and genital tracts. The young are especially susceptible. Candidiasis involving the gastrointestinal tract may result from prolonged antibiotic therapy. Disseminated candidiasis has been reported occasionally in immunocompromised animals and those undergoing prolonged chemotherapy. Natural infections in animals appear to be uncommon, and there are few reports in the literature.

Candida possess adhesins consisting of fibrillar, peptide-mannans which have an affinity for the fibronectin on the surface of cells. The yeast forms are responsible for tissue damage. Inhibition of yeast cell division results in hyphal elements that invade tissues. Possible virulence factors include cell wall glycoprotein, proteases, neuraminidase, chitin, mannoprotein, and lipids. The cell wall glycoproteins appear to have endotoxin-like activity. Both polymorphonuclear leukocytes and macrophages have candidacidal activity and the latter are involved when there is a granulomatous response. Both cell-mediated and humoral immunity are important defense mechanisms.

Puppies, Kittens, Calves, and Foals. Infection of the oral and intestinal mucous membrane is uncommon. Mycotic stomatitis and enteritis result, and white to gray patches representing pseudomembranous inflammation of the mucous membrane are seen. Pyothorax and cystitis in adult cats have been attributed to *C. albicans*.

Swine. Infections of the lower esophagus and esophageal region of the stomach occur. *C. albicans* may be found in stomach ulcers. Diarrhea and cutaneous candidiasis have been reported in swine.

Chickens, Turkeys, and Other Birds. Infections of the mouth, esophagus, and crop occur, with pseudomembranous whitish areas, usually in young animals. Crop mycosis (thrush) may affect a considerable number of young chickens and turkeys.

Humans. The clinical picture varies, depending on the site of infection. The mucous membranes of the mouth, tongue, and genital tract are more commonly involved than the nails and skin. The oral form (thrush), characterized by white patches, occurs frequently in infants. Respiratory tract infec-

261

tions usually involve the lungs. Occasionally endocarditis and bone infections are encountered.

Cows. Mastitis caused by *Candida* is common in cows. Genital infections are rare.

Mares. *Candida albicans* causes metritis and vaginitis.

Stallions and Bulls. Genital candidiasis is seen in stallions and bulls.

ISOLATION AND CULTIVATION

Organisms can frequently be seen in wet mounts (20% KOH, India ink, or lactophenol cotton blue) and in smears stained with Gram's stain (gram-positive), where they appear as oval, thin-walled, budding cells and hyphal fragments (pseudohyphae).

They are readily cultivated on blood agar and Sabouraud agar at 25° C and 37° C. Soft, creamy colonies resembling those of staphylococci are seen in 24 to 48 hours.

IDENTIFICATION

This is accomplished by the demonstration of the large chlamydospores (see Fig. 35–1) or germ tubes characteristic of *C. albicans*. Plates of corn meal or chlamydospore agar are inoculated by cutting into the agar at an angle to the bottom of the plate. If present, the chlamydospores can be seen below the surface in 24 to 48 hours by focusing directly on the line of inoculation.

In order to demonstrate germ tubes, a small amount of fetal bovine serum is inoculated with a light inoculum of growth. After incubation for 2 to 4 hours at 37° C, a drop from the serum sediment is examined microscopically. A germ tube is a filamentous outgrowth from the yeast cell. Unlike pseudohyphae, there is no restriction at the point of origin.

Species of *Candida* other than *C. albicans* are identified by carbohydrate fermentation and assimilation tests. These reactions are used to identify species in several commercial systems. DNA probes are also available for the identification of important species of *Candida*.

ANIMAL INOCULATION

Rabbits and mice are susceptible to intravenous and intraperitoneal inoculation, respectively. Abscesses develop in the kidneys.

SEROLOGY

A number of serologic tests are used in humans to detect *Candida* antigens. They are not used routinely in veterinary diagnostic laboratories.

TREATMENT

Nystatin (mycostatin) is used in ointments for skin infections and locally for oral and genital infections. It is administered in the feed to treat candidiasis in chickens and turkeys, and intestinal and oral candidiasis in swine, dogs, and cats. Very little of the drug is absorbed orally. It has been administered in the mammary gland to treat mastitis caused by *Candida* species.

Amphotericin B is the most effective drug for the treatment of systemic candidiasis. Flucytosine (5-fluorocytosine) has been used with some success.

Ketoconazole and clotrimazole have been effective in the treatment of mucocutaneous candidiasis in human beings.

CRYPTOCOCCOSIS (TORULOSIS)

There are at least 19 species in the genus *Cryptococcus*. Only *Cryptococcus neoformans* is considered potentially pathogenic. There are two varieties, *C. neoformans* var. *neoformans* (serotypes A and D) and *C. neoformans* var. *gattii* (serotypes B and C). *Filobasidiella neoformans* is the telemorphic state of serotypes A and D; *Filobasidiella bacillispora* is the telemorphic state of serotypes B and C. These serotypes are based on differences in capsular antigens. Their reservoir is not known.

Most strains from clinical disease in humans are types A and D. The reservoir of types A and D is the feces of birds, particularly pigeons, and soil contaminated by avian excreta. These types occur in nature and reach high concentrations in pigeon droppings and nests. The pigeon is not infected; the organisms colonize feces after they have been passed. Infections are exogenous and are usually acquired by inhalation. Primary foci are most often in the respiratory system, including the paranasal sinuses, with possible subsequent spread. Animal-to-animal transmission is not known to occur.

PATHOGENICITY

In cattle, only sporadic cases of mastitis have been reported. It is uncommon in sheep and goats.

In the dog and cat, the organisms show a predilection for the central nervous system. Infections of the pharynx and paranasal sinuses are seen, with dissemination to the CNS and other tissues including lungs, kidney, and joints. A form with subcutaneous granulomas is also seen.

In horses, it is most frequently seen as a paranasal infection, which may or may not spread to other tissues, including the brain. Abortion in a mare has also been reported.

In humans, infections involving the lungs and central nervous system (cryptococcal meningitis) are most common.

Cryptococcosis has been reported in the fox, dolphin, monkey, ferret, guinea pig, cheetah and some avian species.

The thick capsule of *C. neoformans*, which is composed mainly of polysaccharide with mannose units, is antiphagocytic and immunosuppressive. Secretion of capsular antigen into body fluids binds antibody before it reaches *C. neoformans* cells. Both humoral and cell-mediated immunity are important defense mechanisms.

DIRECT EXAMINATION

Yeast-like cells can be seen in wet mounts of cerebrospinal fluid and pus. The large capsule can be seen if clinical material is mixed with India ink or nigrosin (see Fig. 35–1). The yeast-like cells are gram-positive and can be seen in stained smears.

ISOLATION AND CULTIVATION

The organism grows at 37° C and 25° C on blood agar and Sabouraud agar; it is inhibited by cycloheximide. Wrinkled, whitish granular colonies usually appear within a week. They become slimy, mucoid, and cream to brownish in color on further incubation. Budding yeast-like cells with large capsules can be seen in wet mounts.

Most saprophytic strains of *Cryptococcus* species do not grow at 37° C.

IDENTIFICATION

Identification is based in part on cultural and morphologic characteristics, especially the presence of the large capsule (see Fig. 35–1). Members of the genus *Cryptococcus* produce urease on Christensen's urea agar, while *Candida* species do not. Several species of *Cryptococcus* possess capsules, but only *C. neoformans* produces brown colonies on bird seed agar. The latter medium, which contains *Guizotia abyssinica* seeds, can also be used as a selective medium for *C. neoformans*. The various species are identified by carbohydrate assimilation tests. Strains of the true yeast *Saccharomyces* can be distinguished from the cryptococci by the presence of ascospores in the former. The ascospores stain well with methylene blue.

Geotrichum and *Trichosporon* both produce true mycelia. The various cryptococcal species can be identified precisely by sugar and nitrate assimilation tests. Commercial kits are available for the identification of most *Cryptococcus* spp.

C. neoformans produces a unique enzyme, diphenol oxidase which is thought to be a virulence factor.

ANIMAL INOCULATION

Mice are susceptible to pathogenic strains. The routes of inoculation are intracerebral or intraperitoneal. Organisms are demonstrable in brain or lung lesions in 1 to 3 weeks.

SEROLOGY

A latex agglutination procedure is available as a test for antigen; it is not ordinarily used in animals.

Tube agglutination, complement fixation, enzyme immunoassay, and indirect fluorescent antibody tests are used in humans but infrequently in animals. False-positive and false-negative reactions are encountered.

TREATMENT

Amphotericin B and flucytosine are the drugs of choice, although imidazole derivatives such as ketoconazole, fluconazole, and itraconazole have shown some promise.

GEOTRICHOSIS

Geotrichosis caused by *Geotrichum candidum* is an uncommon disease rarely diagnosed clinically. This fungus is found widely in nature, and its isolation is not necessarily significant. Two cultural forms occur: (1) the glabrous or yeast-like form and (2) the fluffy form. The latter strains are sometimes given the name *Oospora*. The glabrous form of *G. candidum* is the one usually associated with disease.

PATHOGENICITY

Infections have been reported from cattle, pigs, horse, ocelot, dogs, fowl, and humans. They are usually identified on postmortem examination. The bronchi, lungs, udder (mastitis), and the mucous membranes of the alimentary tract are most frequently affected. The disease is usually mild and is characterized by the formation of granulomas that may suppurate. *G. candidum* is occasionally recovered from otitis externa in the dog.

DIRECT EXAMINATION

Purulent material or scrapings from lesions are examined in wet mounts. The organism appears as rectangular or spherical arthrospores. They are thick-walled, nonbudding, and in stained smears strongly gram-positive.

264 — Fungi

ISOLATION AND IDENTIFICATION

The organisms grow fairly rapidly at room temperature (25° C) on Sabouraud agar. The colonies are membranous, with radial furrows, and soft, with a dry, granular surface. The mycelium is made up of septate hyphae that fragment, producing chains of characteristic rectangular to round arthrospores (see Fig. 35–1). The organism does not grow well on blood agar at 37° C.

Differentiation from other fungi is based upon cultural and morphologic characteristics. *G. candidum* can be distinguished from *Coccidioides immitis* and *Blastomyces dermatitidis* by the fact that the latter two species produce cottony, filamentous colonies at room temperature. *G. candidum* produces a soft, yeast-like colony at room temperature. *G. candidum* does not form blastospores and this differentiates it from *Trichosporon* spp.

TREATMENT

Specific treatment is rarely administered. In vitro tests indicate susceptibility to amphotericin-B and 5-flucytosine.

MALASSEZIA (PITYROSPORUM)

Species of this genus of lipophilic yeasts are associated with the skin of humans and animals. *Malessezia furfur* causes blepharitis, folliculitis, seborrhea, dandruff, and tinea versicolor in human beings. The yeasts that have been called *Pityrosporum canis* and *P. felis* and similar organisms from other animals are now called *M. pachydermatis*.

This species occurs as a commensal on the oily areas of the skin and ears of dogs. Strains may also be recovered from the ears of cats. In some cases of otitis externa, they appear to be present in larger numbers than usual and some veterinarians think they may have etiologic significance. There are reports of chronic dermatitis in the dog caused by this organism.

Malassezia are bottle-shaped, small budding cells that reproduce by a process known as bud fission in which the bud detaches from the parent cell by the production of a septum (see Fig. 35– 1). They can be demonstrated in wet mounts (10% NaOH) of clinical material from dogs' ears. No telemorphic state has been described for this fungus.

They can be readily recovered on Sabouraud agar within 2 weeks of incubation at room temperature. Growth is increased if sterile olive or coconut oil is applied to the surface of the medium. On blood agar greenish discoloration at the site of inoc-ulation may sometimes be the only evidence of growth.

TRICHOSPORONOSIS

Trichosporonosis is caused by the soil-borne yeast *Trichosporon beigelii*. It is an imperfect fungus within the family *Cryptococcaceae* and has been recovered from various infections in animals including a nasal granuloma in a cat, skin infections in the horse and monkey, mastitis in cattle and sheep, and bladder infections in cats. This saprophytic yeast is occasionally a contaminant in clinical specimens. *Trichosporon capitatum* (new name *Blastoschizomyces capitatus*) has been implicated as a cause of bovine mastitis.

OTHER YEASTS

Torulopsis glabrata occurs as a commensal in animals and is found in soil. It has been implicated as the cause of pyelonephritis, pneumonia, septicemia, and meningitis in immunocompromised human patients; mastitis and abortion in cattle; and systemic infections in dogs and monkeys. The fungi *Rhodotorula minuta* and *R. rubra* have been recovered from the canine ear and equine uterus, and associated infrequently with infections in animals.

FURTHER READING

(Note: See also "Further Reading" for Chapter 31.)

Anderson, P.G., and Pidgeon, G.: Candidiasis in a dog with parvoviral enteritis. J. Am. Anim. Hosp. Assoc., 23:27, 1987.

Bistner, S., de Lahunta, A., and Lorenz, M.: Generalized cryptococcosis in a dog. Cornell Vet., 61:440, 1971.

Blanchard, P.C., and Filkins, M.: Cryptococcal pneumonia and abortion in an equine fetus. J. Am. Vet. Med. Assoc., 201:1591, 1992.

Blasi, E., et al.: Early differential molecular response of a macrophage cell line to yeast and hyphal forms of *Candida albicans*. Infect. Immun., 60:832, 1992.

Bowman, P.I., and Ahearn, D.G.: Evaluation of commercial systems for the identification of clinical yeast isolates. J. Clin. Microbiol., 4:49, 1976.

Carter, G.R., and Chengappa, M.M.: Microbial Diseases in North America. *In* Microbial Diseases: A Veterinarian's Guide to Laboratory Diagnosis. Ames, Iowa State University Press, 1993.

Chengappa, M.M., et al.: Isolation and identification of yeasts from clinical veterinary sources. J. Clin. Microbiol., 19:427, 1984.

Chute, H.L., and Richard, J.L.: Fungal infections. *In* Diseases of Poultry. 9th Ed. Edited by B.W. Calnek, et al. Ames, Iowa State University Press, 1991.

Doster, A.R., et al.: Trichosporonosis in two cats. J. Am. Vet. Med. Assoc., 190:1184, 1987.

Dufait, R.: *Pityrosporon canis* as the cause of canine chronic dermatitis. Vet. Med. Sm. Anim. Clinician, 78:1055, 1983.

Foley, G.L., and Schlafer, D.H.: Candida abortion in cattle. Vet. Pathol., 24:532, 1987.

Fulton, R.B., and Walker, R.D.: *Candida albicans* urocystitis in a cat. J. Am. Vet. Med. Assoc., *200*:524, 1992.

Gedek, B., et al.: The role of *Pityrosporum pachydermatis* in otitis externa of dogs. Evaluation of a treatment with miconazole. Vet. Rec., *104*:138, 1979.

Gross, T.L., and Mayhew, I.G.: Gastroesophageal ulceration and candidiasis in foals. J. Am. Vet. Med. Assoc., *182*:1370, 1983.

Hodgin, E.C., Corstvet, R.E., and Blakewood, B.W.: Cryptococcosis in a pup. J. Am. Vet. Med. Assoc., *191*:697, 1987.

Jergens, A.E., Wheeler, C.A., and Collier, L.L.: Cryptococcosis involving the eye and central nervous system of a dog. J. Am. Vet. Med. Assoc., *189*:302, 1986.

Kadel, W.L., Kelley, D.C., and Coles, E.H.: Survey of yeast-like fungi and tissue changes in esophagogastric region of stomachs of swine. Am. J. Vet. Res., *30*:401, 1969.

McCaw, D., et al.: Pyothorax caused by *Candida albicans* in a cat. J. Am. Vet. Med. Assoc., *185*:311, 1984.

Plant, J.D., Rosenkrantz, W.S., and Griffin, C.E.: Factors associated with and prevalence of high *Malassezia pachydermatis* numbers on dog skin. J. Am. Vet. Med. Assoc. *201*:879, 1992.

Rhyan, J.C., Stackhouse, L.L., and Davis, E.G.: Disseminated geotrichosis in two dogs. J. Am. Vet. Med. Assoc., *197*:358, 1990.

Warren, N.G., and Shadomy, H.J.: Yeast of medical importance. *In* Manual of Clinical Microbiology. 5th Ed. Edited by E.H. Lennette, et al. Washington, D.C., American Society for Microbiology, 1991.

34

Subcutaneous Mycoses

There is some confusion in the names used for several of the fungous diseases discussed in this chapter. We have employed the names used by Rippon (see Further Reading).

SPOROTRICHOSIS

Sporotrichosis is caused by *Sporothrix schenckii*, a dimorphic fungus that occurs in nature and is associated with soil, wood, and vegetation. Infections are exogenous and worldwide in distribution. The portal of entry is usually wounds.

PATHOGENICITY

Infections in humans and some animals are characterized by the formation of subcutaneous nodules or pyogranulomas. The organisms usually enter through wounds in the skin, and spread via the lymphatics. The nodules eventually ulcerate and discharge pus. Involvement of bones, joints, and visceral organs with fatal termination is rare but has been reported in the dog, cat, and horse. Infections have been described in humans and in the dog, cat, horse, donkey, mule, camel, cattle, fowl, and rodents. In practice the disease occurs most commonly in the horse in which it is seen most frequently as an ascending lymphocutaneous infection of the leg. Proteases are possible virulence factors of *S. schenckii*.

DIRECT EXAMINATION

In pus and tissue the organism appears as a single-celled cigar-shaped body, usually within neutrophils. These structures (yeast phase) are very difficult to demonstrate in stained smears and wet mounts of pus and tissue scrapings except in feline specimens which contain numerous yeast cells. Fluorescent antibody, Periodic acid-schiff, and Calcofluor White staining of clinical materials frequently yields positive results. Characteristic "asteroid bodies" consisting of clusters of yeast cells with peripheral eosinophilic rays are seen in tissue sections.

ISOLATION, CULTIVATION, AND IDENTIFICATION

Sporothrix schenckii is readily grown on brain heart infusion agar, blood agar (37° C), and Sabouraud agar with cycloheximide and chloramphenicol (25° to 27° C) in 1 to 3 weeks.

Tissue Phase. At 37° C, colonies appear in 3 to 5 days. They are yeast-like, smooth, soft, and cream to tan color.

There is no mycelium. Colonies are composed of the same elements that occur in pus and tissue, i.e., cigar-shaped cells and spherical or oval budding cells. Some large pyriform cells may also be seen (Table 34–1)

Mycelial Phase. At 25° to 27° C colonies appear early, but the characteristic structures are not evident until the aerial mycelium is produced. Colonies are white and soft at first, and then become tan to brown to black. The texture is leathery, wrinkled, and coarsely tufted.

The mycelium consists of fine, branching septate hyphae that bear pyriform or ovoid microconidia, which are borne in clusters from the ends of conidiophores or as sessile forms directly on the sides

266

Table 34–1 Morphologic Elements of Important Dimorphic Fungi

	Growth in tissues at 37°C	Growth on blood agar at 37°C	Growth on Sabouraud's at 25°C
Sporothrix schenckii	Cigar bodies	Yeast cells	Hyphae, microconidia in "flowerette" arrangement
Blastomyces dermatitidis	Yeast cells	Yeast cells	Hyphae, chlamydospores
Histoplasma capsulatum	Small, intracellular yeast cells with a dark central area	Yeast cells	Tuberculate chlamydospores
Coccidioides immitis	Intra- or extracellular spherules containing round endospores	Hyphae, arthrospores with collarettes	Hyphae, arthrospores with collarettes

of hyphae (see Table 34–1). Thick-walled, large, chlamydospores may be seen in old cultures.

The mold phase of *S. schenckii* can be converted to the yeast phase by subculturing the former from Sabouraud agar to brain heart infusion agar with 10% blood. The latter is incubated for 3 to 5 days at 37° C in 5% CO_2.

ANIMAL INOCULATION

Mice are susceptible. Suspected material or cultures are inoculated intraperitoneally. The mice are sacrificed in 3 weeks and if infected, cigar-shaped bodies can be seen in smears from the peritoneal exudate and granulomata.

SEROLOGY

A latex agglutination test and a tube agglutination test are used to detect antibodies in humans. The immunodiffusion test is reliable and easy to perform.

TREATMENT

Potassium iodide is administered orally to the point of producing iodinism. It is continued for several weeks after apparent recovery in order to

prevent recrudescence. Other drugs that have been useful are amphotericin B and 5-fluorocytosine. Itraconazole and fluconazole have been effective experimentally.

PHAEOHYPHOMYCOSIS (CHROMOMYCOSIS)

This name denotes infrequent opportunistic fungal infections of humans, dogs, and horses caused by a wide variety of dematiaceous fungi. The infections, which are characterized by the presence of brown pigmented fungal elements in tissue, begin in wounds or abrasions, result in nodular and frequently ulcerating lesions of the skin of the feet and legs, with regional granulomatous lymphadenitis. Ocular infections and systemic disease in turkeys have been reported. The following species of fungi have been incriminated in animals: *Bipolaris* spp. *Dactylaria gallopava, Exophiala pisciphila, E. salmonis, Scolecobasidium humicola, S. tshawytschae, Drechslera* spp., *Exophilia jeanselmei, E. verrucosa,* and *Fonsecaea pelrosoi.* Many fungi have been implicated in the human disease and no doubt additional fungi may cause phaeohyphomycosis in animals.

DIRECT EXAMINATION

Material from granulomatous or ulcerous lesions is examined in 10% sodium hydroxide. Organisms are single-celled or clustered, spherical, and thick-walled, with a black or dark brown pigment. They multiply by cross-wall formation or splitting rather than budding.

ISOLATION AND CULTIVATION

The organisms will grow on Sabouraud agar at room temperature. Growth is slow, requiring up to a month.

IDENTIFICATION

Identification of the genus is usually not difficult. The aid of a specialist may be required to identify the species.

TREATMENT

Surgical excision may be helpful. Amphotericin B (locally or systemically), thiabendazole, and 5-fluorocytosine have been used in humans; they have not been adequately tested in animals.

PYTHIOSIS (MYCOTIC SWAMP CANCER, FLORIDA HORSE LEECHES, OOMYCOSIS)

This disease was originally called phycomycosis. It is seen mainly in tropical and subtropical areas including Australia, New Guinea, India, Brazil, Colombia, Central America, Japan, and Indonesia; several cases have been reported in southern United States.

It is a chronic skin disease of horses, cattle, and dogs caused by the fungus, *Pythium insidiosum* (formerly called *Hyphomyces destruens*). It gains entrance via wounds involving the hoof, hock, fetlock, head, neck, or lips. There is a pyo- or fibrogranulomatous reaction, with necrosis and the formation of fistulous tracts. Masses of branching, sparsely septated fungi are seen in the yellow necrotic lesions. The disease is progressive but not usually systemic, and there have been no remissions reported in the absence of treatment, which involves radical surgery and administration of amphotericin B.

Direct examination of smears, fresh affected tissue including biopsies, and histopathologic examination of affected tissue may suggest a diagnosis of pithiosis. However, definitive diagnosis requires the isolation and identification of the causal fungus. The presence of characteristic zoospores in cultures will suggest *P. insidosum*. Final identification may require the aid of a mycologist.

An immunodiffusion test is available in some reference laboratories.

EUMYCOTIC MYCETOMA

Eumycotic mycetomas (subcutaneous mycotic abscesses) consist of granulomatous processes produced by a number of species of fungi. According to Rippon the term mycetoma is defined by the triad, tumefaction, draining sinuses and grains. Microcolonies (grains or granules) that frequently are pigmented can sometimes be seen grossly in lesions and exudate. There have been several reports of these infrequent infections in horses, cattle, dogs, and cats. The lesions occur most commonly on the extremities but may also be found involving the nasal mucosa (e.g., bovine nasal granuloma), the peritoneum, and the skin in various locations.

The following species of fungi have been recovered: *Pseudoallescheria boydii, Curvularia geniculata, Cochliobolus spicifer, Madurella mycetomatis,* and *Helminthosporium* spp. These fungi occur in soil and are implanted via wounds.

Incision of the lesions in the case of the dematiaceous fungi reveals discrete brown or black fungal microcolonies embedded in a large mass of granulation tissue.

The first species mentioned above is a "hyaline" nonpigmented fungus, whereas the others are dematiaceous (black or brown pigment) fungi. The first grows rapidly, whereas the others require several weeks. Some additional species and genera have been recovered from human eumycotic mycetomas.

DIRECT EXAMINATION

Scrapings or biopsy tissue are examined grossly for the characteristic microcolonies, which are small (0.5 to 3.0 mm), irregularly shaped, and variously colored. These colonies or "grains" are placed in 10% sodium hydroxide and then pressed out by means of a coverslip and observed microscopically. The grains of maduromycosis reveal mycelia that are usually 2 to 4 μm in width in contrast to the narrower filaments found in the actinomycotic granule. Also of significance is the presence of chlamydospores in the grains.

ISOLATION, CULTIVATION, AND IDENTIFICATION

The species involved grow readily but slowly (two to three weeks) on Sabouraud agar at room temperature. Identification is based upon cultural characteristics and microscopic morphology. Cultures are usually submitted to a mycology laboratory for confirmation of identification.

TREATMENT

Excision of the lesion may effect a cure. Amphotericin B, 5-fluorocytosine, iodides, thiabendazole, and ketoconazole have been effective in some cases.

CHROMOBLASTOMYCOSIS

Chromoblastomycosis occurs in horses, dogs, cats, and humans, but only a small number of cases have been reported in animals. Some of the animal infections reported earlier as chromoblastomycosis were probably phaeohyphomycosis. The fungi enter tissues at the site of some trauma or wound and are generally limited to cutaneous and subcutaneous tissue. There is a hyperplasia with formation of verrucoid, warty cutaneous nodules. The latter are irregular, vegetative, and sometimes pedunculated. Lymphatics may be involved and occasionally there is dissemination to other tissues and organs. The disease is chronic and if not treated it persists and frequently progresses.

The dematiaceous fungi that have been most often implicated are *Fonsecaea pedrosoi, Fonsecaea compacta, Cladosporium carrionii,* and *Phialophora verrucosa.*

Definitive diagnosis is based upon the demonstration of the fungi in tissues and their isolation and identification. Cultures are usually submitted to a mycology laboratory for confirmation of identification.

Treatment is essentially the same as for eumycotic mycetoma.

HYPHOMYCOSIS

This is an uncommon opportunistic fungous disease of animals and humans caused by species of the genera *Penicillium, Beauveria, Acremonium, Fusarium,* and *Paecilomyces.* Many additional fungi have been recovered from human hyphomycosis.

A wide variety of infections have been reported in humans and to a lesser extent in animals. Among the many predisposing causes of these infections are trauma and neoplastic conditions. Infections may be localized or systemic.

Definitive diagnosis requires the isolation and identification of the fungus. Media containing antibacterial agents are helpful in the isolation of these fungi.

EPIZOOTIC LYMPHANGITIS (EQUINE PSEUDOGLANDERS, AFRICAN GLANDERS)

This disease is caused by *Histoplasma farciminosum (Cryptococcus farciminosum).* It occurs in horses, mules, and donkeys in parts of Europe, Africa, and Asia. Although this organism does not correctly belong in the genus *Histoplasma* it has been placed there because its morphology and life cycle are similar to *H. capsulatum.*

PATHOGENICITY

H. farciminosum causes a chronic disease involving the lymph nodes, superficial lymph vessels, and skin mainly of the limbs, back, and neck. It is characterized by the formation of suppurative nodular, ulcerating lesions along the lymphatics of the legs. More than 90% of cases are reported from horses. A pulmonary form has also been described as well as disseminated disease. The mortality rate can reach 15% in fully susceptible animals. Although the organism may occur in nature, most cases are considered to derive from other infected animals. As yet, the natural habitat, other than the horse, is not known. The organism gains entrance via wounds and abrasions. Though rare, respiratory, conjunctival, and gastrointestinal infections have been reported.

DEMONSTRATION AND CULTIVATION

The oval or pear-shaped cells can be seen in pus from fresh lesions. A diagnosis is usually made by demonstration of the characteristic double-contoured yeast cells in wet mounts from typical lesions. The organism is dimorphic, growing in the mycelial phase at room temperature and in the yeast phase at 37° C. Growth of the two phases is often slow, taking up to 8 weeks. Yeast-like cells with some hyphae are seen at 37° C. At room temperature hyphae yield characteristic thick-walled chlamydospores.

An enzyme-linked immunosorbent assay has been developed recently which is claimed to be specific for *H. farciminosum.* Specific antibodies are demonstrable by the indirect fluorescent-antibody test and the presence of antibodies is indicative of infection.

TREATMENT

Iodides orally, and local application of iodine and silver nitrate are reported to be effective. Modern antifungal drugs have not been adequately tested.

RHINOSPORIDIOSIS

The agent that is considered the cause of this disease is *Rhinosporidium seeberi*, a fungus presumed to occur in nature (water), but which has not been cultivated as yet on artificial media; it has been propagated in cell culture.

PATHOGENICITY

R. seeberi causes a chronic, generally benign disease of cattle, horses, mules, dogs, and humans characterized by the formation of polyps on the nasal and ocular mucous membranes. More than 90% of the nasal cases involve male animals. The disease occurs mostly in tropical and subtropical countries. Several cases of the infection have been reported in dogs in the United States.

DIRECT EXAMINATION

Wet mounts from nasal discharge and sections from polyps disclose large sporangia (200 to 300 μm) that contain thousands of endospores. The latter are released when the sporangia rupture. Sporangia develop in tissue from small, globose spores. Typical sporangia are seen in stained sections of biopsy specimens.

TREATMENT

Surgical excision of polyps.

FURTHER READING

(Note: See also "Further Reading" for Chapter 31.)

Allison, N., and Gillis, J.P.: Enteric pythiosis in a horse. J. Am. Vet. Med. Assoc., *196*:462, 1990.

Austwick, P.K.C., and Copland, J.W.: Swamp cancer. Nature, *250*:84, 1974.

Brearley, J.C., et al.: Nasal granuloma caused by *Pseudoallescheria boydii*. Equine Vet. J., *18*:151, 1986.

Bridges, C.H., and Beasley, J.N.: Maduromycotic mycetomas. J. Am. Vet. Med. Assoc., *137*:192, 1960.

Carter, G.R., and Chengappa, M.M.: Microbial Diseases in North America. *In* Microbial Diseases: A Veterinarian's Guide to Laboratory Diagnosis. Ames, Iowa State University Press, 1993.

Davis, H.H., and Worthington, W.E.: Equine sporotrichosis. J. Am. Vet. Med. Assoc., *151*:45, 1964.

Kier, A.B., Mann, P.C., and Wagner, J.E.: Disseminated sporotrichosis in a cat. J. Am. Vet. Med. Assoc., *175*:202, 1979.

Knudtson, W.U., and Kirkbride, C.A.: Fungi associated with bovine abortions in the northern plains states (USA). J. Vet. Diagn. Invest., *4*:181, 1992.

Kurtz, H.J., Finco, D.R., and Perman, V.: Maduromycosis (*Allescheria boydii*) in a dog. J. Am. Vet. Med. Assoc., *157*:917, 1970.

Londerno, A.T., et al.: Two cases of sporotrichosis in dogs in Brazil. Sabouraudia, *3*:273, 1964.

McGinnis, M.R., et al.: Dematiaceous fungi. *In* Manual of Clinical Microbiology. 5th Ed. Edited by E.H. Lennette, et al. Washington, D.C., American Society for Microbiology, 1991.

Mendoza, L., Kaufam, L., and Standard, P.: Antigenic relationship between animal and human pathogen *Pythium insidiosum* and nonpathogenic *Pythium* species. J. Clin. Microbiol., *25*:2159, 1987.

Myers, D.D., Simon, J., and Case, M.T.: Rhinosporidiosis in a horse. J. Am. Vet. Med. Assoc., *145*:345, 1964.

Refai, M., and Loot, A.: The incidence of epizootic lymphangitis in Egypt. Mykosen, *13*:247, 1970.

Rippon, J.W.: Medical Mycology. 3rd Ed. Philadelphia, W.B. Saunders Company, 1988.

Salkin, I.F., et al.: *Scedosporium inflatum* osteomyelitis in a dog. J. Clin. Microbiol. *30*:2797, 1992.

Singh, T.: Studies on epizootic lymphangitis: Study of clinical cases and experimental transmission. Indian J. Vet. Sci., *36*:45, 1966.

Sisk, D.B., and Chandler, F.W.: Phaeohyphomycosis and cryptococcosis in a cat. Vet. Path., *19*:554, 1982.

Smith, J.M.B.: Opportunistic Mycoses of Man and Other Animals. Wallingford, England, CAB International Mycological Institute, 1989.

Stuart, B.P.: Rhinosporidiosis in a dog. J. Am. Vet. Med. Assoc., *167*:941, 1975.

35

Systemic Mycoses

ZYGOMYCOSIS (MUCORMYCOSIS)

Zygomycosis denotes human and animal disease caused by members of the order Mucorales. Earlier names for zygomycosis were mucormycosis, hyphomycosis, and phycomycosis. Zygomycosis is caused by species of *Mucor, Absidia, Rhizopus,* and *Mortierella.* Strains of these genera occur widely in nature.

PATHOGENICITY

The mode of infection is by inhalation or ingestion.

These fungi occasionally infect lymph nodes of the respiratory and alimentary tracts. Lesions are granulomatous and occasionally ulcerative; they are usually localized but may be generalized. Lymph nodes enlarge and become caseocalcareous. Ulceration of stomach and intestines has been attributed to zygomycosis.

Pigs. Lesions are found in mediastinal and submandibular lymph nodes; embolic "tumors" are seen in the liver and lungs. Fungi of this group may be found in gastric ulcers.

Cattle. Lesions are found in the bronchial, mesenteric, and mediastinal lymph nodes; there may be nasal and abomasal ulcers. Abortions are attributed to these fungi. However, it should be kept in mind that placentas are frequently contaminated by some fungi of these genera.

Horses. There are several reports of zygomycosis in this species.

Infections have also been reported in dogs, cats, sheep, mink, guinea pigs, and mice.

The pathogenicity of several specific fungi follows:

Rhizomucor and *Mucor*

Mucor circinelloides has been isolated only rarely from animals.

Rhizomucor pusillus (*M. pusillus*) and *R. meihi* are recognized as pathogenic for animals.

Absidia

Absidia corymbifera is the only pathogenic species recognized in this genus. Most zygomycosis in pigs and cattle are caused by this species.

Rhizopus

The species *R. arrhizus, R. microsporus* and *R. rhizopodoformis* have been reported as causing zygomycosis in animals.

Mortierella

Mortierella wolfii is an important cause of bovine abortion (mycotic placentitis) which is sometimes followed by acute pneumonia and death. *Mortierella hygrophila* and *M. polycephala* have been recovered from zygomycosis in fowl and cattle respectively.

DIRECT EXAMINATION

Fragments and pieces of coarse, nonseptate, branching hyphae are seen. The coarseness or thickness of the pieces is especially significant. These infections are frequently detected in stained tissue sections.

ISOLATION AND CULTIVATION

Fungi of this group grow rapidly at room temperature on Sabouraud agar. Because they are common contaminants, isolation alone is not necessarily considered significant. Repeated isolation, characteristic lesions, and the presence of fungal elements in sections indicate significance.

IDENTIFICATION

All have round sporangia borne on sporangiophores; sporangia contain numerous sporangiospores.

Identification of species may require the aid of a mycologist.

Rhizomucor **species.** These fungi produce a thick, gray mycelium with few if any rhizoids. Sporangiophores are short with black, spherical sporangia.

Mucor **species.** They have thick, colorless mycelium without rhizoids. Sporangiophores are simple or branched, and globose sporangia contain small spores (see Figure 35–1).

Absidia **species.** In this genus the sporangiophores do not arise from the stolons opposite the rhizoids as in *Rhizopus*. However, *Absidia* resemble *Rhizopus* species grossly (Fig. 35–1).

Rhizopus **species.** They have dense, cottony, aerial mycelium that are first white and then turn grey. Sporangiophores arise from the stolons where stolons contact the medium through rhizoids (see Fig. 35–1).

Mortierella **species** *M. wolfii* grows on blood agar and Sabouraud agar at 25° to 27° C and 37° C. The colonies on Sabouraud and blood agars are white, velvety, dense, and characteristically lobulated. The hyphae are hyaline, and sporangia are produced on special media. Definitive identification is based on the morphology of the sporangia and spores.

TREATMENT

Amphotericin B is the preferred drug. Surgical measures may be indicated.

ENTOMOPHTHOROMYCOSIS (BASIDIOBOLOMYCOSIS)

This disease, which affects many animal species, resembles zygomycosis and is caused by fungi in the genera *Basidiobolus* and *Conidiobolus*. These fungi differ somewhat from those in the order *Mucorales* discussed above. *B. ranarum* and *C. coronatus* cause ulcerative granulomas involving subcutaneous tissues and oral and nasal mucous membranes of the mouth and nasal passages. Lesions caused by *B. ranarum* may be large and involve the skin of the head, neck, and chest. There may be fistulous tracts with extension to lymph nodes.

Unlike the *Mucorales*, these fungi produce colonies that are flat and waxy, which later become fuzzy and white. The hyphae are septate and the characteristic conidia and sporangia are used in identification. Final identification is usually made by a mycologist.

Surgical excision and treatment with amphotericin B or ketoconazole have been effective.

ASPERGILLOSIS

The most prevalent pathogenic species of *Aspergillus* is *A. fumigatus*. Other potentially pathogenic species are *A. flavus, A. nidulans,* and possibly *A. niger* and *A. terreus*. Species of *Aspergillus* are widely found in nature and are common contaminants in the laboratory.

PATHOGENICITY

Several manifestations of aspergillosis are seen in chickens, turkeys, and other wild and domestic avian species including penguins in captivity: (1) a diffuse infection of the air sacs; (2) a diffuse pneumonic form; and (3) a nodular form involving the lungs. The disease is called "brooder pneumonia" in chicks and poults; many birds may be affected. The spores are acquired by inhalation from the fungi growing on feed or litter. The principal gross lesion consists of yellow nodules found in the lungs and air sacs.

Cattle. Infections involve the uterus, fetal membranes, and fetal skin, and on occasion result in abortion. Aspergilli occasionally cause bovine mastitis and ocular infections, and diarrhea in calves.

Horses. Infection causes abortion, keratomycosis, occasionally pulmonary aspergillosis, and guttural pouch mycosis mainly in stabled horses.

Other Animals (Including Dogs, Cats, and Sheep). Infrequent infections occur, most often involving the lungs. Nasal aspergillosis is an important disease of dogs. Disseminated aspergillosis with multiple granulomas and infarcts has been reported in dogs. Pulmonary and intestinal aspergillosis occurs infrequently in cats.

Humans. Primary and secondary infections occur in a wide variety of tissues and locations: lungs, skin, nasal sinuses, external ear, bronchi, bones, and meninges. Infections occur most frequently in immunocompromised patients.

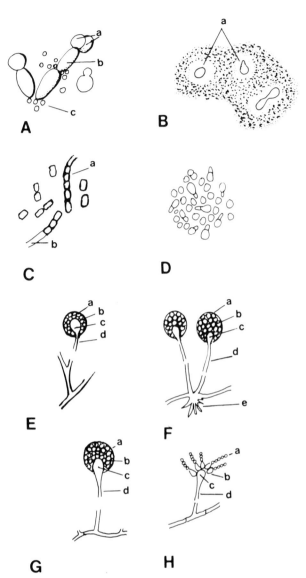

Figure 35–1. A, *Candida albicans:* a. chlamydospore, b. pseudohypha, c. blastospores. B, *Cryptococcus neoformans,* India ink preparation: a. large capsules. C, *Geotrichum candidum:* a. arthrospores, b. hypha. D, *Malassezia (Pityrosporum):* yeast cells showing budding (bottle-shaped). E, *Mucor:* a. sporangium, b. sporangiospores, c. columnella, d. sporangiophore. F, *Rhizopus:* a. sporangium, b. sporangiospores, c. columnella, d. sporangiophore, e. rhizoids. G, *Absidia:* same basic structure as *Mucor.* H, *Aspergillus:* a. conidia, b. sterigmata, c. vesicle, d. conidiophore.

DIRECT EXAMINATION

Small pieces of tissue or deep scrapings are examined in 10% sodium hydroxide. Short pieces of thick, septate hyphae are characteristic. The typical conidial heads are seen only in the lungs and air sacs, where there is access to oxygen.

ISOLATION AND CULTIVATION

Aspergilli grow rapidly on blood and Sabouraud agars at room and incubator temperatures. Colonies are white at first but later turn green to dark green, flat, and velvety. Colony color varies with different species.

IDENTIFICATION

The genus is identified by the presence of the conidiophores with large terminal vesicles bearing sterigmata from which chains of spores or conidia

are produced (see Fig. 35–1). The vesicle of *A. fumigatus* is flask-shaped whereas that of *A. flavus* is globose. Identification of species is based upon colony and microscopic morphology. The assistance of a mycologist may be required for definitive identification.

Because *Aspergillus* occur widely as contaminants repeated isolation or histological demonstration may be required for diagnosis.

SEROLOGY

An agar gel immunodiffusion test has been of value in the diagnosis of nasal aspergillosis in dogs.

TREATMENT

Surgery and drug treatment are used in nasal aspergillosis and guttural pouch mycosis. Ketoconazole, nystatin, amphotericin B, 5-fluorocytosine, and thiabendazole have been used. Avian aspergillosis is not usually treated.

BLASTOMYCOSIS (NORTH AMERICAN)

The causative agent, *Blastomyces dermatitidis*, probably occurs in the soil but its natural habitat has not yet been determined. Blastomycosis is widespread, and in the United States it is most common in the north-central and southeastern states.

PATHOGENICITY

The mode of infection is usually via the respiratory tract, and the initial lesions are found in the lung. Infection via wounds is rare. The disease is characterized by the formation of granulomatous nodules and occurs principally in humans and dogs. It has also been described in the horse, cat, dolphin, ferret, and sea lion, but it is uncommon in these animals. In dogs the lesions are usually found in the lungs and on the skin. Skin lesions and generalized blastomycosis result from hematogenous dissemination from the original pulmonary lesions. The fungus can usually be demonstrated and recovered from all lesions including those involving bone, eyes, brain, and genitalia. Unless treated, the disseminated disease terminates in death. The skin lesions, which are circumscribed and granulomatous, may ulcerate.

DIRECT EXAMINATION

The large, spherical, thick-walled cells (5 to 20 μm in diameter) are readily demonstrable in wet mounts. A single bud connected to the larger mother cell by a wide base is frequently seen. Some cells give a double contoured effect.

ISOLATION, CULTIVATION, AND IDENTIFICATION

The organism grows slowly at 25° C and 37° C on Sabouraud agar and blood agar, respectively.

On Sabouraud agar at 25° C, a moist, greyish, yeast-like colony is seen that develops a white cottony mycelium. As it ages, it becomes tan to dark brown to black. The septate hyphae bear small, oval, or pyriform conidia laterally, close to the point of septation. Older cultures form chlamydospores with thickened walls (see Table 34–1).

On blood agar at 37° C, creamy, waxy, wrinkled colonies, cream to tan in color, are observed. Thick-walled budding yeast cells similar to those in tissue sections and exudate are seen (see Table 34–1).

The sexual or teleomorphic form has been described and is named *Ajellomyces dermatitidis*.

ANIMAL INOCULATION

Guinea pigs, mice, rats, and hamsters can be infected by intraperitoneal inoculation. They usually die within 3 weeks. Yeast-like cells are demonstrable in the peritoneal exudate and nodules.

SEROLOGY

The complement fixation test can be of value; rising titers are significant. A positive immunodiffusion test indicates recent or current infection. Falling antibody titers during the course of the disease indicates a poor prognosis. An ELISA test and counterimmunoelectrophoresis using a commercially available antigen have been effective in diagnosis.

TREATMENT

Amphotericin B is preferred for severe cases. The disseminated disease does not usually respond to treatment. Ketaconazole has been used effectively in human beings and dogs.

HISTOPLASMOSIS

Histoplasmosis is caused by *Histoplasma capsulatum*, a dimorphic fungus that is found in soil and on decaying vegetation. A heavy concentration has been encountered in soils containing the feces of bats and birds, e.g., starlings and pigeons. Infection is exogenous, usually by inhalation and less frequently by ingestion. Apparently, soil with avian and bat feces, i.e., with a high nitrogen content, provides a favorable milieu for multiplication. It only occurs passively in the intestines of live birds. There are many subclinical, transient infections. The heaviest concentration of infections in the United States is in the northeast, central, and south-central states. The disease is worldwide in distribution.

PATHOGENICITY

Clinical histoplasmosis is a generalized disease involving the reticuloendothelial system. The mode of infection is usually via inhalation with primary infection of the respiratory tract. Infection via wounds or ingestion is rare. Infections have been reported from dogs, cattle, nonhuman primates, cats, horses, sheep, swine, humans, and various wild animals. Some of the lesions seen in dogs and cats are ulcerations of the intestinal tract; enlargement of the liver, spleen, and lymph nodes; and necrosis and tubercle-like lesions in the lungs, liver, kidneys, and spleen. Acute and chronic forms are seen. Although the clinical disease is generalized, it usually assumes either a predominantly pulmonary or an intestinal form in animals. Osteomyelitis in cats caused by *H. capsulatum* has been reported in the United States.

DIRECT EXAMINATION

Because *H. capsulatum* is small and rarely found extracellularly, it is extremely difficult to demonstrate in clinical materials. Smears are made from scrapings of ulcers, from cut surfaces of lymph nodes, from biopsies, and from material from sternal puncture and buffy coat. They are stained by the Giemsa or Wright method and examined under oil immersion objective. The organisms occur intracellularly (mononuclear cells) as small, round or oval, yeast-like, single, or budding cells. A clear halo is seen around the darker staining central material. The characteristic small yeast cells can be seen in the cytoplasm of macrophages in stained sections of affected tissues. Fluorescent antibody staining has been used to identify the organism in cultures and clinical specimens.

ISOLATION, CULTIVATION, AND IDENTIFICATION

On Sabouraud agar at 25° C colonies are cottony white to cream at first, later becoming tan to brown. Two kinds of spores are borne on the septate hyphae: (1) small, smooth, round to pyriform microconidia, either on short lateral branches or attached directly by the base; and (2) small and large macroconidia or chlamydospores (7 to 18 μm in diameter) that are round, thick-walled, and may be covered with knob-like projections (tuberculate chlamydospores) (see Table 34–1).

On blood agar at 37° C colonies are small, white, and yeast-like and yield yeast-like cells (see Table 34–1).

ANIMAL INOCULATION

This organism can be recovered from contaminated specimens by mouse inoculation. The route of inoculation is intraperitoneal and infection develops within 2 to 4 weeks. The organism (yeast phase) is cultured from spleen and liver of successfully infected mice, and demonstrated in tissue sections. The mycelial phase of cultures can be converted to the yeast phase by mouse infection.

SEROLOGY

The complement fixation test is useful; rising titers are significant; titers disappear after about 9 months. The immunodiffusion test and counterimmunoelectrophoresis are useful. They are interpreted according to the antigen being used. The skin test is of little value in diagnosis as it may only indicate exposure.

TREATMENT

Amphotericin B is the preferred drug. The azoles, miconazole, ketoconazole and itraconazole are of value. The prognosis in acute and disseminated histoplasmosis is poor.

COCCIDIOIDOMYCOSIS

The causative agent of coccidioidomycosis is *Coccidioides immitis*. It occurs widely in the soil of certain arid areas of the southwestern United States and South America. Its occurrence is infrequent outside the Americas. There are many subclinical, transient infections in humans and animals. The mode of infection is by inhalation.

PATHOGENICITY

The disease is characterized by the formation of nodules or granulomas. The disease is usually minimal and localized. It has been encountered in humans, cattle, sheep, dogs, cats, primates, horses, swine, and various wild animals. The gross lesions in cattle resemble tuberculosis and are usually seen in the bronchial and mediastinal lymph nodes and less frequently in the lungs. Lesions have been found in the lungs, brain, liver, spleen, bones, and kidneys of dogs. Disseminated, progressive disease occurs most frequently in primates and dogs. Abortion and infrequent disseminated infections have been reported in horses.

DIRECT EXAMINATION

In unstained wet mounts the organisms are seen as nonbudding, thick-walled sporangia having diameters varying from 10 to 80 μm. These large sporangia or spherules contain numerous endospores 2 to 5 μm in diameter. The large sporangia burst releasing the endospores and leaving "ghost" spherules.

ISOLATION AND IDENTIFICATION

Caution: C. immitis is highly infectious. It grows readily in 1 to 2 weeks at 25° C and 37° C on Sabouraud and blood agars, respectively. Colonies are flat, moist, and membranous at both temperatures, later developing a coarse, cottony, aerial mycelium, the color of which varies from white to brown. The tissue phase is not seen on artificial media unless a special spherule medium is used with incubation at 40° C. The yeast form can be obtained by inoculating cultures into mice (see Table 34–1).

When stained by lactose phenol cotton blue the culture shows branching septate mycelia that form chains of thick-walled, barrel-shaped arthrospores (2 to 3 μm long) separated by clear spaces, the remnants of empty cells.

ANIMAL INOCULATION

The mouse is inoculated intraperitoneally, and spherules are demonstrable in smears and wet mounts from the peritoneum and various organs 7 to 10 days postinoculation.

SEROLOGY

The complement fixation test is useful; rising titers are significant. Other serologic procedures that have been found useful are immunodiffusion, the tube precipitin test and the latex agglutination test. A positive skin test indicates exposure.

TREATMENT

Amphotericin B is the preferred drug. The imidazole compounds including ketoconazole, fluconazole, and triazole have been effective.

ADIASPIROMYCOSIS (HAPLOMYCOSIS)

Chrysosporium parvum and *C. crescens* cause respiratory infection in many species of rodents and other wild mammals, including insectivores, herbivores, and carnivores. They are soil-borne fungi and infection is caused by inhalation of conidia that do not replicate in vivo; however, the conidia grow to form spherules which do not form endospores. The disease has been reported in humans and in a dog but is probably rare.

Diagnosis is based upon the demonstration of the spherules and conidia in tissue sections and isolation and identification of the fungus on culture media.

This dimorphic fungus grows on blood agar at 37° C and on Sabouraud agar at room temperature. It has a mycelial phase at 25° C, and adiaconidia (yeast form) are produced at 37° C. Additional characteristics for definitive identification are provided in the references.

FURTHER READING

(Note: See also "Further Reading" for Chapter 31.)

Barsanti, J.A., Attleberger, M.H., and Henderson, R.A.: Phycomycosis in a dog. J. Am. Vet. Med. Assoc., *167*:293, 1975.

Breider, M.A., et al.: Blastomycosis in cats: Five cases (1979–1986). J. Am. Vet. Med. Assoc., *193*:570, 1988.

Bridges, C.H., and Emmons, C.W.: A phycomycosis of horses caused by *Hyphomyces destruens*. J. Am. Vet. Med. Assoc., *138*:579, 1961.

Brodey, R.S., et al.: Disseminated coccidioidomycosis in a dog. J. Am. Vet. Med. Assoc., *157*:926, 1970.

Cates, M.B., et al.: Blastomycosis in an Atlantic bottlenose dolphin. J. Am. Vet. Med. Assoc., *189*:1148, 1986.

Cook, W.R., Campbell, R.S.F., and Dawson, C.: The pathology and etiology of gutteral pouch mycosis in the horse. Vet. Rec., *83*:422, 1968.

Cordes, D.O., Dodd, D.C., and O'Hara, P.J. Bovine mycotic abortion. N. Z. Vet. J., *12*:95, 1967.

Dallman, M.J., et al.: Disseminated aspergillosis in a dog with diskospondylitis and neurologic deficits. J. Am. Vet. Med. Assoc., *200*:511, 1992.

DeMartini, J.C., and Riddle, W.E.: Disseminated coccidioidomycosis in two horses and a pony. J. Am. Vet. Med. Assoc., *155*:149, 1969.

Greet, T.R.C.: Outcome of treatment of 35 cases of gutteral pouch mycosis. Eq. Vet. J., *19*:483, 1987.

Hattel, A.L., et al.: Pulmonary aspergillosis associated with acute enteritis in a horse. J. Am. Vet. Med. Assoc., *199*:589, 1991.

Kabay, M.J., et al.: The pathology of disseminated *Aspergillus terreus* infection in dogs. Vet. Pathol., *22*:540, 1985.

Kaufman, L., and Standard, P.G.: Specific and rapid identification of medically important fungi by exoantigen detection. Ann. Rev. Microbiol., *41*:289, 1987.

Kowalewich, N., et al.: Identification of *Histoplasma capsulatum* organisms in the pleural and peritoneal effusions of a dog. J. Am. Vet. Med. Assoc., *202*:423, 1993.

Kramme, P.M., and Ziemer, E.L.: Disseminated coccidioidomycosis in a horse with osteomyelitis. J. Am. Vet. Med. Assoc., *196*:106, 1990.

Lane, J.G., and Warnock, D.W.: The diagnosis of *Aspergillus fumigatus* infection of the nasal chambers of the dog with particular reference to the value of the double diffusion test. J. Sm. Anim. Pract., *18*:169, 1977.

Legendre, A.M., Walker, M., Buyukmihci, N., and Stevens, R.: Canine blastomycosis: A review of 47 clinical cases. J. Am. Vet. Med. Assoc., *178*:1163, 1981.

Lingard, D.R., Gosser, H.S., and Monfort, T.M.: Acute epistaxis associated with gutteral pouch mycosis in two horses. J. Am. Vet. Med. Assoc., *164*:1038, 1974.

Miller, R.I.: Gastrointestinal phycomycosis in 63 dogs. J. Am. Vet. Med. Assoc. *186*:473, 1985.

Ohbayashi, M., and Ishimoto, Y.: Two cases of adiaspiromycosis in small animals. Jpn. J. Vet. Res., *19*:103, 1971.

Ossent, P.: Systemic aspergillosis and mucormycosis in 23 cats. Vet. Rec., *120*: 330, 1987.

Reed, W.M., et al.: Gastrointestinal zygomycosis in suckling pigs. J. Am. Vet. Med. Assoc., *191*:549, 1987.

Rose, M.N.: Aspergillosis in wild and domestic fowl. Avian Dis., *8*:1, 1964.

Spreadbury, C., et al.: Detection of *Aspergillus fumigatus* by polymerase chain reaction. J. Clin. Microbiol., *31*:615, 1993.

Stevens, D.A. (ed.): Coccidioidomycosis. New York, Plenum Publishing Corporation, 1980.

Stock, B.L.: Case report: Generalized granulomatous lesions in chickens and wild ducks caused by *Aspergillus* species. Avian Dis., *5*:89, 1961.

Stockman, L., et al.: Evaluation of commercially available acridium ester-labelled chemiluminescent DNA probes for culture identification of *Blastomyces dermatitidis, Coccidioides immitis, Cryptococcus neoformans,* and *Histoplasma capsulatum*. J. Clin. Microbiol., *31*:845, 1993.

Wolf, A.M.: *Histoplasma capsulatum* osteomyelitis in the cat. J. Vet. Intern. Med., *1*:158, 1987.

Ziemer, E.L., et al.: Coccidioidomycosis in horses: 15 cases (1975–1984). J. Am. Vet. Med. Assoc., *201*:910, 1992.

Part IV

INTRODUCTORY VIROLOGY

36

General Characteristics and Classification of Viruses

It is beyond the scope and the intent of this book to present the vast amount of information that has accumulated on this subject. What will be presented is a brief summary of the general properties of viruses, followed by a brief overview of virus replication. In addition, the current position on classification of viruses will be presented. For readers interested in a more thorough treatment, selected references are provided at the end of this chapter.

CHEMICAL COMPOSITION, STRUCTURE AND SIZE

Viruses consist of protein, nucleic acid and, in some cases, lipid and carbohydrate. The major constituent is protein, which provides a protective coat for the nucleic acid. This coat is composed of protein subunits or capsomeres, and as a whole is referred to as a capsid. Besides its role as a protective container for the nucleic acid, the capsid may also interact with specific host cell receptor sites, thereby determining the host range of a virus.

Viruses contain only one type of nucleic acid, either DNA or RNA. The DNA exists as a single molecule which is usually double-stranded and linear. RNA viruses have a genome which is usually single-stranded; the RNA exists as a single molecule in some viruses, while in others there are multiple copies. Lipid and carbohydrates are only found in enveloped viruses, and in poxviruses. In the former, they are of cellular origin.

Viruses are grouped according to capsidal structure as cubical, helical, and complex. Virions with cubical symmetry are hexagonal in outline with the shape of an icosahedron. Such a figure presents a variable number of equilateral triangular faces with capsomeres situated in regular fashion along the bases of the triangles (Fig. 36–1). Virions with helical symmetry have their capsomeres attached to each other in a ribbon-like pattern in association with the elongated spiral molecule of nucleic acid (Fig. 36–2). The complex structure of the poxviruses includes a central nucleoid mass with multiple angulated stranded structures enveloped by at least two covering membranes.

Viruses vary in size from circoviruses at 15 nm in diameter to poxviruses approaching 300 nm.

VIRUS REPLICATION

Replication of RNA Viruses

Replication of most RNA viruses occurs strictly within the cytoplasm of cells and is independent of nuclear activity. Exceptions are orthomyxoviruses which require host DNA transcription, paramyxoviruses which have a nonobligatory nuclear phase of replication, and retroviruses which replicate via a DNA intermediate.

The first three steps in replication are essentially the same for all RNA viruses. Attachment is an electrostatic interaction between the virus and specific cell receptors. Viruses then enter the cell by viropexis (pinocytosis) or perhaps, in the case of

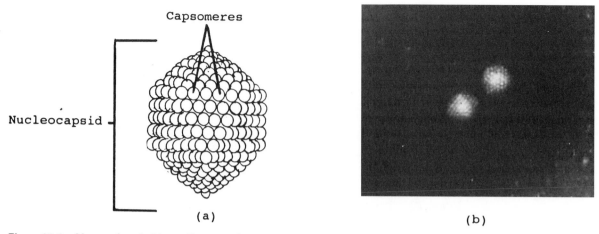

Figure 36–1. Nonenveloped virion with an icosahedral capsid. (*a*) Diagram; (*b*) Electron micrograph.

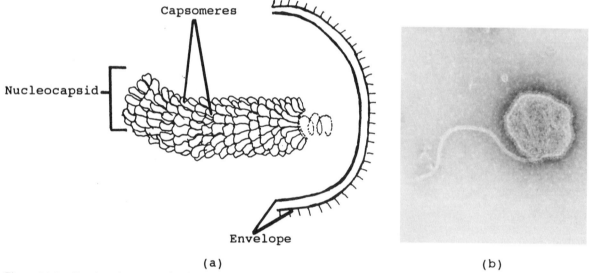

Figure 36–2. Enveloped virion with a helical capsid. (*a*) Diagram; (*b*) Electron micrograph.

enveloped viruses, by fusing with the cell membrane. Release of viral nucleic acid (uncoating) occurs in the cytoplasm, or during passage through the cell membrane, as appears to be the case for picornaviruses. The RNA of reoviruses, however, is never completely uncoated but remains in viral cores.

The RNA of most animal viruses is singlestranded. Exceptions are reoviruses and birnaviruses which have double-stranded RNA. In addition, the genome of some RNA viruses is a single molecule of RNA; in others, the genome is fragmented. The RNA of some animal viruses has messenger function (+ sense) and can be directly translated, whereas the genome in others is antimessage (– sense), and must first be transcribed by a virion-

associated transcriptase. Retroviruses have a "reverse transcriptase" (RNA-dependent DNA polymerase) permitting the formation of a DNA intermediate, which becomes incorporated into the host genome, and is subsequently transcribed into messenger RNA by host DNA-dependent RNA polymerase.

In general, replication of viral RNA is semiconservative and proceeds via a replicative intermediate (RI). The RI consists of parental viral RNA which serves as a template for the transcription of several RNA strands, which eventually "peel off" and serve as templates for the synthesis of viral RNA. Replication of double-stranded RNA of reoviruses is conservative and asymmetrical; only one strand is replicated, unlike double-stranded DNA.

The replication processes require RNA-dependent RNA polymerases (replicases) which are virus coded.

Maturation occurs in the cytoplasm with the viral RNA becoming associated with the capsid. Enveloped viruses complete maturation by budding through the endoplasmic reticulum or through the cell membrane.

Replication of DNA Viruses

Unlike RNA viruses which, for the most part, replicate strictly within the cytoplasm, DNA viruses replicate within the nucleus. Exceptions are poxviruses and iridoviruses which use cytoplasmic "factories." Attachment, penetration, and uncoating are essentially the same as that described for RNA viruses.

The DNA of most animal viruses is linear and double-stranded. Exceptions are papovaviruses, which have circular double-stranded DNA; parvoviruses, which have single-stranded DNA; and circoviruses, which have closed, circular single-stranded DNA. The DNA of hepadnaviruses exists in a circular form, which is partially double-stranded and partially single-stranded. Those DNA viruses that multiply within the nucleus use host DNA-dependent RNA polymerase for transcription. The transcripts are large molecules that are cleaved into smaller messengers, with subsequent addition of polyadenylic acid (poly A) to their 3' end. The presence of poly A is presumably important in the transportation of messenger RNA to the cytoplasm for translation. Poxviruses and iridoviruses have virion-associated transcriptases because they multiply in the cytoplasm, but iridoviruses are still dependent on the host cell nucleus. These viruses, as well as some RNA viruses, also have poly A tracts on their messenger RNAs; the function is unknown.

Replication of viral DNA is semiconservative and symmetrical with both strands being replicated. The replication of papovavirus DNA, which is closed, circular and double-stranded is postulated to be mediated by a "swivel mechanism" consisting of endonuclease and ligase. The endonuclease "nicks" one strand, allowing a short region to be replicated. The nick is then repaired by the ligase. The single-stranded circular DNA of circoviruses is thought to be replicated by a rolling circle method. Host DNA polymerases may be involved in replicating viruses of limited genome, whereas larger viruses may code for their own polymerases.

Maturation of DNA viruses, with the exception of poxviruses and iridoviruses, occurs in the nu-cleus. Structural proteins are transported from the cytoplasm to the nucleus, where they are assembled into capsids that surround the nucleic acid. Enveloped viruses complete maturation by budding through the nuclear membrane, or, in the case of iridoviruses, through the cytoplasmic membrane.

VIRUS CLASSIFICATION

The classification of viruses is constantly evolving, and the schema presented below should not be considered final. However, it is the current position of the International Committee on the Taxonomy of Viruses (ICTV).

The virus families are presented in Tables 36–1 and 36–2 along with the major distinguishing characteristics. Each virus family is also discussed separately.

DNA Viruses

Poxviridae. The Poxviridae consists of two subfamilies, Chordopoxvirinae (poxviruses of vertebrates) and Entomopoxvirinae (poxviruses of insects). Eight genera presently exist for the Chordopoxvirinae. These are *Orthopoxvirus* (smallpox and related viruses), *Parapoxvirus* (pseudocowpox and related viruses), *Capripoxvirus* (goatpox and related viruses), *Avipoxvirus* (fowlpox and related viruses), *Leporipoxvirus* (myxoma and related viruses), *Suipoxvirus* (swinepox), *Molluscipoxvirus* (molluscum contagiosum), and *Yatapoxvirus* (Yaba monkey tumor virus and related viruses).

Poxviruses replicate within the cytoplasm, and thus require a virion-associated transcriptase. The membrane which is not considered an envelope is viral coded and acquired within the cytoplasm. Viruses of this family possess a common nucleoprotein antigen, and some (mainly *Orthopoxviruses*) will agglutinate red blood cells.

Poxviruses infect the epidermis and produce focal lesions which frequently become proliferative and later necrotic. Generalized infections are occasionally fatal. Many poxviruses produce an infection resulting in changes conveniently summarized as papule, vesicle, pustule, and finally scabs or crusts. Secondary bacterial infections are not uncommon. Recovery from infection with poxviruses usually confers long-term immunity.

Many poxviruses can be cultivated on the chorioallantoic membrane of chicken embryos producing focal lesions or "pocks," and most can be grown in cell cultures. Because of their large size, poxviruses can be seen with light microscopy in stained smears. Virus elementary bodies stained by various procedures including Gutstein's and

Table 36–1. RNA Virus Families

Family	Appearance	Virion Size (nm)	RNA Genome	Capsid Symmetry
Orthomyxoviridae*		90–120	single-stranded 7-8 molecules - sense 13-14 kilobase	helical
Reoviridae		60–80	double-stranded 10-12 segments 16-27 kilobase	icosahedral
Rhabdoviridae*		180x70	single-stranded 1 molecule - sense 13-16 kilobase	helical
Retroviridae*		80–100	single-stranded 1 molecule (dimer), + sense 7-10 kilobase	icosahedral
Paramyxoviridae*		100–300	single-stranded 1 molecule - sense 15-16 kilobase	helical
Togaviridae*		60–70	single-stranded 1 molecule + sense 12 kilobase	icosahedral
Coronaviridae*		60–220	single-stranded 1 molecule + sense 27-33 kilobase	helical
Arenaviridae*		110–130	single-stranded 2 molecules - sense, ambisense 10-11 kilobase	helical

Giemsa can be readily seen either as aggregates (acidophilic cytoplasmic inclusions) or singly.

The principal viruses of this family that cause disease of veterinary importance are cow, sheep, swine, and horsepox, papular stomatitis, pseudocowpox, orf, fowlpox (and related viruses), ectromelia, and lumpy skin disease.

Derivation of family and genus names:

Archaic derived: pox from *poc* meaning "pustule"

Greek derived: ortho from *orthos* meaning "straight or correct"

para from *para* meaning "by side of"
entomo from *entomon* meaning "insect"
Latin derived: avi from *avis* meaning "bird"
capri from *caper* meaning "goat"
lepori from *lepus* meaning "hare"
sui from *sus* meaning "swine"
molluscum from *molluscum* meaning "clam"

Parvoviridae. This family consists of three genera: *Parvovirus, Dependovirus,* and *Densovirus.* The former includes those viruses which infect vertebrates and the latter includes those viruses which

Table 36–1.   RNA Virus Families (Continued)

Family	Appearance	Virion Size (nm)	RNA Genome	Capsid Symmetry
Picornaviridae		22–30	single-stranded 1 molecule + sense 7-8 kilobase	icosahedral
Bunyaviridae*		80–100	single-stranded 3 molecules - sense, ambisense 13-21 kilobase	helical
Flaviviridae*		40–60	single-stranded 1 molecule + sense 10-11 kilobase	icosahedral
Birnaviridae		60–70	double-stranded 2 segments 6-7 kilobase	icosahedral
Toroviridae*		120–140	single-stranded 1 molecule + sense 20 kilobase	helical
Caliciviridae		35–39	single-stranded 1 molecule + sense 8 kilobase	icosahedral
Filoviridae*		80x≥800	single-stranded 1 molecule - sense 12-13 kilobase	helical

*Enveloped

infect insects. *Dependoviruses* are those viruses formerly referred to as adeno-associated viruses.

Parvoviruses replicate in the nucleus with the production of intranuclear inclusions. Replication depends upon cellular functions associated with the S phase of cell division. Parvoviruses thus grow best in rapidly dividing cells. Dependoviruses are defective and require an adenovirus (or herpesvirus) "helper" in order to replicate efficiently.

The principal parvoviruses of veterinary importance are feline panleukopenia virus and its host range variants, canine parvovirus, mink enteritis virus, and raccoon parvovirus. Additional important viruses are Aleutian mink disease virus, porcine parvovirus, and goose parvovirus.

Derivation of family and genus names:

Latin derived: parvo from *parvus* meaning "small"
dependo from *dependere* meaning "depending"
denso from *densus* meaning "thick"

Herpesviridae. The Herpesviridae is divided into three subfamilies: Alphaherpesvirinae, Betaherpesvirinae, and Gammaherpesvirinae. Replication occurs in the nucleus with the formation of a nucleocapsid or naked virus. An outer envelope is acquired during the passage from the nucleus to the cytoplasm. There is no common antigen for all members, but some cross reactions do occur.

Table 36–2. DNA Virus Families

Family	Appearance	Virion Size (nm)	DNA Genome	Capsid Symmetry
Poxviridae*		300x240 x200	double-stranded linear 130–260 kilobase	complex
Parvoviridae		18–22	single-stranded linear 5 kilobase	icosahedral
Herpesviridae*		120–200	double-stranded linear 120–220 kilobase	icosahedral
Adenoviridae		70–90	double-stranded linear 36–38 kilobase	icosahedral
Papovaviridae		40–55	double-stranded circular 5–8 kilobase	icosahedral
Iridoviridae*		125–300	double-stranded linear 150–350 kilobase	icosahedral
Hepadnaviridae*		40–50	double-stranded† circular 3.2 kilobase	icosahedral
Circoviridae		15–25	single-stranded circular 1.7–2.3 kilobase	icosahedral

* Enveloped
† Mostly double-stranded with large single-stranded gap

Viruses belonging to the Alphaherpesvirinae have a relatively short replicative cycle (<24 h), a variable host range, and usually cause rapid destruction of cultured cells. Two genera presently exist for this subfamily: *Simplexvirus* and *Varicellovirus*. Most of the common herpesviruses of veterinary importance are members of the *Varicellovirus*.

The Betaherpesvirinae contains two genera, *Cytomegalovirus* and *Muromegalovirus*. Unlike the Alphaherpesvirinae, this group of viruses has a relatively slow replicative cycle (>24 h), a narrow host range, and causes a slow destruction of cultured cells. Infected cells are often greatly enlarged and may contain cytoplasmic as well as nuclear inclusions.

The Gammaherpesvirinae comprises two genera, *Lymphocytovirus* and *Rhadinovirus*. These are herpesviruses that have a narrow host range and are specific for B or T lymphocytes.

The principal diseases caused by herpesviruses are pseudorabies, infectious bovine rhinotracheitis, bovine ulcerative mammillitis, equine rhinopneumonitis, equine coital exanthema, infectious laryngotracheitis, malignant catarrhal fever, and Marek's disease.

Derivation of family name:

Greek derived: herpes from *herpes* meaning "to creep"

Adenoviridae. Viruses of this family are divided into two genera, *Mastadenovirus* (those of mammals) and *Aviadenovirus* (those of birds). Most of the mammalian adenoviruses share a common group specific complement fixation (CF) antigen.

Adenoviruses replicate within the nucleus forming basophilic and/or acidophilic intranuclear inclusions. Many agglutinate red cells of various animal species, and some are capable of oncogenesis when inoculated into laboratory animals. Like the herpesviruses, adenoviruses are often latent.

Adenoviruses have been recovered from a variety of animal species, but do not appear to be important causes of disease in most of these species. The principal adenoviruses causing disease of veterinary significance are canine adenoviruses, equine adenoviruses, and bovine adenoviruses.

Derivation of family and genus names:

Greek derived: adeno from *aden* meaning "gland"
  mast from *mastos* meaning "breast"
Latin derived: avi from *avis* meaning "bird"

Papovaviridae. This family consists of two genera, *Papillomavirus* and *Polyomavirus*. Papillomaviruses have a predilection for surface epithelium causing the production of usually nonmalignant tumors referred to as warts or papillomas. They differ antigenically and are generally host specific. They are larger than the polyomaviruses, being approximately 55 nm in diameter compared to 45 nm. The polyomaviruses are present in their natural hosts as latent infections, but may show oncogenic properties experimentally. For this reason, they are of special interest to viral oncologists.

Some of the viruses, primarily the vacuolating agents which belong to the polyomavirus genus, can be propagated in cell cultures with resulting cytopathic changes and intranuclear inclusions. Many of the papovaviruses will cause "malignant" transformation of cell cultures.

Principal diseases caused by papillomaviruses are canine oral papillomatosis and bovine and equine papillomatosis. A polyomavirus is the cause of a generalized and often fatal infection of psittacine birds.

Derivation of family and genus names:

Papilloma: from *papilla* (Latin) meaning "nipple" and the suffix *oma* (Greek) meaning "tumors"
Polyoma: from *poly* (Greek) meaning "many" and the suffix *oma*
Papova: from the first two letters of the genus names and vacuolating agent which denotes the cytopathic effect viruses of this group have on cultured cells

Iridoviridae. There are presently four recognized genera of the family Iridoviridae. Two of these, *Iridovirus* and *Chloroiridovirus*, are represented by the small iridescent insect viruses and large iridescent insect viruses respectively. The *Ranavirus* includes those iridoviruses which affect amphibians. Viruses of the *Lymphocystivirus* and the goldfish virus group affect fish.

Iridoviruses are similar to the poxviruses in that assembly of virions occurs within the cytoplasm, although the host cell nucleus appears to be required for some DNA transcription and replication.

African swine fever is no longer considered to be a member of this family.

Derivation of family and genus names:

Latin derived: rana from *rana* meaning "frog"
  lympho from *lympha* meaning "water"
Greek derived: chloro from *khloros* meaning "green"
  cysti from *kystis* meaning "bladder or sac"
  irido from *iris* meaning "rainbow (iridescent)"

Hepadnaviridae. Viruses of the Hepadnaviridae have a circular DNA genome which is partially double-stranded and partially single-stranded. One DNA strand is shorter than the other, and the circular form is maintained by base pairing of overlapping cohesive 5' ends of the two strands. Virions contain a DNA polymerase which, during replication, repairs the single-stranded regions to make full-length double-stranded DNA.

Viruses of the Hepadnaviridae are hepatotropic and are placed in genera based on whether they are mammalian viruses (*Orthohepadnavirus*) or avian viruses (*Avihepadnavirus*). Hepatitis B virus of humans and similar viruses which affect woodchucks, ground squirrels, ducks and herons belong to this family.

Derivation of family name: from *hepa*totropism and deoxyribonucleic acid (DNA)

Circoviridae. Circoviridae is the proposed family name for a recently identified group of viruses that have a covalently closed, circular DNA genome which is single-stranded. These viruses are presently the smallest recognized viruses being approximately 15 nm in diameter. They replicate poorly in cell cultures and are probably dependent on cellular functions associated with cell division.

Three viruses are presently recognized for this proposed family. These are porcine circovirus which has not yet been associated with disease, and two disease producing avian viruses, chicken anemia virus and psittacine beak and feather disease.

RNA Viruses

Reoviridae. The Reoviridae consists of eight recognized genera: *Orthoreovirus, Orbivirus, Coltivirus, Rotavirus, Aquareovirus, Cypovirus, Phytoreovirus,* and *Fijivirus.* The latter four genera represent viruses that affect fish (aquaviruses), insects (cypoviruses), and plants (phytoreoviruses and fijiviruses).

Viruses of this family contain ten to twelve segments of linear double-stranded RNA. They replicate in the cytoplasm and some (especially orthoreoviruses) produce large cytoplasmic perinuclear inclusions. Orthoreoviruses can be propagated in cell cultures with relative ease compared to orbiviruses and rotaviruses which are often difficult to cultivate.

Orthoreovirus consists of the classical mammalian reoviruses which, regardless of animal origin, belong to serotypes 1, 2, or 3. It also includes several avian serotypes. Despite the widespread occurrence of mammalian reoviruses in a number of animal species including cats, cattle, dogs, swine, and human beings, they have not been generally accepted as significant causal agents of disease.

Orbivirus includes those viruses of vertebrates that also multiply in insects. The significant diseases caused by orbiviruses are bluetongue, African horse sickness, and equine encephalosis.

Rotavirus includes viruses that cause diarrhea in most mammalian species and in birds. There are six serogroups designated A through F, that have been described:

Group A: mammals and birds in general
Group B: pigs, cattle, sheep, rats, and human beings
Group C: primarily pigs, rarely human beings
Group D and F: poultry
Group E: pigs.

Colorado tick fever virus, which affects human beings, belongs to the *Coltivirus* genus.

Derivation of family and genus names:

Latin derived: orbi from *orbis* meaning "ring"
rota from *rota* meaning "wheel"
aqua from *aqua* meaning "water"
Greek derived: phyto from *phyton* meaning "plant"
Other derivations: reo from *r*espiratory *e*nteric *o*rphan
colti from *Col*orado *ti*ck fever
cypo from *cy*toplasmic *po*lyhedrosis
fiji from the country where virus was first isolated

Birnaviridae. The family Birnaviridae was created to accommodate those double-stranded RNA viruses which did not adequately fit into the family of Reoviridae because their genome contained only two segments of linear double-stranded RNA rather than the ten to twelve segments of the Reoviridae.

Birnavirus is the only genus presently recognized and includes infectious pancreatic necrosis virus of salmonoid fish and infectious bursal disease of chickens.

Derivation of family name: bi from double-stranded and bi-segmented genome, and rna from ribonucleic acid (RNA)

Rhabdoviridae. The Rhabdoviridae consists of two genera, *Vesiculovirus* and *Lyssavirus*; other genera will probably be proposed. These viruses have a cylindrical or bullet shape, and maturation of the complete virus is by budding from the cell membrane.

Diseases of veterinary significance caused by viruses of this family are vesicular stomatitis (*Vesiculovirus*), rabies (*Lyssavirus*) and bovine ephemeral fever (*Lyssavirus*). Numerous other rhabdoviruses have been isolated from a wide variety of vertebrates and invertebrates.

Derivation of family and genus names:

Greek derived: rhabdo from *rhabdos* meaning "rod"
lyssa from *lyssa* meaning "rage"
Latin derived: vesiculo from *vesicula* meaning "bladder or blister"

Retroviridae. The Retroviridae includes those RNA viruses that replicate via a DNA intermediate, and thus contain a reverse transcriptase. The three subfamilies previously recognized, Oncovirinae (RNA tumor viruses), Spumavirinae (foamy agents), and Lentivirinae (visna and related viruses) are no longer considered valid and have been eliminated from the classification scheme.

Current classification groups the retroviruses into seven genera but only two of these have been named, *Spumavirus* and *Lentivirus*. The remaining five genera are referred to as groups viz., mammalian type B, mammalian type C, avian type C, mammalian type D, and HTLV-BLV.

Principal viruses of this family important in diseases of animals are type C viruses, which cause leukemia and sarcoma in cats and fowl, and lentiviruses, which cause equine infectious anemia, feline AIDS, visna/maedi, and caprine arthritis/encephalitis. Bovine leukemia virus is a member of the HTLV-BLV group of retroviruses. The foamy agents, bovine syncytial virus, feline syncytial virus, and simian foamy virus, do not appear to be associated with disease, but may present problems as contaminants in cell cultures.

Derivation of family and genus names:

Latin derived: retro from *retro* meaning "backwards"
  spuma from *spuma* meaning "foam"
  lenti from *lenti* meaning "slow"
Greek derived: onco from *onkos* meaning "tumor"

Paramyxoviridae. Two subfamilies representing three genera are presently recognized in this family. The Paramyxovirinae is comprised of two genera, *Paramyxovirus* and *Morbillivirus*. *Pneumovirus* is the only genus of the Pneumovirinae. Viruses of the Paramyxoviridae replicate in the cytoplasm, but may also have a nonobligatory nuclear phase of replication. Most can be propagated in cell cultures with the production of cytopathic effects including cytoplasmic inclusions. Some viruses, such as parainfluenza 3, also produce intranuclear inclusions.

Principal diseases of veterinary importance caused by viruses of this family are Newcastle disease and parainfluenza-3 (*Paramyxovirus*), canine distemper and rinderpest (*Morbillivirus*), and bovine respiratory syncytial virus (*Pneumovirus*).

Derivation of family and genus names:

Latin derived: morbilli from the plural of *morbillus* meaning "disease"
Greek derived: paramyxo from *para* meaning "by the side of" and *myxa* meaning "mucus"
  pneumo from *pneuma* meaning "breath"

Orthomyxoviridae. The Orthomyxoviridae contains two proposed genera but neither have been assigned names. One proposed genus contains both type A and type B influenza viruses while the other is represented by type C influenza viruses.

Viruses of this family require host-DNA transcription in order to replicate. Thus, unlike the Paramyxoviridae, they are sensitive to the action of actinomycin-D which inhibits DNA-dependent RNA synthesis. Virions are pleomorphic in appearance, occurring as either roughly spherical forms or as filamentous structures. Type A influenza viruses are best propagated in the amniotic cavity of chicken embryos. Types B and C will grow in cell culture, but often without observable cytopathic changes.

The classification and the antigenic relationships of influenza viruses are determined on the basis of the three major virus-coded antigens: the ribonucleoprotein antigen, which determines the type; and the two surface antigens, hemagglutinin and neuraminidase, which determine the subtype or strain. In nature, RNA heterogeneity appears to be a general characteristic of influenza viruses in lower mammals and birds, and it is thought that multiple infections with different subtypes result in genetic reassortment and the possible debut of new strains.

Viruses of this family have a predilection for the respiratory tract, but usually do not cause a serious disease in uncomplicated cases. Principal viruses of veterinary importance are type A influenza viruses which cause equine, swine, and avian influenza.

Derivation of family name:

Greek derived: ortho from *orthos* meaning "straight or correct"
  myxo from *myxa* meaning "mucus"

Togaviridae. The Togaviridae is presently divided into three genera, *Alphavirus*, *Rubivirus*, and *Arterivirus*. Flavivirus, which was once considered a genus, has been given family status, and *Pestivirus* has been moved to the Flaviviridae. In all likelihood, based on the way members process their mRNA, the genus of *Arterivirus* will soon be given family status.

The natural hosts for alphaviruses are primarily wild birds in which they produce an inapparent viremia. They are transmitted to domestic animals and human beings by arthropod vectors, although some types are capable of being transmitted by direct contact with an infected animal. Most can be propagated in cell cultures, or in nursing mice inoculated intracerebrally. Viruses of the other two genera can also be propagated in cell cultures, but often without observable cytopathic changes.

Principal viruses of veterinary importance are those causing the equine encephalitides and equine arteritis. The virus of porcine reproductive and respiratory disease syndrome (PRRS) has many features in common with equine arteritis virus and is a proposed member.

Derivation of family and genus names:

Greek derived: alpha from the letter "A"
Latin derived: toga from *toga* meaning "gown or cloak"
  rubi from *rubeus* meaning "reddish"
Other derivation: arteri from arteritis.

Flaviviridae. The Flaviviridae consists of three genera, *Flavivirus*, *Pestivirus*, and the yet unnamed Hepatitis C virus group. The first two genera were once classified as genera within the Togaviridae, but were reassigned owing to differences in replication. Unlike togaviruses which utilize subgenomic mRNA in their replication cycle and mature by budding through the cell membrane, flaviviruses use the intact viral genome as mRNA and mature into cytoplasmic vesicles.

Members of the *Flavivirus* are group B arboviruses whose natural hosts are wild mammals and birds. They are transmitted to man and domestic animals by the bite of hematophagous arthropods, and are most easily isolated by the intracerebral inoculation of newborn mice. Members of the *Pestivirus* are transmitted by direct and indirect contact; vectors are not involved.

Principal viruses causing diseases in animals are hog cholera, bovine viral diarrhea, border disease, louping ill, and Wesselsbron.

Derivation of family and genus names:

Latin derived: flavi from *flavus* meaning "yellow"
  pesti from *pestis* meaning "plague"

Coronaviridae. The Coronaviridae presently consists of only one genus, *Coronavirus*. The virions are somewhat pleomorphic but roughly spherical, and have surface projections which are petal shaped. Maturation occurs in cytoplasmic vesicles from which the virions obtain an envelope. The viruses can be propagated in cell culture, but often with difficulty.

The principal viruses of veterinary significance are the ones that cause transmissible gastroenteritis in pigs, calf scours, infectious bronchitis of birds, vomiting and wasting disease of pigs (porcine hemagglutinating encephalitis), and feline infectious peritonitis.

Derivation of family name:

Latin derived: corona from *corona* meaning "crown"

Toroviridae. Toroviridae is a newly designated family of viruses that presently consists of one genus, *Torovirus*. Toroviruses are similar to coronaviruses in morphology as well as genome organization and expression. This genomic similarity is also noted with arteriviruses, and it has been proposed that these three groups of viruses be classified under a superfamily. However, the nucleocapsid structure of these viruses, which is important in viral classification, is quite different. The nucleocapsid of coronaviruses is helical, while that of toroviruses is tubular and that of arteriviruses is icosahedral.

There are only two viruses currently recognized as toroviruses and both are pathogens of domestic animals. They are Berne virus and Breda virus associated with diarrhea in horses and calves, respectively.

Derivation of family and genus name:

Latin derived: toro from *torus* meaning "doughnut shaped surface"

Arenaviridae. The Arenaviridae consists of viruses that have in common, among other things, electron-dense granules incorporated within the virion. These granules are apparently cellular ribosomes and glycogen, and give a "grains of sand" appearance to the virion. There is only one genus, *Arenavirus*.

Arenaviruses, which include lymphocytic choriomeningitis virus, are serologically related and are only of minor importance in veterinary medicine.

Derivation of family and genus name:

Latin derived: arena from *arenosus* meaning "sandy"

Picornaviridae. The Picornaviridae presently consists of five genera, *Enterovirus*, *Rhinovirus*, *Cardiovirus*, *Aphthovirus*, and *Hepatovirus*. Enteroviruses and Cardioviruses are stable at acid pH (≤ 5), whereas viruses of the other genera are unstable.

Most picornaviruses can be propagated in cell culture producing a characteristic and rapid cytopathic effect. Exceptions are some rhinoviruses which require a lower temperature and restricted cell types. While most picornaviruses are host specific, aphthoviruses infect most cloven-footed animals.

Principal viruses of this family of veterinary importance are those causing Teschen disease, foot-and-mouth disease, avian encephalomyelitis, swine vesicular disease, and encephalomyocarditis virus. Hepatoviruses have only been described in human beings and other primates.

Derivation of family and genus names:

Italian derived: pico from *pico* meaning "small" plus the abbreviation for ribonucleic acid
Greek derived: entero from *enteron* meaning "intestine"
rhino from *rhinos* meaning "nose"
cardio from *kardia* meaning "heart"
aphtho from *aphtha* meaning "vesicles in the mouth"

Caliciviridae. The Caliciviridae consists of one genus, *Calicivirus*, which was earlier considered a provisional genus of Picornaviridae. The rationale for assigning family status to caliciviruses is based on their distinct differences from picornaviruses. Caliciviruses are approximately 10 nm larger in diameter than picornaviruses, and the average virion molecular weight is about twice as great. The cup-shaped depressions on a spherical capsid surface give caliciviruses a distinctive virion morphology. Caliciviruses have a single major capsid polypeptide while picornaviruses have four. The RNA of caliciviruses and picornaviruses has messenger function. However, unlike picornaviruses whose proteins are derived by cleavage of a single translation product of genomic-size RNA, a subgenomic RNA appears to be the messenger for the capsid protein of caliciviruses, and genomic-size RNA apparently serves as a messenger for nonstructural proteins.

Feline calicivirus, canine calicivirus, and vesicular exanthema virus are the principal viruses of veterinary importance.

Derivation of family and genus names:

Latin derived: calici from *calix* meaning "cup"

Filoviridae. Viruses of the Filoviridae are pleomorphic viruses that may appear as long filamentous forms up to 14,000 nm in length but with a uniform diameter of approximately 80 nm. They may also exist in circular or U-shaped forms. Replication occurs in the cytoplasm of infected cells, and virions mature by budding through the cell membrane.

Filovirus, presently the only genus of this family, comprises two viruses indigenous to Africa. These two viruses, Marburg and Ebola, cause an often fatal hemorrhagic fever in human beings.

Derivation of family and genus name:

Latin derived: filo from *filo* meaning "thread-like"

Bunyaviridae. There are presently five genera assigned to the Bunyaviridae. These are *Bunyavirus*, *Phlebovirus*, *Nairovirus*, *Hantavirus*, and *Tospovirus*. Viruses of the latter genus affect plants. Bunyaviruses have a segmented RNA genome which may undergo genetic reassortment leading to new strains. Most bunyaviruses are transmitted by biting arthropods and, with the exceptions of Cache valley, Rift valley fever, and Nairobi sheep disease, are of limited importance in veterinary medicine.

Derivation of family name:

Locale derived: Bunya from *Bunyamwera* in Africa

Unclassified Viruses

A group of RNA viruses similar to picornaviruses has been associated with enteritis in a number of animal species, including bovine, ovine, and porcine. The viruses are approximately 25 to 30 nm in diameter, and when viewed under the electron microscope appear as circular outlines with a surface structure arranged as a five- or six-pointed star. This latter feature has led investigators to refer to these viruses as astroviruses.

Viroids

Viroids are non-encapsulated, low-molecular-weight nucleic acids that are extremely resistant to heat and ultraviolet and ionizing radiation. The nucleic acid is a single-stranded, closed-circular RNA that exists as a highly base-paired rod-like structure. Viroids cause several plant diseases, the prototype being potato spindle tuber disease. Viroids have not been associated with disease in animals, although the agents causing scrapie in sheep and goats and similar diseases of other mammals were once considered viroid-like. These agents have since been classified as prions and appear to consist entirely of protein.

Prions

Prions are proteinaceous infectious particles associated with transmissible neurodegenerative diseases of human beings and animals. These diseases are characterized by a long incubation period (years), and an insidious development of CNS dysfunction. Owing to the unique histopathologic brain lesions (spongiform changes), these diseases are collectively referred to as "transmissible spongiform encephalopathies" (TSE).

TSEs include scrapie of sheep and goats, transmissible mink encephalopathy, chronic wasting disease of mule deer and elk, bovine spongiform encephalopathy, feline spongiform encephalopathy, and three diseases of human beings: Kuru, Creutzfeldt-Jakob, and Gerstmann-Straussler syndrome.

Brain tissue from diseased animals contains an accumulation of prion proteins associated with fibrils and amyloid plaques. These proteins are thought to be derived by an abnormal post-translational modification of a normal cellular protein, the function of which is unknown. The normal cellular protein is designated as PrP^c, and the prion protein is designated as PrP with a superscript denoting the particular disease, e.g. PrP^{sc} for scrapie prion.

There is some recent evidence that the cause of TSE may actually be a bacterium. Spiroplasma-like organisms have been demonstrated in brain tissue from patients with Creutzfeldt-Jakob disease. Spiroplasmas have slender internal fibrils which are morphologically identical to scrapie fibrils, and these fibrils have been shown to cross react with antibody to scrapie.

FURTHER READING

Bastian, F.O.: Bovine spongiform encephalopathy: Relationship to human disease and nature of the agent. Am. Soc. Microbiol. News, 59:235, 1993.

Conzelmann, K.K., Visser, N., Van Woensel, P., and Thiel, H.J.: Molecular characterization of porcine reproductive and respiratory syndrome virus, a member of the arterivirus group. Virol., 193:329, 1993.

denBoon, J.A., Snijder, E.J., Chirnside, E.D., et al.: Equine arteritis virus is not a togavirus but belongs to the coronavirus superfamily. J. Virol., 65:2910, 1991.

Fields, B.N., and Knipe, D.M. (eds.): Fundamental Virology. 2nd Ed. New York, Raven Press, Ltd., 1991.

Fenner, F.J., Gibbs, E.P.J., Murphy, F.A., et al. (eds.): Veterinary Virology. 2nd Ed. New York, Academic Press, Inc., 1993.

Francki, R.I.B., Fauquet, C.M., Knudson, D.L. and Brown, F. (eds.): Classification and Nomenclature of Viruses. Fifth Report of the International Committee on Taxonomy of Viruses. Arch. Virol. Suppl. New York, Springer Verlag., 1991.

Lai, M.M.C.: RNA recombination in animal and plant viruses. Microbiol. Rev., 56:61, 1992.

Moussa, A., Chasey, D., Lavazza, A. et al.: Haemorrhagic disease of lagomorphs: evidence for a calicivirus. Vet. Microbiol. 33:375, 1992.

Schreuder, B.E.C.: General aspects of transmissible spongiform encephalopathies and hypotheses about the agents. Vet. Quart., 15:167, 1993.

Stahl, N. and Prusiner, S.B.: Prions and prion proteins. FASEB, J. 5:2799, 1991.

Studdert, M.J.: Circoviridae: New viruses of pigs, parrots and chickens. Aust. Vet. J. 70:101, 1993.

Telford, E.A.R., Studdert, M.J., Agius, C.T. et al.: Equine herpesviruses 2 and 5 are γ-herpesviruses. Virol., 195:492, 1993.

Webster, R.G., Bean, W.J., Gorman, O.T. et al.: Evolution and Ecology of influenza A viruses. Microbiol. Rev., 56:152, 1992.

37

Some Methods Used to Study Viruses

INTRODUCTION

Fundamental to the detailed study of viruses is the ability to cultivate them successfully. Since viruses are obligate intracellular parasites, they cannot be propagated on artificial media but require living cells.

Initially, viruses were propagated in the natural host. Nearly 100 years ago mosaic disease of tobacco was transmitted to healthy plants using filtered extracts obtained from diseased plants, and the field of virology was born. Similar studies were done in animals with foot-and-mouth disease a short time later.

There have been several landmark advancements in the study of viruses, especially in recent years, but none with more impact than the in vitro cultivation of cells. Although limited success was obtained in cultivating cells prior to 1940, it was the advent of antibiotics in the 1940s that led to their widespread use, and the era of modern virology.

CULTIVATION OF VIRUSES

Animals

A number of routes are available for the inoculation of experimental animals. The method selected is dependent upon the animal to be used and the virus. Intracerebral inoculation is used for many neurotropic viruses, while the intranasal route is usually recommended for those viruses which attack the respiratory tract. Care must be taken to select animals free of antibodies to the virus being studied.

Natural host animals are almost never used for the purpose of routine cultivation of viruses. They are, however, used to study the pathogenesis of viral infections and to evaluate the efficacy of viral vaccines. Laboratory animals, on the other hand, are occasionally used to help diagnose viral infections. An example is the intracerebral inoculation of suckling mice for rabies diagnosis in those instances where the results of the standard diagnostic method of immunofluorescence is equivocal. At one time, pseudorabies was routinely diagnosed by the subcutaneous inoculation of rabbits with brain suspension of affected animals. If pseudorabies virus was present, the rabbits developed an intense pruritis ("mad-itch") at the injection site.

In addition to serving the purpose of propagating viruses, different experimental animals can be used to differentiate viruses that produce similar lesions. For example, foot-and-mouth disease virus can be distinguished from the virus of vesicular stomatitis by inoculating calves and horses. While calves are susceptible to both viruses, horses are not susceptible to the virus of foot-and-mouth disease.

Chicken Embryos

Fertile eggs, when inoculated by one or more of the various routes, are susceptible to a large number of viruses. The more common routes of inoculation are via the yolk sac, allantoic cavity, and chorioallantoic (CA) membrane. Virus growth may be indicated by clinical signs such as sluggishness or death of the embryo, specific lesions, or by the presence of hemagglutinins in embryonic fluids. Chicken embryos are most commonly used for the propagation of avian viruses, but are particularly useful for growing type A influenza viruses of most animal species.

Besides being useful in propagating viruses, chicken embryos are also useful in the differentiation of viruses that produce diseases that are clinically similar. The virus of cowpox, for example, can be distinguished from pseudocowpox virus by inoculation of the CA membrane. Pocks are formed by cowpox virus and not by pseudocowpox virus.

Fertile chicken eggs for use in the virus laboratory should be obtained from a "disease-free" flock with a known vaccination history or preferably a nonvaccinal status. Embryonated eggs containing antibodies to the prevalent avian viruses are not suitable for the recovery of those viruses.

Cell Cultures

Cell culture monolayers are the most widely used method of cultivating viruses. Cell cultures can be initiated from various tissues by treating finely minced tissue with a proteolytic enzyme such as trypsin. Trypsin disassociates the tissue into individual cells which, when provided with a nutrient medium, will attach to the surface of the culture vessel and grow. These cells will continue to grow until they form a layer of cells which is one cell thick (monolayer) at which time they cease to divide. This postconfluence inhibition is a phenomenon observed with normal cells. In contrast, some neoplastic cells or cells with neoplastic properties may grow in multiple overlapping areas or form areas within the monolayer which are several cells thick (piling up).

Cell monolayers can be removed from the surface of the culture vessel by treatment with trypsin-EDTA solution. These dispersed cells can be collected and transferred to fresh medium and new cultures can be initiated, or they can be resuspended in a "freeze medium" that contains a cryoprotectant such as dimethylsulfoxide. Cryoprotected cells can be stored in liquid nitrogen for an indefinite period of time.

Nutrient media used to cultivate cells are commercially available. They contain a mixture of salts, sugars, amino acids, vitamins, etc., and usually have sodium bicarbonate as a buffer. Serum is normally added as a growth factor at a final concentration of 10%. Although fetal calf serum is principally used, iron-supplemented calf serum can be substi-

tuted for a fraction of the cost with little or no adverse effect on most cells.

Three different types of cell cultures are recognized:

1. Primary cell lines. These are cultures usually initiated from the tissues of healthy embryos. They are considered the most satisfactory cultures for the isolation of viruses from clinical specimens. In primary cultures, a mixture of epithelial and fibroblastic cells is present. After a number of passages the fibroblasts often become predominant.

2. Diploid cell lines. These are serially propagated cell cultures which retain a normal set of chromosomes. They have a finite life span and the number of transfers that can be carried out successfully depends to a large extent on the tissue and the animal species. Some bovine and porcine cultures can be carried through a considerable number of passages while cultures from some other species cannot be transferred more than five or six times.

3. Permanent or serial cell lines. These are cells with an abnormal chromosomal pattern and morphology (heteroploidy) that are capable of being maintained indefinitely in vitro by serial transfer. Such cells may originate from diploid cells that undergo a "malignant transformation" during culture or they may be initiated from cancerous tissue.

Many cell lines have been documented and coded by the American Type Culture Collection (ATCC) and are available for distribution at a nominal fee. A list of some of the more useful cells for cultivating veterinary viruses is presented in Table 37-1.

Light Microscope

Most viruses are so small that they cannot be seen by the highest magnification of the light microscope. An exception occurs in the poxviruses, the elementary bodies of which can be readily seen in suitably stained smears.

While the light microscope is not useful for the studies of viruses per se, it is an invaluable instrument for observing the effect of viruses on cells. When viruses are inoculated onto susceptible cell cultures, virus growth is often accompanied by cell destruction or cytopathic effect (CPE)(Plate 4a,b). This CPE is frequently characteristic of a particular virus group and is an aid in preliminary identification of viruses isolated from clinical specimens. Some types of CPE are:

Table 37–1.   Some ATCC Available Cell Cultures Useful for the Cultivation of Animal Viruses

Culture Name*	Type of Culture	Life Expectancy	Usefulness
CRFK	Feline Kidney	Infinite	Feline viruses, Canine parvovirus Type 2
A-72	Canine tumor	Infinite	Canine viruses
MDCK	Canine kidney	Infinite	Type A influenza
MDBK	Bovine kidney	Infinite	Bovine viruses (not BVD)
BT	Bovine turbinate	Finite	Bovine viruses, especially BVD
EBTR	Bovine trachea	Finite	Bovine viruses, especially BVD, BRSV, & PI3
PK-15	Porcine kidney	Infinite	Porcine viruses (not TGE or parvo)
ST	Swine testes	Infinite	Porcine viruses, including TGE & parvo
E.DERM	Equine skin	Finite	Equine viruses
RK-13	Rabbit kidney	Infinite	Very good for EHV-1 and EVA. Also excellent for EEE.
VERO	Monkey kidney	Infinite	Rotaviruses, EEE, WEE
P-388	Mouse macrophage	Infinite	E. risticii, psittacosis†

* All of these cells except P-388 grow well in EMEM with 10% iron-supplemented calf sera. P-388 cells grow best in RPMI 1640 medium.

† Not viruses, but usually isolated in virology laboratories.

1. Cells round up and aggregate in grape-like clusters as with adenoviruses,
2. Cells round up, shrink, and lyse, leaving much cellular debris as with enteroviruses,
3. Cells become swollen and round up in focal areas as with herpesviruses,
4. Cells fuse producing multinucleated cells (syncytia), as with paramyxoviruses.

The CPE associated with viral growth is usually evident by the low power viewing of unstained inoculated cultures. However, by staining these cultures with a stain such as hematoxylin and eosin (H & E), additional cellular changes are often noted. For example, many viruses produce characteristic inclusion bodies. These inclusion bodies usually represent an accumulation of virions and viral subunits such as nucleic acid and protein. Inclusion bodies may occur in the cytoplasm or nucleus, or occasionally in both. Cytoplasmic inclusions are normally associated with RNA viruses and nuclear inclusions are normally associated with DNA viruses (Plate 4c). Exceptions are poxviruses (DNA viruses), which replicate strictly within the cytoplasm and thus produce cytoplasmic inclusions (Plate 4d); and paramyxoviruses (RNA viruses) which have a nonobligatory nuclear phase of replication and may produce both intranuclear and intracytoplasmic inclusions.

Fluorescence Microscope

The fluorescence microscope is a variation of the conventional light microscope. It is equipped with a more powerful light source and a combination of barrier and exciter filters. When an appropriate fluorochrome is used, the excitation light is ab-sorbed by the molecules of the fluorochrome and they gain energy. These molecules in turn release their energy by emitting light of a longer visible wavelength.

There are two basic types of fluorescence microscopes, transmitted light and reflected light (epifluorescence). With transmitted light, the excitation light is directed through a darkfield condenser and passes through the specimen being examined. In contrast, the excitation light with epifluorescence is directed onto the specimen through the objective. The principal advantage of epifluorescence is that the full emission intensity of the specimen is obtained, and thus the degree of fluorescence is greater, especially at higher magnifications. A distinct advantage of transmitted fluorescence is that the specimen can readily be viewed by routine darkfield microscopy by simply removing the exciter filter. The ease of alternately examining specimens by fluorescence and darkfield is useful in locating specific areas of a specimen not easily discernible by fluorescence microscopy alone. For example, darkfield examination of a section of small intestine will readily determine if the area being viewed is lamina propria, crypt epithelium, villi, etc. Also, certain cells such as granulocytes may autofluoresce. These cells are usually refractile when viewed by darkfield microscopy.

Most epifluorescence microscopes are also equipped with an alternate transmitted light source in addition to the reflected source which can be used for darkfield examination. Some of the better microscopes are equipped for both transmitted and reflected light fluorescence.

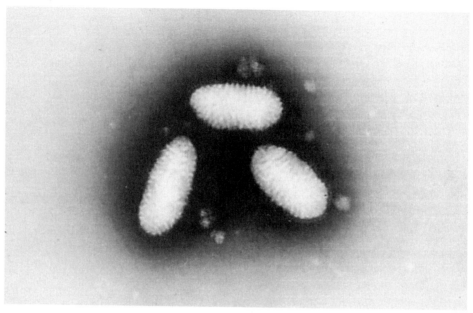

Figure 37–1. Electron micrograph of a parapoxvirus.

The fluorochrome most commonly used in virological studies is fluorescein isothiocyanate (FITC). This fluorochrome can be conjugated with specific antibody resulting in a "fluorescent antibody," which is extremely useful in the rapid diagnosis of viral infections.

Electron Microscope

The development of the electron microscope (EM), which has a resolving power of better then 5 Å as compared to 0.3 μm for the light microscope, has made it possible to study the morphology of viruses in detail. In the EM, electron rays are used instead of light, as in the light microscope, and focusing of the electrons is accomplished by electromagnetic "lenses." As the electrons are invisible, they are focused onto a fluorescent screen. The screen fluoresces in response to the electron bombardment and an image is then visible to the eye.

In preparing material for EM examination, the method of negative staining is simple and rapid. It consists of mixing the specimen, usually purified virus or distilled water lysates of viral infected tissues or cell cultures, with a "stain" of heavy atoms such as sodium phosphotungstate. Under the EM, the electron beam is scattered by the heavy atoms but passes relatively uninhibited through the lighter atoms of the biological specimen. The specimen, as a result, is outlined by the dark material of the stain. This procedure is used for the rapid diagnosis of some viral infections such as skin infections caused by poxviruses (Fig. 37–1), and enteric infections caused by a variety of viruses

including coronavirus and rotavirus (Figs. 37–2 and 37–3).

Another widely used method is to embed small fragments of tissue or cell culture pellets in a plastic such as epon, metacrylate or araldite. After hardening, the embedded material is sectioned in an ultramicrotome using glass or diamond knives. The thin sections are usually stained with a solution of heavy atoms such as lead citrate and uranyl acetate. The atoms of these compounds attach themselves to certain cell structures, and when the section is viewed in the EM, a pattern of electron-opaque regions becomes visible. This method is not useful for the routine diagnosis of viral infections in that it is a time-consuming procedure and extremely difficult to find the virus in clinical specimens. The sections examined are so thin that a single cell can be sectioned numerous times. Thus, looking for viruses in tissues by EM is analogous to looking for the proverbial "needle in the haystack." However, the examination of infected cell cultures is feasible because a large number of these cells are infected. Such studies have contributed much to the understanding of virus entry into cells, viral replication, etc. Other methods of preparing specimens include freeze-etching and shadowing the specimen with heavy atoms.

CONCENTRATION AND PURIFICATION OF VIRUSES

One of the first steps in purification of viral preparations is differential centrifugation. The preparation is centrifuged at a relatively low g force (approximately 2,000) to remove cell debris. This

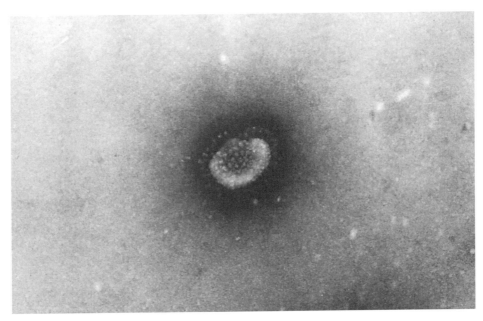

Figure 37–2. Electron micrograph of a coronavirus.

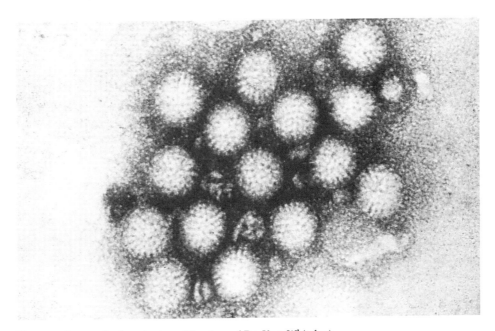

Figure 37–3. Electron micrograph of a rotavirus. (Courtesy of Dr. Kent Whitaker)

clarified suspension is then concentrated by one of several methods, depending upon the circumstances. Small volumes are easily concentrated by centrifugation at high g forces (approximately 40,000 to 80,000) for several hours, whereas large volumes are more conveniently concentrated by other means such as dialysis and precipitation. For example, large volumes of viral suspension can be reduced to small volumes by placing the suspension in a dialysis bag and surrounding the bag with carbowax or dry sucrose, which will draw the aqueous solution through the membrane while leaving the virus inside. The reduced volume is then centrifuged at high g force as described above.

Another convenient way to concentrate large volumes of virus is by cold ($-70°$ C) methanol precipitation. Infectivity of the virus is retained if the methanol-virus mixture is maintained at 2 to 3° C.

Purification steps include chromatography and centrifugation through density gradients. Enveloped viruses which are relatively buoyant, are often purified by velocity sedimentation through sucrose gradients, whereas unenveloped viruses are usually purified by centrifugation through cesium chloride. The area of the gradient in which the virus has settled can be seen as an opaque band that can be removed by a needle and syringe. Centrifugation through cesium chloride is referred to as isopynic centrifugation, which means that the virus will band at an area in the gradient of equal density and will remain at this area despite continued centrifugation.

SENSITIVITY TO LIPID SOLVENTS

The sensitivity of viruses to lipid solvents such as ether and chloroform is of value in taxonomic characterization. The lipids are located in the outer envelope of the virion, and all of the animal viruses that possess envelopes surrounding their nucleocapsids, excepting some poxviruses, are ether sensitive.

IDENTIFICATION OF NUCLEIC ACID TYPE

The most commonly used method for determining the nucleic acid type of a virus is by determining whether nucleic acid synthesis is inhibited in cell cultures by inhibitors of DNA synthesis. For this purpose, the inhibitor 5-bromo-2-deoxyuridine (BUDR) or closely related inhibitors of DNA synthesis are added to the infected cell cultures. If viral DNA synthesis is inhibited, virus multiplication will likewise be decreased. In the event that virus growth is not inhibited, the virus is presumed to contain RNA.

HEMAGGLUTINATION

Some viruses are able to bind to red blood cells (RBCs) of certain animal species, causing them to agglutinate. Binding is accomplished by an interaction of viral proteins (hemagglutinins) located in the outer coat of the virion or virion envelope with receptor sites on the RBC. Agglutination is a result of the bridging effect of one virion binding to two RBCs simultaneously and these in turn being bound to other RBCs by additional virions. The result is a lattice-like aggregate of RBCs. The ability of viruses to agglutinate RBCs is influenced by pH and temperature.

Agglutination of RBCs is useful in the concentration and purification of some viruses, and as a rapid presumptive test for the presence of these viruses in fluids from infected cell cultures and chicken embryos. It is especially useful for assaying viral activity of cell cultures infected with hemagglutinating viruses that produce little or no discernible CPE. Clinical specimens such as feces can also be directly examined for hemagglutinating (HA) activity. For example, a presumptive diagno-

sis of canine parvovirus can be readily made by demonstrating HA activity to porcine RBCs in fecal emulsions. Previous studies have shown that HA activity of 1:32 or greater is almost always a result of parvovirus infection, and titers of greater than 1:4096 are common.

HEMADSORPTION

Membrane-bound viruses such as orthomyxoviruses and paramyxoviruses obtain their outer envelope by budding through the cell membrane. Prior to budding, viral coded proteins (hemagglutinins) are incorporated into the cell membrane. Such cells will adsorb erythrocytes to their surfaces, and the resulting foci of hemadsorption can be detected microscopically.

IMMUNOLOGICAL METHODS

Animals infected with viruses respond by making antibodies. Detection and measurement of these antibodies are useful in planning herd health programs and studying the epidemiology of disease outbreaks.

While detection of antibodies is also useful in disease diagnosis, it is often a time-consuming process requiring the comparative measurements of antibody in acute and convalescent sera, usually collected 10 to 14 days apart. A more rapid approach is to use specific antiviral antibodies to detect viral antigens directly in clinical specimens. These antibodies are usually obtained by hyperimmunizing rabbits or goats with a specific virus. Alternatively, they may be monoclonal in nature.

Monoclonal antibodies are prepared in mice by first exposing the mouse to the viral antigen, which sensitizes B cells of the spleen. These cells are collected and chemically fused with a mouse plasmocytoma cell line that secretes IgG. These hybrid cells are then cloned and the resulting hybridomas, which are derived from a single cell, are analyzed for secretion of the specific antiviral IgG. Selected hybridoma cells are injected back into mice intraperitoneally. These cells grow rapidly in the peritoneal cavity causing an accumulation of ascitic fluid containing a high concentration of monoclonal antibody. Monoclonal antibodies are particularly useful in subtyping viruses. They are normally not used for the routine diagnosis of viral infections because they only recognize a specific antigenic determinant and may not detect different strains of the same virus.

The more common tests used to detect antibodies and antigens are discussed below.

Serum Neutralization Test

Serum neutralization (SN) is the most widely used method of detecting and measuring antibodies to viruses of veterinary importance. This test is generally considered to be the most reliable of all serologic tests, being less prone to variation and less subjective in its interpretation.

The principle of the test is based on the fact that the demonstrable activity of the virus—whether it be cytopathic effect (CPE) in cell culture, clinical signs, lesions, or death in embryonated eggs and animals—can be inhibited by specific antibody to that virus.

Serum neutralization tests are almost always performed using cell cultures. Stock viruses for use in the tests are previously grown, aliquoted, and stored at ultra-low temperature. These viruses are titrated several times to determine the amount of virus present. Performance of the test entails the dilution of test serum in microtiter plates, followed by the addition of an equal volume of virus suspension diluted to contain approximately 100 to 300 infective doses. Following incubation of 1 to 2 hours at room temperature, indicator cell cultures are added. Plates are sealed, incubated at 37° C, and observed daily for development of viral CPE. The presence of specific antibody in the test serum inhibits the production of this CPE.

The SN test is also used to identify unknown viral isolates in essentially the same manner as described above. The only difference is that the antibody is known and the virus is unknown. If a specific antibody inhibits the development of CPE of the unknown virus, then identification is accomplished.

Hemagglutination Inhibition Test

The hemagglutination inhibition (HI) test is similar in principle to SN tests except that the viral activity being inhibited is hemagglutination. HI tests are quite sensitive and highly specific, and are particularly useful for measuring antibody to those hemagglutinating viruses that either grow poorly in cell culture or produce little or no discernible CPE. Examples of such viruses are Type A influenza viruses of most animal species, Newcastle disease virus of birds, and porcine parvovirus.

HI tests are usually performed in microtiter plates. Dilutions of test sera (25 μl) are made, followed by the addition of an equal volume of virus suspension diluted to contain approximately 4 to 8 HA units. The appropriate RBC suspension is then added (50 μl) and the plates are gently mixed and allowed to incubate for 1 to 2 hours at 4° C

(for most viruses). If the specific antibody is present in the test serum, agglutination of RBC will be inhibited and the RBC will settle out in a well-defined "button." Agglutinated cells, in contrast, will settle out in a thin layer over the entire bottom of the test well, or in a rough, irregularly fringed button.

Test sera often contain nonspecific inhibitors of agglutination and must first be adsorbed with RBC prior to testing.

Complement Fixation Test

Complement fixation (CF) tests are most useful as an aid in the diagnosis of acute or recent viral infections, because they primarily detect IgM, the first immunoglobulin class to respond to infection.

The test entails the use of viral antigens, guinea pig complement, and an indicator system of "sensitized" sheep RBCs. The sheep RBCs are sensitized by reacting with antibody directed against themselves. This anti-sheep RBC antibody is referred to as hemolysin and is prepared in rabbits. The antigen and complement are each titrated and diluted to contain approximately two units. A brief summary of the test as it is used for determining the presence of antibody is outlined below.

1. Dilutions of test sera are made in microtiter plates and two units of antigen are added. The complement present in the sera has previously been inactivated by heat.
2. Two units of complement are then added. If the serum contains enough specific antibody, and if the amount of complement is closely related to the amount of antigen as it should be, all the complement will be fixed.
3. After adequate time has been given for combination, the indicator system is added. If no specific antibodies are present in the serum being tested, the complement is left free and will react with the sensitized RBCs, causing lysis. If sufficient antibody is present, the complement will have been fixed by the antigen-antibody reaction in step two and no lysis will occur.

Immunofluorescence

Immunofluorescence or fluorescent antibody (FA) is the single most useful test for routine viral diagnosis. A large number of FA conjugates are available from the National Veterinary Services Laboratory (Ames, IA) for detecting viruses that affect food-producing animals. Some excellent conjugates that detect viruses of dogs and cats are available from American Bioresearch (Seymour, TN).

The principle of immunofluorescence is based upon the fact that antibodies can be labeled (coupled) with fluorescent compounds without interfering with their ability to bind to antigens. The fluorescent compound most commonly used is fluorescein isothiocyanate (FITC). Coupling occurs via a chemical interaction (covalent bonding) between the FITC and lysine residues of the antibody. The resulting conjugated antibody is relatively stable, especially if stored at −20° C or below.

There are two basic types of FA techniques: direct (DFA) and indirect (IFA). In the direct procedure, the antiviral antibody is labeled. This labeled antibody is then used to detect viral antigens in cryostat sections of tissues, scrapings, blood smears, etc. (Plate 4e,f,g,h)

The IFA technique is a two-step procedure. The specimen to be examined is first reacted with an unlabeled antiviral antibody. After sufficient incubation time is allowed for antigen-antibody interaction, the specimen is washed and then reacted with a labeled antibody directed against IgG of the species in which the unlabeled antiviral antibody was prepared. This labeled anti-antibody will attach itself to the viral-bound unlabeled antibody, and if this occurs, fluorescence is observed and the test is considered positive.

There are advantages and disadvantages to both FA procedures. The DFA technique is quicker to perform and is most often used because of the availability of DFA conjugates. The IFA technique, on the other hand, is more time consuming but only requires one labeled antibody if all antiviral antibodies are prepared in a single species.

In practice, the IFA procedure is most often used for detecting antibody. This is usually accomplished by infecting cell cultures with a virus, and then preparing "spot" microscope slides with these infected cells. Sera can then be analyzed for specific antibody by reacting them with the infected cells followed by a reaction with the antispecies IgG conjugate.

Immunoperoxidase

The immunoperoxidase technique is similar in principle to the fluorescent antibody technique, the primary difference being that the antibody is conjugated to the enzyme horseradish peroxidase rather than to a fluorescent compound. Although the enzyme is bound to the antibody, it remains active and, when provided with its substrate, reacts and gives a color reaction. This technique has some advantages over fluorescent antibody in that it does not require a fluorescence microscope, and it

is especially useful for locating viral antigens in histopathologic lesions.

Immunoelectron Microscopy

The negative staining technique of electron microscopy referred to earlier for the demonstration of viruses is also useful for identification. The virus is reacted with immune serum, resulting in clumping that can be seen when viewed under the electron microscope.

Immunodiffusion

The two most commonly used techniques of immunodiffusion are the double-diffusion plate system and immunoelectrophoresis. Both tests are conducted in a semisolid medium, usually agar. The essential difference is that, in the latter method, one of the reagents is electrophoretically fractionated before the second reagent is added. In both methods, the antigen and antibody diffuse against each other, forming a line of precipitation where they react.

The double-diffusion plate system is the more commonly used diagnostic test. The best-known example is the "Coggins test" for equine infectious anemia.

Immunodiffusion tests can be made more sensitive by using a radioactive label, which will permit the detection of antigen-antibody reactions not visible to the naked eye. The radioactive label is usually iodine (^{125}I), and either the antigen or antibody can be labeled. Labeling occurs by ^{125}I coupling to the amino acid tyrosine. The tests are read by covering the plates or slides with an x-ray film that records the radioactive (precipitation) lines.

Radioimmunoassay

There are two basic radioimmunoassay (RIA) systems, liquid phase and solid phase. In the liquid phase system, the antigen-antibody complexes are precipitated by subsequent addition of anti-gammaglobulin. The precipitate is collected by centrifugation and dried. The amount of radioactivity in the precipitate compared to the total radioactivity is a quantitative measure of the antigen-antibody reaction. The labeling is done with ^{125}I (see Immunodiffusion), and any one of the three components can be labeled.

In the solid phase system, the antibody is coated to the inside of a polystyrene tube and then reacted with antigen. The test is performed essentially as follows. The specimen is added to a polystyrene tube previously coated with antiviral antibody. If the antigen is present, it attaches to the bound antibody. Following rinsing, ^{125}I labeled antiviral antibody is added which reacts with the complex giving a "sandwich effect". The tube is washed and the amount of radioactivity is determined.

Enzyme-Linked Immunosorbent Assay

Enzyme-linked immunosorbent assay (ELISA) can be used to detect antigen or antibody. The sensitivity of ELISA is comparable to RIA, and the two procedures are similar in principle.

A solid-phase system is used for most ELISA assays. For virus detection, specific antibody is first adsorbed to the surface of a polystyrene tube, microtiter plate, etc., and sample containing the suspected virus is then added. If the virus is present, it binds to the adsorbed antibody. After rinsing, specific antiviral antibody labeled with an enzyme (usually alkaline phosphatase or horseradish peroxidase) is added. The labeled antibody reacts with the complex, creating a "sandwich effect." Following rinsing, the substrate for the enzyme is added, resulting in a color reaction. Some tests are visually interpreted, but greater sensitivity is obtained by spectrophotometric analysis.

An indirect ELISA procedure is usually used for antibody detection. Antigen is first adsorbed to a solid phase, followed by the addition of the test serum. After rinsing, an enzyme-labeled anti-gammaglobulin is added followed by addition of the enzyme substrate.

Variations of the standard ELISA include competitive ELISA for antibody detection, in which the enzyme labeled anti-gammaglobulin is replaced with enzyme-labeled antiviral antibody. The subsequent color development following the addition of the enzyme substrate is inversely proportional to the level of antibody present in the test sample. In other words, if specific antibody has been bound, the enzyme-labeled antibody will not bind. Thus, positive tests are those with no color reaction or less than that of appropriate controls. Another variation is the kinetic ELISA, in which the reaction is continuously monitored over a period of time, rather than being stopped after a predetermined amount of time.

Latex Agglutination

Latex agglutination (LA) tests are similar in principle to bacterial agglutination in that latex particles coated with antibody will agglutinate when mixed with the corresponding antigen. Conversely, the latex particles can be coated with antigens and used to detect antibody. These tests are easy to perform and provide results within minutes. Commercial kits are available for the detection of antibody to pseudorabies virus, and for the

detection of rotavirus antigen. The latter is designed for "in office" use.

Protection Tests

Protection tests are used primarily in the testing of vaccines and for virus identification where other less involved means are not available. They involve the production of either active or passive immunity in an animal or animals followed by challenge with the agent in question.

An example of a protection test once used is that for the identification of hog cholera virus. The test was carried out by injecting anti-hog cholera serum simultaneously with blood or spleen suspension from the animal suspected of having hog cholera. If the agent was hog cholera virus, the passive immunity provided by the anti-hog cholera serum would protect the pig from the challenge dose.

MOLECULAR BIOLOGICAL TECHNIQUES

Over the years, molecular biology has contributed much to the basic understanding of viruses, and in recent years, many of the newer molecular methods have been applied to clinical situations. Two of these techniques, restriction enzyme analysis and polymerase chain reaction, are particularly useful and will be discussed directly below. Readers interested in a more detailed discussion of these methods and others are referred to selected references at the end of this chapter.

Restriction Enzyme Analysis

Restriction enzymes are bacterial enzymes first discovered in the study of bacteriophage growth restriction in certain strains of bacteria. These enzymes are endonucleases that cut double-stranded DNA at specific recognition sites. These recognition sites are usually specific six-base-pair sequences, but may be as few as four or as many as eight base pairs.

Some of these restriction endonucleases (RE) cut both strands at the exact same position, resulting in a fragment of DNA with "blunt" ends. "Sticky" ends result from REs that cut unevenly, leaving a slight single-stranded overhang at each end of the DNA fragment.

Restriction endonuclease analysis is particularly useful in the "subserotypic" classification of viruses, in the differentiation of modified-live virus of vaccines from virulent virus, and in the epidemiologic tracking of disease outbreaks. Procedurally, the method entails treating viral DNA with one or more REs, and then separating the resulting fragments according to size by polyacrylamide gel electrophoresis. Gels are then soaked in a solution of ethidium bromide, which intercalates the DNA, causing the fragments to fluoresce when exposed to ultraviolet light.

RNA viruses can be similarly analyzed by first making a complementary DNA strand from the RNA using reverse transcriptase, and then amplifying this cDNA by the PCR method described directly below.

Polymerase Chain Reaction

The polymerase chain reaction (PCR), an in vitro method of DNA synthesis, is capable of amplifying targeted DNA segments by more than a million-fold. This is accomplished by creating a reaction mixture that, in addition to sample DNA contains two oligonucleotide primers that complement opposite ends of each strand of the targeted sequence, deoxynucleoside triphosphates, and a thermostable DNA polymerase (Taq polymerase). The first step of the PCR cycle is to denature the sample DNA by heating the reaction mixture to 95° C. Secondly, the mixture is cooled to allow the primers to anneal to the target DNA. Thirdly, the mixture is warmed to 70° C to allow for DNA synthesis by the DNA polymerase. As each cycle of the PCR is repeated, theoretically the number of target sequences doubles. Once the desired number of cycles is completed, the target DNA is separated by gel electrophoresis (described above under restriction enzyme analysis). The DNA is then transferred to nitrocellulose membranes by the method of "Southern blotting," and reacted with a specific DNA probe to verify results.

PCR is applicable to the study of RNA viruses if reverse transcriptase is first used to make cDNA from the target RNA.

It is unlikely that PCR will replace currently available tests such as fluorescent antibody for routine diagnosis of veterinary viruses. However, the technique is well suited for selected viruses that are difficult to cultivate or identify by conventional means. In fact, PCR-based diagnostic tests are currently in use commercially for the detection of two viruses of psittacine birds: psittacine beak and feather disease, and polyoma virus.

FURTHER READING

Belák, S. and Ballagi-Pordány: Application of the polymerase chain reaction (PCR) in veterinary diagnostic virology. Vet. Res. Comm. *17*:55, 1993.

Fenner, F.J., Gibbs, E.P.J., Murphy, F.A. et al. (eds.): Veterinary Virology. 2nd Ed. New York, Academic Press Inc., 1993.

Freshney, R.I. (ed.): Culture of Animal Cells. A Manual of Basic Technique. 2nd Ed. New York, Alan R. Liss, Inc., 1987.

Innis, M.A., Gelfan, D.H., Sninsky, J.J., and White, T.J.: PCR Protocols. A Guide to Methods and Applications. New York, Academic Press, Inc., 1990.

Miller, L.E., Ludke, H.R., Peacock, J.E., and Tomar, R.H. (eds.): Manual of Laboratory Immunology. 2nd Ed. Philadelphia, Lea & Febiger, 1991.

Paul, P.S.: Applications of nucleic acid probes in veterinary infectious diseases. Vet. Microbiol., 24:409, 1990.

38

An Overview of Pathogenesis, Prevention, and Control of Viral Infections

PATHOGENESIS OF VIRAL INFECTIONS

The first step in the disease process is exposure. Exposure may occur by direct contact with an infected animal, by indirect contact with secretions/excretions from an infected animal, or by mechanical or biological vectors. Viruses enter the host through the respiratory tract (aerosolized droplets), the alimentary tract (oral-fecal contamination), the genitourinary tract (breeding), the conjunctivae (aerosolized droplets), and through breaches of the skin (abrasions, needles, insect bites,etc.). Whether or not infection ensues following exposure depends upon the availability of susceptible cells. The susceptibility of cells depends in large part on their surface receptors which allow for attachment and subsequent penetration of the virus.

Following infection, the virus replicates at or near the site of viral entry (*primary replication*). Some viruses remain confined to this initial site of replication and produce *localized infections*, whereas others cause *disseminated infections* by spreading to additional organs via the blood stream, lymphatics, or nerves. The initial spread of virus to other organs by the blood stream is referred to as *primary viremia*. After multiplication in these organs, there may be

a *secondary viremia* with spread to target organs. The preference of a particular virus for a specific tissue or cell type is known as *tropism*.

Virus replication occurs in target organs causing cell damage and clinical manifestation of disease. The interval between initial infection and the appearances of clinical signs is the *incubation period*. Incubation periods are short in diseases in which the virus grows rapidly at the site of entry, e.g., influenza, and longer if infections are generalized, e.g., canine distemper. Some viruses infect animals but cause no overt signs of illness. Such infections are termed *subclinical* or *inapparent*. There are numerous factors that may influence the outcome of viral infections. These include preexisting immunity, age of the animal, and stress related factors such as nutritional status, housing, etc.

The mechanisms by which viruses cause disease are complex. Disease may result from direct effects of the virus on host cells or from indirect effects caused by the immunologic and physiologic responses of the host. The ability of a virus to cause disease is referred to as its *virulence*.

Direct Effect of Viruses on Host Cells

Cells infected with viruses undergo alterations of varying severity depending upon the particular virus. Some viruses exist in cells as an endosymbiotic infection causing no apparent changes, some cause subtle changes that affect the cell's function, and others cause complete cell destruction. Cell destruction occurs when the virus inhibits the synthesis of cellular macromolecules causing damage to lysosomal membranes and subsequent release of hydrolytic enzymes. Cell transformation and resulting neoplasia may occur if the viral genome (or a portion) is incorporated into the host genome.

Indirect Effect of Viruses on Host Cells: The Inflammatory Response

In an effort to ward off the infection, the host initiates an inflammatory response. Principal components of this response include interferons, cytotoxic T lymphocytes, antibody producing B lymphocytes, a variety of effector molecules, and complement. These various components work in concert and augment one another in an attempt to rid the host of the infecting virus.

Interferons (α and β) are produced by viral infected cells. They act to stop further virus replication in the infected cell, and they make other cells less permissive to infection. Interferons also enhance antigen expression on infected cells, thereby making them more recognizable to cytotoxic T cells. Cytotoxic T cells not only kill viral infected cells, they also release an interferon (γ), which enhances the production of antibody producing B lymphocytes. The specific antibodies that are produced neutralize the infectious virions when they are liberated by the cell. Antigen-antibody complexes in turn activate the complement system. Complement aids in the effective neutralization of virus and in the destruction of viral infected cells. The various effector molecules (cytokines) that are produced by B and T lymphocytes have many roles, including the induction of fever and the attraction of other inflammatory cells, e.g., neutrophils and macrophages, to the injured site. In this effort to rid itself of the infecting virus, the inflammatory response causes many of the clinical signs and lesions associated with viral infections.

Some viruses have the ability to abrogate this inflammatory response and cause *persistent infections*. They accomplish this in a number of ways, including the destruction of T lymphocytes causing immunosuppression, the avoidance of immunologic surveillance by altering antigen expression, and by the inhibition of interferon production.

A special type of persistent infection is one in which the virus is maintained in the host in a "nonproductive" state. This type of infection is referred to as *latent*.

Herpesviruses are notorious for causing latent infections. The viral genome is maintained in neurons in a closed circular form, and is periodically activated (often during stressful conditions) resulting in a productive infection.

Latent infections also occur with retroviruses in which the viral DNA transcript is incorporated into the host cell genome. Cell transformation and malignancy may result if the integrated transcript causes a disruption of normal cellular control processes.

PREVENTION AND CONTROL OF VIRAL INFECTIONS

Preventing Infection

The only certain way to prevent viral infection is to prevent exposure. This is accomplished in practice by only allowing those animals without evidence of previous exposure to commingle. This restricted contact is often referred to as "closed herds." To effectively maintain this closed status, all replacement animals and show animals must be isolated from the remaining animals for a period of 2 to 3 weeks. During this time, they are monitored for clinical signs and tested serologically for evidence of exposure. Preventing exposure through restricted contact is quite effective in areas where particular viruses are relatively uncommon, but is impractical in areas where these viruses are enzootic. In such instances, efforts are redirected from preventing infection to preventing disease.

Preventing Disease

Preventing disease is accomplished through vaccination. While vaccination doesn't necessarily prevent infection, the previous "priming" of the host's immune system allows for a quick response and clearance of the virus before disease occurs. There are two principal types of vaccines that are widely used, those made with killed virus and those prepared with modified-live virus.

Killed virus vaccines consist of viruses that have been chemically inactivated, often with formalin or beta-propiolactone. These vaccines frequently contain other ingredients to make them more immunogenic by enhancing the inflammatory response. Such ingredients are referred to as *adjuvants*.

Modified-live virus vaccines consist of viruses that have been attenuated in some fashion so that they are no longer virulent. This is usually accomplished by the serial transfer of the virus through cell cultures, embryonated eggs, or laboratory animals. Viruses can also be attenuated by removing certain genes responsible for virulence. This "genetic engineering" was used to make a commercially available pseudorabies vaccine.

There are particular advantages and disadvantages to killed and modified-live vaccines. The duration of immunity is usually longer with modified-live virus vaccines since these viruses actually cause mild or subclinical infections in the host. Also, a single dose of the vaccine is often sufficient, as opposed to killed vaccines, which usually require multiple doses. Some modified-live virus vaccines can be administered by the oral and nasal routes where they elicit a secretory antibody response (IgA).

There are three principal disadvantages to modified-live vaccines. They contain relatively low amounts of antigen, which is quickly neutralized by preexisting antibody. Thus, they are often ineffective in young animals that have received colostrum. Some may cause lethal infections of the fetus. There is a possibility that the attenuated virus may regain its virulence. In contrast, the virus in killed vaccines cannot revert to virulence, killed vaccines are safe for use in pregnant animals, and their large amounts of antigenic mass often make them more suitable for immunizing neonates that have maternal antibody.

There are several new approaches that are being explored in efforts to make vaccines safer and more effective. These approaches include the use of viral subunits, synthetic peptides, recombinant viruses, and anti-idiotypic antibodies.

Controlling Infection and Disease

Fundamental to controlling viral infections and disease are good management practices. Stress factors play important roles in predisposing animals to infection and in the spread of disease. Particularly important are the stresses associated with poor nutrition, overcrowding, and housing with improper ventilation.

Management practices should include preventative measures to protect the fetus and the newborn. Some viruses that cause mild or inapparent infections in adult animals may cause abortions or serious disease of neonates. Thus, efforts should be made to restrict the contact of pregnant animals and newborns from other animals. It is also important to insure that the newborn receives colostrum.

Another aspect of good management is the need to minimize contact between different species of animals, as some viruses cause inapparent infections in one species but severe disease in others. An example is the virus of pseudorabies, which causes subclinical infections in older pigs but uniformly fatal infections in cattle.

Thorough cleaning and disinfecting (see Chapter 7), and the use of clean coveralls and footbaths, are essential to prevent the spread of viruses by fomites. These aspects of management should be practiced at all times, but especially during disease outbreaks. When a disease outbreak occurs, affected animals should be quarantined and, if indicated, treated symptomatically. For instance, they should receive the necessary supportive therapy, such as fluid replacement in severe cases of diarrhea. In some instances, treatment with antibiotics may be advisable to prevent secondary bacterial infections, but the unnecessary use of antibiotics may exacerbate the illness by destroying normal bacterial flora.

Interferon and *antiviral drugs* are used for the specific treatment of viral diseases. Interferons are low-molecular-weight proteins that exert nonspecific, antiviral activity that is most effective in homologous cells. Interferon genes are present in all mammalian species, but these genes are not usually expressed in normal cells. In the presence of inducers such as viral infections, these genes are transcribed and interferons are produced as a defense mechanism. Interferons have no direct effect on the virus, but they induce the infected cell to make an antiviral protein that appears to block translation of viral messenger RNA. There is some evidence that the antiviral effects may also include inhibition of transcription and alterations in plasma cell membranes, which may inhibit penetration or virus assembly. Interferon diffuses out of infected cells and activates the production of antiviral protein in uninfected cells. These uninfected cells are protected from the virus but they do not make interferon.

Two distinct groups of interferons are presently recognized. The virus type (Type 1) is induced by viruses, is stable at pH 2, and originates from either fibroblasts or leukocytes. Type II (immune) interferon is induced in primed lymphocytes with specific antigens or in unprimed lymphocytes with T-cell mitogens. Accepted nomenclature for these interferons is α (leukocyte), β (fibroblast), and γ (immune).

Interferons appear early in the infection prior to the appearance of antibodies, and play a major role in recovery. The treatment of animals with exogenous interferon is not practiced widely because of the general unavailability of host-species interferons. While interferons are not necessarily host-species specific, their action is dependent upon their ability to bind to specific cell surface receptors. Human α-interferon, which is commercially available as a DNA recombinant, has some cross-species activity and has been used to orally treat cats infected with feline leukemia virus.

Most of the commercially available antiviral drugs are nucleoside analogs which affect the viral DNA polymerase. The more common of these are acycloguanosine (*acyclovir*), dihydroxypropoxymethylquanine (*ganciclovir*), adenine-arabinoside (*vidarabine*), and azidothymidine (*zidovudine*). Azidothymidine (AZT) specifically affects the RNA-dependent DNA polymerase (reverse transcriptase) of retroviruses. The pyrophosphate derivative, *foscarnet*, interacts with both DNA- and RNA-dependent DNA polymerases. *Ribavirin* interferes with protein synthesis by affecting mRNA. *Amantadine* and *rimantadine* are amines that inhibit Type A influenza viruses by preventing penetration, and *chalcone* and *arildone* interfere with decapsidation of rhinoviruses and enteroviruses, respectively.

Antiviral drugs are not widely used in veterinary medicine. Acyclovir is effective against herpesviruses and been used to treat ocular herpesvirus infection of cats. This drug has also been used to prophylactically treat expensive psittacine birds that have been exposed to psittacine herpesvirus.

FURTHER READING

Arnon, R. and Van Regenmortel, M.H.V.: Structural basis of antigenic specificity and design of new vaccines. FASEB J., 6:3265, 1992.

Dimmock, N.J. and Minor P.D. (eds.): Immune Responses, Virus Infections, and Disease. Oxford, IRL Press, 1989.

Fernandez-Botran, R.: Soluble cytokine receptors: their role in immunoregulation. FASEB J., 5:2567, 1991.

Greenspan, N.S., and Bona, C.A.: Idiotypes: structure and immunogenicity. FASEB J., 7:437, 1993.

Hawood, A.M.: Virus receptors: binding, adhesion, strenthening, and changes in viral structure. J.Virol., 68:1, 1994.

Huraux, J.M., Ingrand, D., and Agut, H.: Perspectives in antiviral chemotherapy. Fundam. Clin. Pharmacol., 4:357, 1990.

Kurstuk, E., Marusyk, R.G., Murphy, F.A. and Van Regenmortel, M.H.V. (eds.): Applied Virology Research, Volume 1, New Vaccines and Chemotherapy. New York, Plenum Publishing Corp., 1988.

Mims, C.A.: The pathogenetic basis of viral tropism. Am. J. Pathol., 135:447, 1989.

Mims, C.A.: New insights into the pathogenesis of viral infection. Vet. Microbiol., 33:5, 1992.

Moldoveanu, Z., Novak, M., Huang, Wen-Qiang, et. al.: Oral immunization with influenza virus in biodegradable microspheres. J. Infect. Dis., 167:84, 1993.

Myers, C.D.: Role of B cell antigen processing and presentation in the humoral immune system. FASEB J., 5:2547, 1991.

Noelle, R.J., and Snow, E.C.: T helper cell-dependent B cell activation. FASEB J., 5:2770, 1991.

Oldstone, M.B.A.: Molecular anatomy of viral persistence. J. Virol., 65:6381, 1991.

Trautwein, G. : Immune mechanisms in the pathogenesis of viral diseases: a review. Vet. Microbiol., 33:19, 1992.

Weiss, R.C., Cummins, J.M., and Richards, A.B.: Low-dose orally administered alpha interferon treatment for feline leukemia virus infection. J. Am. Vet. Med. Assoc., 199:1477, 1991.

39

Laboratory Diagnosis of Viral Infections

DIAGNOSTIC APPROACHES

Three general approaches for the laboratory diagnosis of viral infections are: (1) demonstration of the virus or some viral component; (2) isolation of the virus; and (3) measurement of the infected animal's immune response. Each approach has its merits, but demonstration of the virus is the most effective and useful approach for routine diagnosis.

The techniques of viral demonstration are varied, ranging from visualizing the intact virion by electron microscopy to detecting a unique piece of the viral genome using DNA probes. However, the technique most widely used is immunofluorescence or fluorescent antibody.

Fluorescent Antibody. The fluorescent antibody (FA) test detects viral antigens in infected cells via specific antiviral antibody that has been labeled with a fluorescent dye. Fluorescent antibody tests are performed on frozen sections of tissues, blood smears, tissue imprints, and scrapings. Results are available often in less than 1 hour, and these results are accurate provided that appropriate specimens in moderately good condition are tested. Table 39-1 lists the FA tests routinely available in many diagnostic laboratories and appropriate specimens to be submitted. Other commonly used rapid diagnosic tests for demonstrating viruses or viral antigens include electron microscopy, enzyme-linked immunosorbent assays, and latex agglutination. Additional information or special

considerations are presented in subsequent chapters when specific viral diseases are discussed.

Electron Microscopy. In the technique of negative contrast electron microscopy (EM), distilled water lysates of clinical specimens are "stained" with a solution of heavy atoms. This technique is primarily used for the examination of those clinical specimens expected to contain a large number of viral particles, such as feces (coronaviruses, rotaviruses, and parvoviruses) and vesicular and poxlike lesions (herpesviruses and poxviruses). Specimen preparation and EM examination usually can be completed within thirty minutes.

Enzyme-Linked Immunosorbent Assays and Latex Agglutination. Enzyme-linked immunosorbent assays (ELISA) and latex agglutination (LA) systems detect viral antigens by "capturing" them with specific antibody adsorbed to appropriate substrates. These techniques provide for a rapid diagnosis and are often available for "in office" use. Commercially available kits include ELISA and LA kits for detecting rotaviruses in feces from a variety of animal species, and ELISA kits for detecting canine parvovirus in feces and feline leukemia viral antigen in blood.

While the aforementioned techniques of antigen detection are used as the first approach to viral diagnosis, in many instances these techniques are not applicable. For example, appropriate specimens are often not obtainable from live animals for FA testing. Also, rapid antigen detection systems are not available for numerous viral diseases

Table 39–1. *Commonly Performed FA Tests and Preferred Specimens*

Species	Virus	Specimens
Avian		
	Duck viral enteritis	Liver, mesenteric lymph nodes
	Psittacine herpesvirus	Liver, spleen, lung
	Psittacosis*	Liver, spleen, lung
Bovine		
	Infectious bovine rhinotracheitis	Lung, trachea, kidney, lymph nodes, gut
	Bovine viral diarrhea	Lung, trachea, kidney, lymph nodes, gut
	Parainfluenza-3	Lung, trachea
	Respiratory syncytial virus	Lung, trachea
	Bluetongue	Lymph nodes, gut, spleen
	Rotavirus	Gut (spiral colon, ileum)
	Coronavirus	Gut (spiral colon, ileum)
	Pseudocowpox	Lesion and adjacent area
	Herpes mammillitis	Lesion and adjacent area
	Bovine parvovirus	Fetal lung, kidney, liver
	Bovine papular stomatitis	Lesion and adjacent area
Canine		
	Canine parvovirus	Gut, spleen
	Canine coronavirus	Gut
	Canine distemper	Brain, lung, stomach, urinary bladder, conjunctival scrapings, blood smears
Equine		
	Equine herpesvirus Type 1	Fetal lung, liver, spleen, thymus
	Equine adenovirus	Lung
Feline		
	Feline infectious peritonitis	Lung, spleen, liver, kidney, gut
	Feline panleukopenia	Gut, spleen
	Feline herpesvirus	Lung, trachea, conjunctival scrapings
	Feline leukemia	Blood smears
	Feline chlamydia*	Lung, conjunctival scrapings
Miscellaneous		
	Epizootic hemorrhagic disease of deer	Esophagus, spleen, lymph nodes, trachea
	Contagious ecthyma	Lesions and adjacent area
Porcine		
	Pseudorabies	Brain, lung, tonsil, spleen, liver
	Hog cholera	Tonsil, spleen, lymph node
	Porcine parvovirus	Mummified fetus
	Transmissible gastroenteritis	Gut (ileum)
	Rotavirus	Gut (ileum)
	Swine influenza	Lung
	Encephalomyocarditis	Brain, heart
	Hemagglutinating Encephalomyelitis	Brain, gut
	Porcine adenovirus	Gut

* A bacterial disease but usually diagnosed in virology laboratories.

(including unknown viral diseases). In these instances, virus isolation is the method of choice.

Virus Isolation. Viruses are obligate intracellular parasites, and thus require living cells in order to replicate. In the laboratory, living cells are usually provided as cell cultures in which cells obtained by enzymatic digestion of tissues are cultivated on glass or plastic surfaces. When clinical specimens containing virus are inoculated onto susceptible cell cultures, the virus replicates and often produces a characteristic pattern of cell destruction, or cytopathic effect. In some instances, the virus grows without any discernible effect on the cells and must be demonstrated by special stains that reveal viral inclusion bodies or by FA tests to detect viral antigens, etc. The time required to isolate viruses is highly variable, ranging from as little as 24 hours to as long as several weeks.

The clinical manifestations of disease generally guide the selection of appropriate clinical specimens; e.g., nasal and ocular swabs from upper respiratory tract infections, feces from enteric infections, etc.

The acute phase of illness is the best time to demonstrate and isolate viruses. As disease progresses, antibody develops, virus shedding is reduced, and virus is cleared from tissues. During the late stages of illness, evaluating the serum of infected animals for antibodies to specific viruses may be the only means of diagnosis. This is accomplished through a variety of serologic tests.

Serologic Tests. The serologic tests most often used in veterinary diagnostic laboratories to diagnose viral infections are serum neutralization (SN) tests and hemagglutination inhibition (HI) tests. The principle of these tests (see Chapter 37) is based

Table 39–2. Commonly Performed Serological Tests

Species	Virus	Frequency of Positive	Common Titer
Bovine			
	Infectious bovine rhinotracheitis (IBR)	~40%	1:4 –1:32$^{\parallel}$
	Bovine viral diarrhea (BVD)	~60%	1:32 –1:512$^{\parallel}$
	Parainfluenza-3 (PI3)	>90%	1:32 –1:256$^{\parallel}$
	Bovine respiratory syncytial virus (BRSV)	~50%	1:4 –1:32$^{\parallel}$
	Bovine leukemia virus (BLV)*	Highly variable	NA¶
	Bluetongue (BT)†	Highly variable	NA¶
Equine			
	Equine herpesvirus-1 (EHV-1)	>90%	1:8 –1:64$^{\parallel}$
	Equine influenza	~75%	1:8 –1:32**
	Equine viral arteritis (EVA)‡	~4%	1:4 –1:256$^{\parallel}$
	Equine infectious anemia (EIA)	Very low	NA¶
Porcine			
	Pseudorabies (PRV)	Very low	1:4 –1:64$^{\parallel}$
	Porcine parvovirus (PPV)	>90%	1:256–1:2048**
	Transmissible gastroenteritis (TGE)§	Highly variable	1:8 –1:32$^{\parallel}$

* BLV is more common in dairy herds; as many as 90% of cows in a herd may be positive if a clinical case of BLV has occurred. † BT is common in some southeastern states; frequency of positives may be as high as 50%. ‡ EVA is endemic in some Standardbred populations where the frequency of positives may be greater than 50%. Positive stallions of all breeds should be evaluated for carrier status. § Herds with a recent history of TGE will often have a positive rate of greater than 90%. $^{\parallel}$ Serum neutralization, ¶ Agar-gel, ** Hemagglutination inhibition.

on the fact that viral activity can be inhibited by the presence of specific antibody. Dilutions of serum are tested, and results are reported as the reciprocal of the highest dilution in which antiviral activity is noted. Ideally, the results of serum collected during the acute phase of illness are compared with results of serum collected during convalesence. Diagnosis is confirmed if a four-fold increase is noted between these paired samples.

Results from single (non-paired) serum samples are more difficult to interpret. Positive results only mean that the animal has been exposed, either naturally or through vaccination. Interpretation is made easier by testing a percentage of those animals that were sick vs. those that were not, because higher titers are usually more indicative of recent infections. Table 39-2 lists some of the commonly performed serologic tests, frequency of positives, and common titers. The positivity rates referred to in this table may vary depending upon geographic location and are only included to demonstrate the difficulty in drawing conclusions from the results of single samples.

Positive results of regulatory tests are always meaningful regardless of antibody titer. For this reason, other serologic tests more suited to standardization and test kit form have been developed. Examples are the agar gel immunodiffusion test (AGID) for equine infectious anemia and the ELISA and LA tests for pseudorabies. The results of these tests are reported as either positive or negative.

COLLECTION AND SUBMISSION OF SPECIMENS

The laboratory diagnosis of clinical illness depends upon the type and condition of submitted specimens. It also depends upon the practicing veterinarian and laboratory working in close concert. Because many of the laboratory tests are for specific disease agents, an adequate clinical history must accompany all submissions. This will permit laboratory staff to perform additional tests as they deem it necessary.

General guidelines for the collection and submission of specimens are presented below. Most laboratories supply a specimen submission form that should be completed with the available pertinent information. In the absence of a form, the veterinarian should supply as complete a history as possible. Veterinarians should contact the diagnostic laboratory if they have any questions.

Animals. Live, sick animals are preferable to dead animals. Whenever possible, animals should be submitted directly to the diagnostic laboratory for complete necropsy examination. If a herd problem exists, more than one animal should be submitted. Bus and courier service may be used to ship small animals provided they are packaged in leakproof insulated containers with sufficient ice or cold packs. *Do not freeze* animals submitted for necropsy.

Tissues. To minimize contamination during necropsy, it is best to collect a routine set of tissues prior to thorough examination. Recommended tissues are lung, kidney, liver, spleen, small intestine, large intestine, and mesenteric lymph node. Brain tissue should also be collected if central nervous system disease is suspected. Other tissues containing abnormalities noted during the thorough examination should also be collected. Table 39-1 lists the preferred tissues for the common FA tests used to diagnose viral infections.

A portion of these tissues should be placed in leakproof plastic bags and placed under refrigeration. While it is recommended that each tissue be placed in a separate bag, it is absolutely essential that intestine be separated from other tissues. Otherwise, bacteriologic examinations will be compromised. Tissues should be brought directly to the laboratory, or shipped under refrigeration by overnight mail, bus, or courier service. Tissues collected during the latter part of the week should be frozen and shipped on Monday.

Since many viruses produce characteristic microscopic lesions, small pieces (1/4 inch thick) of each tissue should be placed in ten percent buffered formalin for histopathologic examination. An entire longitudinal half of the brain should be submitted. These samples should *not be frozen*.

Feces. Feces should be collected from acutely ill animals and placed in leakproof containers. While well saturated swabs are adequate for many individual virologic examinations, several milliliters or grams of feces permit a more complete diagnostic workup including bacteriologic and parasitologic examinations. Samples should be submitted to the laboratory using cold packs as coolant.

Swabs. Nasal and ocular swabs are useful for isolating viruses from animals with upper respiratory tract infections. These swabs should be collected from acutely ill animals and placed directly into screw-capped tubes containing a viral transport medium. The sampling of several animals in different stages of the illness increases the likelihood of isolating the causative agent.

Swabs are also useful for the sampling of vesicular lesions. Fresh vesicles should be ruptured and the swab saturated with the exuding fluid. Two swabs should be collected, one for virus isolation and one for electron microscopy. The swab for virus isolation should be placed in viral transport medium and the swab for electron microscopy should be placed in a screw-capped tube containing one or two drops of distilled water. Scab material from more advanced lesions should also be submitted.

There are several commercially available viral transport media that help maintain the viability of viruses during shipment to the laboratory. Most of these transport media are balanced salt solutions containing a high protein content and antibiotics to prevent bacterial overgrowth. Many diagnostic laboratories provide their own version of transport medium to practicing veterinarians upon request.

Slides. A number of infectious diseases can be diagnosed by examining slides prepared from blood and tissues. Blood smears are used for diagnosing feline leukemia, while blood smears and conjunctival scrapings are used to diagnose canine distemper. Conjunctival scrapings are particularly useful for diagnosing herpesvirus and chlamydial infections in cats. Imprints made from liver, spleen, and lung are especially useful for diagnosing chlamydia and herpesvirus infections of psittacine birds.

Slides should have sufficient cells to allow thorough examination, but should not be so thick as to cause difficulty in staining. A conjunctival scraper or some other device (blunt end of scalpel blade) should be used to scrape the conjunctiva; cotton swabs are not adequate. Matted eyes should be cleaned and flushed prior to scraping the conjunctiva. Tissue imprints should be made by lightly touching the microscope slide with fresh cuts of tissue previously blotted with a paper towel to absorb some of the blood.

Slides should be air-dried and sent to the laboratory in slide holders to prevent breakage. Several slides permit a more thorough diagnostic workup, including cytologic examinations.

Serum. Blood samples should be collected in sterile tubes containing no anticoagulants. These should be submitted to the laboratory in specially designed styrofoam holders to avoid breakage. Blood samples should *not be frozen or allowed to overheat*. If samples cannot be delivered to the laboratory within a reasonable time, serum should be removed and refrigerated or frozen.

FURTHER READING

Castro, A.E., and Heuschele, W.P. (eds.): Veterinary Diagnostic Virology. A Practitioner's Guide. St. Louis, Mosby-Year Book Inc., 1992.

Fenner, F.J., Gibbs, E.P.J., Murphy, F.A., et al. (eds.): Veterinary Virology. 2nd Ed. New York, Academic Press, 1993.

Galasso, G.J., Whitley, R.J., and Merigan, T.C. (eds.): Practical Diagnosis of Viral Infections. New York, Raven Press Ltd., 1993.

McNulty, M.S., and McFerran, J.B. (eds.): Recent Advances in Virus Diagnosis. Boston, Martinus Nijhoff Publishers, 1984.

Part V

SURVEY OF VIRAL INFECTIONS

40

Viral Infections of Cattle

INFECTIONS OF THE RESPIRATORY SYSTEM

Infectious Bovine Rhinotracheitis

Synonyms. Summer pinkeye, rednose, infectious pustular vulvovaginitis, infectious pustular balanoposthitis, bovine herpesvirus Type 1 (BHV-1).

Cause. *Varicellovirus* (Family: Herpesviridae. Subfamily: Alphaherpesvirinae).

Distribution and Transmission. Infectious bovine rhinotracheitis (IBR) virus affects cattle throughout the world. Infection occurs via the respiratory and genital routes. Direct contact, aerosol droplets, and fomites are important means of spread.

Pathogenicity. Six clinical manifestations of IBR have been described, with the respiratory form being the most common. There are also the conjunctival form, the genital form, the abortion form, the encephalitic form, and the enteric or generalized form in young calves. The latter two are relatively uncommon. The virus has also been associated with mastitis. Three subtypes of IBR (BHV-1) virus have been defined based on restriction enzyme analysis. These are designated BHV-1.1 (respiratory subtype), BHV-1.2 (genital subtype), and BHV-1.3 (encephalitic subtype). It has been proposed recently that BHV-1.3 be reclassified as BHV-5. Although BHV-1.1 is referred to as the respiratory subtype, it is also associated with abortion and encephalitis. Subtype BHV-1.2 is further divided into BHV-1.2a and BHV-1.2b. The former may cause abortion, whereas the latter does not.

The respiratory form has a sudden onset with high temperature. There is congestion and severe inflammation of the mucous membranes with serous ocular and nasal discharges. The morbidity is high in unvaccinated (nonimmune) herds but mortality is generally low. Recovery is usually uneventful in well managed herds within about 14 days. Under stressful conditions (e.g., feedlots), secondary bacterial infections may lead to a severe tracheitis (diphtheritic membrane) and bronchopneumonia. Abortion or stillbirths may occur 1 to 3 months postinfection.

The genital form of IBR is characterized by inflammation of the genital mucosa and development of small pustules that coalesce and ulcerate. Infections may be mild or subclinical.

Diagnosis. Clinical specimens: Nasal and ocular swabs; vaginal and preputial swabs; trachea and lung; fetal liver, kidney, and lung; acute and convalescent sera.

A presumptive diagnosis is often made on the basis of clinical signs and lesions. A definitive diagnosis requires demonstration of viral infected cells by immunofluorescence, isolation, and identification of the virus, or the demonstration of a significant increase in IBR antibody levels between acute and convalescent serum samples. Immunofluorescence is the preferred method for the diagnosis of IBR abortions because the virus is often nonviable owing to advanced autolysis of fetal tissues. The virus is easily isolated from other clinical specimens by the inoculation of cell cultures of bovine origin.

Prevention and Control. Modified live and killed vaccines often are available in combination with other bacterial and viral antigens. The modified live vaccines are of two types, one that is administered intramuscularly (IM) and one that is given intranasally (IN). The IM vaccine should not be used in pregnant cows.

Malignant Catarrhal Fever

Synonym. Snotsiekte (Africa), gangrenous coryza.

Cause. Herpesvirus (Family: Herpesviridae. Subfamily: Gammaherpesvirinae).

Additional Hosts. Wildebeest, hartebeest, and other wild ruminants. Sheep are subclinically infected.

Distribution and Transmission. Malignant catarrhal fever (MCF) occurs worldwide, but the incidence is not high. Except for feedlots, there are usually only one or two cases in a herd at one time. The method of transmission is uncertain, but appears to require close contact with infected animals. There are apparently at least three distinct herpesviruses associated with MCF. Two of these are named for the Bovidae subfamily (Alcelaphinae) of animals from which they were isolated. *Alcelaphine herpesvirus* Type 1 (AHV-1) was isolated from the wildebeest and AHV-2 was isolated from the hartebeest. A herpesvirus that is antigenically related to AHV-1 is carried by sheep. This virus is thought to be responsible for MCF in cattle of Europe and North America, and the disease is usually referred to as "sheep associated" MCF.

Pathogenicity. Four forms of MCF have been described:

1. Peracute.
2. Intestinal.
3. Head (brain) and eye.
4. Benign.

Most affected animals have a combination of these forms and display fever, depression, anorexia, and rhinitis with nasal discharge that becomes mucopurulent and encrusted. The skin of the muzzle becomes eroded, and there is stomatitis, pharyngitis, laryngitis, and parotitis with salivation. After a short febrile period, most cattle with the severe disease die within 10 days.

In addition to the lesions giving rise to the above, there may be edema of the meninges, perivascular cuffing in other areas of the brain, enteritis, general lymphoid hyperplasia, and corneal opacity. Gray foci may be seen in the kidneys and liver. The anterior cervical and retropharyngeal lymph nodes may be hemorrhagic and edematous. Vasculitis is a characteristic histologic change that may be present in any tissue.

Diagnosis. Clinical specimens: Fresh leukocytes (buffy coat), fresh thyroid and adrenal tissue, serum.

Diagnosis is usually based on clinical signs and pathologic changes. The usual sporadic nature of the disease helps distinguish MCF from bovine virus diarrhea and rinderpest. The history of sheep associated with cattle supports a diagnosis.

Laboratory confirmation of MCF is difficult. Serologic tests, virus isolation, and molecular techniques (polymerase chain reaction) are used, but these procedures are not available in most diagnostic laboratories.

Prevention and Control. Vaccines are not available. Cattle should be separated from sheep.

Parainfluenza-3

Cause. *Paramyxovirus* (Paramyxoviridae).

Additional Hosts. Sheep.

Distribution and Transmission. Parainfluenza-3 (PI3) virus infections occur in cattle throughout the world. Droplet infection, contact, and fomites are important in transmission.

Pathogenicity. The PI-3 virus is prevalent and most cattle have antibodies as a result of exposure. Exposure generally results in mild or subclinical respiratory infection. Environmental stresses, including those incidental to transportation, may lead to secondary bacterial infections with resulting pneumonia. The most important complicating bacteria are *Pasteurella haemolytica* and *P. multocidia*. This complex of a predisposing viral infection with subsequent bacterial infection is often referred to as "shipping fever" or bovine pneumonic pasteurellosis.

Diagnosis. Clinical specimens: Nasal swabs, lung, and acute and convalescent sera.

The virus can be isolated in cell cultures of bovine origin in which it produces cytopathic effects characterized by the production of both cytoplasmic and intranuclear inclusions. Examination of cryostat sections of lung tissue by immunofluorescence provides for a rapid diagnosis of PI-3 infection in animals that have died.

A fourfold increase in antibody titer (serum neutralization or hemagglutination inhibition) indicates that an infection has been sustained. Many cattle possess antibodies to PI-3 virus; thus, paired sera are important.

Prevention and Control. Killed and live attenuated PI-3 virus vaccines of cell culture origin are available, usually in combination with other viral and bacterial antigens.

Efforts should be made to minimize stress associated with marketing by allowing calves to adjust to weaning and dehorning before they are subjected to the rigors of sale barns, transportation, and feedlots.

Antibiotic therapy is used to control secondary bacterial infections.

Bovine Respiratory Syncytial Virus

Synonym. Atypical interstitial pneumonia.
Cause. *Pneumovirus* (Paramyxoviridae).
Additional Hosts. Sheep and goats.
Distribution and Transmission. Bovine respiratory syncytial virus (BRSV) is widely distributed in cattle throughout the world. Infected cattle shed virus in respiratory secretions, and susceptible cattle become infected by direct and indirect contact.
Pathogenicity. The morbidity is generally high in fully susceptible herds, but the mortality is low. Many cattle experience mild to subclinical infections, but some develop acute lower respiratory tract infections characterized by coughing, nasal discharge, and fever. Severely affected animals may display signs of dyspnea and mouth breathing. In the absence of secondary bacterial infections, recovery occurs in 1 to 2 weeks.
Diagnosis. Clinical specimens: Slide preparations from nasal and conjunctival scrapings, nasal and conjunctival swabs, lung, and acute and convalescent sera.

A rapid diagnosis sometimes can be achieved by the fluorescent antibody (FA) examination of cytologic preparations of nasal and conjunctival epithelia collected early in the course of disease. Similarly, FA examination is used to demonstrate viral infected cells in cryostat sections of lung tissue in animals that have died. In these animals, histopathologic lesions are helpful in making a diagnosis of BRSV infection, especially if syncytial cells containing cytoplasmic inclusions are observed.

The virus, which is antigenically related to human respiratory syncytial virus, can be isolated in cell cultures of bovine origin in which it produces cytopathic effects consisting of syncytia and eosinophilic cytoplasmic inclusions. Owing to the lability of the virus, isolation attempts are apt to be negative unless the specimens are exceedingly fresh.

A serologic diagnosis can be made by the demonstration of a significant increase in antibody levels between acute and convalescent sera.

Rhinoviruses

Rhinoviruses (Picornaviridae) comprising several serologic types have been isolated from calves and older cattle with mild to acute respiratory infections. It is likely that these viruses have a primary role in some cases of "shipping fever" pneumonia in cattle. Rhinoviruses can be isolated using primary cell cultures of bovine kidney. Nasal swabs are the appropriate clinical specimens.

Bovine Herpesvirus Type 4

There are several different strains of bovine Herpesvirus Type 4 (BHV-4), including DN 599 and Movar 33/63. These viruses have often been referred to as "slow herpesviruses" because of the longer time required (as compared with BHV-1) to cause cytopathic effects in cell culture.

The role of BHV-4 as a cause of disease is unclear. The virus appears to be ubiquitous in cattle, having been recovered from both "normal" and clinically ill animals. The virus has also been isolated from other ruminants including sheep, and from cats with urolithiasis. The recovery of this virus from animals other than cattle must be viewed with some caution because such isolates may only represent contaminant bovine viruses present in fetal calf serum used in cell culture media.

The molecular biology of BHV-4 indicates a close genomic relationship with herpesviruses of the subfamily gammaherpesvirinae.

Adenoviruses

Adenoviruses have been associated with various clinical illnesses in cattle, including respiratory tract disease, epizootic pneumoenteritis, and weak calf syndrome. At present, 10 serotypes are recognized, and it has been proposed that they be divided into two groups. Serotypes 1 through 3 have characteristics similar to human adenoviruses and would be classed as Group 1. The remaining serotypes are similar in their properties to avian adenoviruses and would be placed in Group 2. The viruses can be cultivated in cell cultures of bovine origin, although those of Subgroup 2 often require numerous subpassages before cytopathic effects are evident. Also, viruses of Subgroup 2 are more readily isolated in cell cultures derived from bovine testes.

INFECTIONS OF THE DIGESTIVE SYSTEM

Bovine Virus Diarrhea

Synonyms. Mucosal disease.
Cause. *Pestivirus* (Flaviviridae).
Additional Hosts. Possibly sheep and deer.
Distribution and Transmission. Bovine virus diarrhea (BVD) virus infections occur in cattle throughout the world. Transmission is by contact

and fomites; the mode of infection is by ingestion and inhalation. *In utero* infections also occur.

Pathogenicity. There are two biotypes of BVD virus, one that causes cytopathic effects in cell cultures and one that does not. Most cattle infected with either biotype develop subclinical infections or only a mild clinical illness of short duration. A severe disease results when cattle are infected with both biotypes. This occurs when cattle persistently infected with a noncytopathic strain of BVD virus (a result of *in utero* infection) are superinfected with a cytopathic strain; or perhaps, as recent evidence suggests, when cytopathic virus develops from the infecting noncytopathic virus as a result of insertions of cellular sequences into the viral genome. This severe and uncommon disease is often referred to as "mucosal disease." Leukopenia, anorexia, loss of condition, and pyrexia are common signs. Temperatures range from 104 to 106° F and most animals develop a severe diarrhea with the feces containing mucus and streaks of blood. Salivation and a thick, stringy nasal discharge may be evident and shallow erosions of the oral and nasal mucosa are frequent. The skin of the muzzle may be eroded and crusty. Frequent necropsy findings are erosions and ulcerations of the upper respiratory and digestive tracts; characteristic ulcers are seen in the esophagus and involving Peyer's patches. The virus has an affinity for lymphoid tissues resulting in depression of the cell-mediated immune response.

Infections of pregnant cows in early gestation may result in fetal death and resorption of the fetus leading to infertility and repeat breeding. Abortions may occur during the first and second trimester, but fetuses infected during the third trimester usually suffer no ill effects. Fetuses that survive infections during early gestation may be born with congenital anomalies such as ocular defects, alopecia, arthrogryposis, and cerebellar hypoplasia. Persistent infections may result if fetuses are infected between 2 and 4 months of gestation. These animals are often "poor doers" and frequently die from secondary bacterial infections because of an impaired immune system.

A strain of non-cytopathic BVD virus has been reported to cause severe disease in cattle in the absence of cytopathic BVD virus. This highly virulent strain of BVD virus was associated with disease characterized by fever, diarrhea, hemorrhage, and death. Affected cattle were thrombocytopenic and leukopenic.

Diagnosis. Clinical specimens: Nasal discharge, feces, blood, blood smears, spleen, kidney, lymph nodes, turbinate, intestine, acute and convalescent sera, and fetal liver and kidney.

The most convenient way to diagnose BVD infections is by fluorescent antibody (FA) examination of blood smears and cryostat sections of diseased tissues. The virus is easily isolated in cell cultures of bovine turbinate but most strains are noncytopathic. The presence of virus in inoculated cultures is confirmed by FA examination.

A diagnosis can be inferred from the demonstration of a fourfold increase in the level of BVD antibody between acute and convalescent serum samples.

Persistently infected animals are identified by the isolation of BVD virus from the serum or by the demonstration of viral infected leukocytes by FA. The latter often can be achieved through the examination of blood smears, but the isolation and culturing of monocytes (from freshly collected EDTA blood) for several days prior to FA examination increases the chance of accurately identifying infected animals. These cells should be cultured in a medium containing nonbovine serum (e.g., horse serum) because bovine serum may be contaminated with noncytopathic strains of BVD virus.

Prevention and Control. Both modified live and killed vaccines are available to help prevent and control BVD infections. Modified live vaccines are generally safe, but may cause disease in animals persistently infected with BVD. Modified live vaccines should not be used in pregnant cows.

Calf Scours

Causes. *Rotavirus* (Reoviridae) and *Coronavirus* (Coronaviridae).

Distribution and Transmission. Rotaviruses and coronaviruses occur in cattle throughout the world. The viruses are transmitted by contact and fomites; the mode of infection is ingestion. Dams may carry the viruses and infect neonatal calves.

Pathogenicity. The viruses affect calves usually within the first 3 weeks of age. Rotavirus is seldom found in calves over 7 days old, whereas coronavirus is often seen in calves as old as 3 weeks and as young as 1 day. Both viruses produce a disease characterized clinically by profuse, watery diarrhea of sudden onset leading to exteme dehydration. Morbidity is often near 100% and mortality may range from 0 to >50%. Damage to the intestinal mucosa including loss of villous absorptive cells results in malabsorption.

Bovine coronavirus can be recovered from the respiratory tract but its role in respiratory disease is unclear. The virus has also been incriminated as a cause of "winter dysentery" in adult cattle.

Diagnosis. Clinical specimens: Fresh feces and segments of intestine including spiral colon, ileum, and jejunum.

There are several convenient and rapid methods used to diagnose rotavirus and coronavirus infections, including the electron microscopic examination of distilled water lysates of feces and fluorescent antibody examination of fecal smears and frozen sections of intestine. Commercial antigen detection test kits (ELISA and Latex agglutination) designed for "in office" use are available for the diagnosis of rotavirus infections. There are several distinct groups of rotaviruses, designated A through F. Most rotaviruses affecting calves belong to Group A, although rare infections apparently occur with rotaviruses of Groups B and C. Viruses belonging to these latter groups would not be detected using current antigen detection systems, although virus particles would still be observed by electron microscopy.

Both rotaviruses and coronaviruses can be cultivated in cell cultures of bovine origin but often with some difficulty.

Prevention and Control. Commercial vaccines are available for rotavirus and coronavirus but their efficacy is questionable. Good management practices important in control include cleaning, disinfecting, the use of footbaths, and provision of colostrum.

Vesicular Stomatitis

Cause. *Vesiculovirus* (Rhabdoviridae).

Additional Hosts. Swine, horses, human beings, and a variety of wild animals, including deer and raccoons. Most human cases have occurred in laboratory workers, although infections probably occur in the field as well. Human infections resemble influenza and are characterized by sore throat and fever.

Distribution and Transmission Vesicular stomatitis (VS) virus is enzootic in cattle, swine, and horses in certain areas of Central and South America and Mexico; and in feral swine on Ossabaw Island off the coast of Georgia. Occasional outbreaks occur throughout the United States, the most recent being the 1982 outbreak in cattle and horses in several western states. The mode of transmission is uncertain but is thought to occur by contact, fomites, and probably by biting insects.

Pathogenicity. Two distinct serotypes of VS virus are recognized. They are represented by the Indiana and New Jersey strains, of which there are several subtypes. The disease, which may occur as extensive epizootics, resembles foot-and-mouth disease in cattle but is considerably milder. Lesions most commonly involve the mouth and teats. These vesicular lesions occur on the lips, tongue, and oral mucosa, and affected cattle display clinical signs of hypersalivation, depression, and anorexia. Teat lesions often lead to decreased milk production and mastitis in lactating cows. The disease usually runs a benign course with complete recovery within 2 to 3 weeks. Mouth lesions are the most common clinical manifestation of VS in horses, whereas lesions of the feet are most often seen in affected swine.

Diagnosis. Clinical specimens: Vesicular fluid, saliva, and affected mucous membranes collected early in the disease.

The virus is easily isolated in cell cultures derived from various animal species. Identification is accomplished using a variety of serologic procedures, including complement fixation and serum neutralization. A rapid presumptive diagnosis can be achieved by the electron microscopic demonstration of rhabdovirus in distilled H_2O lysates of lesion material. Vesicular stomatitis can be differentiated from other vesicular diseases by the inoculation of animals listed in Table 40–1.

Prevention and Control. Vaccination is not practiced. State and federal regulatory officials should be notified if vesicular stomatitis is suspected.

Foot-and-Mouth Disease

Synonyms. Aphthous fever.

Cause. *Aphthovirus* (Picornaviridae).

Additional Hosts. All cloven-footed animals, including swine, sheep, goats, deer, and water buffalo. Guinea pigs, rabbits, mice, and other species can be infected experimentally. Contact with infected animals may result in infection of human beings, which is characterized by the development of lesions on the hands, feet, and in the mouth.

Distribution and Transmission. Foot-and-mouth disease (FMD) is widespread, occurring in South America, Africa, Europe, the Middle East, and Asia. North America, New Zealand, Australia, and the United Kingdom are free at present, although a recent outbreak in Britain was traced to frozen lamb introduced from Argentina. The Canadian outbreak of 1952 was traced to a European immigrant. The disease is spread by contact, fomites, and migratory birds. The mode of infection is by inhalation and ingestion.

A total of seven different serologic types of FMD virus have been recognized. These are O, A, C, SAT 1, SAT 2, SAT 3, and Asia 1. The first three types of FMD are often referred to as European types, because they were first isolated in France

Table 40–1. *Differentiation of Vesicular Diseases by Animal Inoculation*

	Cattle*	Swine**	Horse*	Guinea Pig†
Foot-and-mouth disease	+	+	–	+
Vesicular stomatitis	+	+	+	+
Vesicular exanthema	–	+	+	+
Swine vesicular disease	–	+	–	–

* Intradermal-tongue.
** Intramuscular.
† Intradermal.

and Germany, although they do occur in other countries. The SAT types were isolated in "Southern African Territories" and are restricted to Africa. The Asia type has only been reported in various parts of Asia.

Pathogenicity. The FMD virus produces a highly contagious disease of cloven-hoofed animals and is characterized by the production of vesicular lesions in the mouth, muzzle, interdigital space, and on the coronary band of the foot after a usual incubation period of 2 to 5 days. Vesicular lesions may also be found on the udder and teats of cows, and the snout of swine. The most common and characteristic sign is excessive salivation; the saliva is sticky, foamy, and stringy.

The vesicles, which are pronounced on the buccal mucous membrane and tongue, break, erode, ulcerate, and eventually heal. Myocardial degeneration may be seen in the malignant form, and pregnant animals may abort. Morbidity is high. Mortality is low in mature animals but may be high in calves and lambs. Secondary bacterial infections may lead to worse complications than those seen in the primary disease. Lameness and marked loss of condition are frequent sequelae.

Diagnosis. Clinical specimens include vesicular fluid, affected mucous membranes, blood, and serum.

The FMD virus can be isolated in a variety of cell cultures, including those derived from bovine kidney and thyroid. Viral growth with accompanying cytopathology occurs best in primary cell cultures. Identification is accomplished by serum neutralization and complement fixation tests.

Foot-and-mouth disease can be differentiated from other vesicular diseases by the inoculation of cattle, swine, horses, and guinea pigs as outlined in Table 40–1.

Prevention and Control. State and federal regulatory officials should be contacted if FMD is suspected. Confirmed outbreaks are dealt with by strict quarantine and slaughter.

In areas where the disease is enzootic, vaccination is practiced using killed vaccines containing the appropriate serotypes of virus for the region.

Rinderpest

Cause. *Morbillivirus* (Paramyxoviridae).

Additional Hosts. Water buffalo, sheep, goats, deer, camels, and swine.

Distribution and Transmission. Rinderpest occurs in remote parts of Asia and Africa, and for centuries has been the cause of severe epizootics with enormous losses of cattle. It has not occurred in North America, and has not been reported in Europe since World War I.

Transmission is usually by food, water, and litter contaminated with secretions and excretions from infected animals.

Pathogenicity. Rinderpest is a highly fatal, contagious, febrile disease of cattle and water buffalo. The disease is usually less severe in other hosts, and subclinical infections occur in swine. The incubation period is 4 to 9 days followed by high fever and acute inflammation of the mucous membranes of the digestive and upper respiratory tracts. There is ultimately diarrhea with blood-stained feces, a characteristic arching of the back, and rapid loss of condition. A milder disease may be seen where the disease is enzootic and less susceptible species are involved.

Characteristic necropsy lesions are congestion and hemorrhage of intestinal epithelium with occasional necrosis of Peyer's patches. Erosions are found in the mouth and upper respiratory tract.

Diagnosis. Clinical specimens: Urine, blood, nasal discharge, feces, lymph nodes, and spleen collected in the acute phase of the disease; serum from surviving animals.

Tissues from suspected cases are inoculated into known susceptible and immune or passively protected calves.

Cytopathic changes, including cytoplasmic and nuclear inclusions, are produced in primary bovine kidney cell cultures and in the Vero cell line. Extracts of tissues can be used as sources of antigen in complement fixation and agar gel precipitin tests. Serum neutralization tests in cell cultures can be done on the sera of animals that have survived long enough to produce antibodies.

Prevention and Control. In those countries where the disease does not occur, outbreaks are dealt with by a strict slaughter and quarantine policy.

Modified live vaccines are commonly employed in countries where the disease is enzootic.

INFECTIONS OF THE INTEGUMENTARY SYSTEM

Cowpox

Cause. *Orthopoxvirus* (Family: Poxviridae. Subfamily: Chordopoxvirinae).

Additional Hosts. Human beings and various animals, including large zoo cats, domestic cats, anteaters, and rodents. The latter are thought to be the natural reservoir hosts.

Distribution and Transmission. Cowpox occurs sporadically in various countries of Western and Eastern Europe, but the disease is thought to be nonexistent in the United States. Transmission occurs by contact and fomites.

Pathogenicity. Cowpox virus produces what is usually a benign infection of the udder and teats. Papules are first seen, followed by vesicles, which rupture leading to scab formation. Scabs drop off in about 2 weeks. Losses in milk production result from the soreness of affected teats and also from secondary bacterial infection, which may complicate the disease and contribute to development of mastitis.

Vaccinia virus, the virus used in smallpox vaccines, was once responsible for some outbreaks of cowpox-like infections in cattle as a result of contact with recently vaccinated human beings. Although original smallpox vaccines were prepared from virus isolated from the teats of cows with "cowpox," the virus of vaccinia is distinctly different from that of cowpox. Although the origin of vaccinia remains a mystery, it is likely that the virus evolved from cowpox virus, or as a recombinant of cowpox virus and smallpox virus.

Diagnosis. Clinical specimens: Vesicular fluid, scabs, and scrapings from lesions.

It is difficult to clinically distinguish cowpox from pseudocowpox and other infections of the teats. Diagnosis is most easily confirmed by the examination of distilled H_2O lysates of lesion material by electron microscopy. Virions are characteristic of other orthopoxviruses, being "brick-shaped" as opposed to the virions of pseudocowpox (a parapoxvirus), which are ovoid in appearance.

Cowpox virus can be cultivated in cell cultures of bovine and human origin, and on the chorioal-

lantoic (CA) membrane of chicken embryos. The latter method of cultivation also provides a means to differentiate cowpox virus from pseudocowpox virus, which does not grow on the CA membrane.

Prevention and Control. Vaccination is not practiced. Control is best accomplished by good milking management practices.

Pseudocowpox

Synonyms. Milker's nodules, paravaccinia.

Cause. *Parapoxvirus* (Family: Poxviridae. Subfamily: Chordopoxvirinae).

Additional Hosts. Human beings.

Distribution and Transmission. Pseudocowpox is a widespread disease that is transmitted by contact and fomites.

Pathogenicity. Pseudocowpox is characterized by the formation of papules, vesicles, scabs, and nodules on the udder and teats of cows, with a course of several weeks. The disease may spread to milkers, producing lesions that begin as papules, then develop to nodules up to 2 cm in diameter.

Diagnosis. Clinical specimens: Vesicular fluid, scabs, and scrapings from lesions.

A rapid laboratory diagnosis can be achieved by the examination of distilled H_2O lysates of lesion material by electron microscopy. The virus grows in a variety of cell cultures but, unlike cowpox virus, it can not be propagated on the CA membrane of chicken embryos.

Prevention and Control. Vaccination is not practiced. Good milking practices help control the disease.

Papular Stomatitis

Cause. *Parapoxvirus* (Family: Poxviridae. Subfamily: Chordopoxvirinae).

Distribution and Transmission. Papular stomatitis occurs worldwide and is a widespread disease in North America. Transmission occurs by direct contact and fomites.

Pathogenicity. Papular stomatitis is a mild disease of cattle usually up to 2 years of age and is characterized by proliferative, reddish, raised papules on the epithelium of the mouth, muzzle, and in the nostrils. Lesions may also be noted in the esophagus, abomasum, and rumen. Histologically there is hyperplasia of the mucosa with intracytoplasmic inclusions. The major importance of bovine papular stomatitis is that the clinical signs may be confused with those of foot-and-mouth disease and other kinds of stomatitis.

Diagnosis. Clinical specimens: Scrapings from lesions.

Diagnosis is usually based on gross and microscopic lesions. A rapid laboratory confirmation can be obtained by the electron microscopic examination of distilled H_2O lysates of lesion material. The virus grows in a variety of bovine cell cultures producing cytopathic changes, including cytoplasmic inclusions.

Prevention and Control. None practiced.

Bovine Papillomatosis

Synonym. Common warts of cattle.

Cause. *Papillomavirus* (Papovaviridae).

Distribution and Transmission. Papillomaviruses occur in cattle throughout the world. Transmission is thought to be by direct contact and fomites.

Pathogenicity. There are presently six recognized types of bovine papillomaviruses that are associated with the production of papillomas of various sites in cattle. The most common sites affected are the head, neck, and shoulders. The skin thickens, becomes rough and nodular followed by alopecia. Warts may be large, pendulant, and cauliflower in shape. They may occur on the penis of the bull and in the vaginal mucosa of the female, resulting in breeding difficulty. Two papillomavirus types have a predilection for the skin of teats, and one type has been associated with lesions of the alimentary tract.

Diagnosis. Diagnosis is based on gross and microscopic examination.

Prevention and Control. Commercial wart vaccines and autogenous wart vaccines are used but their efficacy is questionable. Affected animals should be isolated.

Bovine Ulcerative Mammillitis

Synonyms. Bovine herpes mammillitis, Pseudolumpy skin disease, Allerton virus, Bovine herpesvirus Type 2.

Cause. *Simplexvirus* (Family: Herpesviridae. Subfamily: Alphaherpesvirinae).

Distribution and Transmission. Distribution of bovine herpesvirus Type 2 is probably worldwide. Transmission is thought to occur by direct contact, fomites, and mechanically by biting insects.

Pathogenicity. Bovine herpesvirus Type 2 (BHV-2) primarily affects dairy cattle causing an ulcerative mammillitis resulting in a marked loss of milk production. Clinically, this sporadic disease is characterized by edema of teats followed by vesicle formation and subsequent erosion of the teat and udder epithelium. Vesicles usually rupture within 24 hours and yield a serous exudate.

Scabs begin to form at 4 days, and healing occurs under the scab with recovery usually in 3 to 4 weeks. Milking may prevent scab formation and consequently delay healing. Face and muzzle lesions may occur in nursing calves. The Allerton strain of BHV-2 was originally isolated in Africa from cattle with generalized skin infections.

Diagnosis. Clinical specimens: Vesicular fluid, scabs, and scrapings of lesion material.

A rapid diagnosis of herpes mammillitis can be achieved by the electron microscopic demonstration of herpesvirus in distilled H_2O lysates of lesion material. The virus can be isolated in cell cultures of bovine origin but grows best at reduced temperature. Identification is accomplished by serum neutralization and fluorescent antibody tests.

Prevention and Control. Vaccines are not available. Control is best accomplished by good milking practices.

Lumpy Skin Disease

Synonym. Neethling virus.

Cause. *Capripoxvirus* (Family: Poxviridae. Subfamily: Chordopoxvirinae).

Additional Hosts. Buffalo, giraffe, and impala.

Distribution and Transmission. Lumpy skin disease occurs on the African continent and is thought to be spread mechanically by biting insects.

Pathogenicity. The incubation is about 2 to 4 weeks. Some animals may be subclinically infected or only show a mild febrile response with few skin lesions, whereas others may develop numerous nodules over large areas of the skin and on mucous membranes of the eye, nose, mouth, and genitalia. Nodules may become necrotic leading to secondary bacterial infections. Morbidity may be quite high but mortality is generally low.

Diagnosis. Clinical specimens: Biopsies (fresh and fixed) from lesions.

Gross and microscopic findings are suggestive. The finding of typical poxviruses in lesion material by electron microscopy is supportive, but confirmation requires isolation and identification of the virus.

Prevention and Control. State and federal regulatory officials should be contacted if lumpy skin disease is suspected. Modified live virus vaccines are used in Africa.

INFECTIONS OF THE NERVOUS SYSTEM

Sporadic Bovine Meningoencephalitis

Sporadic bovine meningoencephalitis (SBME) is a disease of low incidence, and is similar to the human disease, subacute sclerosing panencephalitis (SSPE), caused by measles virus. SBME is an inflammatory disease; pathological changes in the brain include perivascular cuffing, diffuse infiltration of lymphocytes, and neuronal loss. A paramyxovirus, closely related to the distemper-measles-rinderpest group, was isolated from a young heifer with SBME.

Pseudorabies

Pseudorabies is an infrequent sporadic and fatal disease of cattle. Cattle acquire the infection through close contact with pigs. The virus gains entry through abrasions of the skin and affected cattle display clinical signs of "mad-itch" followed by rapid death. Pseudorabies virus is discussed in detail under its principal host, the pig (see Chapter 41).

Rabies

Rabies virus is discussed in detail under viral infections of dogs (see Chapter 44). The disease in cattle is usually nonexcitive or "dumb." Clinical signs of pharyngeal paralysis may be confused with choking, and owners and veterinarians are often exposed while trying to remove a nonexistent object.

Louping-Ill

The virus of louping-ill causes an encephalomyelitis principally of sheep but occasionally of cattle in close contact with infected sheep. The virus is discussed in detail in Chapter 42.

Malignant Catarrhal Fever

The virus of malignant catarrhal fever is associated with a variety of clinical syndromes in cattle. The head or brain form was discussed earlier in this chapter.

INFECTIONS OF THE REPRODUCTIVE SYSTEM

Infectious Bovine Rhinotracheitis

The virus of infectious bovine rhinotracheitis (IBR), which was discussed in detail earlier in this chapter, causes abortion, usually during the second half of gestation. There are no consistent gross lesions observed in aborted fetuses, but focal necrosis is observed microscopically in a variety of tissues, including liver, kidney, spleen, and adrenal. Vaccination is effective in preventing abortion "storms," but sporadic abortions are common. The virus of IBR also causes genital infections in cows and bulls.

Bovine Viral Diarrhea

The effect of bovine viral diarrhea virus on the fetus is dependent upon the age of the fetus at the time of infection. Infection during the first trimester may lead to death and fetal resorption, mummification or abortion. Fetuses infected between 2 and 4 months may be born persistently infected ("poor doers"), whereas those infected after 4 months usually suffer no ill effects. Bovine viral diarrhea is discussed in detail elsewhere.

Bluetongue

Bluetongue virus (BT) (see Chapter 42) usually causes a subclinical infection in adult cattle and rare infections of the fetus. Mummification, abortion, and fetuses born with congenital defects have been associated with bluetongue infections early in gestation. Many cattle in the United States, particularly those in Southeastern states, have antibodies to BT virus.

Akabane Disease

Synonyms. Congenital arthrogryposis-hydraencephaly.

Cause. *Bunyavirus* (Bunyaviridae).

Additional Hosts. Sheep and goats.

Distribution and Transmission. Akabane disease occurs in Australia, Japan, Argentina, South Africa, and countries of the Middle East. The causative virus is transmitted to susceptible animals by biting insects.

Pathogenicity. There are no overt clinical signs in adult animals exposed to Akabane virus other than an early febrile response. Fetal infections, which result in deformities of the fetus, may occur if pregnant cows are infected during the first trimester of gestation. There may be abortions, stillbirths, mummified fetuses, and premature live births. Arthrogryposis is the most common deformity noted, affecting a single joint in one limb to multiple joints in all limbs and the vertebral column. Severely affected animals may suffer difficult deliveries. Hydranencephaly is noted less frequently.

Diagnosis. Clinical specimens: Placenta and fetus.

A presumptive diagnosis is based on clinical history and gross lesions observed in affected fetuses. The virus can be isolated by the intracerebral inoculation of young mice and in various cell cultures.

Prevention and Control. Killed vaccines are available. Akabane disease does not occur in the United States, and state and federal regulatory officials should be notified if the disease is suspected.

Chuzan Disease

Cause. *Orbivirus* (Reoviridae).

Additional Hosts. Sheep, goats, and probably other ruminants.

Distribution and Transmission. Chuzan disease occurs in Southeast Asia and Japan. The virus is transmitted to susceptible animals by hematophagous arthropods.

Pathogenicity. Adult cattle infected with Chuzan virus develop a transient, mild leukopenia but otherwise remain clinically normal. Infection of pregnant cows may result in congenital anomalies characterized by hydronencephaly and cerebellar hypoplasia. Development of these anomalies appears to be related to the age of the fetus at the time of infection, and are thought to occur most often when the fetus is infected at about 4 months of age. Affected calves may be blind and display seizures and opisthotonos. Beef cattle are more often affected than dairy cattle.

Diagnosis. Clinical specimens: Brain, spleen, serum.

Diagnosis is usually based on clinical history, microscopic lesions, and supportive serologic results.

Prevention and Control. Vaccines are not available. This disease does not occur in the United States.

Bovine Leukemia

Synonyms. Enzootic bovine leukosis, bovine viral leukosis, adult form of bovine leukosis, bovine lymphosarcoma.

Cause. HTLV-BLV retrovirus group (Retroviridae).

Distribution and Transmission. The virus causing bovine leukemia is widely distributed in cattle of many countries. Susceptible cattle are infected by direct contact with blood from an infected animal. Fetal infections also occur but are relatively uncommon.

Pathogenicity. Although susceptible cattle of all breeds can be infected at any age with bovine leukemia virus (BLV), most infections occur in dairy cattle over 2 years of age. The fact that disease is seldom seen in younger animals is related to the presence of protective maternal antibody and the separation of younger animals from the remaining herd until they reach sexual maturity.

Most animals infected with BLV remain clinically normal. Those that develop disease (approximately 2%) ultimately die. Initial clinical signs are often those of weight loss and reduced milk production, but may be quite varied depending on the site of tumor development. The organs most commonly affected are the lymph nodes, heart, abomasun, uterus, and spleen.

A sporadic form of leukemia occurs in calves and young adults, but this disease is not associated with BLV infection.

Diagnosis. Clinical specimens: Affected tissues (fixed) and serum.

Diagnosis of disease associated with BLV infection is often based on the finding of tumors upon clinical and gross necropsy examination. Microscopic examination of affected tissues is required to confirm the disease.

Specific antibody may be detected in the serum of infected cattle by a variety of serological tests, the most common being the agar gel immunodiffusion (AGID). Many cattle have antibodies to BLV but most never develop disease.

Prevention and Control. Vaccines to prevent BLV infections are not available. In herds free of BLV infection, prevention is best accomplished by the quarantine and serologic testing of any replacement animal. Control of BLV in infected herds is based on the removal of serologically positive animals and good management practices to prevent spread of the virus during blood sampling, clinical examinations, castration, dehorning, etc.

Bovine Immunodeficiency-Like Virus Infection

Synonyms. Bovine AIDS-like virus infection.

Cause. *Lentivirus* (Retroviridae).

Bovine immunodeficiency-like (BIV) virus was originally isolated from an adult dairy cow with persistent lymphocytosis. Although isolation of this virus was reported in 1972, only recently have additonal isolations been made. Few studies of pathogenesis have been done and none of these has been long term. Thus, the relationship of BIV infection and disease has not been adequately determined. Experimentally infected cattle have exhibited lymphoid proliferation and decreased cell mediated cytotoxicity. Serologic studies have indicated a prevalence rate of about 4%.

Bovine Ephemeral Fever

Synonyms. Bovine epizootic fever, three-day sickness.

Cause. *Lyssavirus* (Rhabdoviridae).

Additional Hosts. Water buffalo.

Distribution and Transmission. The virus of bovine ephemeral fever is widely distributed in many countries of Africa and Asia, and is present in Australia but not in Europe or North and South America. Natural transmission is thought to occur by insect vectors.

Pathogenicity. Bovine ephemeral fever is generally a mild disease characterized by a biphasic febrile response, depression, anorexia, muscle twitching, and generalized stiffness. The respiratory rate may be increased and some infected animals may have ocular and nasal discharges. Recovery is usually rapid and uneventful.

Diagnosis. Clinical specimens: Blood.

Diagnosis is often based on clinical signs and history. The finding of gross necropsy lesions consisting of fibrin-rich fluid in the pleural and peritoneal cavities and in joint capsules is supportive. Diagnosis is best confirmed by the intravenous inoculation of susceptible cattle with infected blood.

Prevention and Control. Modified-live virus and killed vaccines are available.

Bovine Spongiform Encephalopathy

Synonym. Mad cow disease.

Cause. Prion (proposed).

Distribution and Transmission. More than 99% of the laboratory confirmed cases of bovine spongiform encephalopathy (BSE) have occurred in Great Britain. Transmission occurs orally through the eating of feed supplemented with BSE contaminated ruminant-derived offal. There is no evidence of horizontal or vertical transmission.

Pathogenicity. Following exposure to the agent of BSE, there is a long incubation period in infected cattle prior to development of clinical signs. The average time appears to be about 4 years. Affected cattle display clinical signs associated with progressive CNS dysfunction, including behavioral changes, incoordination, and hypersensitivity to various stimuli. The disease is uniformly fatal within 1 to 6 months after the onset of signs.

Diagnosis. Clinical specimens: Formalin-fixed brain tissue.

Diagnosis of BSE is based on clinical signs and the subsequent demonstration of spongiform changes in the brain by histopathologic examination.

Prevention and Control. Prevention is best accomplished by the exclusion of ruminant-derived protein from cattle feed. Affected cattle are destroyed.

FURTHER READING

Baker, J.C.: Human and bovine respiratory syncytial virus: immunopathologic mechanisms. Vet. Quart., 13:47, 1991.

Barr, B.C., and Anderson, M.L.: Infectious diseases causing bovine abortion and fetal loss. Vet. Clin. North. Am. Food Anim. Pract. 9:343, 1993.

Bolin, S.R., and Ridpath, J.F.: Differences in virulence between two noncytopathic bovine viral diarrhea viruses in calves. Am. J. Vet. Res. 53:2157, 1992.

Carpenter, S., Miller, L.D., Alexandersen, S., et al.: Characterization of early pathogenic effects after experimental infection of calves with bovine immunodeficiency-like virus. J. Virol. 66:1074, 1992.

Castro, A.E., and Heuschele, W.P. (eds.): Veterinary Diagnostic Virology. A Practitioner's Guide. St. Louis, Mosby-Year Book, 1992.

Denny, G.O., Wilesmith, J.W., Clements, R.A., and Hueston, W.D.: Bovine spongiform encephalopathy in Northern Ireland: epidemiological observations 1988–1990. Vet. Rec. 130:113, 1992.

d'Offay, J.M., Mock, R.E., and Fulton, R.W.: Isolation and characterization of encephalitic bovine herpesvirus type 1 isolates from cattle in North America. Am. J. Vet. Res. 54:534, 1993.

Ferris, D.H. (ed.): Foreign Animal Disease Reference Manual. 4th Ed. National Veterinary Services Laboratories, Science and Technology, Animal and Plant Health Inspection Service, United States Department of Agriculture, P.O. Box 844, Ames, IA, 1984 (Revised 1990).

Flaming, K., Van der Maaten, M., Whetstone, C., et al.: Effect of bovine immunodeficiency-like virus infection on immune function in experimentally infected cattle. Vet. Immunol. Immunopathol. 36:91, 1993.

Gibbs, C.J., Bolis, C.L., Asher, D.M., et al.: Recommendations of the international roundtable workshop on bovine spongiform encephalopathy. J. Am. Vet. Med. Assoc. 200:164, 1992.

Heamon, J.A.: Focus on Chuzan disease. Foreign Animal Disease Report No. 19,2:10, 1991.

Ja Goe, S., Kirkland, P.D., and Harper, P.A.W.: An outbreak of Akabane virus-induced abnormalities in calves after agistment in an endemic region. Aust. Vet. J. 70:56, 1993.

Koopmans, M., van Wuijekhuise-Sjouke, L., Schukken, Y.H., et al.: Association of diarrhea in cattle with torovirus infections on farms. Am. J. Vet. Res. 52:1769, 1991.

Liggitt, H.D., and DeMartini, J.C.: The pathomorphology of malignant catarrhal fever. I. Generalized lymphoid vasculitis. Vet. Pathol. 17:58, 1980.

Meyers, G., Tautz, N., Stark, R. et al.: Rearrangement of viral sequences in cytopathogenic pestiviruses. Virology 191:368, 1992.

Miller, J. M., Whetstone, C.A., and Van der Maaten, M.J.: Abortifacient property of bovine herpesvirus type 1 isolates that represent three subtypes determined by restriction endonuclease analysis of viral DNA. Am. J. Vet. Res. 52:458, 1991.

Mirangi, P.K.: Attempts to immunize cattle against virulent African malignant catarrhal fever virus (alcelaphine herpesvirus-1) with a herpesvirus isolated from American cattle. Vet. Microbiol. 28:129, 1991.

Monke, D.R., Rohde, R.F., Hueston, W.D., and Milburn, R.J.: Estimation of the sensitivity and specificity of the agar gel immunodiffusion test for bovine leukemia virus: 1,296 cases (1982–1989). J. Am. Vet. Med. Assoc. 200:2001, 1992.

Prusiner, S.B., Füzi, M., Scott, M., et al.: Immunologic and molecular biologic studies of prion proteins in bovine spongiform encephalopathy. J. Infect. Dis. 167:602, 1993.

Qi, F., Ridpath, J.F., Lewis, T., et al.: Analysis of the bovine viral diarrhea virus genome for possible cellular insertions. Virology 189:285, 1992.

Saif, L.J., Brock, K.V., Redman, D.R., and Kohler, E.M.: Winter dysentery in dairy herds: electron microscopic and serological evidence for an association with coronavirus infection. Vet. Rec. 128:447, 1991.

Suarez, D.L., Van der Maaten, M.J., Wood, C., and Whetstone, C.A.: Isolation and characterization of new wild-type isolates of bovine lentivirus. J. Virol. 67:5051, 1993.

Timoney, J.F., Gillespie, J.H., Scott, F.W., and Barlough, J.E. (eds.): Hagan and Bruner's Microbiology and Infectious Diseases of Domestic Animals. 8th Ed., Ithaca, NY, Comstock Publishing Associates, 1988.

Wilesmith, J.W., Ryan, J.B.M., and Atkinson, M.J.: Bovine spongiform encephalopathy: epidemiological studies on the origin. Vet. Rec. 128:199, 1991.

41

Viral Infections of Swine

INFECTIONS OF THE RESPIRATORY SYSTEM

Swine Influenza

Synonyms. Swine flu, hog flu.

Cause. Influenza virus A (Orthomyxoviridae).

Additional Hosts. Human beings, other mammals, and birds.

Distribution and Transmission. Swine influenza is widespread, occurring most commonly in the fall and winter. Aerosol droplets, contact, and fomites are means of spread. In swine herds where the virus is enzootic, young susceptible pigs are continually infected, thereby maintaining the virus. Explosive outbreaks of acute disease occur when the virus is introduced into susceptible herds.

Pathogenicity. Morbidity is high but the mortality is only 2% or less. Virus infection is mild without secondary bacteria. In a typical outbreak, there is an incubation period of about 3 days followed by an acute onset of respiratory distress with rapid respiration, coughing, anorexia, and prostration. The course is usually 2 to 6 days with rapid recovery in uncomplicated cases. Necropsy in acute cases discloses edematous mediastinal lymph nodes and pneumonic lesions usually limited to the apical and cardiac lobes. Affected areas are firm and purplish in color and there is often a sharp line of demarcation between normal and affected tissue. Exudative bronchitis and interstitial pneumonia are common microscopic findings.

Diagnosis. Clinical specimens: Nasal swabs and lungs, acute and convalescent sera.

A presumptive diagnosis is made on the basis of clinical and pathologic findings. Confirmation requires isolation of the virus, demonstration of seroconversion, or detection of viral infected cells in frozen sections of lung tissue by immunofluorescence. Swine influenza virus is most easily isolated by the inoculation of embryonated eggs via the allantoic cavity.

Prevention and Control. Swine influenza virus is usually introduced into herds via replacement stock or show animals. Thus, prevention is best accomplished by the good management practices of separation and quarantine. Vaccination is not practiced. In the event the disease is particularly severe, antibiotics may be used to control secondary bacteria.

Recovery from swine influenza infection confers immunity, but the duration of this immunity is not known. The virus is quite sensitive and does not survive long outside living cells. It is easily inactivated by disinfectants including sodium hypochlorite (bleach).

Cytomegalovirus of Swine

Synonyms. Inclusion body rhinitis.

Cause. *Muromegalovirus* (Family: Herpesviridae. Subfamily: Betaherpesvirinae).

Distribution and Transmission. Cytomegalovirus of swine (suid herpesvirus Type 2) is widely distributed throughout the world. The virus is shed in nasal secretions and transmission is by contact with aerosol droplets.

Pathogenicity. Inclusion body rhinitis of swine is a common but usually minor disease of young pigs. It is most severe in swine up to 2 weeks of age. The virus affects the mucosa of the nasal passages and upper respiratory tract with varying severity. Clinically inapparent, generalized infections occur in which epithelial cells of other organs, particularly the kidney, are involved. Infection is via the respiratory tract and pigs may exhibit clinical signs, principally sneezing, at any time up to 10 weeks of age.

Diagnosis. Clinical specimens: Nasal swabs or scrapings and lung tissue.

The disease is usually diagnosed histologically by demonstrating large basophilic intranuclear inclusions in sections or scrapings from the nasal mucosa. The inclusion bodies can also be demonstrated in exfoliated epithelial cells obtained with nasal swabs. Electron microscopy is useful for demonstrating the virus in negative stained distilled water lysates of nasal mucosa. The virus can be propagated in primary cell cultures of pig lung producing cytopathic changes, including large intranuclear inclusions within 11 to 18 days postinoculation. Since the virus is strongly cell associated, the initiation of cell cultures from infected tissues may be a more successful method of isolation.

Prevention and Control. There are no vaccines available for the prevention of cytomegalovirus of swine. The virus is often enzootic in swine herds and poses little threat to well managed operations. Efforts should be made to differentiate inclusion body rhinitis from atrophic rhinitis. The latter is a more serious bacterial disease.

Porcine Reproductive and Respiratory Syndrome. See Infections of the Reproductive System.

Porcine Respiratory Coronavirus. Porcine respiratory coronavirus is a variant of transmissible gastroenteritis (TGE) virus and probably occurs worldwide. It is widespread in Europe. The virus is spread by aerosol droplets, and infection is usually subclinical, although mild interstitial pneumonitis may occur. Cross-reaction with TGE virus occurs and may cause confusion in the interpretation of serologic results. Otherwise, the virus appears to be of little consequence.

INFECTIONS OF THE DIGESTIVE SYSTEM

Transmissible Gastroenteritis

Cause. *Coronavirus* (Coronaviridae).

Additional Hosts. Transmissible gastroenteritis (TGE) virus is relatively host-specific for pigs, but it can infect dogs subclinically. The virus is serologically related to porcine respiratory coronavirus, canine coronavirus, and feline infectious peritonitis virus.

Distribution and Transmission. The virus is probably worldwide in its occurrence. Transmission is by contact. The virus is present in feces and nasal secretions, and may also be present in the milk of infected sows. The majority of outbreaks occur during the colder months of the year.

Pathogenicity. In previously unexposed swine herds, TGE is highly fatal to pigs less than 10 days old and usually spreads rapidly through the whole herd. Young pigs have a severe diarrhea with a watery, whitish or whitish-green stool. Vomiting is common. Dehydration is especially marked, and deaths occur in 2 to 5 days after onset of signs. The TGE virus selectively multiplies and destroys absorptive epithelial cells of the villi, giving rise to villous atrophy and impaired absorption (malabsorption). The disease in older animals may be manifested by elevated temperature, poor appetite, mild diarrhea, and depression. Vomiting may also occur in some cases. In herds where the virus is enzootic, clinical signs are milder and mortality is relatively low. Clinical signs are often seen in these pigs during the postweaning period when passive immunity has declined.

Although clinical signs of respiratory infection are not common, the virus can be recovered from lung tissue. TGE virus has been shown to persist in the intestine and lungs of pigs for extended periods of time, and it has been suggested that many animals that have recovered from the disease may actually be carriers. A variant form of TGE virus does affect the respiratory tract.

Diagnosis. Clinical specimens: Portions of jejunum and ileum.

Clinically and pathologically, TGE may be confused with colibacillosis, rotaviral diarrhea, and diarrhea caused by porcine epidemic diarrhea virus (also a coronavirus). Thus, a presumptive diagnosis of TGE based on clinical signs and pathologic findings must be confirmed by laboratory tests.

The laboratory method most often used to diagnose TGE infections is fluorescent antibody examination of cryostat sections or scrapings of affected intestine. The virus can be cultivated in cell cultures of swine origin, but may produce little or no discernible cytopathology.

Prevention and Control. Both live attenuated and killed vaccines are available for the immunization of sows prior to farrowing. Their value seems to depend on their capacity to produce colostral and lactogenic immunity. Greater immunity is achieved via natural infection, and one procedure employed to control the disease has been to feed intestines from known positive cases to pregnant sows about a month before farrowing.

Prevention is best accomplished by maintaining closed herds. Replacement stock and show animals should be isolated and tested serologically before they are introduced into the herd.

Rotavirus Infection

Synonyms. White scours, milk scours, and 3-week-old scours.

Cause. *Rotavirus* (Reoviridae).

Distribution and Transmission. Rotaviral infection is widespread in swine herds throughout the world. Transmission is by contact and pigs are infected by the oral/fecal route. The virus is present in feces up to 3 weeks after infection.

Pathogenicity. Rotavirus is enzootic in many swine herds. Disease seems to occur when the immune status of the pig is lowered and there is an overwhelming buildup of the virus. The mature epithelial cells of the distal half of the villi of the small intestine appear to be especially susceptible to rotavirus infection. This selective destruction of villous cells leads to villous atrophy, malabsorption, and diarrhea. The diarrhea usually occurs in pigs 1 to 4 weeks of age. The severity of the infection is influenced by concurrent infection with other agents or by stress such as chilling.

Diagnosis. Clinical specimens: Portions of small intestine.

Rotaviral diarrhea resembles the enzootic form of TGE clinically and histopathologically. Specific diagnosis is best accomplished by fluorescent antibody examination of frozen sections of intestine or by electron microscopic examination of feces and intestinal contents. Propagation of rotavirus using conventional cell culture systems is difficult; the use of enzymes such as trypsin enhances growth.

Prevention and Control. Rotavirus appears to be present in most swine herds. Modified live and killed vaccines are available. Keeping pigs warm and dry, insuring that they get adequate colostrum and milk, and providing good sanitation reduce the severity of the disease.

Porcine Epidemic Diarrhea

Synonyms. Epidemic viral diarrhea, enteric coronavirus (CV-777).

Cause. *Coronavirus* (Coronaviridae).

Distribution and Transmission. Porcine epidemic diarrhea virus appears to be distributed throughout much of Europe, but has not been reported in the United States. Infection occurs by the oral or oronasal route.

Pathogenicity. There is an incubation period of about 1 to 3 days following exposure. The principal clinical sign is that of watery diarrhea and all ages of pigs may be affected.

The clinical disease is somewhat similar to TGE but differs in that spread of the virus throughout the herd is slower, vomiting is not a clinical sign, and mortality is lower. In addition, older pigs are occasionally more severely affected than younger ones.

The virus infects the epithelial cells of the small intestinal villi, causing histopathologic lesions similar to but milder than those caused by TGE virus.

Diagnosis. Clinical specimens: Portions of small intestine.

The virus can be propagated in cell cultures (Vero) if trypsin treatment is utilized. Diagnosis is usually accomplished by the immunofluorescence examination of cryostat sections of affected intestine or by immune electron microscopic examination of feces or intestinal contents.

Prevention and Control. Porcine epidemic diarrhea virus has not been reported in the United States. Vaccines are not yet available for use in those countries where the virus does occur.

Swine Vesicular Disease

Cause. *Enterovirus* (Picornaviridae).

Additional Hosts. Human beings.

Distribution and Transmission. This disease was first reported in feeder pigs in Italy in 1966. It has since been reported in Great Britain (declared free in 1980), several European countries, and Asia. Transmission is by contact and fomites. Several outbreaks have been traced to improperly cooked garbage.

Pathogenicity. The disease is clinically indistinguishable from foot-and-mouth disease (FMD), vesicular stomatitis (VS), and vesicular exanthema (VE). Epithelial tissue is initially involved, followed by a generalized infection of lymphoid tissues and viremia. The first signs are reduced feed intake, lameness and tenderness of the feet, fever up to 106° F, and the formation of vesicles on the feet, snout, tongue, mouth, nostrils, and teats. The prognosis is favorable, but in most countries infected animals are slaughtered. Experimentally infected pigs may show central nervous sytem involvement.

The SVD virus is closely related to the human enterovirus, Coxsackie B-5. Mild infections of SVD virus have been reported in several laboratory workers.

Diagnosis. Clinical specimens: Vesicular fluid, affected skin and mucous membranes, blood with anticoagulant, and serum.

The procedures for the diagnosis of this disease are the same as those recommended for FMD, VS, and VE. See Table 40–1 for the differentiation of SVD from the other vesicular diseases by animal inoculation. The virus can be propagated in cell cultures of porcine kidney, including the PK-15 cell line. Cytopathic changes typical of picornavirus are produced within 2 to 4 days after inoculation.

State and federal regulatory officials should be contacted if SVD is suspected. They will collect appropriate clinical specimens to be tested at the federal laboratory using procedures that are not available to other diagnostic laboratories. Among the tests used is an ELISA to detect viral antigen in vesicular material.

Prevention and Control. There is no vaccine available to prevent SVD. Because of the similarity of SVD to FMD, strict measures of control are implemented, including the elimination of infected hogs by slaughter and the prevention of spread by quarantine of the premises.

Vesicular Exanthema

Synonym: San Miguel sea lion virus disease.
Cause. *Calicivirus* (Caliciviridae).
Additional Hosts. Horses, dogs, and hamsters can be infected experimentally.

Distribution and Transmission. The disease, with the exception of isolated outbreaks in Hawaii and Iceland, has only been seen in the continental United States and it has not been reported since 1956. A virus closely related or identical to VE virus was isolated from sea lions along the California coast. It was capable of producing vesicular lesions in pigs experimentally. There are several serotypes of this virus that affect other marine mammals, and antibodies to these viruses have been detected in a variety of terrestrial mammals on the West coast.

Vesicular exanthema virus is transmitted by contact and fomites. The virus is present in the saliva and feces of infected pigs.

Pathogenicity. The disease in swine resembles foot-and-mouth disease. Vesicles appear on the snout, the mucous membranes of the mouth, the feet, and the udder of nursing sows about 48 hours after viremia. Mortality is usually low.

Diagnosis. Clinical specimens: Vesicular fluid, affected mucous membranes, blood with anticoagulant, and serum.

The virus can be cultivated in swine embryonic kidney cells in which cytopathic changes are noted. The virus can be identified by neutralization tests in animals and cell cultures, and by immunofluorescence.

Differentiation from the other vesicular diseases can be carried out by means of animal inoculation, as shown in Table 40–1.

Prevention and Control. The disease is now considered eradicated from swine, although the possibility of infection from marine mammals must be kept in mind. If VE appears in swine, it should be handled with the same strict measures used to control other vesicular diseases.

ECSO Viruses

Acronym. ECSO (*e*nteric *c*ytopathic *s*wine *o*rphan).

A number of enteroviruses have been recovered from the alimentary tract of apparently healthy pigs. These are not considered to produce overt disease, and have thus been classified as "orphan."

INFECTIONS OF THE NERVOUS SYSTEM

Pseudorabies

Synonyms. Aujeszky's disease, mad itch, infectious bulbar paralysis, porcine herpesvirus Type 1.
Cause. *Varicellovirus* (Family: Herpesviridae. Subfamily: Alphaherpesvirinae).
Additional Hosts. Cattle, cats, dogs, horses, sheep, rats, mink, and other subhuman mammals. Rabbits are particularly susceptible to experimental inoculation. Swine are the only known reservoir host.

Distribution and Transmission. The disease is widespread but often regional in distribution. Direct contact between infected and susceptible swine appears to be the most important means of spread. The virus is also spread by aerosol droplets and fomites. Infection in species other than swine is via skin or mucous membranes, and by ingestion.

Pathogenicity. The severity of the disease in swine is inversely related to the animal's age. The morbidity in pigs up to 1 month old is very high and the mortality may be nearly 100%. The young pigs usually have high temperature and nervous signs such as incoordination of hind limbs, paddling movements, and convulsions. Older pigs, up to 6 months old, are less susceptible and the mortality is usually less than 10%. They may show respiratory and nervous signs.

Adult hogs may have an inapparent infection or may develop anorexia and mild signs of respiratory infection. Pregnant gilts and sows may experience reproductive failure, including abortions and stillbirths.

In cattle, sheep, dogs, cats and other subhuman mammals, the disease is highly fatal but noncontagious. These animals are called dead-end hosts. There is an intense itching at the site of infection if infection is via the skin, followed by mania, encephalitis, paralysis, coma, and death.

Diagnosis. Clinical specimens: Brain, lung, tonsil, spleen, kidney, liver, and serum. In animals other than pigs, a portion of the subcutaneous tissue taken from the site of pruritis and spinal cord.

Gross necropsy lesions consisting of small focal areas of necrosis is sometimes noted in the liver and spleen of aborted fetuses and baby pigs infected with PRV. Microscopic examination of these tissues reveals the presence of intranuclear inclusions typical of herpesvirus. A nonsuppurative meningoencephalitis is the most common microscopic finding in pigs experiencing CNS signs.

Fluorescent antibody tests on frozen sections of tissue are used for rapid diagnosis. Inoculation of infectious material subcutaneously into the rabbit produces an intense pruritus at the site followed by death, usually in 3 to 6 days.

The virus can be propagated readily on the chorioallantoic membrane of chicken embryos, and in pig kidney and other cell cultures producing cytopathic changes as early as 16 hours postinoculation. The virus may be identified by virus neutralization and fluorescent antibody tests.

Serum neutralization, latex agglutination, and ELISA tests are used for the detection of antibody.

Prevention and Control. Efforts should be made to keep herds free of PRV by purchasing replacement stock only from certified free herds. Show animals and new additions should be isolated and serologically tested before introduction to the herd.

Gene-deleted vaccines are used in areas where the virus is enzootic. The advantage of gene-deleted vaccines over other modified live or killed PRV vaccines is that special ELISA tests can be used to differentiate vaccine induced antibody from antibody resulting from natural infection.

Teschen and Teschen-Like Diseases

Synonyms. Porcine encephalomyelitis, porcine polioencephalomyelitis, Talfan disease, porcine enterovirus Type 1.

Cause. *Enterovirus* (Picornaviridae).

Distribution and Transmission. There are a number of serologically closely related strains of porcine enterovirus Type 1 that cause encephalomyelitis in pigs. Some strains are more virulent than others. Teschen disease, a severe form of porcine encephalomyelitis, only occurs in Europe and Africa. The less severe form, Talfan disease, probably occurs worldwide. The virus is shed in feces and saliva; infection is by ingestion.

Pathogenicity. These viruses usually cause an infrequent disease in young pigs. The incubation period is approximately 10 days and in epizootics, pigs of all ages are affected. The most serious outbreaks (Teschen) have been reported from Europe. Clinical signs are elevated temperature (104 to 106° F), ataxia, stiffness, tremors, dog-sitting position, nystagmus, convulsions, and prostration. Deaths usually occur within a few days after onset of signs. Mortality is 50 to 75% or higher in young pigs. The disease may be confused with pseudorabies, hog cholera, and hemagglutinating encephalomyelitis virus (HEV) infection.

Diagnosis. Clinical specimens: Brain, spinal cord, and intestine.

These viruses can be propagated in cell cultures of swine kidney and swine testes in which they produce cytopathic changes. Identification is accomplished by neutralization tests using specific antisera.

Prevention and Control. Animals that recover are immune. Live modified virus and an inactivated virus vaccine are employed with success in Europe.

Vomiting and Wasting Disease

Synonyms. Hemagglutinating encephalomyelitis virus (HEV) infection, viral encephalomyelitis of piglets.

Cause. *Coronavirus* (Coronaviridae).

Distribution and Transmission. Hemagglutinating encephalomyelitis virus is widespread in North America and Europe. Transmission occurs by direct contact with infected pigs and by aerosol droplets.

Pathogenicity. Swine less than 2 weeks old are more susceptible, but most infections are subclinical. Clinical disease that occurs in some pigs consists of anorexia, rapid loss of weight, and depression. Vomiting and constipation may follow. Neurologic signs, such as muscle tremors, incoordination, and paddling movements, may develop later in the course of the disease. Mortality rate may reach 100% in baby pigs.

Diagnosis. Clinical specimens: Tonsil, lungs, stomach, small intestine, brain, spinal cord, and acute and convalescent sera.

Clinically, HEV infection may resemble some of the neonatal diseases of pigs, such as TGE, colibacillosis, and clostridial enterotoxemia; the absence of diarrhea and the irregularity of vomiting may help in differentiation. The neurologic signs may be confused with pseudorabies, hog cholera, erysipelas, and salt poisoning.

Laboratory diagnosis is required to confirm HEV infection. Laboratory methods of diagnosis include fluorescent antibody tests on frozen sections of tissue (brain stem) and virus isolation. Histopathologic examination of brain stem may reveal nonsuppurative encephalitis. The virus is cultivated best in early passage porcine thymic cell cultures in which it produces syncytia. Hemadsorption can be demonstrated on infected cells. The virus of HEV agglutinates chicken, sheep, rabbit, rat, mouse, and hamster erythrocytes.

Prevention and Control. The virus is widespread and most infections are subclinical. There is no vaccine available and no control measures are practiced.

Adenoviruses

Adenoviruses recovered from pigs have usually not been shown to be pathogenic. An exception is the isolation of an adenovirus (Type 4) from the brain of a pig with encephalitis. This virus produced CNS disease in experimentally infected pigs. Porcine adenoviruses have been isolated frequently from feces of "healthy" pigs and adenoviral inclusions have been noted in a variety of tissues, including lung and intestine.

Adenoviruses can be propagated in cell cultures of swine kidney in which they produce cytopathic changes, including intranuclear inclusions. Several passages may be necessary before typical cellular destruction occurs, but intranuclear inclusions can often be detected on initial isolation attempts.

Porcine Paramyxovirus Infection

Synonym. Swine "blue eye" disease.

Cause. *Paramyxovirus* (Family: Paramyxoviridae. Subfamily: Paramyxovirinae).

Distribution and Transmission. Swine "blue eye" disease has only been reported in Mexico. Transmission occurs by direct contact with infected animals and by indirect contact with secretions/excretions from infected animals.

Pathogenicity. Swine "blue eye" disease is most severe in pigs less than 3 weeks of age, and is characterized clinically by sudden onset of fever,

depression, and progressive CNS signs. Affected pigs are weak and ataxic, and may have rigidity of the hind legs and tremors. Dilated pupils, nystagmus, and conjunctivitis may be noted in some pigs, and approximately 1 to 10% of affected pigs develop corneal opacity. The mortality rate may approach 90%.

In older pigs, clinical signs are principally those associated with respiratory infection, including sneezing, coughing, anorexia, and fever. Central nervous system signs are rare in pigs more than 30 days old and mortality rates are low.

In adult swine, most infections are subclinical, although corneal opacity is occasionally observed. Reproductive problems may be noted in pregnant sows. Orchitis and epididymitis may occur in boars.

Gross necropsy lesions are minimal and nonspecific. Microscopic lesions are those of a nonsuppurative encephalomyelitis and interstitial pneumonitis.

Diagnosis. Clinical specimens: Brain, lung, tonsil, and affected eyes.

A presumptive diagnosis is often made on the basis of clinical signs and histopathologic lesions. Confirmation requires isolation and identification of the virus. The virus can be cultivated in cell cultures of swine origin (PK-15 cell line) in which it causes a cytopathology characterized by syncytia. The virus agglutinates erythrocytes of various animal species including those of chicken.

Prevention and Control. Prevention is best accomplished by maintaining closed herds. All replacement animals should be isolated and serologically tested.

INFECTIONS OF THE REPRODUCTIVE SYSTEM

Porcine Parvovirus Infection

Cause. *Parvovirus* (Parvoviridae).

Distribution and Transmission. Porcine parvovirus (PPV) is widespread in swine of the United States, Canada, and some countries in Europe. Transmission is mainly by contact with water and food containing feces and other infectious discharges. The mode of infection is probably by ingestion. Clinically normal but latently infected boars may transmit the virus to sows through semen.

Pathogenicity. Infection with PPV is common in most swine herds, and may result in reproductive failure in nonimmune pregnant gilts and sows if they are infected early in gestation. There are no premonitory clinical signs. Most notable reproductive failures include sows returning to estrus (following death and resorption of the fetus) and fetal mummification. If pregnant sows and gilts are infected after 70 days of gestation when the fetus is immune competent, reproductive failure is uncommon.

The virus occasionally has been recovered from pigs with vesicular skin lesions.

Diagnosis. Clinical specimens: Mummified fetuses and skin lesions.

Diagnosis is most easily accomplished by fluorescent antibody examination of cryostat sections of fetal liver and lung. The virus can be propagated in cell cultures of swine testes and swine kidney, although several subcultures may be required before cytopathic changes are evident. Examination of fluid extracted from fetal tissues for hemagglutinating activity or for antibodies is also useful. The virus agglutinates guinea pig erythrocytes.

Prevention and Control. Porcine parvovirus is common in swine, and generally no attempts are made to maintain virus free herds. Management practices normally include the vaccination of breeding stock and boars with modified live or killed vaccines.

Porcine Reproductive and Respiratory Syndrome

Synonyms. Mystery pig disease, blue ear disease, swine infertility and respiratory syndrome (SIRS), porcine epidemic abortion and respiratory syndrome (PEARS), and Lelystad virus.

Cause. *Arterivirus*[1] (Togaviridae).

Distribution and Transmission. The virus of porcine reproductive and respiratory syndrome (PRRS) is widely distributed in North America and Europe. Transmission is by aerosol, contact, and fomites. Infected boars shed virus in their semen, but the duration of shedding is unknown.

Pathogenicity. There is an incubation period of about 2 to 7 days following exposure. Clinical signs in adult swine are nonexistent to mild consisting of a slight febrile response and anorexia of short duration. A bluish discoloration of the ears has been associated with PRRS outbreaks in Europe. Pregnant sows may abort late in gestation or deliver prematurely. Abortions and/or stillbirths may reach epizootic proportions in fully susceptible herds.

Young pigs infected with PRRS virus exhibit depression, anorexia, and rapid respiration with some coughing and sneezing. Mortality may be as high as 50% in nursing pigs, but is low in older

pigs. Secondary bacterial infections may result in poor growth and performance.

Gross necropsy lesions are minimal in the uncomplicated respiratory form of PRRS, but interstitial pneumonitis is a consistent histopathologic finding. There are no gross or histopathologic lesions noted in aborted or stillborn fetuses.

Diagnosis. Clinical specimens: Nasal swabs, blood, serum, lung tissue, and aborted fetuses.

The PRRS virus can be cultivated in porcine alveolar macrophages and in a continuous cell line (MARC) derived from a clone of MA 104 cells (African green monkey kidney). Identification is most easily accomplished by indirect fluorescent antibody (IFA) examination of infected cultures.

Infection can also be diagnosed by using the IFA test on frozen sections of lung and fetal tissues or by the demonstration of seroconversion in affected pigs or sows that have aborted. Antigenic differences have been noted among different isolates.

Prevention and Control. Prevention is best accomplished by good management practices, including the quarantine and testing of replacement stock and show animals. The possibility that previously infected boars might shed virus in their semen for extended periods of time should be considered. Appropriate antibiotic therapy may be warranted to control secondary bacterial infections. A vaccine has recently been developed.

SMEDI Viruses

Cause. *Enteroviruses* (Picornaviridae).

Pathogenicity. The viruses are designated by the name SMEDI (*s*tillbirth, *m*ummification, *e*mbryonic *d*eath, *i*nfertility) and have been isolated from stillborn pigs, "3-day" dead pigs, and fetuses found dead in the uterus in midpregnancy after hysterectomy. Herds from which these enteroviruses were recovered generally had small litter sizes and low survival rates.

Sows were immune after infection but the disease manifestations frequently appeared cyclically every 2 to 3 years, perhaps because of the susceptibility of new gilts. The typical disease manifestations of this group of viruses were produced experimentally. The five SMEDI virus groups reported fell into four groups of serologically related viruses. At least six other enterovirus groups have been identified that are not associated with reproductive problems in sows.

Porcine parvovirus is considered to be the primary viral cause of reproductive problems in swine and little significance is given to the SMEDI viruses.

---

[1]The genus of *Arterivirus* will likely be upgraded to family status.

Diagnosis. Clinical specimens: Tissue from fetuses and stillborn pigs.

The viruses can be cultivated in primary pig kidney cell cultures; however, the frequency of isolations has been low, mainly because of the absence of viable virus at the time clinical disease becomes apparent.

Prevention and Control. There are usually no attempts to prevent or control enterovirus infections in swine.

Getah Virus Infection

Cause. *Alphavirus* (Togaviridae).

Getah virus infection in swine is widespread in Japan. Most infections are subclinical but fetal deaths have been reported. See Chapter 43 for a more complete description of Getah virus.

INFECTIONS OF THE INTEGUMENTARY SYSTEM

Swinepox

Cause. *Suipoxvirus* (Family: Poxviridae. Subfamily: Chordopoxvirinae).

Pathogenicity. The disease is worldwide in distribution but the clinical incidence in the United States is low. The morbidity is generally high in young pigs. The virus is mechanically transmitted by the hog louse, *Hematopinus suis*, and by contact. A transient low-grade fever occurs early in the course of the disease. The typical pox lesions (papule, vesicle, pustule, and scab) are seen involving the skin of abdomen, back, and side. On the lower abdomen, lesions with hemorrhagic dark centers are characteristic. The disease will usually run its course without deaths or other serious effects. Rare congenital infections occur with typical lesions on the skin and in the oral cavity of newborns.

Diagnosis. The disease is usually diagnosed clinically, but it may be confused with other skin diseases, e.g., mange. Confirmation of swinepox infection is easily accomplished by the electron microscopic examination of distilled water lysates of lesions. The virus can be cultivated in swine kidney cell cultures, but not on the chorioallantoic (CA) membrane of chicken embryos. Eosinophilic cytoplasmic inclusion bodies are seen in epithelial cells of affected animals.

In some countries, vaccinia virus causes a disease of swine that closely resembles "true" swinepox. This virus can be distinguished from "true" swinepox virus by serologic means, and by the fact that it can be grown on the CA membrane of chicken embryos.

Prevention and Control. Vaccination is not practiced. Delousing and good sanitation are the primary control measures.

MISCELLANEOUS INFECTIONS

Hog Cholera

Synonym. Swine fever.

Cause. *Pestivirus* (Flaviviridae).

Distribution and Transmission. Hog cholera virus is widely distributed in swine throughout the world. The eradication program initiated in the United States in 1962 has resulted in complete eradication of the disease. Other countries free of the virus include Canada, Great Britain, New Zealand, Australia, Iceland, and Switzerland.

The virus is present in saliva, nasal secretions, feces, blood, and urine. Transmission is by direct and indirect contact, and pigs are infected by ingestion or inhalation; birds and hematophagous arthropods may be mechanical vectors. The disease has been spread by consumption of uncooked pork scraps.

Pathogenicity. In susceptible swine, the disease is usually acute and characterized by a high temperature, depression, and anorexia. The morbidity is high and the mortality is usually about 90%. Neurological signs are not uncommon, and abortions and stillbirths may occur.

Typical hog cholera is frequently complicated with secondary bacterial infections. The two most common are *Pasteurella multocida* and *Salmonella choleraesuis*. Thus, affected animals often have bronchopneumonia and severe enteritis. Leukopenia is common. The changes observed in affected pigs are related to the strong affinity of the virus for the vascular system. Among the more commonly described lesions are: petechial and ecchymotic hemorrhages involving all serous surfaces; petechial hemorrhage of the kidney ("turkey egg kidney"), hemorrhagic lymphadenitis ("strawberry" lymph nodes), and the so-called "button" ulcers of the intestinal mucosa. The most striking microscopic change observed is the accumulation of lymphocytes in the perivascular spaces. Infection of fetuses may result in malformations, such as cerebellar hypoplasia and microencephalopathy.

A less severe chronic form of the disease may be seen that often escapes detection and makes eradication difficult. This may be owing to some immunity, or to a less virulent strain of virus.

Diagnosis. Clinical specimens: Kidney, spleen, tonsil, lymph nodes, brain, and blood.

The diagnosis is based on clinical signs, gross and microscopic lesions, and laboratory tests. The fluorescent antibody (FA) test on frozen sections of spleen, tonsil, and lymph nodes is the simplest and most reliable means of diagnosis. The virus can be cultivated in cell cultures of swine origin (PK-15 cell line) but grows without discernible CPE. Cell culture coverslips are stained with specific FA to confirm the presence of virus.

Prevention and Control. Countries free of hog cholera have strict importation and quarantine requirements to prevent virus entry. Modified live vaccines are used in countries where the virus is enzootic in an effort to control clinical disease.

African Swine Fever

Cause. Unclassified virus (previously classified as a member of the Iridoviridae).

Additional Hosts. Feral swine, warthogs, and bush pigs can be immune carriers.

Distribution and Transmission. African swine fever (ASF) virus presently exists in swine of Africa, Portugal, Spain, and Italy. Outbreaks have occurred in the Caribbean and South America. Transmission is by direct and indirect contact; the mode of infection is principally by ingestion but also by tick vectors that may remain infectious for long periods. Warthogs and bush pigs may provide a reservoir. The virus may be present in uncooked pork products and may be spread by the feeding of garbage.

Pathogenicity. The ASF virus causes an acute, highly contagious disease in swine resembling hog cholera, with mortality of 95 to 100%. Gross and microscopic lesions closely resemble those of hog cholera, and the vascular system is severely affected. In contrast to hog cholera, however, button ulcers are not usually seen, and severe edema of the lungs is present, with marked increases in pericardial, pleural, and peritoneal fluids. Infections with some strains of the virus may result in mild or subclinical disease.

Diagnosis. Clinical specimens: Blood, spleen, tonsil, and lymph nodes.

Presumptive diagnosis is usually based on clinical features and pathologic changes; however, definitive diagnosis requires isolation and identification of the virus in cell cultures of porcine macrophages or by fluorescent antibody examination of affected tissues. The ELISA test is considered the most useful serologic test for detecting antibodies to ASF.

Prevention and Control. Effective immunization procedures have not been developed. Strict quarantine and slaughter are recommended. Gar-bage from international flights and ships should be incinerated.

Encephalomyocarditis

Cause. *Cardiovirus* (Picornaviridae).

Additional Hosts. Rodents, squirrels, raccoons, monkeys, elephants, and several other vertebrate species.

Distribution and Transmission. Encephalomyocarditis (EMC) virus is present in many countries throughout the world. Rats and mice are considered to be the natural hosts and principal reservoir for the virus, and pigs are thought to be infected by eating feed contaminated with rodent urine and droppings.

Pathogenicity. The virus causes a sporadic disease in young pigs characterized primarily by sudden deaths. Premonitory clinical signs may include anorexia, depression, and difficulty breathing. Mortality may be high in very young pigs but is usually subclinical in weaned pigs and adults. *In utero* infection may occur leading to fetal death.

Diagnosis. Clinical specimens: Heart and brain.

Gross necropsy lesions may reveal an enlarged heart with pale areas on the right ventricle. Confirmation of EMC infection is best accomplished by fluorescent antibody examination of cryostat sections of affected tissue. The virus can be cultivated in a variety of cell cultures and in young mice inoculated intracerebrally.

Prevention and Control. Rodent control is the primary means of controlling EMC on swine farms. An inactivated vaccine is available, but its effectiveness in preventing EMC infections is not clear.

FURTHER READING

Borst, G.H.A., Kimman, T.G., Gielkens, A.L.J., and van der Kamp, J.S.: Four sporadic cases of congenital swine pox. Vet. Rec. *127*:61, 1990.

Castro, A.E., and Heuschele, W.P. (eds.): Veterinary Diagnostic Virology. A Practitioner's Guide. St. Louis, Mosby-Year Book. 1992.

Christianson, W.T., Collins, J.E., Benfield, D.A., et al.: Experimental reproduction of swine infertility and respiratory syndrome in pregnant sows. Am. J. Vet. Res. *53*:485, 1992.

Conzelmann, Karl-Klaus, Visser, N., Van Woensel, P., and Thiel, Heinz-Jürgen: Molecular characterization of porcine reproductive and respiratory syndrome virus, a member of the arterivirus group. Virology *193*:329, 1993.

Ferris, D.H. (ed.): Foreign Animal Disease Reference Manual. National Veterinary Services Laboratories, Science and Technology, Animal and Plant Health Inspection Service, United States Department of Agriculture, P.O. Box 844, Ames, IA, 1984 (Revised 1990).

Lehman, J.R., Weigel, R.M., and Siegel, A.W., et al.: Progress after one year of a pseudorabies eradication program for large swine herds. J. Am. Vet. Med. Assoc. *203*:118, 1993.

Leman, A.D., Straw, B.E., Mengeling, W.L., et al. (eds.): Diseases of Swine. 7th Ed. Ames, IA, Iowa State University Press, 1992.

Meulenberg, J.J.M., Hulst, M.M., deMeijer, E.J., et al.: Lelystad virus, the causative agent of porcine epidemic abortion and respiratory syndrome (PEARS), is related to LDV and EAV. Virology *192*:62, 1993.

Pijpers, A., van Nieuwstadt, A.P., Terpstra, C., and Verheijden: Porcine epidemic diarrhoea virus as a cause of persistent diarrheoa in a herd of breeding and finishing pigs. Vet. Rec. *132*:129, 1993.

Shibata, I., Hatano, Y., Nishimura, M., et al.: Isolation of Getah virus from dead fetuses extracted from a naturally infected sow in Japan. Vet. Microbiol. *27*:385, 1991.

Simkins, R.A., Weilnau, P.A., Bias, J., and Saif, L.J.: Antigenic variation among transmissible gastroenteritis virus (TGEV) and porcine respiratory coronavirus strains detected with monoclonal antibodies to the S protein of TGEV. Am. J. Vet. Res. *53*:1253, 1992.

Stephano, H.A., Gay, G.M., and Ramirez, T.C.: Encephalomyelitis, reproductive failure and corneal opacity (blue eye) in pigs, associated with a paramyxovirus infection. Vet. Rec. *122*:6, 1988.

Stephano, H.A.: Focus on swine blue eye disease. In Foreign Animal Disease Report. No. *18-1*:11, Spring 1990.

Studdert, M.J.: Circoviridae: new viruses of pigs, parrots and chickens. Aust. Vet. J. *70*:101, 1993.

Timoney, J.F., Gillespie, J.H., Scott, F.W., and Barlough, J.E. (eds.): Hagan and Bruner's Microbiology and Infectious Diseases of Domestic Animals. 8th Ed. Ithaca, NY, Comstock Publishing Associates, 1988.

Wensvoort, G., Terpstra, C., Pol, J.M.A., et al.: Mystery swine disease in the Netherlands: the isolation of Lelystad virus. Vet. Quart. *13*:121, 1991.

Wesley, R.D., Woods, R.D., and Cheung, A.K.: Genetic analysis of porcine respiratory coronavirus, an attenuated variant of transmissible gastroenteritis virus. J. Virol. *65*:3369, 1991.

42

Viral Infections of Sheep and Goats

INFECTIONS OF THE RESPIRATORY SYSTEM

Ovine Progressive Pneumonia

Synonyms. Visna/Maedi, Montana progressive pneumonia, progressive pneumonia of sheep.

Cause. *Lentivirus* (Retroviridae).

Hosts. Sheep.

Distribution and Transmission. Ovine progressive pneumonia (OPP) is thought to occur in sheep throughout the world. The virus of OPP is shed in nasal secretions and in the milk of infected ewes.

Pathogenicity. The virus of OPP is associated with a number of different clinical syndromes including respiratory disease (Maedi), central nervous system (CNS) disease (Visna), arthritis, and mastitis. Although sheep remain infected for life, few develop clinical disease. In those that do, there is a protracted incubation period of a year or longer.

The various disease manifestations, which progress over a period of months, are most often seen in sheep over 2 years of age. The pulmonary form is characterized by a slow and progressive weight loss and dyspnea upon exertion. Sheep afflicted with the CNS form develop ataxia of the hind quarters and ultimately paralysis. Chronic active inflammation is noted histologically in affected tissues. Lung lesions are those of interstitial pneumonitis and lymphoid hyperplasia. Leukoencephalo-myelitis with focal demyelination and lymphocytic perivascular cuffing are observed in the brain. Affected mammary glands are fibrotic with lymphocytic infiltrates, and affected joints are characterized by proliferative changes in the synovial membrane.

Diagnosis. Clinical specimens: Serum and live, clinically ill sheep.

Diagnosis is usually based on clinical signs and histopathologic lesions with supporting serologic evidence of exposure as determined by the agar gel immunodiffusion test (AGID). The virus of OPP is closely related antigenically to the virus of caprine arthritis encephalitis and current AGID test kits will detect antibodies to both viruses.

Prevention and Control. No vaccines are available. Prevention is best accomplished by maintaining closed flocks. All replacement stock should be quarantined and tested serologically. Control of OPP infection within a flock requires periodic serologic testing and subsequent removal of seropositive animals. Lambs should not be allowed to suckle seropositive dams.

Pulmonary Adenomatosis

Synonym. Jaagsiekte.

Cause. Herpesvirus (Family: Herpesviridae. Subfamily: Gammaherpesvirinae).

Hosts. Sheep.

Distribution and Transmission. The disease has been reported in Europe, Africa, Asia, and

South America. Experimental transmission by pulmonary or intravenous inoculations and by inhalation of infected droplets has been demonstrated. Vertical transmission also occurs.

Pathogenicity. Pulmonary adenomatosis is a chronic pneumonia of sheep characterized by progressive adenomatous proliferation of alveolar and bronchiolar epithelium resulting in coughing, nasal discharge, and difficulty breathing, leading eventually to emaciation and death. The incubation period may be as long as several years. Clinically the disease may be confused with ovine progressive pneumonia, but lung lesions are distinctly different. Grossly, there are widespread nodular growths throughout the lung that are microscopically adenomas or adenocarcinomas.

Diagnosis. Clinical specimens: Formalin fixed lung tissue.

Diagnosis is based on gross and microscopic lung lesions.

Prevention and Control. No vaccines are available. Affected sheep should be removed from the flock. There is no test to detect subclinically infected animals.

Paramyxovirus Infections

Cause. *Paramyxovirus* and *Pneumovirus* (Paramyxoviridae).

Parainfluenza virus-3 (*Paramyxovirus*) and bovine respiratory syncytial virus (*Pneumovirus*) cause respiratory diseases in sheep and goats clinically similar to the respective diseases in cattle. The viruses are discussed in detail in Chapter 40.

INFECTIONS OF THE DIGESTIVE SYSTEM

Bluetongue

Cause. *Orbivirus* (Reoviridae).

Hosts. Sheep, cattle, and wild ruminants.

Distribution and Transmission. Bluetongue (BT) is a vector transmitted disease that was first described in South Africa. The disease has been reported in many countries, including the United States, Spain, Portugal, Japan, Australia, and India. Various species of culicoides are the common vector for BT viruses, of which there are twenty-four serologic types.

Pathogenicity. The incubation period following exposure of sheep to the virus of BT is about 6 to 10 days. Although some sheep may experience only mild disease, typical infections are characterized by acute onset with high fever, depression, anorexia, nasal and ocular discharge, salivation, and ulcers on the lips, tongue, and dental pad. Swelling and tenderness of the coronary region of the hoof may result in lameness. Principal lesions observed at necropsy are the oral lesions, a generalized edema, and hemorrhages of skeletal and cardiac muscles. Pregnant ewes may abort or deliver lambs with hydranencephaly.

Bluetongue infection in cattle is usually subclinical, but pregnant cows infected early in gestation may abort or deliver calves with birth defects. Bluetongue is a devastating disease of white-tailed deer and pronghorn antelope.

Diagnosis. Clinical specimens: Whole blood, spleen, serum.

A presumptive diagnosis is based on clinical signs and gross necropsy lesions with supportive serologic evidence of exposure. Confirmation requires isolation of the virus, which is best accomplished initially by the intravenous inoculation of chicken embryos and subsequently in cell cultures, e.g., Vero cell line.

The serologic tests most often used to determine exposure are the agar gel immunodiffusion and a competitive enzyme-linked immunosorbent assay. The latter is considered to be more sensitive and specific.

Prevention and Control. Modified-live virus vaccines are used in Africa but not in the United States. Although BT infections occur widely in ruminants of the United States, import restrictions are enforced in an attempt to prevent introduction of new serotypes.

Rinderpest

Cause. *Morbillivirus* (Paramyxoviridae).

Rinderpest virus infects sheep and goats, and causes disease similar to that seen in cattle. The disease is discussed in detail in Chapter 40.

Peste des Petits Ruminants

Synonyms. Pseudorinderpest, Kata.

Cause. *Morbillivirus* (Paramyxoviridae).

Hosts. Sheep and goats.

Distribution and Transmission. The virus of peste des petits ruminants (PPR) is closely related antigenically to the virus of rinderpest, and is enzootic in sheep and goats of West Africa. Transmission occurs by direct contact with infected animals and by indirect contact with food, water, litter, etc. contaminated with secretions/excretions from infected animals.

Pathogenicity. The virus of PPR causes a disease in sheep and goats clinically similar to the disease caused by rinderpest virus. Following an incubation period of about 5 days, infected animals become febrile and anorectic. They quickly develop a necrotic stomatitis, and nasal and ocular discharge, followed by severe diarrhea. Goats are more severely affected than sheep, and the mortality rate may approach 90% in young kids. The overall mortality rate varies from about 10 to 90%. The virus of PPR causes a subclinical infection of cattle.

Diagnosis. Clinical specimens: Oral lesions, whole blood, spleen, intestine, and acute and convalescent sera.

A presumptive diagnosis is made on the basis of clinical signs and history. Confirmation requires isolation and identification of the virus or the demonstration of a significant increase in antibody levels between acute and convalescent sera. The virus can be cultivated in a variety of cell cultures, including Vero cells, in which cytopathic changes characterized by syncytial formation are observed. The virus of PPR can be differentiated from the virus of rinderpest by cross neutralization studies, or by the inoculation of goats and cattle. The latter do not develop clinical disease with PPR virus.

Prevention and Control. Vaccines are not available for PPR, but vaccines prepared with the closely related rinderpest virus have been used. In those countries where the disease does not occur, outbreaks are dealt with by strict quarantine and slaughter.

Nairobi Sheep Disease

Cause. *Nairovirus* (Bunyaviridae).
Hosts. Sheep, goats, and human beings.
Distribution and Transmission. Nairobi sheep disease is a tick-transmitted viral disease of sheep and goats in East Africa.
Pathogenicity. The disease is characterized clinically by high fever, depression, anorexia, nasal discharge, and a severe hemorrhagic gastroenteritis. Pregnant animals are likely to abort. The disease is more severe in sheep; mortality rates range from 30 to 90%.
Diagnosis. Clinical specimens: Whole blood, acute and convalescent sera, spleen, mesenteric lymph nodes.

A presumptive diagnosis is made on the basis of clinical signs and history. Confirmation requires isolation and identification of the virus or the demonstration of a significant increase in antibody levels between acute and convalescent sera. The virus is most easily isolated by the intracerebral inoculation of infant mice. The virus also grows in a variety of cell cultures, including those of hamster origin (BHK-21 cell line).

Prevention and Control. In countries where the disease is enzootic, dipping of animals to eliminate ticks is widely practiced. Outbreaks in countries free of disease are dealt with by strict quarantine and slaughter.

INFECTIONS OF THE REPRODUCTIVE SYSTEM

Border Disease

Synonyms. "Hairy shaker" disease.
Cause. *Pestivirus* (Flaviviridae).
Hosts. Sheep and cattle.
Distribution and Transmission. Border disease occurs in sheep flocks of Great Britain, New Zealand, Australia, and other countries, including the United States and Canada. Transmission occurs by direct contact with infected animals or through indirect contact with virus laden excretions/secretions from infected animals.
Pathogenicity. The virus of border disease is antigenically closely related to the viruses of bovine viral diarrhea (BVD) and hog cholera. The virus causes no overt clinical signs in adult sheep, but infection of pregnant ewes prior to 80 days of gestation results in fetal infections with much the same consequences observed in bovine fetuses infected with BVD virus (see Chapter 40). Fetal resorption, abortion, and the birth of persistently infected animals are common sequelae. Persistently infected lambs often have abnormally hairy birthcoats and congenital tremors resulting from defective myelination of CNS. Persistently infected lambs that are severely affected usually die. Those minimally affected may live and provide a source of infection for other animals.
Diagnosis. Clinical specimens: Whole blood and serum. Affected lambs for necropsy examination.

Clinical signs and history are suggestive. The histological finding of nerve fibers with defective myelin sheaths is supportive. The virus can be propagated in a variety of cell cultures but without observable cytopathic effects. Viral antigen can be demonstrated in infected cell cultures, blood smears, and affected tissues by immunofluorescence using BVD conjugates.
Prevention and Control. No specific vaccines are available. Prevention is best accomplished by maintaining closed flocks. Efforts to control the disease are directed at identifying and removing persistently infected animals.

Akabane

Cause. *Bunyavirus* (Bunyaviridae).

Akabane virus, which causes fetal anomalies in sheep and goats, is discussed in detail under Reproductive Diseases in Cattle (see Chapter 40).

Cache Valley

Cause. *Bunyavirus* (Bunyaviridae).

Cache Valley virus has been associated with congenital malformations in sheep. These defects, which are principally arthrogryposis and hydraencephaly, are virtually indistinguishable from those observed with Akabane disease. Serologic evidence indicates that the virus is widely distributed in the United States and that numerous mammalian species are susceptible to infection.

INFECTIONS OF THE NERVOUS SYSTEM

Scrapie

Cause. *Prion* (proposed).

Hosts. Sheep and goats.

Distribution and Transmission. Scrapie is enzootic in the United Kingdom and Europe, but it has been eradicated from Australia and New Zealand. The disease was first diagnosed in the United States in Michigan in 1947. The agent of scrapie is transmitted both vertically and horizontally.

Pathogenicity. Scrapie is a nonfebrile, insidious disease with a long incubation period (1 to 5 years). Initial signs are restlessness, excitability, and grinding of the teeth. Later signs are tremors, pruritus resulting in shedding of wool and laceration of the skin, and convulsions. Death occurs from several weeks to several months after onset of signs.

Scrapie is one of several "slow diseases" observed in a number of different animal species. These diseases are all characterized by an insidious development of central nervous system dysfunction and ultimately death. Histological lesions in the brain from diseased animals are essentially identical, consisting of characteristic spongiform changes. Although the relationship of the causative agents is unclear, these diseases are collectively referred to as spongiform encephalopathies.

Diagnosis. Clinical specimens: Brain and spinal cord.

Clinical signs are suggestive of scrapie but definitive diagnosis requires histological examination of brain tissue.

Prevention and Control. Prevention is best accomplished by maintaining closed flocks. Affected flocks are quarantined and depopulation is recommended.

Visna

Cause. *Lentivirus* (Retroviridae).

Visna is a disease manifestation caused by the same virus which causes ovine progressive pneumonia. This form of disease is characterized by chronic degeneration and demyelination of the central nervous system resulting in stiffness, paralysis, and ultimately death. The virus is discussed in detail under Infections of the Respiratory System.

Louping Ill

Synonyms. Ovine encephalomyelitis.

Cause. *Flavivirus* (Flaviviridae).

Hosts. Sheep, cattle, deer, horses, pigs, wild rodents, and human beings.

Distribution and Transmission. Louping ill is a tick-borne disease, principally of sheep, that occurs in England, Ireland, and Scotland.

Pathogenicity. Louping ill is characterized clinically by a biphasic fever and progressive central nervous system dysfunction. Initial clinical signs are those of high fever and depression of about 24 to 48 hours duration. A second febrile response occurs a few days later accompanied by signs of central nervous system dysfunction, including excitability, incoordination, muscular tremors, and paralysis. The mortality rate is high in those animals that develop central nervous system disease.

Louping ill causes similar central nervous system diseases in cattle, horses, and pigs.

Diagnosis. Clinical specimens: Fresh and formalin-fixed brain tissue.

A presumptive diagnosis is based on clinical signs and history. Histologic lesions of meningoencephalomyelitis are supportive. The virus can be isolated in young mice inoculated intracerebrally.

Prevention and Control. Inactivated vaccines are used in areas where the virus is enzootic. Animals are dipped, sprayed, etc. in an effort to prevent tick feeding.

Borna Disease

Cause. Unclassified virus.

Hosts. Sheep and horses.

The virus of Borna disease causes a central nervous system disease in sheep that is clinically similar to the disease in horses. The virus is discussed in detail in Chapter 43.

Caprine Arthritis-Encephalitis

Synonyms. Leukoencephalomyelitis of goats, caprine encephalomyelitis.

Cause. *Lentivirus* (Retroviridae).

Hosts. Goats.

Distribution and Transmission. Caprine arthritis-encephalitis (CAE) virus is widely distributed in goat herds throughout the world. Young kids are most commonly infected through the ingestion of milk from infected does. Horizontal transmission is thought to occur by direct contact with secretions/excretions from infected goats and through breeding.

Pathogenicity. The virus of CAE causes a chronic connective tissue disease affecting the joints of mature goats, and a leukoencephalomyelitis of young goats; and less commonly, mastitis and pneumonia. The arthritic form is characterized by a proliferative synovitis of the carpal, fetlock, hock, and stiffle joints. Joints are enlarged, especially the carpal joints, and common histological lesions are those of synovial cell proliferation and inflammatory cell infiltration (lymphocytes, plasma cells, and macrophages). The arthritis may remain static or become progressively worse with development of fibrinous concretions, necrosis, and mineralization.

Central nervous system disease is principally seen in young kids between 2 and 4 months of age, and is characterized by a progressive ascending paralysis. Microscopically, the central nervous system lesions resemble those of Visna in sheep and include lymphocytic cell infiltration and demyelination of the white matter.

Some infected goats may develop an interstitial pneumonitis and some infected does may develop swollen, fibrotic mammary glands.

Diagnosis. Clinical specimens: Serum.

Diagnosis of CAE associated disease is usually made on the basis of clinical signs and supportive serologic evidence of exposure. The serologic test most often used is agar gel immunodiffusion.

The virus can be propagated in caprine cell cultures derived from synovial membranes, but isolation is time consuming and rarely attempted.

Prevention and Control. Goats infected with CAE virus remain infected for life. Prevention is best accomplished by maintaining closed herds. All replacement animals should be isolated and tested serologically. Control of CAE in herds where the virus is enzootic is difficult. If economically feasible, test and removal is the preferred method. Otherwise, serologically positive animals should be segregated from negative animals. Young kids should be removed from positive does at birth. Milk from infected does should not be fed unless it has been pasteurized.

DISEASES OF THE INTEGUMENTARY SYSTEM

Contagious Ecthyma

Synonyms. Soremouth, orf, contagious pustular dermatitis.

Cause. *Parapoxvirus* (Family: Poxviridae. Subfamily: Chordopoxvirinae).

Hosts. Sheep, goats, various wild ruminants, and human beings.

Distribution and Transmission. Contagious ecthyma is a widely occurring disease of sheep and goats that is spread by contact.

Pathogenicity. The disease is characterized clinically by the development of pox-like lesions on the lips and nose; and, less frequently, in other parts of the mouth and on the udder, teats, vulva, and coronet of the feet. Losses are rare but may occur in young lambs because of difficulty in feeding and lameness.

Veterinarians and sheep handlers should avoid contact with infectious material. The lesions in human beings, although more proliferative, are similar to those in sheep and occur most frequently on the hands, forearms, and face and take up to 2 months to heal. Regional lymph nodes may be sore and swollen.

Diagnosis. Clinical specimens: Lesion material.

Diagnosis is usually made on the basis of clinical examination. Laboratory confirmation is most easily and rapidly obtained by the demonstration of parapoxvirus in lesion material by electron microscopy. The virus can be propagated in a variety of cell cultures in which it produces a slowly developing cytopathic effect, including the production of cytoplasmic inclusions.

Prevention and Control. Sheep and goats can be effectively immunized with a live virus vaccine derived from scab material. The vaccine is administered via scarification of the thigh. Care should be exercised when using the vaccine as it is infectious for humans.

Sheep and Goatpox

Cause. *Capripoxvirus* (Family: Poxviridae. Subfamily: Chordopoxvirinae).

Distribution and Transmission. Sheep and goatpox virus occurs in sheep and goats in Africa, the Middle East, Asia, and the Mediterranian islands. Transmission occurs by contact.

Pathogenicity. Sheep and goatpox is the most severe pox disease of domesticated animals. The infection is generalized, and mortality rates may exceed 50% in young lambs and kids. Pox lesions occur on the skin and on mucous membranes of the respiratory and digestive tracts. Severely affected animals frequently develop pneumonia.

Diagnosis. Clinical specimens: Lesion material.

A presumptive diagnosis is based on clinical signs and history. Confirmation is most easily and rapidly obtained by the electron microscopic demonstration of poxvirus in distilled H_2O lysates of lesion material. The virions are morphologically similar to the orthopoxviruses, being "brick" shaped as opposed to the virions of contagious ecthyma (a parapoxvirus), which are ovoid in appearance.

The virus can be propagated in a variety of cell cultures derived from goats, sheep, and cattle.

Prevention and Control. Both modified live virus and killed virus vaccines are used in areas where the virus is enzootic. In areas where the disease does not occur, outbreaks are dealt with by strict quarantine and slaughter.

MISCELLANEOUS INFECTIONS

Caprine Herpesvirus Infections

Cause. Herpesvirus (Family: Herpesviridae. Subfamily: Alphaherpesvirinae).

Herpesviruses have been isolated from young kids with a severe, generalized infection and also from does with vulvovaginitis.

The generalized infection is clinically similar to that seen in young pups with canine herpesvirus infection. It is characterized by rapid onset, acute abdominal pain, poor appetite, and rapid, shallow breathing. The mortality rate is high. Gross lesions are limited to the gastrointestinal tract, and are most severe in the cecum and colon; intranuclear inclusions are found in connective tissue and epithelial cells. Experimentally, the virus has caused abortion, but the virus could not be recovered from fetal tissue because of severe autolysis. Only a mild or clinically inapparent infection has been produced in adult goats, and the virus was not pathogenic for lambs or calves.

The genital disease in does is clinically similar to the genital form of infectious bovine rhinotracheitis virus observed in cattle, and is characterized by hyperemic and edematous mucous membranes of the vulva and vagina, with subsequent development of papular eruptions, vesicles, and ulcers. Recovery is uneventful, and takes about 1 week.

The relationship of the herpesviruses associated with these two clinical syndromes has not been determined.

Rift Valley Fever

Cause. *Phlebovirus* (Bunyaviridae).

Hosts. Sheep, goats, cattle, and human beings.

Distribution and Transmission. Rift Valley fever occurs in Africa and the Middle East. The virus is transmitted by mosquitoes.

Pathogenicity. Infection is most severe in young animals, and is characterized by a high fever, anorexia, weakness, and rapid death. Some affected animals may have nasal discharge and hemorrhagic diarrhea. Adult animals are less severely affected, but pregnant animals are likely to abort. The mortality rate may exceed 70% in young animals but is considerably less in adults. Human beings may become infected through contact with diseased tissues. Infections are "flu-like," and infrequently are severe and fatal.

A consistent and characteristic necropsy finding is severe liver necrosis.

Diagnosis. Clinical specimens: Liver and spleen.

A presumptive diagnosis is made on the basis of clinical signs and gross and microscopic lesions observed in the liver. Confirmation requires isolation and identification of the virus. The virus is most easily isolated by the intracerebral inoculation of infant mice.

Prevention and Control. Modified live virus and killed virus vaccines are used in countries where the virus is enzootic. The modified live vaccine should not be used in pregnant animals. Mosquito control reduces the chances of infection. In countries where the disease does not occur, outbreaks are dealt with by strict quarantine and slaughter.

Wesselsbron

Cause. *Flavivirus* (Flaviviridae).

Hosts. Sheep, cattle, and human beings.

Distribution and Transmission. Wesselsbron virus, which is transmitted by mosquitoes, occurs in sheep and cattle of South Africa.

Pathogenicity. The disease in sheep is characterized by high fever and death in newborn lambs and abortion in pregnant ewes. Infection of pregnant cattle may result in abortions and congenital anomalies of the central nervous system. Flu-like symptoms are noted in human beings.

Diagnosis. Clinical specimens: Liver and spleen.

The virus can be propagated in cell cultures of ovine origin and in chicken embryos inoculated via the yolk sac.

Prevention and Control. Modified live virus vaccines are used in areas where the virus is enzootic. Mosquito control reduces the chances of infection.

Adenoviral Infection of Sheep and Goats

Cause. *Mastadenovirus* (Adenoviridae).

There are six recognized adenoviral serotypes that occur in sheep, but their role as disease producing agents appears to be minor. They have been recovered from animals with mild respiratory disease and enteritis.

Adenoviruses have been isolated from goats on relatively few occasions. They have been associated with enteritis, severe conjunctivitis, and cholangiohepatitis.

Enzootic Nasal Tumor of Sheep

Synonyms. Nasal adenocarcinoma, infectious nasal adenopapilloma.

Cause. Probably Retrovirus (Retroviridae).

Hosts. Sheep and goats.

Nasal adenopapilloma is an infectious disease of sheep and goats that is thought to be caused by a type D retrovirus. The disease is characterized clinically by serous to mucopurulent nasal discharge and open-mouthed breathing. The tumors originate from the mucosa of the lateral mass of the ethmoid bone and may be unilateral or bilateral. The nasal passages may become completely occluded, and the tumorous growths may extend into the sinus, cranial cavity, and pharynx.

Diagnosis is based on gross and microscopic lesions.

FURTHER READING

Berrios, P.E. and McKercher, D.G.: Characterization of a Caprine Herpesvirus. Am. J. Vet. Res. *36*:1755, 1975.

Bird, P. Blacklaws, B., Reyburn, H.T., et al.: Early events in immune evasion by the lentivirus maedi-visna occurring within infected lymphoid tissue. J. Virol. *67*:5187, 1993.

Carlsson, U.: Border disease in sheep caused by transmission of virus from cattle persistently infected with bovine viral diarrhea virus. Vet. Rec. *128*:145, 1991.

Castro, A.E., and Heuschele, W.P. (eds.): Veterinary Diagnostic Virology. A Practitioner's Guide. St. Louis, Mosby-Year Book, Inc., 1992.

Chung, S.I., Livingston, C.W., Edwards, J.F., et al.: Congenital malformations in sheep resulting from in utero inoculation of Cache Valley virus. Am. J. Vet. Res., *51*:1645, 1990.

Cutlip, R.C., Lehmkuhl, H.D., Sacks, J.M., and Weaver, A.L.: Prevalence of antibody to caprine arthritis-encephalitis virus in goats in the United States. J. Am. Vet. Med. Assoc., *200*:802, 1992.

De las Heras, M., Sharp, J.M., Ferrer, L.M., et al.: Evidence for a type D-like retrovirus in enzootic nasal tumour of sheep. Vet. Rec. *132*:441, 1993.

Foote, W.C., Clark, W., Maciulis, A., et al.: Prevention of scrapie transmission in sheep, using embryo transfer. Am. J. Vet. Res. *54*:1863, 1993.

Gibbs, E.P.J., Taylor, W.P., and Lawman, M.J.P.: The isolation of adenoviruses from goats affected with peste des petits ruminants in Nigeria. Res. Vet. Sci. *23*:331, 1977.

Grewal, A.S. and Wells, R.: Vulvovaginitis of goats due to a herpesvirus. Aust. Vet. J. *63*:79, 1986.

Kelling, C.L., Kennedy, J.E., Stine, L.C., et al.: Genetic comparison of ovine and bovine pestiviruses. Am. J. Vet. Res. *51*:2019, 1990.

Njoku, C.O., Shannon, D., Chineme, C.N., and Bida, S.A.: Ovine nasal adenopapilloma: incidence and clinicopathologic studies. Am. J. Vet. Res. *39*:1850, 1978.

Pommer, J., and Schamber, G.: Isolation of adenovirus from lambs with upper respiratory syndrome. J. Vet. Diagn. Invest. *3*:204, 1991.

Reddington, J.J., Reddington, G.M., and MacLachlan, N.J.: A competitive ELISA for detection of antibodies to the group antigen of bluetongue virus. J. Vet. Diagn. Invest. *3*:144, 1991.

Rimstad, E., East, N.E., Torten, M., et al.: Delayed seroconversion following naturally acquired caprine arthritis-encephalitis virus infection in goats. Am. J. Vet. Res. *54*:1858, 1993.

Rowe, J.D., East, N.E., Thurmond, M.C., et al.: Cohort study of natural transmission and two methods for control of caprine arthritis-encephalitis virus infection in goats on a California dairy. Am. J. Vet. Res. *53*:2386, 1992.

Sawyer, M.M., Schore, C.E., Menzies, P.I., and Osburn, B.I.: Border disease in a flock of sheep: epidemiologic, laboratory, and clinical findings. J. Am. Vet. Med. Assoc. *189*:61, 1986.

Timoney, J. F., Gillespie, J.H., Scott, F.W., and Barlough, J.E. (eds.): Hagan and Bruner's Microbiology and Infectious Diseases of Domestic Animals. 8th Ed. Ithaca, NY, Comstock Publishing Associates, 1988.

Watt, N.J., King, T.J., Collie, D., et al.: Clinicopathological investigation of primary, uncomplicated maedi-visna virus infection. Vet. Rec. *131*:455, 1992.

Wells, G.A.H., and McGill, I.S.: Recently described scrapie-like encephalopathies of animals: case definitions. Res. Vet. Sci. *53*:1, 1992.

Wood, J.N.L., Done, S.H., Pritchard, G.C., and Wooldridge, M.J.A.: Natural scrapie in goats: case histories and clinical signs. Vet. Rec. *131*:66, 1992.

Woods, L.W., Waters, N.G., and Johnson, B.: Cholangiohepatitis associated with adenovirus-like particles in a pygmy goat kid. J. Vet. Diagn. Invest. *3*:89, 1991.

43

Viral Infections of Horses

INFECTIONS OF THE RESPIRATORY SYSTEM

Equine Influenza

Cause. Influenza virus A (Orthomyxoviridae).

Additional Hosts. Donkey and mule.

Distribution and Transmission. Equine influenza is a frequently occurring disease of horses throughout the world. Transmission occurs by direct and indirect contact. Droplet infection is the primary means of spread.

Pathogenicity. Exposure of susceptible horses to equine influenza virus results in clinical signs in about 1 to 3 days. The most common clinical signs are fever, depression, anorexia, and coughing. Most infected horses exhibit some degree of ocular discharge and photophobia, and some infected horses develop edema of the legs. Pneumonia occasionally occurs if the infection is complicated with secondary bacterial infection. In the absence of stress and bacterial complications, recovery is uneventful in about 7 to 10 days, although the ability to work may be impaired for several weeks.

There are two distinct strains of equine influenza virus, designated as Type 1 or A Equi-1 (Prague) and Type 2 or A Equi-2 (Miami). A new strain of influenza virus was isolated from horses in China in 1989. The virus spread rapidly in the horse population of China during 1989 and 1990, causing a relatively severe respiratory disease. Outbreaks have not occurred since 1990. Molecular biological studies indicated that this strain of virus was an avian influenza virus that was introduced into the equine population. Whether or not it will continue to afflict horses in China or other countries remains to be seen.

Diagnosis. Clinical specimens: Nasal and ocular swabs, acute and convalescent sera.

Equine influenza is often diagnosed clinically based on its sudden onset, rapid spread, high fever, and coughing.

Laboratory confirmation is obtained by isolation of the virus in embryonated chicken eggs or by the demonstration of a significant increase in specific antibody between acute and convalescent sera using hemagglutination inhibition tests.

Prevention and Control. Killed bivalent vaccines are used to prevent disease. Clinically ill animals should be isolated and quarantined.

Equine Herpesvirus Type 4 Infection

Synonym. Equine rhinopneumonitis, Equine herpesvirus Type 1, Subtype 2.

Cause. *Varicellovirus* (Family: Herpesviridae. Subfamily: Alphaherpesvirinae).

Distribution and Transmission. Equine herpesvirus Type 4 (EHV-4) occurs in horses throughout the world. Animals are infected via the respiratory route and spread occurs by contact, aerosol droplets, and fomites.

Pathogenicity. Clinical disease associated with EHV-4 infection is a mild respiratory disease principally observed in young horses up to 2 years of age. Following exposure, the incubation period is about 2 to 10 days. Affected horses are febrile and display clinical signs of mild depression, nasal discharge, and rhinitis. In the absence of secondary bacterial infections, recovery is usually uneventful in 1 to 3 weeks. On extremely rare occasions, infec-

339

tion of pregnant mares with EHV-4 may result in abortion.

Diagnosis. Clinical specimens: Nasal swabs, whole blood, and acute and convalescent sera.

Diagnosis of EHV-4 infection is confirmed by isolation of the virus in cell cultures of equine origin or by the demonstration of a significant increase in specific antibody between acute and convalescent sera. The virus of EHV-4 is antigenically related to EHV-1 and conventional serologic tests do not differentiate between the two. Monoclonal antibodies are available to type specific isolates of the virus.

A presumptive method to differentiate EHV-4 from EHV-1 is the inoculation of cell cultures of equine (equine dermal cell line) and rabbit (RK-13 cell line) origin. The virus of EHV-1 grows in both cell types, but EHV-4 only grows in equine cells.

Prevention and Control. Modified live and killed virus vaccines are available for prophylaxis. These vaccines are usually given at 3 to 4 months of age, with subsequent boosters at frequent intervals, especially while horses are young and most susceptible.

Risk of infection can be minimized by good management practices. Newly purchased horses and horses returning from shows and racetracks should be quarantined for several weeks.

Adenoviral Infection

Cause. *Mastadenovirus* (Adenoviridae).

Distribution and Transmission. Adenoviral infection occurs in horses worldwide. The principal mode of infection is aerosol droplets.

Pathogenicity. Adenoviruses cause only subclinical or mild upper respiratory tract infections in most horses. However, in Arabian foals, from which most isolates have been recovered, the infection is characterized by progressive pneumonia and subsequent death. The severity of the infection in Arabian foals is related to an immunodeficiency resulting from a genetic defect. Adenoviruses have also been associated with cauda equina neuritis and foal diarrhea, but their role in these diseases has not been established.

Diagnosis. Clinical specimens: Nasal and ocular swabs, and lung tissue.

Finding typical intranuclear inclusion bodies in conjunctival scrapings and tissue sections of lung and various other tissues is diagnostically significant. However, care must be taken in evaluating conjunctival scrapings, as inclusion bodies produced by "slow-herpesviruses" generally are indistinguishable from those produced by adenoviruses.

The virus can be propagated in cell cultures of equine kidney producing typical adenoviral cytopathic effects, including large intranuclear inclusions.

Prevention and Control. The subclinical nature of most adenoviral infections do not warrant efforts of prevention and control.

Slow-Herpesvirus Infection

Synonym. Equine cytomegalovirus.

Cause. Herpesvirus (Family: Herpesviridae. Subfamily: Gammaherpesvirinae).

Distribution and Transmission. Slow-herpesvirus infection is prevalent in horses throughout the world. Transmission occurs by direct and indirect contact.

Pathogenicity. The role of slow-herpesviruses in equine respiratory disease is not clear. They have been recovered from nasal and ocular swabs, leukocytes, and various tissues from clinically ill horses and from a large percentage of "normal" horses. There are two distinct antigenic types of slow-herpesviruses. These are designated as equine herpesvirus Type 2 and equine herpesvirus Type 5.

Diagnosis. Clinical specimens: Nasal and ocular swabs, and blood.

The viruses can be propagated in various cell cultures of equine origin. Cytopathic effects are slow in developing (thus, the name), usually requiring at least 5 days and often considerably longer. Large intranuclear inclusions are present in infected cells.

Slow-herpesviruses may present a problem as common contaminants of cell cultures derived from equine tissue.

Prevention and Control. There is no vaccine available, and the development of one is not warranted.

African Horse Sickness

Cause. *Orbivirus* (Reoviridae).

Additional Hosts. Mules, donkeys, zebras, elephants, goats, and dogs.

Distribution. African horse sickness (AHS) was first described in Africa. The causative virus subsequently spread to the Middle East, India, and Spain. The virus of AHS is transmitted by insect vectors (*Culicoides* species), although dogs may also be infected from eating infected horse meat.

Pathogenicity. African horse sickness is a febrile disease that may assume one of several forms. There is a severe pulmonary form with acute onset of paroxysmal coughing, labored breathing, high temperature, and edema of the respiratory tract.

A more chronic form occurs that is characterized by hydropericardium, and hemorrhage and edema of the subcutis of the head and neck regions. Some horses may exhibit signs of both pulmonary and cardiac disease, whereas others may only experience a mild transient infection.

The mortality may range from 20 to 95%. The lesions observed at necropsy vary according to the form of the disease and may include edema of the lungs, hydrothorax, and gelatinous exudates in the subcutaneous, interlobular, and intramuscular tissues and lymph nodes.

Diagnosis. Clinical specimens: Freshly collected and refrigerated whole blood.

A tentative diagnosis is made on the basis of clinical signs and pathologic changes. Laboratory confirmation is obtained by isolation of the virus in 1-day-old mice inoculated intracerebrally or in various cell cultures (e.g., Vero cells). There are nine different antigenic types of the virus that can be identified by serum neutralization tests.

Prevention and Control. Strict import regulations are enforced to prevent introduction of AHS virus into countries free of the disease. Modified live polyvalent virus vaccines are used in countries where the disease is enzootic.

Equine Rhinovirus Infection

Cause. *Rhinovirus* (Picornaviridae).

Distribution and Transmission. Equine rhinoviruses are probably present in horses throughout the world. Susceptible horses are infected via the respiratory route through direct and indirect contact with secretions or excretions of infected horses.

Pathogenicity. Rhinoviruses cause a mild, upper respiratory tract infection characterized by pharyngitis, rhinitis, and lymphadenitis after about 3 to 7 days incubation. Many infections are subclinical.

Diagnosis. Clinical specimens: Nasal swabs.

Equine rhinoviruses can be propagated in cell cultures derived from various animals including the horse and rabbit.

Prevention and Control. Equine rhinovirus infections are generally so mild as not to warrant preventive or control measures.

INFECTIONS OF THE DIGESTIVE SYSTEM

Equine Rotavirus Infection

Cause. *Rotavirus* (Reoviridae).

Distribution and Transmission. Rotaviruses are widely distributed in horses throughout the world. Infection occurs by the oral or oronasal route.

Pathogencity. Rotavirus infections are a primary cause of diarrhea in foals less than 3 months of age. Affected foals are depressed, reluctant to suckle, and have watery diarrhea. The disease is usually mild and of short duration, but may be complicated by concurrent *Salmonella* infection. Severely affected foals should receive fluid replacement therapy.

Diagnosis. Clinical specimens: Feces.

Diagnosis is most easily achieved by the electron microscopic demonstration of rotavirus in distilled H_2O lysates of feces, or by commercial test kits (ELISA and Latex), which are available for "in office" use. Rotaviruses can be cultivated in various cell cultures but usually with difficulty.

Prevention and Control. Good management practices are essential in preventing and controlling rotavirus infections in foals. Foaling areas should be restricted, and the use of clean coveralls and footbaths by attendants should be mandatory. Insuring that foals receive colostrum is important. Affected foals should be isolated.

Equine Torovirus Infection

Synonym. Berne Virus Infection.

Cause. *Torovirus* (Toroviridae).

Although the Berne virus was originally isolated from a horse with fatal enteritis and liver necrosis, most torovirus infections in horses appear to be subclinical. Serologic evidence indicates widespread exposure of horses in European countries (particularly Switzerland). Infections probably occur in horses throughout the world.

Vesicular Stomatitis

Cause. *Vesiculovirus* (Rhabdoviridae).

Vesicular stomatitis virus infection of horses is characterized clinically by oral lesions most often involving the tongue. The virus is discussed in detail in Chapter 40.

INFECTIONS OF THE NERVOUS SYSTEM

Equine Encephalomyelitis

Synonyms. Equine encephalitis and virus encephalitis.

Cause. *Alphavirus* (Togaviridae).

There are three principal alphaviruses that cause encephalomyelitis of horses: Western equine encephalomyelitis (WEE), Eastern equine encephalomyelitis (EEE), and Venezuelan equine encephalo-myelitis (VEE).

Additional Hosts. Human beings and a number of domestic animals.

Various animals serve as reservoir hosts. Western equine encephalomyelitis virus and EEE virus are maintained in nature by a variety of wild birds, whereas VEE virus is maintained by several small forest rodents.

Distribution and Transmission. In the United States, EEE occurs mainly in Eastern and Southern states and WEE occurs primarily in states west of the Mississippi river. Epizootic types of Venezuelan encephalomyelitis virus infection of horses have not been reported in the United States since the 1971 outbreak in Texas. An enzootic type of VEE virus is present in the Florida everglades. Transmission of the viruses occurs via the bite of an hematophagous arthropod. Mosquitoes of various genera are the principal vectors. The virus of VEE is shed in oral secretions, and contact transmission may occur.

Pathogenicity. Infections are most common during summer and early fall when mosquito populations are high. After exposure, there is an incubation period of about 1 to 7 days followed by clinical signs of fever, depression, anorexia, sopor, pharyngeal paralysis, head pressing, incoordination, paralysis of the legs; and death frequently occurs in 2 to 7 days. The mortality rate is especially high in horses infected with EEE (80 to 100%) but less so with WEE (10 to 40%) and VEE (40 to 70%).

Diagnosis. Clinical specimens: Whole blood collected during the febrile stage and brain tissue from horses that have died. Acute and convalescent sera.

A presumptive diagnosis is often based on clinical signs and microscopic brain lesions, which consist of an inflammatory cell infiltrate with perivascular cuffing, and congestion and edema of the meninges. A neutrophilic inflammatory cell response is characteristic of EEE virus infection. Confirmation requires isolation and identification of the virus. The viruses can be propagated in various cell cultures and in young mice inoculated intracerebrally.

A definitive diagnosis can also be obtained by demonstrating a significant increase in specific antibody between acute and convalescent sera. A presumptive diagnosis can be made on the basis of results of a single serum sample if those results are positive and the horse has not been vaccinated.

Prevention and Control. Inactivated bivalent (EEE and WEE) vaccines are used in the United States. Mosquito control reduces the chances of exposure.

Borna Disease

Cause. An unclassified virus.

Additional Hosts. Sheep.

Distribution and Transmission. Borna disease has been reported in Germany and Switzerland. Transmission is thought to occur by contact.

Pathogenicity. Following a protracted incubation period (weeks), the virus of Borna disease causes a meningoencephalomyelitis of horses with resulting clinical signs that are similar to those produced by EEE, WEE, and VEE viral infections. Affected horses usually die. Intranuclear inclusions may be present in neuronal cells of the hippocampus and olfactory lobes.

Diagnosis. Clinical specimens: Brain.

A presumptive diagnosis is often made on the basis of clincial signs and the finding of typical inclusions in brain tissue by histopathologic examination. Confirmation requires isolation and identification of the virus. Isolation may be accomplished by the inoculation of embryonated chicken eggs via the chorioallantoic membrane or by the intracerebral inoculation of rabbits. The virus also grows in a variety of cell cultures but without observable cytopathic effects.

Prevention and Control. Modified live virus vaccines are available.

Japanese Encephalitis Virus Infection

Cause. *Flavivirus* (Flaviviridae).

The virus of Japanese encephalitis is present in the Orient and causes disease in human beings and various animals, including horses. The disease in horses is clinically similar to EEE, WEE, VEE, and Borna disease, but the mortality rate is relatively low (0 to 10%).

Rabies

Cause. *Lyssavirus* (Rhabdoviridae).

Rabies in horses may result in clinical signs that are quite variable, including self-mutilation (biting) and general excitement with vicious behavior; or, affected horses may even appear to be afflicted with colic. Rabies is discussed in detail in Chapter 44.

Equine Encephalosis

Cause. *Orbivirus* (Reoviridae).

This little-studied viral disease of horses has only been reported in Africa. It has been called encephalosis because infections are usually subclinical and not accompanied by CNS signs. However, a few peracute cases have been described with signs of CNS involvement. The fact that horses stabled at night do not contract the disease suggests that it is transmitted by biting insects.

Louping Ill

Cause. *Flavivirus* (Flaviviridae).

The virus of louping ill causes a central nervous system disease in horses. Clinically, the disease is similar to the disease in sheep, which is the principal host. Louping ill is discussed in detail in Chapter 42.

INFECTIONS OF THE REPRODUCTIVE SYSTEM

Equine Herpesvirus Type-1

Synonyms. Equine herpesvirus Type-1, Subtype 1, equine abortion, equine rhinopneumonitis.

Cause. *Varicellovirus* (Family: Herpesviridae. Subfamily: Alphaherpesvirinae).

Distribution and Transmission. Equine herpesvirus Type-1 (EHV-1) occurs in horses throughout the world. The mode of transmission is by direct contact and droplet infection.

Pathogenicity. Although EHV-1 virus may cause mild respiratory tract infections in horses, most herpesviral associated respiratory disease is caused by EHV-4 (formerly EHV-1, Subtype 2). The virus of EHV-1 is principally associated with abortion and occasionally with neurologic disease. Most EHV-1 induced abortions occur after 7 months of gestation and about 2 to 4 weeks following exposure of the pregnant mare. Aborted fetuses are freshly expelled and often contain characteristic gross necropsy lesions of edematous lungs and small tan areas of focal necrosis most readily observed in the liver, lungs, and spleen. Some infected foals are born live but usually exhibit loss of muscle tone, weakness, and the inability to stand. Affected foals generally die within a matter of days.

Central nervous system dysfunction is a relatively rare complication of EHV-1 infection. Affected horses may display clinical signs characterized by mild to severe ataxia. Recovery is usually uneventful, but some affected horses may remain permanently impaired.

Diagnosis. Clinical specimens: Fetal liver, lung, spleen, and thymus. Nasal swabs, whole blood, cerebrospinal fluid, acute and convalescent sera, brain, and spinal cord from horses with central nervous system disease.

A presumptive diagnosis of EHV-1 abortion is often made on the basis of gross lesions observed at necropsy. The finding of intranuclear inclusions in fetal tissues by histopathologic examination is supportive. Confirmation is most easily and rapidly obtained by the demonstration of viral infected cells by immunofluorescence examination of cryostat sections of affected tissue. The virus can be propagated in a variety of cell cultures, including those derived from the horse and rabbit (RK-13 cell line). The ability to propagate EHV-1 in cell cultures of nonequine origin provides a means to differentiate EHV-1 from EHV-4, which only grows in equine cells.

Diagnosis of EHV-1 associated central nervous system disease is more difficult. The virus may be isolated from nasal swabs and blood from acutely affected horses, but the virus is difficult to isolate from central nervous system tissue. Infection may be assumed if a significant increase in specific antibody can be demonstrated between acute and convalescent sera. The histopathologic finding of vasculitis in central nervous system tissue is suggestive.

Prevention and Control. Modified live and killed virus vaccines are available, but only the killed product is labeled as a prophylaxis for abortion.

Pregnant mares should be separated from other horses, and any mares that abort or develop respiratory disease should be isolated. The use of footbaths and clean coveralls by attendants is advised.

Equine Viral Arteritis

Synonyms. Equine abortion, pinkeye, epidemic cellulitis.

Cause. *Arterivirus** (Togaviridae).

Additional Hosts. Donkeys and mules.

Distribution and Transmission. Equine viral arteritis (EVA) was first reported in the United States but is thought to occur in horses throughout the world. The virus is more prevalent in certain breeds of horses (especially Standardbred) in the United States. The virus is shed in excretions/secretions and transmission occurs by indirect and direct contact, including breeding.

Pathogenicity. Horses infected with EVA virus may have no overt signs of disease or they may display a host of clinical signs, including fever, depression, anorexia, and nasal and ocular discharge. Affected horses often have hind limb and scrotal edema and some develop a skin rash over various parts of the body. Pregnant mares are likely to abort. Infected stallions recover clinically, but

---

*Arterivirus is presently a genus of the virus family, Togaviridae, but it is likely that this genus will be upgraded to family status, i.e., Arteriviridae.

often remain persistently infected and spread the virus during breeding.

Diagnosis. Clinical specimens: Nasal swabs, ocular swabs, whole blood, serum, fetal tissues, and semen from stallions suspected to be carriers.

Diagnosis is usually made on the basis of virus isolation or by the demonstration of a significant increase in specific antibody between acute and convalescent sera. The virus can be propagated in a variety of cell cultures, including those derived from the horse and rabbit (RK-13 cell line). The serologic test most often used to measure antibody response is the serum neutralization test conducted in the presence of 10% guinea pig complement.

Prevention and Control. A modified live vaccine is available, but is not used in pregnant mares. Prevention is best accomplished by isolation and quarantine of new additions and horses returning from race tracks and shows. Serologically positive stallions should be evaluated as to carrier status through virus isolation attempts on the sperm-rich fraction of semen or by a program of test breeding of seronegative mares.

Pregnant mares should be isolated from other horses.

Equine Coital Exanthema

Synonyms. Equine herpesvirus Type 3.

Cause. *Varicellovirus* (Family: Herpesviridae. Subfamily: Alphaherpesvirinae).

Distribution and Transmission. Equine coital exanthema (ECE) has been reported in Canada, Australia, Europe, South America, and the United States. The causative virus is spread by coitus and possibly by flies feeding on infectious vaginal discharge.

Pathogenicity. The disease in horses is clinically similar to infectious pustular vulvovaginitis (IPV) and infectious pustular balanoposthitis (IPB) of cattle. The latter two diseases are caused by the herpesvirus, which also causes infectious bovine rhinotracheitis. Secondary bacterial infections are common, but without complications the disease runs its course in less than 2 weeks. Animals recovering from ECE may be carriers.

Lesions produced by ECE virus are similar to those observed with IPV and IPB of cattle. Pustular vesicles and ulcers occur on the mucosa of the vulva, vagina, penis, and prepuce.

Diagnosis. Clinical specimens: Scraping from the affected mucosa of the vulva and penis. Acute and convalescent sera.

The disease is usually diagnosed clinically. Confirmation requires isolation of the virus or the demonstration of a significant increase in specific anti-

body between acute and convalescent sera. The virus can be propagated in cell cultures of equine origin but grows best at reduced temperature.

Prevention and Control. Vaccines are not available. Affected horses should be isolated.

INFECTIONS OF THE INTEGUMENTARY SYSTEM

Equine Papillomatosis

Synonym. Common wart virus of horses.

Cause. *Papillomavirus* (Papovaviridae).

Distribution and Transmission. The virus of equine papillomatosis is thought to occur in horses throughout the world. Transmission occurs by direct and indirect contact. The virus gains entrance through abrasions of the skin.

Pathogenicity. Papillomatosis is most often seen in horses up to 3 years of age. The warts, which generally occur on the nose and lips, vary in size and number and usually disappear within 3 months. Congenital papillomatosis has been reported but occurs rarely. A different papillomavirus is associated with genital lesions in both male and female horses.

Diagnosis. Clinical specimens: Formalin-fixed tissue.

Diagnosis is usually based on clinical lesions. Histologic examination of affected tissue provides confirmation.

Prevention and Control. Autogenous formalin-inactivated wart vaccines are employed on occasion but their value is questionable; repeated doses are recommended. Surgical removal of warts may be helpful. Equine warts, like the warts of other species, will frequently disappear spontaneously.

Sarcoid

Cause. Unknown.

Pathogenicity. The sarcoid is the most common tumor of the horse. These cutaneous tumors, which occur most commonly on the head and neck regions, lower legs, and genitalia, are relatively benign. However, they persist and can only be removed surgically. Even after surgical removal they often recur. The cause of sarcoids is unknown but there is some evidence that bovine papillomavirus Types 1 and 2 may be involved. This is based on the demonstration of viral DNA sequences in sarcoid tissue, and the fact that horses are susceptible to experimental infection with these viruses.

Diagnosis. Clinical specimens: Formalin-fixed tissue.

Sarcoids are diagnosed clinically and histologically.

Prevention and Control. Vaccines are not available.

Horsepox

Synonyms. Contagious pustular stomatitis and "grease-heel."

Cause. *Orthopoxvirus* (Family: Poxviridae. Subfamily: Chordopoxvirinae).

Distribution and Transmission. Horsepox is a disease that has been reported in several European countries. The virus, which is closely related or identical to cowpox virus, is spread by contact and such fomites as combs, saddles, harness, etc.

Pathogenicity. Papules, vesicles, and pustules occur on the skin of lips, nares, pastern, and fetlock regions, and on buccal mucous membranes. Lesions may also occur on the back and are aggravated by the harness and saddle.

Diagnosis. Clinical specimens: Vesicular fluid, scabs, and scrapings from lesions.

Diagnosis is most easily achieved by the electron microscopic demonstration of poxvirus in distilled H_2O lysates of lesion material.

Prevention and Control. The disease is so rare that methods for prevention and control are not practiced.

MISCELLANEOUS DISEASES

Equine Infectious Anemia

Synonym. Swamp fever.

Cause. *Lentivirus* (Retroviridae).

Additional Hosts. Other members of the Equidae.

Distribution and Transmission. Equine infectious anemia (EIA) occurs most commmonly in the United States in low-lying swampy areas. The disease has been reported in South America and in various countries, including Japan, Germany, Italy, and Australia. Transmission occurs mechanically when blood from an infected horse is introduced into a susceptible horse via hematophagous insects, hypodermic needles, and surgical instruments.

Pathogenicity. The incubation period following exposure to EIA virus is generally 2 to 6 weeks. Resulting disease may be acute or chronic. The acute form is characterized by sudden onset of fever, depression, anorexia, thirst, progressive weakness, petechial hemorrhages, ventral edema, and death in 2 to 4 weeks.

Chronic forms of EIA are the most common. Affected horses are intermittently febrile and anemic. They experience weight loss and often have edema of the limbs and abdomen. Some affected horses may exhibit signs of ataxia, and on rare occasions ataxia may be the only notable clinical sign.

Diagnosis. Clinical specimens: Serum, cerebrospinal fluid from ataxic horses.

Since EIA infection is persistent, the demonstration of specific antibody is the most practical and rapid method of diagnosis. This is accomplished by the agar gel immunodiffusion test (AGID) or by a competitive enzyme linked-immunosorbent assay (ELISA). The AGID test is the most commonly used test and is often referred to as the "Coggins" test, so named for the person who first described the test.

Prevention and Control. Vaccines are not available. Routine serologic testing is performed to detect positive horses. These horses should be destroyed, confined to vector proof installations, or segregated from other horses at pasture by at least 200 yards to prevent mechanical spread by biting insects.

Getah Virus Infection

Cause. *Alphavirus* (Togaviridae).

An outbreak of Getah virus infection occurred in racehorses in Japan in 1978. The infection was mild, and characterized by fever, edema of the hind legs, and urticaria. Recovery was uneventful in about 1 week. Transmission was thought to be by mosquitoes principally.

Getah virus has been isolated from mosquitoes in Japan, Southeast Asia, and Australia. Serologic studies indicate that infections occur in a number of other animal species, including cattle and especially pigs. The virus has been incriminated as a cause of fetal death in infected sows.

The virus can be propagated in cell cultures of rabbit (RK-13 cell line) and monkey (Vero cell line) origin, and in mice inoculated intracerebrally.

FURTHER READING

Castro, A.E., and Heuschele, W.P. (eds.): Veterinary Diagnostic Virology. A Practitioner's Guide. St. Louis, Mosby-Year Book, Inc., 1992.

Chambers, T.M.: Cross-reactivity of existing equine influenza vaccines with a new strain of equine influenza virus from China. Vet. Rec. *131*:388, 1992.

Crabb, B.S., and Studdert, M.J.: Epitopes of glycoprotein G of equine herpesviruses 4 and 1 located near the C termini elicit type-specific antibody responses in the natural host. J. Virol. *67*:6332, 1993.

de la Torre, J.C., Carbone, K.M., and Lipkin, W.I.: Molecular characterization of the Borna disease agent. Virol. *179*:853, 1990.

Dwyer, R.M., Powell, D.G., Roberts, W., et al.: A study of the etiology and control of infectious diarrhea among foals in central Kentucky, in Proc. 36th Annu. Conv. Am. Assoc. Equine Practnr. 337, 1990.

Giles, R.C., Donahue, J.M., Hong, C.B., et al.: Causes of abortion, stillbirth, and perinatal death in horses: 3,527 cases (1986–1991). J. Am. Vet. Med. Assoc. *203*:1170, 1993.

Graham, R.R.: Venezuela equine encephalomyelitis (VEE) review. Foreign Animal Disease Report No. *19*,4:5, 1992.

Guo, Y., Wang, M., Kaqaoka, Y., et al.: Characterization of a new avian-like influenza A virus from horses in China. Virology *188*:245, 1992.

Held, J.P., McGavin, M.D., and Geiser, D.: Ataxia as the only clinical sign of cerebrospinal meningitis in a horse with equine infectious anemia. J. Am. Vet. Med. Assoc. *183*:324, 1983.

Henson, J.B., and McGuire, T.C.: Immunopathology of equine infectious anemia. Am. J. Clin. Pathol. *56*:306, 1971.

Kamada, M., Ando, Y., Fukunaga, Y., et al.: Equine Getah virus infection: isolation of the virus from racehorses during an enzootic in Japan. Am. J. Trop. Med. Hyg. *29*:984, 1980.

Lory, S., von Tscharner, C., Marti, E., et al.: In situ hybridisation of equine sarcoids with bovine papilloma virus. Vet. Rec. *132*:132, 1993.

Shibata, I., Hatano, Y., Nishimura, M., et al.: Isolation of Getah virus from dead fetuses extracted from a naturally infected sow in Japan. Vet. Microbiol. *27*:385, 1991.

Telford, E.A.R., Studdert, M.J., Agius, C.T., et al.: Equine herpesviruses 2 and 5 are γ-herpesviruses. Virology *195*:492, 1993.

Timoney, J.F., Gillespie, J.H., Scott, F.W., and Barlough, J.E. (eds.): Hagan and Bruner's Microbiology and Infectious Diseases of Domestic Animals. 8th Ed. Ithaca, NY, Comstock Publishing Associates, 1988.

Timoney, P.J., McCollum, W.H., Murphy, T.W., et al.: The carrier state in equine arteritis virus infection in the stallion with specific emphasis on the venereal mode of virus transmission. J. Reprod. Fert. Suppl. *35*:95, 1987.

Walton, T.E.: Arboviral encephalomyelitides of livestock in the western hemisphere. J. Am. Vet. Med. Assoc. *200*:1385, 1992.

Webster, R.G., Bean, W.J., Gorman, O.T., et al.: Evolution and ecology of influenza A viruses. Microbiol. Rev. *56*:152, 1992.

Wong, F.C., Spearman, J.G., Smolenski, M.A., and Loewen, P.C.: Equine parvovirus: initial isolation and partial characterization. Can. J. Comp. Med. *49*:50, 1985.

44

Viral Infections of Dogs

INFECTIONS OF THE RESPIRATORY SYSTEM

Canine Distemper

Cause: *Morbilivirus* (Family: Paramyxoviridae. Subfamily: Paramyxovirinae).

Additional Hosts. Wolves, foxes, coyotes, raccoons, ferrets, mink, weasels, dingoes, and skunks. Some of the other wild and exotic animals susceptible to canine distemper are listed in Table 47–1.

Distribution and Transmission. Canine distemper is worldwide in distribution. Spread is by direct and indirect contact and the mode of infection is by ingestion or inhalation (droplets). Food, water, litter, etc., are readily contaminated with infectious discharges and secretions.

Pathogenicity. Distemper is usually an acute, febrile disease, especially of young dogs, although older unprotected dogs are susceptible. The first clinical manifestation of distemper is a diphasic febrile response. The first response may be overlooked, but the second generally occurs 2 to 3 days later in conjunction with other clinical signs, which initially include congested mucous membranes of the eyes and nose with subsequent serous to mucopurulent discharges. Pneumonia, depression, anorexia, vomiting, and diarrhea usually follow. Neurologic disturbances, such as neuromuscular tics, "chewing gum" seizures, and paresis are frequent sequelae in dogs that recover from acute disease. Hyperkeratosis of the digital pads ("hard pad") develops in some cases.

Gross necropsy lesions include pneumonia and enteritis. Thymic atrophy may be noted in young dogs. Microscopic lesions are widespread in visceral organs and the brain, and characteristic viral inclusion bodies are commonly found in brain, lung, stomach, and urinary bladder.

Diagnosis. Clinical specimens: Conjunctival scrapings, blood smears, lung, urinary bladder, stomach, and brain.

The most convenient way to diagnose canine distemper viral infection is the demonstration of viral infected cells by immunofluorescence. Examination of conjunctival scrapings and blood smears is useful during early stages of the illness, but false negative results are likely to occur as the disease progresses. Tests are highly accurate when performed on appropriate necropsy tissues.

Microscopic lesions of demyelination in the cerebellum and characteristic inclusion bodies in various tissues are diagnostically significant. The inclusions are primarily intranuclear in the brain and intracytoplasmic in other tissues.

Prevention and Control. Modified live vaccines are administered to dogs between 6 and 16 weeks of age, usually at 2- to 3-week intervals. This multiple dose regimen is necessary because the presence of maternal antibody in puppies greatly hampers the efficacy of vaccination by neutralizing the viral antigen.

Dogs older than 3 months with unknown immune status should be vaccinated twice, 2 to 4 weeks apart. All dogs should receive periodic boosters. Pregnant bitches should not be vaccinated with modified live vaccines.

Supportive treatment, including antibiotic therapy, may be useful in dogs with respiratory illness. The prognosis is poor for dogs with CNS disease.

Kennel Cough

Synonyms. Tracheobronchitis; infectious canine laryngotracheitis.

Cause. *Paramyxovirus* (canine SV-5) and *Adenovirus* (canine adenovirus II), principally; reoviruses, canine herpesvirus, canine distemper virus, and canine adenovirus I have occasionally been associated with kennel cough.

Distribution and Transmission. "Kennel cough" is a common disease most often found in animal hospitals and kennels where a number of dogs are housed in close confinement. Transmission is by direct and indirect (aerosol) contact.

Pathogenicity. Common clinical signs are nasal discharge accompanied by intermittent paroxysmal coughing. Canine SV-5 (parainfluenza virus Type 2) appears to be the primary agent of kennel cough. Mycoplasmas and bacteria (*Bordetella bronchiseptica*) may increase the severity of clinical signs.

Lesions of rhinitis, tracheobronchitis, and exudative pneumonia are often found in affected animals.

Diagnosis. Clinical specimens: Nasal and pharyngeal swabs, trachea, lung, and retropharyngeal lymph nodes.

Diagnosis is usually based on clinical signs and history. The principal viruses associated with kennel cough, canine SV-5, and canine adenovirus II, can be cultivated in cell cultures of canine origin producing CPE characteristic of their respective virus families. Identification is accomplished by virus neutralization.

Prevention and Control. A combination vaccine consisting of live attenuated canine parainfluenza virus and live attenuated *B. bronchiseptica* is widely used to prevent kennel cough. The vaccine is administered intranasally.

Antibiotic therapy is used to control secondary bacterial infections.

INFECTIONS OF THE DIGESTIVE SYSTEM

Canine Coronavirus Infection

Cause. *Coronavirus* (Coronaviridae).

Distribution and Transmission. Canine coronavirus is worldwide in distribution, and transmission is by direct and indirect contact. Virus is shed in the feces and infection occurs via the oral or oronasal route.

Pathogenicity. The virus is highly contagious, affecting dogs of all ages, but the disease in puppies is more severe. Initially, clinical signs are anorexia, depression, and loose stools, followed by vomiting and diarrhea. Feces often contain mucus (seldom blood) and have a fetid odor. Affected puppies may become dehydrated. Asymptomatic infections are commmon, especially in older dogs.

Recovery usually occurs in 1 to 2 weeks and fatal infections in uncomplicated cases are rare. Gross necropsy lesions are those of a nonspecific enteritis; microscopic lesions consist of atrophy and fusion of intestinal villi.

Diagnosis. Clinical specimens: Fresh feces and intestine.

Histopathologic lesions of atrophy and fusion of intestinal villi are suggestive.

Diagnosis is best accomplished by the electron microscopic demonstration of coronavirus in feces, or by the fluorescent antibody examination of cryostat sections of intestine.

The virus, which is antigenically related to transmissible gastroenteritis of pigs and feline infectious peritonitis, can be isolated in cell cultures of canine origin.

Prevention and Control. Inactivated vaccines are available. Puppies are generally vaccinated twice during the first 1 to 2 months of life and thereafter on a yearly basis.

Good sanitation and the use of effective disinfectants (sodium hypoclorite—"Clorox") help control the disease in kennels.

Severely affected dogs may require fluid therapy.

Canine Parvoviral Enteritis

Cause. *Parvovirus* (Parvoviridae).

Synonym. Canine parvovirus Type 2, CPV-2.

Distribution and Transmission. The disease is seen worldwide. The virus is shed in the feces and the mode of infection is by ingestion. Transmission occurs by direct contact and fomites.

Pathogenicity. Dogs of all ages are susceptible, but puppies less than 6 months of age are the most severely affected. The disease may be peracute, with death ensuing after a short course; however, in the more common, less severe form of the disease, the mortality averages about 10%. Among the more common clinical signs are anorexia, depression, pyrexia, vomiting, and bloody diarrhea. Severely affected dogs rapidly become dehydrated and die quickly without electrolyte replacement therapy. Deaths may occur within 48 to 72 hours after onset. Leukopenia is often present.

The cardinal necropsy finding is a hemorrhagic enteritis frequently involving the entire intestinal tract. Grossly, the intestine is often dilated and has a "ground glass" appearance. Microscopically, there is necrosis of the epithelium and dilation of crypts. Lesions resemble those found in cats with panleukopenia.

Sudden death caused by a myocardial form of the disease may be seen in puppies up to 3 months of age. These dogs are usually infected during late gestation or as newborns. A lymphocytic myocarditis and intranuclear inclusion bodies in cardiac myofibrils are noted histologically.

Subclinical infections are common, especially in older dogs.

Diagnosis. Clinical specimens: Fresh feces, intestine, spleen, and heart.

Necropsy findings are suggestive, but lesions may be confused with poisoning. Histopathologic lesions are characteristic.

A rapid diagnosis can be made by electron microscopic examination of fecal samples or by fluorescent antibody examination of fecal smears and frozen sections of intestine and heart. Hemagglutination activity (porcine or Rhesus monkey RBC) of greater than 1:32 in fecal emulsions is considered significant. Antigen detection kits are available for "in office" use. False negative results are not uncommon when these kits are used on feces collected in late stages of the illness or after the dog has died. This is owing to developing antibody complexing with the virus.

The virus, which is thought to have originated as a variant of the closely related feline panleukopenia virus, can be isolated in cell cultures of canine and feline origin (CRFK). Since CPV-2 was first described in 1978, there have been minor genetic changes that have led to replacement biotypes in nature. The current biotype is designated CPV-2b. Canine parvovirus Type 1 (CPV-1), originally referred to as "minute virus of canines" is unrelated to CPV-2 and is not considered to be an important cause of enteric disease, although the presence of this virus in the feces of dogs may cause some confusion in interpreting electron microscopic results.

Prevention and Control. Affected dogs should be isolated from other dogs immediately. Canine parvovirus can survive for weeks in contaminated cages and kennels, and thorough disinfection ("Clorox" solution 1:30) is necessary before uninfected dogs are admitted.

Killed and modified live vaccines are available and are usually administered to young dogs at 4 week intervals from 8 to 16 weeks of age. Young puppies up to 3 months of age are particularly susceptible to CPV-2 infection because maternal antibody may interfere with successful vaccination and yet be insufficient to prevent natural infection.

Thus, an effort should be made to minimize contact between these young puppies and other dogs during this highly vulnerable period.

Other Viruses Associated with Enteritis of Dogs

A number of other viruses, including rotaviruses, reoviruses, astroviruses, and caliciviruses, have been observed in the feces of both clinically ill and asymptomatic dogs. Their relative importance as causes of enteric disease is unclear.

INFECTIONS OF THE NERVOUS SYSTEM

Rabies

Cause. *Lyssavirus* (Rhabdoviridae).

Synonym. Hydrophobia.

Hosts. All mammals; fowl can be experimentally infected.

Distribution and Transmission. The disease is widely distributed, although some countries, including the British Isles, Australia, and West Indian Islands, are free. Rabies is frequently enzootic in wild mammals, e.g., in the skunk, fox, and raccoon (see Chapter 47). Transmission to humans and animals is almost always by bites. Vampire bats and insectivorous bats also transmit the virus by bites. Asymptomatic salivary gland infections occur in bats, resulting in a prolonged viremia. There are reports of human inhalation infections in bat-infected caves; the rabies virus has been recovered from the air of caves harboring bats.

Pathogenicity. The incubation period in dogs is a minimum of 10 days with an average of 20 to 60 days, and rarely as long as 6 months. The virus reaches the brain and cord via nerve trunk pathways (centripetal) and then spreads from the former via peripheral, sensory, and motor nerves (centrifugal) to non-neural tissues, including the salivary gland.

The disease is seen in two forms: (1) furious, and (2) dumb or paralytic. In the furious type, the excitive stage is dominant. Signs include restlessness, depraved appetite, hiding, wandering, aggressive biting, excessive salivation, staggering, paralysis, and finally death, usually 3 to 4 days after signs develop. In the dumb form, frequently there is a short period of excitement, followed by incoordination, paralysis, dehydration, loss of condition, and death.

The most significant histopathologic finding is the presence of eosinophilic cytoplasmic inclusions, called Negri bodies, in affected neurons. Negri bodies are of great diagnostic significance and are most readily found in the hippocampus major.

Diagnosis. Clinical specimens: Brain.

The fluorescent antibody procedure (FA) is widely used and is the preferred method for rabies diagnosis. It is used on animals that have died, and is recommended for the immediate examination of wild animals that cannot be readily held for observation. Smears of the hippocampus major are usually employed. The FA test is highly accurate and provides for a rapid diagnosis.

The FA test is used occasionally on formalin fixed brain tissue (when fresh tissue is unavailable) to confirm a rabies diagnosis based on the microscopic finding of Negri bodies.

Rabies virus can be propagated in cell cultures and in mice inoculated intracerebrally.

Prevention and Control. Prevention is best accomplished by insuring that dogs are properly vaccinated with either modified live or killed vaccines. Modified live vaccines are usually administered to puppies at 3 months of age and when they are 1 year old, and thereafer every 3 years. Some killed vaccines require yearly boosters.

Vaccinated dogs bitten by a known rabid animal should be given a booster vaccination and confined for 90 days; unvaccinated dogs should be euthanized.

A healthy dog or cat that bites a human being should be confined and observed for 10 days. Any wild animal that bites (unprovoked) a human being should be destroyed immediately and tested for rabies.

Individuals at high risk of exposure should be vaccinated with the currently recommended human diploid cell culture vaccine. This vaccine and human rabies immune globulin are used for post-exposure treatment.

Pseudorabies

This disease, which is discussed in detail in Chapter 41, occurs sporadically in dogs that acquire the infection through ingestion. Clinical signs resemble those observed in other animals (excluding pigs). The most characteristic sign is that of intense pruritus (mad itch), most often involving the head region. Self-mutilation is common and animals usually die within 24 to 72 hours after the onset of signs.

INFECTIONS OF THE INTEGUMENTARY SYSTEM

Canine Oral Papillomatosis

Cause. *Papillomavirus* (Papovaviridae).

Synonym. Common wart virus of dogs.

Pathogenicity. The virus commonly affects the mucous membrane of the mouth, lips, tongue, and pharnyx of young dogs, resulting in numerous warts. Warts may occasionally involve the eyelid. Skin warts are seen in older dogs and may be caused by a different papillomavirus.

Diagnosis. The disease is clinically characteristic. The virus is transmissible to young dogs by inoculation of the scarified oral mucosa.

Prevention and Control. Recovered dogs are immune, and dogs more than 2 years of age are usually immune. The treatment of affected dogs with autogenous wart vaccines is of questionable merit. Warts usually regress spontaneously.

MISCELLANEOUS INFECTIONS

Infectious Canine Hepatitis

Cause. *Mastadenovirus* (Adenoviridae).

Synonym. Canine Adenovirus I.

Additional Hosts. The fox, in which the virus causes encephalitis.

Distribution and Transmission. Infectious canine hepatitis (ICH) occurs worldwide. Transmission is by inhalation and ingestion.

Pathogenicity. Dogs less than 1 year of age are most often affected. Clinical signs include depression, fever, vomiting, diarrhea, and discharges from the nose and eyes. Because of a tendency to bleed, hematomas may be seen in the mouth.

The principal tissue changes involve the endothelium and hepatic cells. Damaged endothelium results in widespread petechial hemorrhages. The liver may be enlarged or normal in size but usually is mottled because of focal areas of necrosis. Microscopically, the most significant changes are found in the liver, where centrolobular necrosis is noted and typical adenoviral inclusion bodies are observed in Kupffer cells and parenchymal cells. Recovered dogs may develop a transient corneal opacity ("blue eye").

Diagnosis. Clinical specimens: Liver, urine, nasal swabs.

Diagnosis of ICH is usually made on the basis of clinical signs and gross and microscopic lesions. The virus can be cultivated in cell cultures of canine origin.

Prevention and Control. Recovery from ICH results in lasting immunity. Modified live and killed vaccines are used, often in combination with canine distemper vaccine. Modified live vaccines induce a longer lasting immunity, but a small percentage of vaccinated dogs may develop ocular or renal lesions.

Canine Herpesvirus Infection

Cause. *Varicellovirus* (Family: Herpesviridae. Subfamily: Alphaherpesvirinae).

Distribution and Transmission. The disease is widespread. Infection of puppies is considered to take place transplacentally or by contact during or shortly after parturition.

Pathogenicity. Canine herpesvirus produces a brief but severe illness of puppies characterized by a viremia with an 80% mortality in puppies under 1 week old. The severity of the illness in these young puppies is related to their inability to adequately regulate body temperature or to mount a febrile response to infection. Once these functions develop (2 to 3 weeks of age), puppies become resistant to generalized infections because the virus does not grow well above 36° C. The principal lesions noted in fatal infections are disseminated necrosis and hemorrhage involving the kidney, liver, and lungs. Intranuclear inclusion bodies are observed in the alveolar and interstitial cells of the lung, and in cells adjacent to the areas of necrosis in the liver and kidney.

The virus has also been associated with tracheobronchitis, genital infection, and abortion.

Diagnosis. Clinical specimens: Lung, kidney.

Petechial hemorrhages on the surface of the kidneys and pulmonary edema are characteristic. The finding of typical inclusion bodies is diagnostically significant. A rapid diagnosis can be achieved by the fluorescent antibody examination of cryostat sections of affected tissues. The virus can be propagated in cell cultures of canine origin.

Prevention and Control. Vaccination is not practiced. Prevention is best accomplished by reducing stress and minimizing contact between pregnant bitches and other dogs. Newborn puppies should be maintained in a warm environment.

FURTHER READING

Castro, A.E., and Heuschele, W.P. (eds.): Veterinary Diagnostic Virology. St. Louis, MO, Mosby-Year Book, Inc., 1992.

Chang, S.F., Sgro, J.Y., and Parrish, C.R.: Multiple amino acids in the capsid structure of canine parvovirus coordinately determine the canine host range and specific antigenic and hemagglutination properties. J. Virol. 66:6858, 1992.

Fishbein, D.B., and Robinson, L.E.: Rabies. N. Engl. J. Med. 329:1632, 1993.

Keenan, K.P., Jervis, H.R., Marchwicki, R.H., and Binn, L.N.: Intestinal infection of neonatal dogs with canine coronavirus 1-71: studies by virologic, histologic, histochemical, and immunofluorescent techniques. Am. J. Vet. Res. 37:247, 1976.

Krebs, J.W., Strine, T.W., and Childs, J.E.: Rabies surveillance in the United States during 1992. J. Am. Vet. Med. Assn. 203:1718, 1993.

Mochizuki, M., Kawanishi, A., Sakamoto, H., et al.: A calicivirus isolated from a dog with fatal diarrhoea. Vet. Rec. 132:221, 1993.

Okuda, Y., Ishida, K., Hashimoto, A., et al.: Virus reactivation in bitches with a medical history of herpesvirus infection. Am. J. Vet. Res. 54:551, 1993.

Parrish, C.R., Aquadro, C.F., Strassheim, M.L., et al.: Rapid antigenic-type replacement and DNA sequence evolution of canine parvovirus. J. Virol. 65:6544, 1991.

Raw, M.E., Pearson, G.R., Brown, P.J., and Baumgärtner, W.: Canine distemper infection associated with acute nervous signs in dogs. Vet. Rec. 130:291, 1992.

Tennant, B.J., Gaskell, R.M., Jones, R.C., and Gaskell, C.J.: Studies on the epizootiology of canine coronavirus. Vet. Rec. 132:7, 1993.

Timoney, J.F., Gillespie, J.H., Scott, F.W., and Barlough, J.E. (eds.): Hagan and Bruner's Microbiology and Infectious Diseases of Domestic Animals. 8th Ed. Ithaca, NY, Comstock Publishing, Associates, 1988.

Truyen, U., and Parrish, C.R.: Canine and feline host ranges of canine parvovirus and feline panleukopenia virus: distinct host cell tropisms of each virus in vitro and in vivo. J. Virol. 66:5399, 1992.

45

Viral Infections of Cats

INFECTIONS OF THE RESPIRATORY SYSTEM

Feline Viral Rhinotracheitis

Synonyms: Feline rhinotracheitis, feline coryza, feline influenza, feline herpesvirus Type 1.

Cause. *Varicellovirus* (Family: Herpesviridae. Subfamily: Alphaherpesvirinae).

Distribution and Transmission. Feline herpesvirus is enzootic in the cat population. The virus is transmitted by direct contact and the mode of infection is considered to be inhalation.

Pathogenicity. Feline rhinotracheitis virus affects cats most often between 3 and 18 months of age. The incubation period is usually 2 to 5 days. Clinical signs include fever, anorexia, depression, violent sneezing, conjunctivitis, and nasal discharge. Frontal sinusitis and empyema may occur as sequelae. The virus may cause a generalized infection in young kittens similar to that seen in young pups infected with canine herpesvirus. Abortion, ulcerative keratitis, and bronchopneumonia have been reported.

Common lesions are focal necrosis with occasional ulceration involving nasal passages and turbinates. Intranuclear inclusions are seen in epithelial cells of nasal septum, tonsil, epiglottis, trachea, and nictitating membrane. Cats that recover from the infection should be considered potential carriers.

Diagnosis. Clinical specimens: Conjunctival scrapings and swabs, nasal swabs, lung and trachea from necropsied cats.

The finding of intranuclear inclusions in epithelial cells of affected mucous membranes is diagnostically significant. A rapid definitive diagnosis can be obtained by the demonstration of viral infected cells in conjunctival scrapings or in frozen sections of tissues by immunofluorescence. The virus can be cultivated in cell cultures of feline origin, in which it produces cytopathic changes including intranuclear inclusions. Confirmation of herpesvirus infections associated with chronic ophthalmic conditions is difficult.

Prevention and Control. Attenuated virus and killed virus vaccines are available. Immunity is of short duration and several doses of vaccine are advised for young animals. Annual revaccination of adults is recommended. Killed vaccines are used for pregnant queens.

Feline Calicivirus Infection

Synonym. Feline picornavirus infection.

Cause. *Calicivirus* (Caliciviridae).

Distribution and Transmission. Feline calicivirus infection occurs worldwide, and rivals feline viral rhinotracheitis (FVR) in frequency of occurrence. Transmission is by direct and indirect contact and the mode of infection is by inhalation.

Pathogenicity. The incubation period, course, and clinical manifestations resemble FVR. Clinical signs include fever, mild rhinitis and conjunctivitis, palatine or glossal ulcerations, and, in some instances bronchopneumonia. There is a great variation in severity of the disease, probably owing to variability in the pathogenicity of different strains of the virus. The fatality rate may be substantial in young kittens and older cats with the pneumonic form. Immune complexes are thought to be responsible for a transient "limping" syndrome.

A carrier state may persist for months after recovery with shedding of infectious virus.

Diagnosis. Clinical specimens: Nasal, oropharyngeal, and ocular swabs; lung and trachea from necropsied cats.

Isolation and identification of the virus are required for a definitive diagnosis. The virus can be propagated in cell cultures of feline origin, in which it produces a rapid cytopathic effect. The virus is identified by neutralization tests.

Prevention and Control. Feline calicivirus is strongly immunogenic, and killed and modified live vaccines of cell culture origin are available, often in combination with other viruses. A theoretical limiting factor in the efficacy of FCI vaccine is the occurrence of a number of different antigenic types of the virus.

Feline Reovirus Infection

Feline reovirus infection is a mild upper respiratory tract infection that appears to be widespread in the United States. Clinically, the disease is of short duration and usually confined to the eyes, causing conjunctivitis and lacrimation. The virus can be cultivated in cell cultures of feline kidney, and appears to be reovirus Type 3 or a closely related strain.

INFECTIONS OF THE DIGESTIVE SYSTEM

Feline Panleukopenia

Synonyms. Feline infectious enteritis, cat distemper, feline agranulocytosis.

Cause. *Parvovirus* (Parvoviridae).

Additional Hosts. Members of the felidae: tiger, lion, etc. A number of nonfeline animals are susceptible to feline panleukopenia virus or to its closely related host range variants. They are listed in Table 47-1.

The virus of panleukopenia is immunologically closely related to canine parvovirus Type 2.

Distribution and Transmission. The disease is worldwide in distribution and highly contagious. The virus is present in nasal secretions, urine, and feces. Transmission is by contact (direct and indirect) and infection is mainly by ingestion. Fetuses are infected transplacentally.

Pathogenicity. The disease is seen most commonly in young cats, 3 to 5 months of age. The incubation period is about 1 week. Clinical signs include fever, anorexia, depression, vomiting, diarrhea, nasal discharge, and conjunctivitis. Severe and prolonged leukopenia is commonly found. The mortality rate may be as high as 90% without supportive therapy. Asymptomatic infections may occur in older cats.

The FPL virus can cross the placenta, resulting in abortions, stillbirths, early neonatal deaths, and cerebellar hypoplasia. The latter condition does not become apparent until kittens are 2 to 3 weeks old, when they develop incoordination and ataxia.

Among the changes seen at necropsy are dehydration and emaciation, acute enteritis (particularly of the small intestine), swollen mesenteric lymph nodes, and splenic enlargement. Aplastic bone marrow may be noted. The superficial layer of the intestinal mucosa is eroded in many areas. The crypts are dilated and filled with mucus, and inflammation of the lamina propria is observed. Intranuclear eosinophilic inclusion bodies may be present in epithelial cells adjacent to eroded areas.

Diagnosis. Clinical specimens: Small intestine, mesenteric lymph nodes, and spleen.

Clinical signs and a severe leukopenia are suggestive of FPL. Lesions of the intestine and lymph nodes, and the presence of inclusion bodies are characteristic. A rapid definitive diagnosis is obtained by fluorescent antibody examination of affected intestine and spleen. The virus can be cultivated in cell cultures of feline origin but often without obvious cytopathic changes.

Prevention and Control. Recovery confers immunity. Inactivated and modified live vaccines are available. Two doses of the inactivated vaccines are required, whereas one dose of live attenuated virus vaccine is sufficient. Live vaccines should not be administered to pregnant cats or to kittens less than 4 weeks of age.

The virus is able to survive on fomites for months. Thus, premises should be thoroughly cleaned and disinfected before cats are reintroduced. Clorox solution (1:30) is an effective disinfectant.

Other Viruses Associated with Enteritis of Cats

Astroviruses and rotaviruses have been observed in feces of cats with and without clinical disease. Their respective roles as causes of enteric disease are unclear. Feline enteric coronavirus (see FIP) causes a mild enteritis in young kittens.

INFECTIONS OF THE NERVOUS SYSTEM

Rabies

Rabies is discussed in detail in Chapter 44. The disease in cats is usually the furious form.

Pseudorabies

Pseudorabies is discussed in detail in Chapter 41. The disease seen in cats is similar to that seen in other animal species (excluding pigs), in which the principal clinical signs are neurologic in origin and manifested by "mad itch" and self-mutilation. Cats usually acquire this fatal infection through ingestion.

INFECTIONS OF THE INTEGUMENTARY SYSTEM

Poxvirus Infection

Poxvirus infections have been reported in zoo cats (lions, cheetahs, pumas, etc.) and domestic cats in Eastern and Western Europe. The causative virus appears to be cowpox (or a closely related virus), and it is thought that cats become infected from contact with wild rodents, which are presumed to be the natural reservoir hosts. Affected cats generally have typical pox lesions randomly distributed over the body. Recovery is usually uneventful in about 4 to 6 weeks, although the virus occasionally has been associated with a severe and fatal pulmonary illness.

MISCELLANEOUS INFECTIONS

Feline Leukemia

Synonyms. Feline lymphosarcoma.

Cause. Mammalian Type C Retrovirus (Retroviridae).

Distribution and Transmission. The disease, which is encountered worldwide, is a major malady of cats. The feline leukemia virus (FeLV) is present in respiratory and oral secretions and in urine and feces of infected cats. Saliva is particularly infectious, and biting and mutual grooming are common means of spread.

Pathogenicity. The majority of cats infected with FeLV mount an effective immune response and recover completely without any overt clinical signs. In those cats in which the immune response is ineffective, FeLV is associated with a number of neoplastic and non-neoplastic diseases.

Lymphosarcoma is the most common neoplastic condition noted in cats infected with FeLV. General signs of lymphosarcoma are lethargy, anorexia, and weight loss. Other clinical signs are related to the anatomical location of the tumor, which may be alimentary, multicentric, or thymic. In the alimentary form, the cat may display vomiting and diarrhea. Generalized adenopathy, renal lymphosarcoma, splenomegaly, and hepatomegaly may be found in the multicentric form. In the thymic form, coughing, dysphagia, and dyspnea are common signs, and cyanosis may be present in advanced cases.

The clinical signs associated with FeLV-induced leukemias and myeloproliferative diseases are characterized by anemia. Leukemias are classified according to which hematopoietic cell line has been affected, e.g., lymphoblastic leukemia, erythroleukemia, or myelogenous leukemia.

Infertility, greater susceptibility to infection owing to thymic atrophy, and glomerulonephritis owing to antigen-antibody complexes affecting glomerular basement membrane are examples of non-neoplastic diseases associated with FeLV.

Diagnosis. Clinical specimens: Blood smears, tumors, bone marrow, and serum.

When feline leukemia is suspected, a number of diagnostic procedures are available, including histopathologic examination of biopsies, cytologic examination of thoracic and abdominal fluids, bone marrow examinations, and examination of blood smears by indirect fluorescent antibody (IFA). The latter is a practical and rapid test, and is considered reliable. An enzyme-linked immunoassay (ELISA) system, which detects FeLV antigen in serum, is available to practitioners for in-office testing. The results of IFA and ELISA compare favorably, but false positive results occur more frequently with ELISA. Both tests detect the major core protein, p27, of the FeLV virion. The virus can be propagated in feline lymphoid and fibroblastic cells and in similar cells from dogs and other animals.

Prevention and Control. Prevention and control of FeLV is best accomplished by testing and elimination of positive cats. Vaccines are available but are not entirely efficacious.

Feline Immunodeficiency Virus

Synonyms. Feline T-Lymphotropic virus, Feline AIDS.

Cause. *Lentivirus* (Retroviridae).

Distribution and Transmission. Feline immunodeficiency virus (FIV) occurs in cats throughout the world. Transmission occurs primarily by bites, and male free-roaming cats have the highest incidence of infection.

Pathogenicity. Clinical signs appear 1 to 2 months following infection and consist of depression, fever, and a generalized lymphadenopathy. Signs of illness disappear after a few weeks or months but cats remain viremic for life. A period of clinical normalcy may last for several months to years, but infected cats eventually succumb to various chronic infections as a result of an impaired immune system. Chronic infections may result in stomatitis, gingivitis, rhinitis, conjunctivitis, pneumonitis, enteritis, and dermatitis. Some cats display clinical signs of neurologic dysfunction and some develop lymphosarcoma.

Diagnosis. Clinical specimen: Serum.

Since cats infected with FIV remain persistently infected for life, the detection of antibody to FIV is considered to be the most reliable and convenient means of diagnosis. Antibody may be detected by an indirect fluorescent antibody test or by an ELISA. ELISA test kits are available commercially and are considered to be highly sensitive and specific.

Prevention and Control. Prevention is best accomplished by confining cats indoors. Control is accomplished by test and removal. There is no vaccine.

Feline Infectious Peritonitis

Synonym. Granulomatous disease complex.
Cause. *Coronavirus* (Coronaviridae).
Additional Hosts. Wild Felidae.
Distribution and Transmission. The disease is widespread. The morbidity rate is low, and although a number of cats in a household or colony may be affected, most cases are sporadic. The virus is present in blood and exudates of infected animals. Transmission requires close contact with infected cats, and is thought to occur by the oral route and through inhalation of aerosol droplets.

Pathogenicity. Feline infectious peritonitis (FIP) is a progressive debilitating febrile disease affecting cats of all ages, although most cases occur in cats less than 1 year of age. Following infection, there is an incubation period that may be as short as 2 weeks or as long as several months. The disease has been divided into two forms, "wet" and "dry," but a definite distinction between them cannot always be made.

In the "wet" or effusive form, the initial clinical signs consist of anorexia, high temperature, and depression followed by progressive emaciation. The abdomen is often enlarged as a result of the accumulation of fibrinous fluid in the abdominal

cavity. Dyspnea is a common sign when fluid accumulates in the thoracic cavity. In the "dry" form, there is little or no fluid buildup and a febrile response may be the only initial overt sign of infection. Ocular involvement (anterior uveitis) and CNS dysfunction are more commonly seen with the dry form. Both forms are generally fatal, but death ensues much more rapidly with the wet form. Experimentally, a more rapid development of clinical disease ("accelerated" FIP) occurs in cats with preexisting FIP antibody.

There is considerable variation in the virulence of FIP viral isolates, and most cats with serologic evidence of FIP never develop the disease. The extremely closely related feline enteric coronavirus (FeCV) is endemic in the cat population and is associated with mild enteric disease in young cats. Circumstantial evidence suggest that virulent FIP viruses arise as mutants of FeCV. The FIP virus is also relatively closely related to transmissible gastroenteritis virus of swine and canine coronavirus.

Diagnosis. Clinical specimens: Abdominal and thoracic fluids, lung, kidney, liver, spleen, and brain.

The disease is often diagnosed by gross and histopathologic examinations. In the "wet" form, there are various quantities of characteristic straw-colored fluid in the abdominal and/or thoracic cavities and fibrinous adhesions are present on visceral organs, particularly the spleen and liver. Multifocal grayish-white granulomatous-like lesions are usually noted on the surfaces of various organs. These granulomatous-like lesions are usually larger and penetrate the tissue more deeply in cats with the dry form of FIP. Fibrinonecrosis and pyogranulomas are noted histologically.

Viral infected cells can be demonstrated in cryostat sections of affected tissues by immunofluorescence. Infected cells are usually restricted to or near the surface of affected tissues, and in and around the granulomatous lesions. Failure to sample appropriate areas may result in false negative results.

Antemortem diagnosis is difficult. Hyperproteinemia is suggestive. Positive immunofluorescence results on cells collected from effusions are definitive. Serologic test results are considered to be of little value in diagnosis.

Prevention and Control. A modified live virus vaccine is available but it is not entirely efficacious.

Feline Syncytial Virus

Cause. *Spumavirus* (Retroviridae).
The disease producing ability of feline syncytial virus (FSV) is undetermined. Virus has been recov-

ered from "normal" cats and from cats with respiratory tract infection, neoplasms, peritonitis, and other disorders including chronic progressive polyarthritis. Experimentally, FSV causes no observable illness. The virus appears to be more important to laboratory workers in that it may be present in tissues used to derive cell cultures. Its presence causes degeneration of the cells.

Feline sarcoma virus (FeSV) and R.D. 114 virus (feline endogenous virus) are other retroviruses found in cats. The feline endogenous virus is transmitted vertically in germ cells and is not associated with disease, and FeSV is defective and only causes disease in the presence of a FeLV helper virus.

FURTHER READING

Ackley, C.D., Yamamoto, J.K., Levy, N., et al.: Immunologic abnormalities in pathogen-free cats experimentally infected with feline immunodeficiency virus. J. Virol. *64*:5652, 1990.

Bennett, M., Gaskill, C.J., Gaskell, R.M., et al.: Poxvirus infection in the domestic cat: some clinical and epidemiological observations. Vet. Rec. *118*:387, 1986.

Callanan, J.J., Thompson, H., Toth, S.R., et al.: Clinical and pathological findings in feline immunodeficiency virus experimental infection. Vet. Immunol. Immunopathol. *35*:3, 1992.

Castro, A.E., and Heuschele, W.P. (eds.): Veterinary Diagnostic Virology. A Practitioner's Guide. St. Louis, Mosby-Year Book, Inc., 1992.

Greene, C.E. (ed.): Infectious Diseases of the Dog and Cat. Philadelphia, W.B. Saunders Co., 1990.

Harbour, D.A., Howard, P.E., and Gaskell, R.M.: Isolation of feline calicivirus and feline herpesvirus from domestic cats 1980 to 1989. Vet. Rec. *128*:77, 1991.

Hardy, W.D., and Zuckerman, E.E.: Ten-year study comparing enzyme-linked immunosorbent assay with the immunofluorescent antibody test for detection of feline leukemia virus infection in cats. J. Am. Vet. Med. Assoc. *199*:1365, 1991.

Hoover, E.A., and Mullins, J.I.: Feline leukemia virus infection and diseases. J. Am. Vet. Med. Assoc. *199*:1287, 1991.

Knowles, J.O., Meardle, F., Dawson, S., et al.: Studies on the role of feline calicivirus in chronic stomatitis in cats. Vet. Microbiol. *27*:205, 1991.

Nasisse, M.P., Guy, J.S., Davidson, M.G., et al.: Experimental ocular herpesvirus infection in the cat. Invest. Ophthalmol. Vis. Sci. *30*:1758, 1989.

Nasisse, M.P., Guy, J.S., Stevens, J.B., et al.: Clinical and laboratory findings in chronic conjunctivitis in cats: 91 cases (1983–1991). J. Am. Vet. Med. Assoc. *203*:834, 1993.

Olsen, C.W.: A review of feline infectious peritonitis virus: molecular biology, immunopathogenesis, clinical aspects, and vaccination. Vet. Microbiol. *36*:1, 1993.

Pedersen, N.C., and Barlough, J.E.: Clinical overview of feline immunodeficiency virus. J. Am. Vet. Med. Assoc. *199*:1298, 1991.

Robinson, W.F., Shaw, S.E., Alexander, R., and Robertson, I.: Feline immunodeficiency virus. Aust. Vet. J. *67*:278, 1990.

Rojko, J.L., and Olsen, R.G.: The immunobiology of the feline leukemia virus. Vet. Immunol. Immunopathol. *6*:107, 1984.

Sparkes, A.H., Gruffydd-Jones, T.J., and Harbour, D.A.: Feline infectious peritonitis: a review of clinicopathological changes in 65 cases and a critical assessment of their diagnostic value. Vet. Rec. *129*:209, 1991.

Sparkes, A.H., Gruffydd-Jones, T.J., Howard, P.E., and Harbour, D.A.: Coronavirus serology in healthy pedigree cats. Vet. Rec. *131*:35, 1992.

Tenorio, A.P., Franti, C.E., Madewell, B.R., and Pedersen, N.C.: Chronic oral infections of cats and their relationship to persistent oral carriage of feline calici-, immunodeficiency, or leukemia viruses. Vet. Immunol. Immunopathol. *29*:1, 1991.

Timoney, J.F., Gillespie, J.H., Scott, F.W., and Barlough, J.E. (eds.): Hagan and Bruner's Microbiology and Infectious Diseases of Domestic Animals. 8th Ed. Ithaca, NY, Comstock Publishing Associates, 1988.

Weiss, R.C., Cummins, J.M., and Richards, A.B.: Low-dose orally administered alpha interferon treatment for feline leukemia virus infection. J. Am. Vet. Med. Assoc. *199*:1477, 1991.

46

Viral Infections of Poultry and Other Birds

INFECTIONS OF THE RESPIRATORY SYSTEM

Newcastle Disease

Synonyms. Avian pneumoencephalitis, Avian paramyxovirus Type 1.

Cause. *Paramyxovirus* (Family: Paramyxoviridae. Subfamily: Paramyxovirinae).

Hosts. Chickens, other fowl, and wild and caged birds. Human beings are occasionally infected, resulting in a mild influenza-like disease with conjunctivitis. Hamsters, mice, Rhesus monkeys, and pigs can be infected experimentally.

Distribution and Transmission. Newcastle disease (ND) is a highly contagious malady that occurs throughout the world. Transmission is by droplet infection, fomites, and via the egg.

Pathogenicity. The incubation period following exposure to ND virus is about 5 days. Clinical signs vary greatly depending on the virus strain (and the avian species), from subclinical infections (lentogenic strains), to acute respiratory disease with central nervous system signs (mesogenic strains), to severe generalized infections with high mortality (velogenic strains).

Infection with mesogenic strains is characterized by sudden onset, dullness, with coughing and sneezing and reduced egg production. Clinical signs are usually mild in adult chickens with few if any deaths, but young chicks may be severely affected with mortality as high as 50%. Neurologic

signs may also develop in young chicks shortly after respiratory signs appear. Nervous signs include wing droop, abnormal positioning of the head and neck, and paralysis.

In the velogenic form of ND, also referred to as the viscerotropic velogenic form, clinical signs are severe and include marked respiratory distress and diarrhea. Adult chickens and chicks die rapidly after the onset of clinical signs, and mortality may reach 100%. Some velogenic strains of ND virus are principally neurotrophic, causing paralysis of the legs and wings, twisting of the head and neck, circling, trembling, and walking backward. Similar central nervous system signs may be noted in chickens that survive acute viscerotropic forms of ND.

There are no pathognomonic necropsy lesions associated with ND virus infections. The respiratory system may show hyperemia and congestion with mucus in the trachea. Air sacs may be thickened and cloudy and may contain yellow exudate. These lesions are most severe in velogenic forms of ND. Hemorrhages and necrotic areas involving the proventricular and intestinal mucosa are also noted with velogenic forms of ND.

Diagnosis. Clinical specimens: Lung, trachea, liver, spleen, brain, and serum.

Newcastle disease virus is easily isolated by the inoculation of embryonated chicken eggs via the allantoic cavity. The pathogenicity for embryos varies widely with strains; time of death may vary from more than 100 to less than 50 hours after inoculation. Allantoic fluids containing ND virus

357

agglutinate red cells of chickens, guinea pigs, mice, and humans. The virus can be identified by hemagglutination inhibition and virus neutralization tests, and antibodies in sera can be detected and measured by these same procedures.

Prevention and Control. Prevention is best accomplished by maintaining closed flocks. Any additions should be subjected to testing and quarantine.

Both live virus (low virulence) and killed vaccines are widely used. Live virus vaccines are administered in drinking water and by aerosol sprays, whereas killed vaccines are given by injection.

Newcastle disease outbreaks should be reported to state and federal regulatory officials. Confirmed outbreaks of velogenic forms of ND are dealt with by strict quarantine and slaughter.

Other Avian Paramyxoviruses

Paramyxoviruses have been isolated from birds, and have been shown to be antigenically distinct from Newcastle disease virus. Examples of these isolates are the Yucaipa virus (avian paramyxovirus Type 2) recovered from chickens and ducks exhibiting mild respiratory disease, and the parainfluenza virus (avian paramyxovirus Type 3) isolated from turkeys with severe respiratory infection in Wisconsin and Ontario. Serologic studies indicate that both paramyxoviruses are common in domestic poultry (especially turkeys) in North America. These viruses have been recovered from wild birds in which they are thought to be enzootic. At least six other serotypes of paramyxoviruses have been isolated from a variety of wild and exotic birds.

Infectious Laryngotracheitis

Cause. Herpesvirus (Family: Herpesviridae. Subfamily: Alphaherpesvirinae).

Hosts. Chickens and pheasants.

Distribution and Transmission. The virus of infectious laryngotracheitis (ILT) is widespread geographically. It is transmitted by direct contact and droplet infection.

Pathogenicity. The virus causes a mild to severe respiratory disease in young adult and older adult birds, usually in the fall and winter months. Infection involves principally the larynx and trachea, resulting in coughing, gasping, and dyspnea. Infected birds may cough up blood-stained mucus. Morbidity is high but mortality does not usually exceed 15%.

There is marked congestion and hyperemia of the larynx and trachea. In the advanced disease considerable caseous exudate is seen in the larynx and trachea; caseous cores and diphtheritic membranes may also be present. Intranuclear inclusion bodies are seen in the epithelial cells of the trachea. The tracheal lesions are similar to those seen in the diphtheritic form of fowl pox. Infection with less virulent strains of ILT virus may only result in mild sinusitis and conjunctivitis.

Diagnosis. Clinical specimens: Trachea and lung.

The finding of typical herpesvirus intranuclear inclusions and characteristic gross lesions are diagnostically significant. Electron microscopic examination of distilled H_2O lysates of tracheal scrapings, and fluorescent antibody examination are used for rapid diagnosis.

The virus grows readily on the chorioallantoic membrane of embryonated chicken eggs. The membrane becomes thickened and white plaques are noted.

Prevention and Control. Prevention is best accomplished by maintaining closed flocks. Modified live vaccines administered in drinking water or by aerosol sprays are widely used to control the disease in areas where the virus is enzootic.

Birds that recover from the disease may remain latently infected.

Infectious Bronchitis

Cause. *Coronavirus* (Coronaviridae).

Host. Chicken.

Distribution and Transmission. Infectious bronchitis (IB) is probably worldwide in distribution. The virus is present in respiratory discharges and transmission is by droplet infection and fomites.

Pathogenicity. Infectious bronchitis is a highly contagious disease of sudden onset and high morbidity. The disease is most severe in chicks and young birds; older birds are susceptible, although the disease is mild. Mortality may be high in baby chicks infected with nephrotropic strains.

The most apparent clinical signs are coughing and gasping. Lesions such as cloudiness of the air sacs, exudative bronchitis, and excess serous or catarrhal exudate in the trachea are characteristic. The principal loss in IB is the lowered egg production. The egg-laying capacity of survivors may be permanently impaired; eggs may be misshapen, rough, and soft shelled. Some strains of IB virus are nephrotropic, causing interstitial nephritis and sudden death.

Diagnosis. Clinical specimens: Trachea, lungs, and kidneys.

The virus can be cultivated in susceptible chicken embryos and in chicken epithelial cell cultures. Serotype identification is accomplished by virus neutralization tests with specific antisera.

The changes occurring in the inoculated embryos are usually seen after several passages. They are characterized by death or dwarfing, curling of the embryo, and urate deposits in the mesonephrons.

Fluorescent antibody tests on tracheal scrapings from infected birds have been used for rapid diagnosis.

Prevention and Control. Vaccination is practiced widely. A live attenuated virus is usually administered to birds at 1 to 2 weeks of age via drinking water with revaccination 3 to 4 weeks later, often with a killed vaccine injected subcutaneously. Since there are numerous strains of IB virus, the vaccine used should include the appropriate virus strain(s) for a given area.

Avian Influenza

Synonyms. Fowl pest, fowl plague.
Cause. Influenza virus A (Orthomyxoviridae).
Hosts. Principally chickens, ducks, and turkeys; it is less common in other fowl.

Distribution and Transmission. Influenza virus infection of poultry occurs worldwide. Transmission is by droplet infection and fomites. Migratory waterfowl are a source of infection for domestic poultry.

Pathogenicity. There are numerous strains or subtypes of avian influenza virus. Most of these viruses are associated with subclinical or mild to moderate respiratory infections, characterized by coughing and sneezing. Sinusitis may develop, and infected birds often experience decreased egg production. Concurrent bacterial infections exacerbate the disease.

The highly pathogenic forms of avian influenza (fowl plague) cause severe generalized disease with high mortality. Deaths may occur as early as 24 to 48 hours after onset of clinical signs. Clinical signs are similar in many respects to velogenic viserotrophic Newcastle disease, including occasional neural disturbances. Comb and wattles are cyanotic and there may be edema of the head region with coughing, gasping, blood-stained oral and nasal discharges, and diarrhea. Lesions include hemorrhages and congestion of serous and mucous membranes, consolidation of lungs, and caseation involving the air sacs. Focal necrosis may be noted in the skin and internal organs.

Diagnosis. Clinical specimens: Whole birds killed *in extremis* or lung, trachea, air sac, kidney, spleen, and serum.

The virus is isolated using embryonated eggs, and identified using virus neutralization and hemagglutination inhibition tests. Differentiation from Newcastle disease is carried out with specific immune sera. Sera may be tested for antibody using an agar gel diffusion test.

Isolates of avian influenza virus may be sent to the National Veterinary Services Laboratory in Ames, IA for serotyping and pathogenicity studies.

Prevention and Control. Prevention is best accomplished by maintaining closed flocks. Any additions to the flock should be isolated first and tested serologically. Appropriate antibiotic therapy may be beneficial in controlling secondary bacterial infections in mild forms of avian influenza.

Outbreaks of avian influenza should be reported to state and federal regulatory officials. Confirmed outbreaks of highly virulent avian influenza (fowl plague) are dealt with by strict quarantine and slaughter.

Quail Bronchitis

Cause. *Aviadenovirus* (Adenoviridae).
Hosts. Bobwhite quail.

Distribution and Transmission. The virus occurs in bobwhite quail of the United States. Infected quail shed virus in respiratory secretions and feces. Transmission is via the egg and by direct contact and fomites.

Quail bronchitis virus is indistinguishable from the chicken adenovirus, CELO (chicken embryo lethal orphan) virus. CELO virus is widespread in chickens but is not associated with disease.

Pathogenicity. Quail bronchitis is an acute, highly contagious disease of quail under 4 weeks of age.

Signs of the disease consist of sneezing, coughing, and tracheal rales. Mortality is usually about 50%, but may reach 100%.

Diagnosis. Clinical specimens: Whole birds killed *in extremis.*

A presumptive diagnosis is made on the basis of clinical signs and high mortality. Histopathologic lesions of tracheitis and bronchitis with intranuclear inclusions are supportive.

Confirmation requires isolation of the virus in cell cultures of chicken embryonic liver or kidney, or by the inoculation of chicken embryos via the yolk sac. Several passages may be necessary before the virus causes death of embryos. Dead embryos usually have necrotic foci in the liver and urate accumulation in the mesonephrons. The virus is identified by neutralization tests.

Prevention and Control. There are no commercial vaccines available. Prevention is best accomplished by strict isolation procedures to prevent introduction of the virus.

INFECTIONS OF THE DIGESTIVE SYSTEM

Duck Plague

Synonyms. Viral enteritis of ducks, duck viral enteritis.

Cause. Herpesvirus (Family: Herpesviridae. Subfamily: Alphaherpesvirinae).

Hosts. Wild waterfowl (ducks, geese, and swans).

Distribution and Transmission. The disease has resulted in great losses in ducks in the Netherlands, China, and India. It was first reported in the United States in 1967. Transmission is by direct and indirect contact.

Pathogenicity. The mortality rate may be as high as 90%. Signs of photophobia, depression, inappetence, thirst, and watery diarrhea may be observed.

Diagnosis. Clinical specimens: Whole ducks *in extremis* or liver and mesenteric lymph nodes.

A presumptive diagnosis is made on the basis of clinical signs and high death losses. Lesions noted at necropsy are supportive. Characteristic lesions are widespread hemorrhages affecting many organs, including the heart, liver, and intestine. Small white areas of focal necrosis may also be noted in the liver. The finding of intranuclear inclusions upon histopathologic examination is highly suggestive.

Fluorescent antibody tests on frozen sections of affected tissues are used for rapid diagnosis. The virus can be propagated on the chorioallantoic membrane of duck embryonated eggs, which die approximately 4 days after infection. One-day-old ducklings are susceptible to experimental infection.

Prevention and Control. A modified live vaccine is available but its use requires authorization by regulatory officials.

Prevention is best accomplished by the avoidance of contact between domestic ducks and wild waterfowl.

All suspected outbreaks of duck viral enteritis should be reported to state and federal regulatory officials. Confirmed outbreaks are usually dealt with by strict quarantine and slaughter.

Coronaviral Enteritis of Turkeys

Synonym. Bluecomb disease, mud fever, transmissible enteritis of turkeys.

Cause. *Coronavirus* (Coronaviridae).

Distribution and Transmission. The disease occurs widely and transmission is by direct and indirect contact. The mode of infection is ingestion.

Pathogenicity. Coronaviral enteritis of turkeys is a highly infectious disease of sudden onset. Clinical signs are anorexia, diarrhea, and marked dehydration. Sick birds may show darkening of the head. The mortality rate varies depending on the age of the flock and may approach 100% in young poults. Catarrhal enteritis with villous atrophy is the principal lesion observed in necropsied birds.

Diagnosis. Clinical specimens: Feces and intestine.

Diagnosis is usually based on clinical signs and gross and microscopic lesions. Electron microscopic examination (negative staining) of intestinal contents and fluorescent antibody examination of frozen sections of intestine provide for rapid diagnosis.

The virus can be propagated in embryonated turkey eggs.

Prevention and Control. Affected birds and those that have recovered should be isolated. Good management is important in reducing losses. Preventing secondary bacterial infection by antibiotic therapy is often beneficial. Vaccines are not available.

Hemorrhagic Enteritis of Turkeys

Synonym. Bloody gut.

Cause. *Aviadenovirus* (Adenoviridae).

Distribution and Transmission. The disease occurs widely throughout the world and is responsible for losses of several million dollars annually in the poultry industry in the United States. The virus is transmitted by ingestion.

Pathogenicity. The disease is of sudden onset, and occurs most often in young turkey poults between 4 and 16 weeks of age. The disease is characterized by bloody diarrhea, depression, and death. The mortality may be as little as 1%, or may exceed 60%. Affected layers may produce thin and soft-shelled eggs.

The principal lesion is the hemorrhagic enteritis. The spleen may be enlarged and mottled, resembling marble spleen disease of pheasants and adenoviral splenomegaly of chickens. Similar microscopic changes, including intranuclear inclusions are seen in all three diseases. The viruses of hemorrhagic enteritis, marble spleen disease, and adenoviral splenomegaly of chickens are closely related group II avian adenoviruses that share a common group specific antigen.

Diagnosis. Clinical specimens: Intestine and spleen.

The disease is usually diagnosed clinically, and by gross and microscopic lesions. The finding of typical inclusion bodies (poults examined early in the course of the disease are better) is significant.

Prevention and Control. A commercial vaccine is available. Appropriate antibiotic therapy to prevent secondary colisepticemia is advised.

Reovirus and Rotavirus Associated Enteritis

Reoviruses have been incriminated as a cause of diarrhea in young turkey poults and a malabsorption syndrome in chickens. The reovirus associated enteritis of turkeys was seen in young poults, 2 to 3 weeks old, and was characterized by a yellowish-tan diarrhea and dehydration. The malabsorption syndrome of chickens was characterized by necrosis of the proventriculus and diarrhea.

Rotaviruses have been recovered from the feces of chickens, turkeys, and pheasants with and without clincal signs of disease. Mild to severe diarrhea has been noted in experimentally infected chickens and turkeys.

INFECTIONS OF THE INTEGUMENTARY SYSTEM

Fowlpox

Cause. *Avipoxvirus* (Family: Poxviridae. Subfamily: Chordopoxvirinae).

Hosts. Chickens, turkeys, grouse, pheasants, canaries, pigeons, and other avian species. These are not necessarily affected by identical viruses, but all are antigenically related.

Distribution and Transmission. Fowlpox is worldwide in distribution. Transmission occurs by contact with infected birds or contaminated litter. Virus enters the skin (cutaneous form) through minor abrasions or by the bite of mosquitoes; or, entry may occur through the oral mucous membranes via aerosal droplets leading to the diphtheric form of fowlpox.

Pathogenicity. This is an important, widespread disease of many avian species. It affects adult and young chickens and turkeys most often during the fall and winter. Mortality is usually low but may be as high as 50% with the diphtheric form. Lesions that resemble those of other pox diseases are normally present on the comb, wattles, around eyelids, and on other featherless areas. Birds usually recover within 1 month. The diphtheric form is more severe and is often complicated by secondary bacteria. Lesions involve the mouth, pharynx, trachea, orbit, and sinuses. This form of the disease may be confused with infectious laryngotracheitis as typical cutaneous pox lesions may not be seen.

Diagnosis. Diagnosis is usually based on typical clinical and pathologic findings. Demonstration of acidophilic cytoplasmic inclusions called Bollinger (aggregates) and Borrel (single) bodies in tissue scrapings and sections is diagnostically significant. The virus can be readily cultivated on the chorioallantoic membrane of chicken embryos, producing focal or diffuse pock lesions. The electron microscopic examination of distilled water lysates of lesions is a rapid means of diagnosis.

Prevention and Control. Vaccination is widely practiced in high-risk flocks. The most widely used and safest product for chickens is the pigeonpox virus, which is highly immunogenic, but is of low pathogenicity for chickens. It is propagated in embryonated eggs and administered by the wing-web stick method or by brushing defeathered follicles. Vaccination during the first few weeks of life, with revaccination at 8 to 12 weeks is recommended. Turkeys are usually vaccinated at 2 to 3 months of age with a fowlpox vaccine by the thigh stick method.

Canarypox

Infections with poxvirus occur occasionally in many avian species; however, the form seen in canaries is particularly severe, with mortality sometimes reaching 100%. The disease is frequently systemic, and inclusion bodies may be seen in the liver, salivary glands, pancreas, and other organs. There is no effective vaccine.

INFECTIONS OF THE NERVOUS SYSTEM

Avian Encephalomyelitis

Synonym. Epidemic tremor.

Cause. *Enterovirus* (Picornaviridae).

Hosts. Chickens, pheasants, turkeys, and quail. The virus can be experimentally transmitted to other gallinaceous species.

Distribution and Transmission. Avian encephalomyelitis is worldwide in distribution. The virus is transmitted via the egg and by the oral/fecal route.

Pathogenicity. Avian encephalomyelitis is principally a disease of young chicks during the first 6 weeks of age. The typical clinical disease usually occurs between 1 to 3 weeks of age. In laying birds, clinical signs are not apparent other than a decline in egg production, which may last 2 to 3 weeks.

Clinical signs in young birds include tremor of the head, incoordination, and leg weakness with loss of condition followed frequently by prostration and death. Average mortality rate is about 20%. Some infections are asymptomatic and are only diagnosed by the finding of brain lesions. The lesions in the brain and spinal cord consist of loss of neurons and perivascular cuffing that is mainly observed in the cerebellum, medulla, and pons. Diffuse lymphoid nodular hyperplasia is observed in the proventriculus, spleen, pancreas, and liver.

Diagnosis. Clinical specimens: Brain and spinal cord.

A presumptive diagnosis can be made clinically. Finding the typical microscopic lesions is supportive. Definitive diagnosis depends upon the demonstration of the virus by the intracerebral inoculation of day-old susceptible chicks. If virus is present, "epidemic tremor" develops in 10 to 12 days, and the brains can be harvested for histopathologic examination. Another diagnostic method is the inoculation of brain suspension into chicken embryos via the yolk sac; signs of encephalomyelitis infection in the chicks are observed after hatching. Tissues from these birds should be examined histologically after the signs appear.

The virus can be cultivated in primary whole embryo cell cultures. Antibodies can be demonstrated by means of neutralization tests in chicken embryos employing embryopathogenic strains of the virus. An ELISA kit is available commercially for the serologic monitoring of chicken flocks.

Prevention and Control. A live virus vaccine is administered in the drinking water to 10- to 16-week-old birds. Killed vaccines are used to revaccinate breeders with poor antibody response. These vaccines are administered by the wing-web stick method.

MISCELLANEOUS INFECTIONS

Marek's Disease

Synonyms. Neural lymphomatosis, range paralysis, fowl paralysis.

Cause. Herpesvirus (Family: Herpesviridae. Subfamily: Alphaherpesvirinae).

Hosts. Domestic fowl and turkeys.

Distribution and Transmission. Marek's disease occurs worldwide. Maturation of the virus occurs in the epithelial cells of feather follicles, and copious amounts of infectious virus are shed in dust and dander. Susceptible birds are infected via the respiratory tract through contact with viral contaminated airborne dust particles.

Pathogenicity. Marek's disease occurs most often in birds 8 to 20 weeks of age. The most common clinical sign associated with "classical" Marek's disease is motor paralysis resulting from the effect of the virus on peripheral nerves. Depending on which peripheral nerves are affected, there may be signs of progressive paralysis in the neck, wings, or legs. In the acute form of the disease, visceral tumors are common and birds may die without obvious signs of paralysis.

Characteristic necropsy lesions noted with "classical" Marek's disease are enlarged peripheral and autonomic nerves that appear yellow and translucent. Visceral tumors may or may not be present. In the acute form of the disease, visceral tumors are common and often involve multiple organs. The most common organs affected are gonad, kidney, liver, lung, muscle, and skin. Nerve lesions may not be noted grossly in the acute form of the disease.

Microscopically, an infiltrate of mononuclear cells is seen in affected tissues. Occasionally the eye may be affected, resulting in blindness. This form of the disease is referred to as gray-eye or ocular lymphomatosis.

Diagnosis. Clinical specimens: Whole birds *in extremis.*

Diagnosis is usually based on clinical signs and necropsy examinations. Marek's disease is diagnosed if clinical signs of paralysis or paresis are noted and if peripheral nerves are enlarged. If only visceral tumors are noted, the disease must be differentiated from lymphoid leukosis by microscopic examination of tissues. With Marek's disease, there is usually perivascular cuffing in the white matter of the cerebellum and an infiltration of mononuclear cells in peripheral nerves. These lesions are absent with lymphoid leukosis. Also the cytologic appearance of the lymphoid cells is different. With Marek's disease, there is a mixture of mature and immature pleomorphic cells, whereas with lymphoid leukosis the cells are uniformly "blast" cells. Differential features of Marek's disease and lymphoid leukosis are summarized in Fig. 46–1.

Virologic and serologic procedures are usually not performed because the virus is present in most chicken flocks. There are three serotypes of the virus. Types 1 and 2 occur in chickens and Type 3 occurs in turkeys. Type 1 virus is oncogenic, whereas Types 2 and 3 are nononcogenic. These viruses can be propagated in chicken embryo kidney cells and in duck embryo fibroblasts.

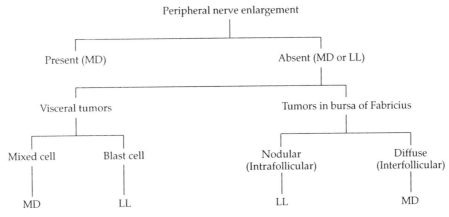

Figure 46–1. Differential Features of Marek's Disease (MD) and Lymphoid Leukosis (LL).

Prevention and Control. Marek's disease is usually controlled through vaccination of flocks at hatching using the serotype 3 Marek's disease virus (turkey herpesvirus). Chicks should be reared in a clean environment for 10 to 14 days until immunity is well established.

Avian Leukosis/Sarcoma

Cause. Avian Type C Retrovirus Group (Retroviridae).

The avian leukosis/sarcoma group of viruses is comprised of seven subgroups, which are lettered A through G.

Hosts. Chickens (Subgroups A through E); Pheasants (Subgroups F and G).

Distribution and Transmission. Diseases associated with avian leukosis/sarcoma viruses occur worldwide. Although transmission may occur by contact, the principal route of transmission is via the egg.

Pathogenicity. All avian leukemia/sarcoma viruses are oncogenic except those viruses belonging to Subgroup E. The pathogenic mechanisms involved in the development of neoplastic conditions are complex and are dependent upon such factors as age, sex, and genetic factors of the host; and whether or not the virus is replication competent or defective. Viruses of Subgroups A through D are associated with a variety of neoplastic conditions in chickens, including lymphoid leukosis, erythroblastosis, myeloblastosis, myleocytoblastosis, osteopetrosis, nephroblastomas, hemangiomas, and sarcomas. The more common conditions are described directly below.

Lymphoid leukosis is the most prevalent disease manifestation associated with avian leukosis/sarcoma viruses. The disease is most often seen in chickens at least 16 weeks of age, and occurs more commonly in females. Clinical signs may be absent or birds may appear unthrifty with pale combs. The abdomen may be enlarged because of massive tumor growth in the liver.

Osteopetrosis is a sporadic disease that occurs primarily in males. The shafts of the long bones are thickened, often resulting in a stilted gait. Affected birds may be anemic and have lesions of lymphoid leukosis.

Erythroblastosis may be manifested in one of two forms, anemic or proliferative, with the latter form being the more common. Clinical signs are similar for both forms. Chickens become depressed, emaciated, and dehydrated. With the anemic form, there are few circulating erythroblasts and chickens appear pale, as opposed to cyanotic with the proliferative form in which circulating erythroblasts are present in large numbers.

Myeloblastosis is similar clinically to erythroblastosis. There is an abnormal proliferation of myeloblasts resulting in severe leukemia.

Diagnosis. Clinical specimens: Whole birds *in extremis.*

Diagnosis of the neoplastic conditions caused by avian leukosis/sarcoma viruses is usually based on clinical signs and gross and histopathologic lesions, but lymphoid leukosis may be confused with the acute form of Marek's disease in older birds. Differential features, which are summarized in Fig. 46–1, include: nodular tumors in the bursa of Fabricius as opposed to diffuse enlargement with Marek's disease; intrafollicular cell proliferation in the bursa of Fabricius as opposed to interfollicular cell proliferation with Marek's disease; and the cytologic appearance of lymphoid cells that are uniformly "blast" cells with lymphoid leukosis but a mixture of mature and immature pleomorphic cells with Marek's disease.

Isolation of the virus or the demonstration of antibody is not considered to be of value in diagnosis because avian leukosis/sarcoma viruses are ubiquitous in chickens.

Prevention and Control. There is no vaccine available and eradication is the preferred method of control. Since the viruses are primarily transmitted via the egg, virus infected breeders are detected by testing the egg albumin for viral antigen by an ELISA method. Positive birds are eliminated.

Reticuloendotheliosis

Cause. Avian Type C Retrovirus Group (Retroviridae).

Hosts. Chickens, turkeys, ducks, and quail.

Distribution and Transmission. Although reticuloendotheliosis is a sporadic disease, the associated viruses are widespread in chickens and turkeys. Transmission occurs through contact and via the egg.

Pathogenicity. Reticuloendotheliosis (RE) viruses represent a group of serologically related avian retroviruses that are distinctly different from the leukosis/sarcoma group of retroviruses. Representative members include reticuloendotheliosis virus of turkeys (REV-T), chick syncytial virus (CSV), and spleen necrosis virus (SNV) of ducks.

A runting syndrome, characterized by atrophy of the thymus and bursa, occurs in chickens experimentally infected with certain strains of the virus. Natural disease outbreaks have been associated with RE viral contaminated vaccines. Chronic lymphoma syndromes, which mimic lymphoid leukosis and Marek's disease, can be produced experimentally.

In turkeys, RE virus has been associated with natural outbreaks of visceral lymphomas usually involving the liver and spleen, although bursal tumors and nerve involvement may be noted.

Diagnosis. Clinical specimens: Whole birds *in extremis*.

The virus can be cultivated in a variety of avian cells but often without cytopathic effects. Identification is accomplished by immunofluorescence or other serological tests, such as ELISA and complement fixation. Antibody may be detected in similar fashion.

Prevention and Control. No vaccines are available. The sporadic nature of the disease does not warrant control measures.

Duck Viral Hepatitis

Cause. *Enterovirus* (Picornaviridae).

Hosts. Young waterfowl and ducklings.

Distribution and Transmission. The disease is widespread. The virus is shed in the feces and is spread by direct contact and fomites.

Pathogenicity. This is an acute, widespread, often highly fatal disease of young waterfowl usually less than 4 weeks of age. It is characterized by a short incubation period (1 to 2 days); the birds stop moving, fall on their sides, have paddling movements and opisthotonos, and die within a few hours. The mortality rate may reach 95%. Deaths usually occur within 1 week of onset of clinical signs. Lesions consist of an enlarged liver with numerous hemorrhages of various sizes, necrosis, and edema. The spleen and kidneys may be enlarged.

Diagnosis. Clinical specimens: Whole birds *in extremis* or liver.

The history and lesions are characteristic. The virus can be propagated in chicken and duck embryos, and identified by virus neutralization. One-day-old ducklings can be inoculated intramuscularly with liver suspension. If duck hepatitis virus is present, opisthotonos develops followed by death within 72 hours postinoculation.

Prevention and Control. A modified live virus vaccine prepared by repeated passages in chicken embryos can be used in young ducklings and breeder ducks. The route of vaccination is via the foot web. Ducklings hatched from eggs laid by immune birds are passively immune, and thus may not respond to vaccination until this passive immunity declines. In the face of an outbreak, immune serum is administered to young ducklings.

Infectious Bursal Disease

Synonym. Gumboro disease.

Cause. *Birnavirus* (Birnaviridae).

Hosts. Chickens.

Distribution and Transmission. Infectious bursal disease (IBD) is worldwide in distribution. The virus is shed in the feces and transmission is by direct contact and fomites.

Pathogenicity. The disease is highly contagious for young chickens (usually 3 to 14 weeks), and is characterized by swelling and edema of the bursa of Fabricius. Clinical signs include diarrhea, anorexia, depression, vent picking, and prostration. Mortality ranges from 0 to about 20%. The principal loss is usually owing to poor weight gains of broilers. Although clinical signs are not usually present in very young birds, the immune system may be permanently impaired.

Lesions in lymphoid tissues are characterized by degeneration of lymphocytes in medullary areas.

On occasion, IBD has been confused with a nephrosis syndrome now considered to be caused by variant strains of infectious bronchitis virus.

Diagnosis. Clinical specimens: Bursa of Fabricius, liver, spleen, kidney, lungs, and blood.

Infectious bursal disease is suspected in cases of swollen and hemorrhagic bursae of Fabricius in young chickens. The virus can be propagated on the chorioallantoic membrane of chicken embryos obtained from flocks free of IBD. Death of embryos usually occurs in 3 to 5 days. Identification is made by virus neutralization.

Prevention and Control. Killed oil adjuvant vaccines are used in breeders. Attenuated live virus vaccines of chicken embryo origin are administered by eye instillation or drinking water to chicks during the first 1 to 2 weeks of age, but vaccination may not be effective if passively acquired immunity is high. Commercial ELISA kits are available for monitoring the immune status of flocks.

Viral Hepatitis of Turkeys

Cause. Probably an *Enterovirus* (Picornaviridae).

This virus causes an infection of turkeys that is usually subclinical, although very young poults may die suddenly without premonitory clinical signs. Focal areas of liver necrosis are noted during necropsy examination.

The virus can be recovered from affected livers by the inoculation of 5- to 7-day-old embryonated turkey or chicken eggs. The virus has not been adequately characterized.

Marble Spleen Disease

Cause. *Aviadenovirus* (Adenoviridae).
Hosts. Pheasants.

Marble spleen disease is a peracute and fatal infection of ringneck pheasants. Among the few clinical signs are depression, bloody droppings, and sudden death. Grayish-tan, mottled, and enlarged spleens are characteristic. Intranuclear inclusions are seen in the reticuloendothelial cells of affected tissue.

The virus, which closely resembles that of hemorrhagic enteritis of turkeys, has been successfully propagated in the turkey B-lymphoblastoid cell line (MDTC-RP19).

Inclusion Body Hepatitis

Synonyms. Hemorrhagic anemia syndrome.
Cause. *Aviadenovirus* (Adenoviridae).
Hosts. Chickens.

Inclusion body hepatitis (IBH), which varies greatly in severity, is seen most often in chickens 6 to 9 weeks of age. Infected chickens may appear anemic and weak, but specific clinical signs are absent. The most consistent lesions are found in the liver, which is enlarged, friable, and yellowish in color. Numerous small hemorrhages are usually observed. Characteristic intranucleur inclusions are found in infected cells. There is some evidence that IBH only occurs in birds that are immunosuppressed, perhaps from an earlier infection with the virus of infectious bursal disease or the virus associated with chicken anemia.

The virus can be propagated on the chorioallantoic membrane of chicken embryos or in avian kidney cell cultures.

Viral Hepatitis of Geese

This is an acute and fatal disease of geese and Muscovy ducks caused by a parvovirus that primarily affects young birds. Affected birds may have anorexia, polydipsia, conjunctivitis, and nasal discharge. Death usually ensues within a few days. Principal lesions are an enlarged liver, ascites, and acute degeneration of both striated and smooth muscle. The virus can be propagated in cell cultures and goose embryos.

Viral Arthritis

Viral arthritis is primarily a disease of broiler chickens caused by an orthoreovirus. Birds 4 weeks old are most often affected, but the disease may also be seen in older birds. Transmission is by the oral/fecal route.

Acute infection is accompanied by lameness with enlargement of the areas of the gastrocnemius tendon or the digital flexor tendon. In chronic cases, immobilization of the hock joints may be observed. Lesions consist of synovitis, edema, and hardening of the tendon sheaths. The virus can be isolated in cell cultures of chick liver or by the yolk sac inoculation of 5- to 7-day-old chicken embryos.

Chicken Anemia Agent

Cause. *Circovirus* (Circoviridae).
Hosts. Chickens.
Distribution and Transmission. The virus is present in chicken flocks throughout the world. Transmission may occur vertically or horizontally, with horizontal transmission occurring by the alimentary and respiratory routes.

Pathogenicity. Chicken anemia agent (CAA) may infect chickens of all ages but only causes overt disease in young chicks within the first 2 to 3 weeks of life. Affected birds display clinical signs of depression and anorexia, and may appear pale as a result of anemia. Necropsy lesions often noted are subcutaneous and muscle hemorrhages, pale visceral organs, an abnormal fatty-appearing bone marrow, and thymic atrophy. Consistent microscopic lesions are found in the bone marrow, where erythrocytes and other cells are replaced by fat cells, and in the thymus, which is depleted of lymphocytes.

Diagnosis. Clinical specimens: Whole chicken, serum.

Diagnosis is often based on clinical signs and gross and microscopic lesions.

The virus can be cultivated in a lymphoblastoid cell line (MDCC-MSBI), but multiple subcultures may be required before cytopathic effects are evident. Antibody to CAA may be detected in chicken sera by an indirect fluorescent antibody test using antigen substrate slides prepared from CAA infected cell cultures.

Prevention and Control. Commercial vaccines are not presently available.

Psittacine Beak and Feather Disease

Cause. *Circovirus* (Circoviridae).
Hosts. Psittacine birds.
Distribution and Transmission. The disease is widespread. Transmission is thought to occur by the alimentary and respiratory routes.

Pathogenicity. The virus of psittacine beak and feather disease (PBFD) affects many species of psittacine birds, causing beak deformities and abnormal feathering. The beak deformities are characterized by palatine necrosis and elongated and easily fractured beaks. Abnormal feathering is progressive, becoming more evident with each molt, and usually occurs in a symmetrical fashion with normal feathers being replaced by dystrophic feathers that cease to grow shortly after emerging from the follicle. The immune system is suppressed and secondary bacterial infections are common.

An acute form of PBFD occurs in which beak and feather lesions may not be evident. The acute form is seen most often in young birds and is characterized clinically by lethargy, anorexia, and diarrhea. Affected birds often die.

Diagnosis. Clinical specimens: Whole birds and infected feathers.

Diagnosis is usually based on clinical signs and histopathologic examination of affected tissues. Intranuclear and intracytoplasmic inclusion bodies are commonly found in feathers, beak, and bursa of Fabricius. A test has been developed to detect PBFD viral nucleic acid in diseased and asymptomatic birds. This test is available commercially. The virus has not been successfully propagated in embryonated eggs or cell cultures.

Prevention and Control. There are no vaccines currently available to prevent PBFD. Prevention is best accomplished by good management practices. New additions to aviaries should only be pur-

chased from reliable sources. These birds should be isolated and quarantined for several weeks and tested for the presence of PBFD.

Psittacine Herpesvirus

Synonym. Pacheco's parrot disease.
Cause. Herpesvirus (Family: Herpesviridae. Subfamily: Alphaherpesvirinae).
Hosts. Psittacine birds.
Distribution and Transmission. The virus is widely distributed, and transmission occurs by the oral or oronasal route.

Pathogenicity. Diseased birds may display clinical signs of weakness and diarrhea followed by coma and death, or they may die suddenly without premonitory clinical signs. Gross necropsy lesions consist of an enlarged and mottled liver, and often an enlarged spleen. Microscopic examination of these tissues reveal focal areas of necrosis and the presence of intranuclear inclusions.

Diagnosis. Clinical specimens: Whole birds or liver, spleen, and lung.

Gross necropsy lesions are suggestive, but similar lesions may be observed in birds that die from chlamydia and polyomavirus infections. The finding of typical herpesviral intranuclear inclusions is diagnositically significant.

The virus can be isolated in cell cultures of chick embryo liver, and in embryonated chicken eggs inoculated via the chorioallantoic membrane.

Diagnosis is most conveniently made by direct fluorescent antibody examination of cryostat sections of liver, lung, and spleen, or from imprints of these tissues.

Prevention and Control. Prevention is best acomplished by good management practices. Avoid mixing birds of different species and minimize stress. New additions should only be purchased from reliable sources, and these birds should be isolated and quarantined for several weeks.

A killed vaccine is commercially available. The antiviral drug, Acyclovir, is effective if sick birds are treated early.

Polyomavirus Infection

Synonym. Budgerigar fledging disease.
Cause. *Polyomavirus* (Papovaviridae).
Hosts. Psittacine birds and finches.
Distribution and Transmission. Distribution of the virus is worldwide. Transmission is thought to occur via the egg and by the alimentary and respiratory routes.

Pathogenicity. Polyomavirus infection causes clinical disease primarily in young psittacine birds that are hand raised. The mortality rate is high (30 to 100%), and birds may die suddenly without overt clinical signs. The clinical signs, when present, are somewhat different in affected budgerigars from those observed in other birds. Affected budgerigars often have a distended abdomen, reddened skin, and abnormal feather development. Birds that survive appear stunted, and are frequently unable to fly because of dystrophic flight feathers.

Common clinical signs observed in other psittacine birds are depression, anorexia, diarrhea, and dehydration. Feather abnormalities rarely occur.

Necropsy examination frequently reveals an enlarged liver and spleen. Microscopically, focal hepatic necrosis is noted and cells with enlarged nuclei containing clear basophilic inclusions are present in a variety of tissues, but especially the spleen.

Diagnosis. Clinical specimens: Whole birds or liver, spleen, and kidney.

Diagnosis is usually based on clinical signs and gross and microscopic lesions. The virus can be propagated in cell cultures derived from budgerigar embryos.

Prevention and Control. There are no vaccines currently available to prevent polyomavirus infection. Prevention is best accomplished by good management practices. Avoid stressful conditions and the mixing of birds of different species. Any new additions of birds to an aviary should be quarantined and tested for the presence of polyomavirus. A test to detect the shedding of polyomavirus from asymptomatic birds is available commercially.

Eastern Equine Encephalomyelitis Virus

Some species of wild birds are the reservoir hosts for eastern equine encephalomyelitis (EEE). The virus also infects many other avian species, but usually without overt clinical signs. In some species, there is an age-related resistance and only young birds are clinically affected. Severe losses occasionally occur in pen-raised bobwhite quail and pheasants that display clinical signs of central nervous system disturbance. A viscerotrophic form of the disease has been reported in whooping cranes.

A viscerotrophic form of the disease also occurs in emus, which frequently die without premonitory clinical signs. Clinical signs, when present, are those of depression and severe hemorrhagic diarrhea. Virus can be recovered from a variety of tissues, including gut, liver, and brain although brain lesions are not observed histologically. Natural infections of other ratities (ostrich and rhea) have not been reported.

See Chapter 43 for a more complete discussion of EEE.

FURTHER READING

Alexander, D.J., and Parsons, G.: Avian paramyxovirus type 1 infections of racing pigeons: 2 pathogenicity experiments in pigeons and chickens. Vet. Rec. *114*:466, 1984.

Alexander, D.J., Campbell, G., Manvell, R.J., et al.: Characterisation of an antigenically unusual virus responsible for two outbreaks of Newcastle disease in the Republic of Ireland in 1990. Vet. Rec. *130*:65, 1992.

Brown, T.P., Roberts, W., and Page, R.K.: Acute hemorrhagic enterocolitis in ratites: isolation of eastern equine encephalomyelitis virus and reproduction of the disease in ostriches and turkey poults. Avian Dis. *37*:602, 1993.

Castro, A.E., and Heuschele, W.P. (eds.): Veterinary Diagnostic Virology. A Practitioner's Guide. St. Louis, Mosby-Year Book. 1992.

Chettle, N.J., Eddy, R.K., Saunders, J., and Wyeth, P.J.: A comparison of serum neutralization, immunofluorescence and immunoperoxidase tests for the detection of antibodies to chicken anaemia agent. Vet. Rec. *128*:304, 1991.

Dein, F.J., Carpenter, J.W., Clark, G.G., et al.: Mortality of captive whooping cranes caused by eastern equine encephalitis virus. J. Am. Vet. Med. Assoc. *189*:1006, 1986.

Gaskin, J.M.: Psittacine viral diseases: a perspective. J. Zoo Wild. Med. *20*:249, 1989.

Kingston, R.S.: Budgerigar fledgling disease (papovavirus) in pet birds. J. Vet. Diagn. Invest. *4*:455, 1992.

Lumeij, J.T., and Stam, J.W.E.: Paramyxovirus disease in racing pigeons. Vet. Quart. *7*:60, 1985.

Magee, D.L., Montgomery, R.D., Maslin, W.R., et al.: Reovirus associated with excessive mortality in young bobwhite quail. Avian Dis. *37*:1130, 1993.

Parede, L., and Young, P.L.: The pathogenesis of velogenic Newcastle disease virus infection of chickens of different ages and different levels of immunity. Avian Dis. *34*:803, 1990.

Pope, C.R.: Chicken anemia agent. Vet. Immunol. Immunopathol. *30*:51, 1991.

Ritchie, B.W., Harrison, G.J., and Harrison, L.R. (eds.): Avian medicine: Principles and Application. Lake Worth, FL, Wingers Publishing, Inc., 1994.

Ritchie, B.W., Niagro, F.D., Latimer, K.S., et al.: Avian polyomavirus: an overview. J. Assoc. Avian Vet. *5*:147, 1991.

Ritchie, B.W., Niagro, F.D., Latimer, K.S., et al.: Routes and prevalence of shedding of psittacine beak and feather disease virus. Am. J. Vet. Res. *52*:1804, 1991.

Sandhu, T.S., Calnek, B.W., and Zeman, L.: Pathologic and serologic characterization of a variant of duck hepatitis type 1 virus. Avian Dis. *36*:932, 1992.

Sharma, J.M.: Hemorrhagic enteritis of turkeys. Vet. Immunol. Immunopathol. *30*:67, 1991.

Spenser, E.L.: Common infectious diseases of psittacine birds seen in practice. Vet. Clin. North Am. Small Anim. Pract. *21*:1213, 1991.

Ture, O., Tsai, H.J., and Saif, Y.M.: Studies on antigenic relatedness of classic and variant strains of infectious bursal disease viruses. Avian Dis. *37*:647, 1993.

Wages, D.P., Ficken, M.D., Guy, J.S., et al.: Egg-production drop in turkeys associated with alphaviruses: eastern equine encephalitis virus and Highlands J virus. Avian Dis. *37*:1163, 1993.

Whiteman, C.E., and Bickford, A.A. (eds.): Avian Disease Manual. American Association of Avian Pathologists, Poultry Pathology Laboratory, Univ. of PA, New Bolton Center, 382 West Street Rd., Kennett Square, PA 19348, 1988.

47

Viral Infections of Laboratory Rodents, Rabbits, and Other Mammals

VIRAL INFECTIONS OF LABORATORY RODENTS

There are a vast number of viruses that occur in laboratory rodents. Their importance, other than their usefulness as disease models, is in the fact that they may compromise experiments in which rodents are used. Prevention and control measures are essentially the same for all of these viruses. Such measures include the purchasing of animals from sources known to be free of disease, barrier maintenance, rigid sanitation, and serologic monitoring. The more important viruses of laboratory rodents are discussed briefly below.

Ectromelia

Synonym. Mousepox.
Cause. *Orthopoxvirus* (Family: Poxviridae. Subfamily: Chordopoxvirinae).
Hosts. Mice.

Outbreaks of ectromelia are relatively infrequent in mouse colonies, but when they do occur the effects can be devastating. Susceptible mice become infected via abrasions of the skin. The virus causes subclinical infections in some strains of mice and highly fatal systemic disease in others. With systemic disease, there is extensive necrosis of the spleen and liver, and mice often die suddenly without premonitory clinical signs. Those that live may develop an ulcerative skin rash. A chronic form of disease may occur in less susceptible strains of mice. The chronic form is characterized by ulcerative pox-like lesions particularly on the feet, ears, and tail.

Diagnosis is often based on clinical signs and gross necropsy lesions. The histopathologic finding of inclusions typical of poxvirus in liver and spleen is diagnostically significant. Confirmation requires isolation of the virus or the demonstration of poxvirus in tissues or lesions by electron microscopy. The virus can be propagated in various cell cultures and in embryonated chicken eggs inoculated via the chorioallantoic membrane. The virus of ectromelia is antigenically related to vaccinia virus, and the latter virus has been used to vaccinate mouse colonies against ectromelia. However, vaccination compromises surveillance testing and may suppress clinical disease in some strains of mice.

Epizootic Diarrhea of Infant Mice

Synonym. Infantile viral diarrhea of mice.
Cause. *Rotavirus* (Rotaviridae).
Hosts. Mice.

Rotavirus infection of mice is similar to rotavirus infection of other animal species in that only the young are affected clinically. Affected mice are usually less than 2 weeks of age. Diarrhea may be mild in some mice but severe in others. A mustard colored feces that stains the rear quarters is characteristic. Mortality is generally low but may result during convalescence when dried feces blocks the anus and causes impaction.

Diagnosis is usually based on clinical signs. The histopathologic finding of swollen and vacuolated villous epithelial cells is supportive. Confirmation is most easily achieved by the electron microscopic demonstration of rotavirus in distilled H_2O lysates of feces.

Pneumonia Virus of Mice

Cause. *Pneumovirus* (Family: Paramyxoviridae. Subfamily: Pneumovirinae).

Hosts. Mice, rats, hamsters, guinea pigs, and gerbils.

Pneumonia virus of mice is enzootic in many mouse colonies and most infections are subclinical. Clinically affected mice may be anorexic and have decreased respiratory rates. An interstitial pneumonitis is noted histologically.

The virus can be propagated in a variety of cell cultures but often without cytopathic changes. Infected cells can be demonstrated by hemadsorption with mouse erythrocytes.

Sendai

Cause. *Paramyxovirus* (Family: Paramyxoviridae. Subfamily: Paramyxovirinae).

Hosts. Mice, rats, hamsters, and guinea pigs.

Sendai virus is enzootic in many mouse colonies and most infections are subclinical. If the virus is introduced into a fully susceptible (naive) colony, the virus spreads rapidly and causes respiratory distress, which is most severe in neonates. Pneumonia with a sharp demarcation between normal and affected areas is noted at necropsy.

The virus can be propagated in various cell cultures including those derived from hamster tissue (BHK-21 cell line).

Mouse Hepatitis

Cause. *Coronavirus* (Coronaviridae).

Hosts. Mice.

There are several strains of mouse hepatitis virus (MHV), which are enzootic in mouse colonies. Some strains of MHV are associated with inapparent respiratory infections, but, under certain stressful conditions, these viruses may cause hepatitis or encephalitis. Other strains of MHV are associated with enteric infections, which are usually mild or subclinical in adult mice, but may cause a relatively severe enteric disease of infant mice. One such strain of MHV is referred to as lethal intestinal virus of infant mice.

The viruses can be propagated in cell cultures of mouse origin producing cytopathic effects characterized by syncytia.

Lactic Dehydrogenase Virus of Mice

Cause. *Arterivirus** (Togaviridae).

Hosts. Mice.

Mice infected with lactic dehydrogenase (LDH) virus remain persistently infected for life. They have no overt signs of illness but plasma LHD levels are elevated, not as a result of increased production but as a consequence of impaired clearance. Mice are most often infected during experimental procedures (e.g., common needles, transplantation studies, etc.). Natural transmission appears to require close contact with contaminated blood or tissue, and is more common in males that fight.

Mouse Poliomyelitis or Encephalomyelitis

Synonym. Theiler's Disease.

Cause. *Enterovirus* (Picornaviridae).

Hosts. Mice.

The virus of mouse poliomyelitis is enzootic in many mouse colonies and is usually associated with subclinical infections of the intestinal tract. Rarely, the virus invades the central nervous system and causes limb paralysis, which may be permanent; or, the virus (depending on the strain) may cause a fatal encephalitis.

The virus can be propagated in a variety of cell cultures including those derived from hamster tissue (BHK-21 cell line) in which it produces a rapidly developing cytopathic effect characteristic of other enteroviruses.

Minute Virus of Mice

Cause. *Parvovirus* (Parvoviridae).

Hosts. Mice.

Minute virus of mice is widespread in mouse colonies but is not associated with disease. Mice become infected at about 8 to 12 weeks of age (when maternal antibody declines) through contact with virus-laden urine and feces from infected mice.

---

*The genus, *Arterivirus*, will likely be upgraded to family status.

The virus can be propagated in cell cultures of mouse and rat origin with little or no accompanying cytopathic effect other than the production of large intranuclear inclusions.

Mouse Mammary Carcinoma

Synonym. Bittner agent.
Cause. Mammalian type B retrovirus (Retroviridae).
Hosts. Mice.

There are several different strains of mouse mammary tumor viruses. Some of these are exogenous strains that are transmitted from dam to offspring via milk, whereas others are endogenous. Mammary tumors usually appear as round or nodular masses in the subcutaneous tissue. Histologically, most of these are adenocarcinomas.

Lymphocytic Choriomeningitis

Cause. *Arenavirus* (Arenaviridae).
Hosts. Mice, rats, hamster, guinea pig, other animals, and human beings.

The virus of lymphocytic choriomeningitis is transmitted vertically and horizontally. Those mice infected *in utero* remain persistently infected, but usually without overt signs of illness until months later when they develop glomerulonephritis owing to immune complexes. Choriomeningitis is rare in natural infections, but can be produced by intracerebral inoculation. Acute infections may occur in immunocompetent mice. These mice do not remain persistently infected but recover completely or die.

Clinically, infection in human beings resembles influenza.

Murine Leukemia

Cause. Mammalian type C retrovirus (Retroviridae).
Hosts. Mice.

There are several strains of murine leukemia virus that cause an array of leukemias dependent upon which hematopoietic cell is affected. These include erythroblastic leukemia, lymphoblastic leukemia, and myeloblastic leukemia.

Rat Cytomegalovirus

Synonym. Rat salivary gland disease, Murid herpesvirus 2.
Cause. *Muromegalovirus* (Family: Herpesviridae. Subfamily: Betaherpesvirinae).
Hosts. Rats.

There are no overt clinical signs associated with rat cytomegalovirus infection. Infections are only noted during histologic examination of salivary glands. Affected salivary glands contain large (cytomegalic) cells with eosinophilic intranuclear inclusions.

Rat Sialoadenitis

Cause. *Coronavirus* (Coronaviridae).
Hosts. Rats.

Rat sialoadenitis virus affects the salivary and lacrimal glands causing nasal and ocular discharge and swelling of the neck region. Infections are self-limiting and mortality is low. Cytomegalic cells may be noted upon histopathologic examination, but these cells do not contain inclusions.

Kilham Rat Virus

Cause. *Parvovirus* (Parvoviridae).
Hosts. Rats.

Kilham rat virus infections are usually subclinical, especially in adults. Congenital infections may result in cerebellar hypoplasia and hepatic necrosis.

Rotavirus Infection of Rats

Synonym. Infectious diarrhea of infant rats.
Cause. *Rotavirus* (Rotaviridae).
Hosts. Rats.

Rotavirus infection of rats is similar to rotavirus infection of other animal species in that only the young are clinically affected. Diarrhea is usually mild and of short duration. The mortality rate is low and most affected rats recover completely, although there may be a transient retardation of growth.

Guinea Pig Cytomegalovirus Infection

Synonym. Caviid Herpesvirus 1.
Cause. *Muromegalovirus* (Family: Herpesviridae. Subfamily: Betaherpesvirinae).
Hosts. Guinea pigs.

There are usually no overt clinical signs associated with guinea pig cytomegalovirus infection. Infections are only noted during histologic examination of salivary glands. Affected salivary glands contain large (cytomegalic) cells with eosinophilic intranuclear inclusions. Two other distinct herpesviruses have been isolated from spontaneously degenerating cell cultures derived from guinea pig tissues.

VIRAL INFECTIONS OF RABBITS

Myxomatosis

Cause. *Leporipoxvirus* (Family: Poxviridae. Subfamily: Chordopoxvirinae).

Distribution and Transmission. The poxvirus causing myxomatosis is enzootic in several species of wild rabbits (*Sylvilagus*) in some areas of North and South America and in some wild rabbit populations of the genus *Oryctolagus*, in Europe, South America, and Australia. Transmission occurs by direct contact, and mechanically by biting insects.

Pathogenicity. In rabbits of the genus, *Sylvilagus*, the virus only causes localized skin tumors, but in the European rabbit (*Oryctolagus cuniculus*) it produces a severe generalized infection with high mortality. Initial clinical signs are swelling around the eyes and conjunctivitis, followed by nasal discharge and swellings around the nose, mouth, and other body orifices. These tumorous swellings (myxomata) may eventually appear over the entire body. Histologically, myxomata are connective tissue tumors that consist of large stellate cells ("myxoma cells") embedded in a soft mucoid matrix.

Diagnosis. Clinical specimens: Fresh and formalin-fixed skin nodules.

Diagnosis is usually based on clinical signs and the characteristic gross and histopathologic lesions. The virus can be propagated in a variety of cell cultures and in embryonated eggs inoculated via the chorioallantoic membrane. The virus is antigenically related to the viruses of rabbit and squirrel fibroma.

Prevention and Control. Prevention is best accomplished by housing domestic rabbits in screened areas to prevent mechanical introduction of the virus by biting insects. Vaccination with the closely related rabbit fibroma virus (Shope fibroma) is practiced in Europe.

Rabbit Fibroma

Synonym. Shope fibroma.

Cause. *Leporipoxvirus* (Family: Poxviridae. Subfamily: Chordopoxvirinae).

Distribution and Transmission. The virus of rabbit fibroma is enzootic in wild cottontail rabbits but rarely occurs in domestic rabbits. Transmission occurs mechanically by biting insects.

Pathogenicity. Rabbit fibroma is a benign disease characterized by the development of one or more raised nodules on the skin that usually regress after 1 to 3 months. Histologically, these nodules are connective tissue tumors characterized by immature fibroblasts although some areas of the tumor may have features that resemble myxoma. A severe generalized infection may occur in neonates.

Diagnosis. Clinical specimens: Fresh and formalin-fixed skin nodules.

Diagnosis is usually based on the typical gross lesions. The virus can be propagated in a variety of cell cultures.

Prevention and Control. Domestic rabbits are rarely affected so no attempt is made to prevent or control the disease.

Hare Fibroma

Cause. *Leporipoxvirus* (Family: Poxviridae. Subfamily: Chordopoxvirinae).

Hare fibroma has only been reported in Europe. The virus, which is related antigenically to the virus of myxomatosis, causes multiple nodules on the skin of the face and ears of affected hares. These nodules (fibromas) are grossly and histologically similar to those observed with Shope fibroma.

Malignant Rabbit Fibroma

Cause. *Leporipoxvirus* (Family: Poxviridae. Subfamily: Chordopoxvirinae).

Hosts. Rabbits.

The virus of malignant rabbit fibroma was isolated from rabbits in a laboratory colony during experimental studies with Shope fibroma virus, and is thought to be a myxoma-fibroma recombinant. The virus causes fibromas similar to those caused by Shope fibroma virus; but, unlike Shope fibroma virus, this virus severely impairs the immune system. Tumors fail to regress and rapidly metastasize to multiple sites. Affected animals usually die from the multiple tumors and secondary bacterial infections.

Rabbit Hemorrhagic Disease

Synonym. Necrotic hepatitis of rabbits.

Cause. *Calicivirus* (Caliciviridae).

Distribution and Transmission. Rabbit hemorrhagic disease (RHD) occurs in China, Korea, and in various countries in Europe. The disease was recently eradicated from Mexico. The virus of RHD is spread by direct contact and indirect contact with secretions/excretions from infected animals. European brown hare syndrome (EBHS), a disease clinically similar to RHD, has been reported in several European countries. The causative agent is a calicivirus that is antigenically related to the calicivirus that causes RHD.

Pathogenicity. Rabbit hemorrhagic disease is a highly contagious disease of domestic rabbits. Infections are characterized by acute onset and rapid death often without premonitory clinical signs. Some affected rabbits may have signs of respiratory distress, such as dyspnea, abdominal respiration, and mild nosebleed. Swollen, congested, and hemorrhagic viscera are noted during necropsy examination. Histologically, the most characteristic lesion is a coagulative hepatic necrosis. There are hemorrhages in the lung and focal areas of necrosis in the spleen and heart. Severe crypt necrosis may be noted in the small intestine.

Diagnosis. Clinical specimens: Liver, spleen, and lung.

A presumptive diagnosis is made on the basis of the peracute nature of the disease. Histopathologic lesions are highly suggestive. The virus will agglutinate human type O erythrocytes, and this hemagglutinating activity can be demonstrated in tissue emulsions. The virus has not been propagated in cell cultures.

Prevention and Control. Rabbit hemorrhagic disease does not occur in the United States. Outbreaks are dealt with by strict quarantine and slaughter.

Rabbit Oral Papillomatosis

Cause. *Papillomavirus* (Papovaviridae).

Oral papillomatosis is a relatively rare disease of domestic rabbits. Affected rabbits have small warts in the mouth that are normally confined to the underside of the tongue. These warts usually regress after a period of months. The causative virus is antigenically distinct from Shope papilloma virus, which causes cutaneous warts.

Rabbit Papillomatosis

Synonym. Common wart virus of rabbits, Shope papilloma.

Cause. *Papillomavirus* (Papovaviridae).

Shope papilloma virus occurs naturally in cottontail rabbits of North America causing warts of the skin, most often in areas of the shoulder, neck, and abdomen. The virus is antigenically distinct from the virus of rabbit oral papillomatosis.

Rabbit Kidney Vacuolating Virus

Cause. *Polyomavirus* (Papovaviridae).

Rabbit kidney vacuolating virus occurs in cottontail rabbits but is not associated with disease. The virus may occur as a contaminant in cell cultures derived from rabbit tissues in which it causes cytopathic changes characteristic of its name.

Herpesvirus Sylvilagus Infection

Cause. *Lymphocrytovirus* (Family: Herpesviridae. Subfamily: Gammaherpesvirinae).

Herpesvirus sylvilagus causes a lymphoproliferative disease of cottontail rabbits characterized clinically by a generalized lymphadenopathy. An enlarged spleen and kidney with nodular infiltrates are noted at necropsy. Microscopically, these infiltrates are principally immature lymphocytes. Infiltrates are also noted in other organs and may be accompanied by inflammatory changes.

Herpesvirus sylvilagus is antigenically distinct from herpesvirus cuniculi, which was isolated from spontaneously degenerating primary rabbit kidney cell culture. Herpesvirus cuniculi is not associated with disease.

VIRAL INFECTIONS OF OTHER MAMMALS

Rabies

Cause. *Lyssavirus* (Rhabdoviridae).

Almost all warm-blooded animals are susceptible to rabies, but raccoons, skunks, and foxes are particularly important in the epizootiology of rabies in the United States. These three animals account for more than 90% of all confirmed rabies in wild animals. Bats are responsible for most of the remaining cases.

There are presently five recognized antigenic varieties of rabies virus that are distributed among wildlife species of the United States. The principal regional reservoir host for these strains is as follows: raccoon in Eastern states; skunk in North Central states and in California and gray fox and coyote in Texas; skunk in South Central states; gray fox in Arizona; and, Arctic fox and red fox in the Northeastern states. The reservoir origin of rabies infection can be determined through the use of monoclonal antibodies. A number of different rabies virus variants occur in bats, and these are distributed throughout the United States.

Canine Distemper

Cause. *Morbillivirus* (Family: Paramyxoviridae. Subfamily: Paramyxovirinae).

Many wild and exotic animals are susceptible to canine distemper virus (CDV), and these are listed in Table 47–1. Ferrets are particularly susceptible to the virus, and natural outbreaks may result in mortality rates that approach 100%. The neurologic signs associated with CDV infection in wild animals, especially raccoons, skunks, and foxes may be confused with rabies. Canine distemper is discussed in detail in Chapter 44.

Parvovirus Enteritis

Cause. *Parvovirus* (Parvoviridae).

Feline panleukopenia (FPL) virus and/or its host range variants of mink enteritis virus, canine parvovirus, and raccoon parvovirus affect a wide variety of wild and exotic animals, causing an enteric

Table 47–1. Some Exotic and Wild Animals Affected by Both Canine Distemper and Feline Panleukopenia Virus and/or Its Host Range Variants*

Canidae	Procyonidae	Mustelidae
Coyote	Bassariscus	Ferret
Dingo	Coati	Fisher
Domestic	Kinkajou	Grison
Fox	Lesser panda	Marten
Jackal	Raccoon	Mink
Wolf		Otter
Cape hunting dog		Sable
Raccoon dog		Wolverine
		Badger
		Skunk

*Host range variants of feline panleukopenia virus include canine parvovirus, mink enteritis, and raccoon parvovirus.

disease much like that observed in dogs and cats. A list of these wild and exotic animals is provided in Table 47–1. Canine parvovirus and FPL are discussed in detail in Chapters 44 and 45, respectively.

Fox Encephalitis

Cause. *Mastadenovirus* (Adenoviridae).

Fox encephalitis is caused by the adenovirus, which causes infectious canine hepatitis (see Chapter 44). The disease is often characterized by peracute deaths without premonitory clinical signs. Some affected animals are lethargic and may have episodes of convulsions. Outbreaks on fur ranches may result in substantial losses.

Aleutian Disease in Mink

Cause. *Parvovirus* (Parvoviridae).
Hosts. Mink, ferrets and striped skunks.
Distribution and Transmission. Aleutian disease is seen principally in ranch-raised Aleutian mink. The virus is present in the urine, feces, and blood, and it is likely that the natural modes of infection are ingestion, inhalation, and transplacental.
Pathogenicity. The parvovirus causing Aleutian disease (AD) is antigenically distinct from feline panleukopenia virus and its host range variants. Mink are the natural host for AD virus, but ferrets and striped skunks are also susceptible. The virus causes a chronic, progressive wasting disease with high mortality in some mink, and an inapparent but persistent infection in others.

The disease is most severe in the fur color mutant strain of mink called Aleutian. These mink have abnormalities of leukocyte granules and are unable to destroy immune complexes. Viral antibody complexes remain infectious and continually stimulate the immune system, leading to hypergammaglobulinemia. Deposits of virus-antibody-complement complexes in the kidney result in glomerulonephritis and renal failure. Lesions noted at necropsy include enlarged kidneys, spleen, and lymph nodes, and a yellowish-brown mottling of the liver.

Diagnosis. Diagnosis is usually based on clinical signs and lesions. The virus can be cultivated in cell cultures of mink testes and kidney but a reduced temperature is required for initial isolation.

Prevention and Control. Prevention and control measures on mink ranches are based on the serologic testing and removal of all positive animals.

Transmissible Encephalopathy of Mink

Cause. Prion (proposed).

Transmissible encephalopathy of mink (TEM) is an insidious neurologic disease characterized by a long incubation period (8 months or longer) and clinical signs of hyperirritability, loss of weight, ataxia, compulsive biting, somnolence, and ultimately death in about 2 to 6 weeks. There are no gross necropsy lesions, but characteristic spongiform changes in the brain are noted histologically. These spongiform changes are essentially identical to those observed in the brain of sheep with scrapie, and with the spongiform encephalopathies of other animals, including cattle. Mink are thought to be infected by eating contaminated meat from ruminants. Cannibalism and fighting may spread the agent among other mink.

Epizootic Hemorrhagic Disease of Deer

Cause. *Orbivirus* (Reoviridae).
Distribution and Transmission. There are seven serotypes of epizootic hemorrhagic disease (EHD) virus, but only two of these (New Jersey and Alberta) occur in the United States. The virus is transmitted by the biting gnat, *Culicoides variipennis*.
Pathogenicity. The virus of EHD causes disease in white-tailed deer. The disease may be subclinical, peracute, acute, or chronic. The peracute form is characterized by severe edema of the head and

neck regions, including the tongue and conjunctiva, and rapid death. Edematous lungs are noted at necropsy but there are few if any signs of hemorrhage. Hemorrhages are more evident in animals that live longer (acute form), and are usually present in the heart, rumen, and intestine. There are also ulcerations on the tongue and dental pad and in the rumen and omasum. The chronic form is characterized by lameness. Bluetongue virus may cause similar disease manifestations.

The virus of EHD may infect cattle, but most infections are subclinical. One strain of EHD (Ibaraki) occurs in Southeast Asia and causes a disease in cattle clinically similar to bluetongue.

Diagnosis. Clinical specimens: Fresh heparinized blood, serum, and spleen.

Diagnosis of EHD is often made on the basis of clinical signs and lesions. Confirmation requires isolation and identification of the virus. The virus can be propagated in embryonated chicken eggs inoculated intravenously and in various cell cultures, including the BHK-21 cell line. Fluorescent antibody tests may be used on frozen sections of affected tissues.

A high percentage of deer in the Southeastern United States have antibodies to EHD virus as determined by the agar gel immunodiffusion test.

Squirrel Fibroma

Cause. *Leporipoxvirus* (Family: Poxviridae. Subfamily: Chordopoxvirinae).
Hosts. Squirrels.

The virus of squirrel fibroma is antigenically related to the virus of rabbit fibroma. It causes usually a benign disease that is characterized by the development of raised nodules on the skin. These fibromas may be small or grow to a size of 25 mm in diameter. The virus is mechanically transmitted by biting insects.

FURTHER READING

Aasted, B., and Leslie, R.G.Q.: Virus-specific B-lymphocytes are probably the primary targets for Aleutian disease virus. Vet. Immunol. Immunopathol. *28*:127, 1991.

Bhatt, P.N., Jacoby, R.O., Morse III, H.C., and New, A.E. (eds.): Viral and Mycoplasmal Infections of Laboratory Rodents. Effects on Biomedical Research. New York, Academic Press, Inc., 1986.

Davidson, W.R., and Nettles V.F.: Field Manual of Wildlife Diseases in the Southeastern United States. Southeastern Cooperative Wildlife Disease Study, Department of Parasitology, College of Veterinary Medicine, The University of Georgia, Athens, GA 30602, 1988.

Darai, G. (ed.): Viral Diseases in Laboratory and Captive Animals. Boston, Martinus Nijhoff Publishing, 1988.

Fisbein, D., and Robinson, L.E.: Rabies. N. Engl. J. Med. *329*:1632, 1993.

Hesselton, R.M., Yang E.C., Medveczky, P., and Sullivan, J.L.: Pathogenesis of herpesvirus sylvilagus infection in cottontail rabbits. Am. J. Pathol. *133*:639, 1988.

Moussa, A., et al.: Haemorrhagic disease of lagomorphs: evidence for a calicivirus. Vet. Microbiol. *33*:375, 1992.

Krebs, J.W., Strine, T.W., and Childs, J.E.: Rabies surveillance in the United States during 1992. J. Am. Vet. Med. Assoc. *203*:1718, 1993.

Ueda, K., Park, J.H., Ochiai, K., and Itakura, C.: Disseminated intravascular coagulation (DIC) in rabbit haemorrhagic disease. Jpn. J. Vet. Res. *40*:133, 1992.

Wirblich, C., et al.: European brown hare syndrome virus: relationship to rabbit hemorrhagic disease virus and other caliciviruses. J. Virol. *68*:5164, 1994.

GLOSSARY

This glossary includes only those terms not explained in the text. Some pathologic, clinical, and immunologic terms are included for those students who have not had instruction in pathology and immunology. An asterisk indicates that the term is defined in the glossary.

Adjuvant. A substance or compound that enhances the immune response when injected (usually) with an antigen. There are a number of adjuvants, e.g., alumina adjuvants,* Freund's adjuvants,* saponin.

Agar. A relatively inert polysaccharide, derived from seaweed and used as a solidifying compound, mainly in culture media. It gels at room temperature.

Agar gel immunodiffusion test. (see **Immunodiffusion test**).

Agglutination. The clumping of particulate antigen, such as bacteria or erythrocytes, by antibody or electrostatic forces. Agglutination tests, in which the antigen is constant and the serum concentration is varied, are carried out in tubes, glass plates, and microtiter plates to measure antibody.

Alopecia. Loss of hair, feathers, or wool.

Alum precipitated. (see **Alumina adjuvants**).

Alumina adjuvants. A number of compounds of aluminum are used to absorb protein antigens, both bacterial and viral, from solution. When these "precipitated" antigens are injected into animals they form a depot from which the antigen is slowly released, thus providing an adjuvant immune effect.

Analogues. Chemical compounds with similar structure but differing in respect to a certain component.

Angström (Å). A unit of length equal to one tenbillionth (10^{-10}) of a meter.

Anorexia. Loss or lack of appetite.

Antigen. A molecule or substance that is recognized by an animal as foreign (nonself) and elicits an immune response (antibodies or immune cells).

Antigen-antibody complexes. (see **Immune complexes**).

Antigenic determinant. (see **Epitope**).

Antiserum. A serum containing antibodies.

Antitoxin. An antibody capable of combining with and neutralizing a toxin.

Aplastic anemia. An anemia in which the bone marrow fails to produce adequate numbers of peripheral blood elements.

Arthrogryposis. Permanent flexure or contracture of a joint.

Asepsis. A state of sterility (absence of potentially harmful microorganisms) or near sterility.

Ataxia. Lack of muscular coordination.

Atrophy. The decrease in the size of an organ, tissue, or cell.

Attenuated. Made less virulent for a particular host. Attenuated strains of some pathogenic bacteria and viruses are used as vaccines.

Autoagglutination. Agglutination in a solution containing saline without the addition of specific antiserum. Some bacteria in the R (rough) phase of growth have a tendency to autoagglutinate.

Autogenous bacterin. A bacterin* prepared from bacteria causing disease in an individual or herd, and used in the same individual or herd to elicit protection.

Avirulent. Lacking in the capacity to produce disease. Some pathogenic microorganisms give rise to avirulent mutants.

Bacteremia. The presence of viable bacteria in the blood.

Bacterin. A preparation, usually a suspension, of killed bacteria used for immunization. Dilute formalin is frequently used to kill the bacteria.

Biopsy. The selection and removal of a small portion of tissue from an animal for diagnostic purposes.

Biotypes. These are closely related varieties within a species that are distinguished by one or more biochemical reactions.

Blepharitis. Inflammation of the eyelids.

B lymphocyte. This cell of the immune system differentiates into cells that produce an immunoglobulin* (antibody).

Bubo. The inflammatory enlargement of a lymph node, as in bubonic plague.

Buffy coat. The layer of white cells and platelets that appear above the red cells when blood settles or is centrifuged.

Capnophilic. This term is used for those microorganisms that prefer an incubation atmosphere with increased carbon-dioxide concentration.

Carbuncle. A local, purulent, necrotic, inflammatory process involving the skin and deeper tissues with multiple openings from which pus is discharged.

Caseous. Resembling cheese or curd.

Cauda equina neuritis. A neuritis involving the upper sacral nerves at the first lumbar vertebra; these nerves form a bundle of filaments within the spinal canal resembling a horse's tail.

Cell-mediated immunity. A specific immunity mediated by T lymphocytes (T cells*) and expressed via macrophages.*

Cellular immunity. (see **Cell-mediated immunity**).

Cellulitis. Diffuse inflammation of connective tissue, particularly that of the subcutis.

Cholangiohepatitis. An inflammation of the bile vessels.

Choriomeningitis. Cerebral meningitis with lymphocytic infiltration of the chorioid plexus.

Cirrhosis. Disease of the liver with loss of normal lobular structure with replacement fibrosis and nodular regeneration.

Coagglutination. The agglutination of protein A containing *Staphylococcus aureus* when coated with antibody and exposed to the corresponding antigen.

Competitive enzyme-linked immunosorbent assay. A type of ELISA that measures the competition in binding of antibody between a fixed amount of labeled antigen and an unknown quantity of unlabeled antigen (e.g., antigen in a clinical sample). This assay can be reversed and the antibody measured.

Complement. A complex of approximately 15 proteins found in the blood that acts with specific antibody in certain kinds of antigen-antibody reactions; they result in various biological sequences including opsonization* and lysis of microorganisms.

Congenital. Acquired during development in the uterus; not owing to heredity.

Coombs' test. This is a procedure that uses antibody to immunoglobulins (bovine, porcine, human, etc.) in order to agglutinate particles or microorganisms carrying nonagglutinating antibody (incomplete antibody) on their surface.

Counter immunoelectrophoresis. The detection of antigen or antibody by a precipitin reaction that occurs in a gel or paper. An electric current is used to carry the reactants toward each other.

Cystitis. Inflammation of the urinary bladder, almost always caused by infection.

Dalton. A unit of mass roughly equal to the weight of a hydrogen atom. It is equivalent to 1.657×10^{-24} g.

Debridement. The surgical removal of damaged, contaminated, or devitalized tissue.

Delayed-type hypersensitivity. A slowly developing skin reaction (24 to 48 hours), mediated by T-cells,* after injection of antigen. An example is the reaction seen with a positive tuberculin test.

Demyelination. Destruction of the sheath of a nerve or nerves involving the removal and loss of myelin.

Diphtheria. Although it denotes a specific human disease, the term is also used in a general sense for an infectious process involving the throat.

Diphtheritic membrane. Similar to the pseudo- or false membrane that is characteristic of diphtheria. It resembles a living membrane but consists of coagulated fibrin with leukocytes, other dead cells, and bacteria.

Diskospondylitis. Inflammation involving an intervertebral disk.

DNA fingerprinting. This involves cleavage of chromosomal DNA by restriction enzymes and the separation of the segments into bands by electrophoresis. The bands obtained can be used to identify varieties of microorganisms.

Dysentery. An infectious diarrhea with the passage of mucus and blood.

Dyspnea. Difficult or labored breathing.

Dystrophic. A dystrophic condition is one caused by defective nutrition to an organ or tissue.

Edema. An excess of serous fluid in tissues.

Embolus. A solid, liquid, or gaseous mass of undissolved material, often a blood clot, traveling in the blood.

Empyema. An accumulation of pus* in a body cavity, most frequently the thorax or abdomen.

Encephalitis. Inflammation of the brain.

Encephalomyelitis. Inflammation of the brain and spinal chord.

Encephalosis. A degenerative brain disease as opposed to a true encephalitis.

Endocarditis. An inflammation of the lining (endocardium) of the heart and its valves.

Endometritis. Inflammation of the mucous membrane (endometrium) lining the uterus.

Endosymbiosis. A state achieved between a virus and its host cell in which cell division is inhibited but the cell is not destroyed.

Enteritis. An inflammation of the intestines.

Epitope (Antigenic determinant). The local chemical configuration on the antigen molecule that elicits specific antibody.

Filamentous. The threadlike morphology of some microorganisms.

Fistula. An abnormal passage leading from an abscess to the body or organ surface and permitting the passage of fluids, frequently pus.

Folliculitis. Inflammation of hair follicles.

Fomites. Inanimate objects that, when contaminated with infectious agents, serve to transmit them.

Freund's adjuvants. Freund's complete adjuvant is a water-in-oil emulsion containing killed mycobacteria. It stimulates both cell-mediated and humoral immunity. Freund's incomplete adjuvant is identical to the complete adjuvant except that it does not contain mycobacteria. The adjuvant effect with both preparations is obtained by the delayed release of antigen.

Furuncle. A localized inflammatory process of the skin and subcutis, that discharges pus, caused by an infection of a skin gland or hair follicle.

Furunculosis. A condition in which furuncles* develop.

Fusiform. Spindle-shaped.

Gangrene. Necrosis of tissue with putrefaction as a result of bacterial invasion.

Gas-liquid chromatography. A procedure for separating compounds in which the volatile phase flows through a heated column with a carrier gas. The identity of the compounds is determined by measuring the time required to reach the end of the column.

Gastroenteritis. Inflammation of the lining or mucous membrane of the stomach and intestine.

Granuloma. An aggregation and proliferation of mainly macrophages* in response to certain chronic infections and foreign bodies. The macrophages, when compressed, are called epithelioid cells; they may fuse to form giant cells. Dead cells, lymphocytes, plasma cells*, and microorganisms may be present.

Granulomatous. (see **Granuloma**).

Hemagglutination. The agglutination or clumping of red blood cells caused by some viruses, high molecular weight polysaccharides, some bacteria, and antibodies (when the red cells are coated with antigen).

Hemaglobinuria. The presence of free hemoglobin, as opposed to red cells, in the urine.

Hematogenous. Spread by way of the blood stream.

Hematophagous. A hematophagous animal is one that subsists on the blood of another animal.

Hematuria. The presence of blood in the urine.

Histamine. An amine released by mast cells* and basophils that cause dilatation of capillaries and plays a major role in allergic reactions.

Horizontal transmission. The transmission of infectious agents from animal to animal by means other than vertical transmission (from female to its offspring).

Humoral immunity. This is immunity mediated by antibodies.

Hydranencephaly. Complete or almost complete absence of the cerebral hemispheres. The space left is occupied with cerebrospinal fluid.

Hydrothorax. An abnormal amount of serous fluid in the pleural cavity.

Hyperplasia. An increase in the number of normal cells in a tissue or organ.

Hypoplasia. The underdevelopment of an organ or tissue, usually caused by a decrease in the number of cells.

Icterus. A yellow discoloration of the sclera, skin, and mucous membrane caused by the deposition of bilirubin in these tissues.

Idiotype. A unique variable region on an antibody molecule that determines the epitope* (specific part) of an antigen that will react with the antibody.

Immune complexes. These are conglomerates of combined antigen and antibody that can give rise to tissue damage. They can be small and soluble or large and precipitating, depending on the proportion of antigen to antibody.

Immunodiffusion test. A procedure for the detection of antigen or antibody by observing the line of precipitation formed in a semisolid gel when homologous antigens and antibodies are allowed to diffuse toward each other from "wells" and react.

Immunoglobulin. A class of proteins called antibodies, of which there are distinct varieties designated by letters, e.g., IgA, IgE, IgG, IgM, etc.

Infarct. An area of necrosis in a tissue or organ owing to deficiency in the blood supply.

Infarction. An obstruction of the blood supply within an organ or tissue resulting in the formation of an infarct.*

Inspissation. When applied to pus, it involves making the latter thick by the absorption or loss of fluid.

Iridocyclitis. Inflammation of the iris and of the ciliary body.

Ischemia. Deficiency of blood in tissue caused by actual obstruction or functional constriction of a blood vessel.

Jaundice. (see **Icterus**).

Keratitis. Inflammation of the cornea of the eye.

Keratoconjunctivitis. Inflammation of the cornea and the conjunctiva of the eye.

Laminitis. Inflammation involving the sensitive laminae of the hoof, mainly of horses, but also occasionally of cattle, sheep, goats, and swine.

Lateral transmission. (see **Horizontal transmission**).

Leukocytosis. An elevated white blood cell count.

Leukoencephalomyelitis. An encephalomyelitis characterized by inflammation of the white matter.

Leukopenia. A lower than normal white blood cell count.

Lymphadenitis. An inflammation of lymph nodes.

Lymphadenopathy. Disease of the lymph nodes.

Lymphokines. These are glycoprotein mediators, produced by lymphocytes, which regulate various aspects of the immune response.

Lysosomes. These are cytoplasmic vesicles present in many animal cells. They contain hydrolytic enzymes (hyaluronidase, β-glucuronidase, lipase, etc.) that play a role in the intracellular digestion of microorganisms.

Lysozyme. An enzyme, also known as muramidase, present in many body fluids, that breaks down murein, a component of the cell walls of many gram-positive bacteria.

Macrophages. These are large mononuclear phagocytes which include wandering and fixed cells. The latter are present in various tissues and are given various names, e.g., Kupffer cells in the liver.

Malignant carbuncle. The carbuncle seen in anthrax. (see **Carbuncle**).

Mast cell. A large tissue cell with basophilic granules containing vasoactive amines, which when released, are involved in inflammatory processes.

Mega-. When used with a particular unit it indicates 1 million times that unit, e.g., a megadalton = one million daltons.

Megadalton. (See **Mega-**).

Meningitis. Inflammation of the meninges, the membranes that cover the spinal chord and brain.

Mesenteric. This refers to the mesentery, a membrane that covers the stomach and intestine.

Metastatic. In microbiology, the spread of an infectious agent from a primary focus to various locations via the bloodstream or lymphatic system.

Metritis. Inflammation of the uterus.

Microaerophilic. An organism that requires a level of oxygen less than that in the atmosphere.

Microbiota. The normal microscopic flora and fauna of plants and animals.

Micrometer. A unit of length equal to one-millionth of a meter or 10,000 Å. It is represented by the symbol μm. It is roughly equal to 1/25,400 of an inch. Micrometer has replaced the earlier unit, the micron.

Mitogen. A substance that induces mitosis, particularly lymphocyte transformation.

Morbidity. The morbidity rate of a disease refers to the number affected by the disease.

Mordant. A chemical, such as iodine, in the Gram stain that fixes the dye, e.g., gentian violet, thus forming an insoluble compound.

Mucosa. Mucous membrane.

Myocarditis. Inflammation of the myocardium, the middle muscular layer of the heart.

Myonecrosis. Death of muscle cells.

Myositis. Inflammation of voluntary muscle.

Nanogram. A unit of weight equal to one-billionth of a gram.

Nares. External orifices of the nose.

Necrosis. The pathologic death of cells or a portion of an organ or tissue. The damage is irreversible.

Neonatal. The first 4 weeks after birth.

Nephritis. Inflammation of the kidney.

Nephrotoxic. Toxic to the kidney.

Neurotrophic. Having an affinity for nervous tissue.

Nictitating membrane. A transparent fold of skin (the third eyelid) that may be drawn over the front of the eyeball. It occurs in the horse and some other animals.

Nosocomial. Infections acquired in the hospital or clinic.

Obligate aerobes. Microorganisms that require oxygen for growth.

Obligate anaerobes. Microorganisms that do not grow in the presence of oxygen.

Oil adjuvant. (see **Freund's adjuvant**).

Omphalitis. Inflammation of the umbilicus.

Omphalophlebitis. Inflammation of the umbilical veins.

Opisthotonus. Spasm of the lower muscles of the back that causes the head and lower limbs to bend backward and the trunk to arch forward.

Opsonization. The process of phagocytosis involving specific antibody and complement. This "engulfment" of microorganisms is an important defense mechanism.

Osteomyelitis. An infectious inflammatory disease of the bone often characterized by necrosis and separation of tissue.

Otitis. Inflammation of the ear.

Paired serum samples. This refers to acute and convalescent sera collected for antibody determination. The acute serum is taken early in the disease before appreciable antibody is produced. The convalescent serum is taken when the animal is recovering and an antibody response has occurred. A fourfold increase in titer is considered evidence that there has been an infection.

Papilloma. A benign tumor, usually small, derived from epithelium.

Parenteral. Administered by means other than via the alimentary tract. It usually refers to administration via intravenous, subcutaneous, intradermal, intraperitoneal, or intramuscular routes.

Pathogenesis. The development of a disease.

Pericarditis. Inflammation of the pericardium, the membranous covering of the heart.

Perivascular cuffing. The formation of a cuff-like accumulation of leukocytes (usually lymphocytes) around a blood vessel.

Petechial hemorrhages. Minute hemorrhages seen as very small reddish or purplish spots.

Peyer's patch. A large oval aggregation of lymphoid tissue in the wall of the small intestine.

Plasma cell. A mature, antibody producing, B lymphocyte.

Pleomorphic. Having different morphologic forms.

Pneumonia. Inflammation of the lungs with consolidation.

Pneumonitis. Inflammation of the lungs.

Polioencephalomalacia. A noninfectious neurological disease of ruminants characterized by extensive necrosis of the gray matter and associated with intensive farming practices.

Polyserositis. Inflammation of serous membranes, most frequently the pleura, peritoneum, and pericardium.

Postparturient. After birth.

Precipitin test. A test used to detect antigen by allowing a specific antibody to diffuse toward antigen in a liquid or gel until precipitation (antigen-antibody complex) results.

Premonitory. Forewarning. Premonitory clinical signs are the early signs suggesting an impending disease.

Prognosis. The prediction as to the probable outcome of a disease.

Prophylaxis. Preventive treatment.

Pseudomembrane. A false membrane, sometimes called a diphtheritic membrane, composed mainly of fibrin and necrotic cells, on the surface of an inflamed mucous membrane.

Purulent. Containing pus.

Pus. A fluid, resulting from inflammation, that contains cellular debris, white blood cells, and often bacteria.

Pyelonephritis. An inflammation of the kidney including the renal (kidney) pelvis. It usually results from infection.

Pyemia. A bacteremia* or septicemia,* often with abscesses, involving pus-forming bacteria, such as staphylococci and streptococci.

Pyoderma. A skin inflammation with lesions caused by pus-forming bacteria.

Pyogenic. Pus-forming.

Pyometra. An accumulation of pus in the uterus.

Pyometritis. An inflammation of the uterus in which pus is produced.

Pyosepticemia. A septicemia* involving pus-forming bacteria.

Pyrexia. Fever, i.e., an abnormal elevation of body temperature.

Reservoir. The source from which infectious microorganisms may be spread; e.g., the principal reservoir of *Mycobacterium bovis* is cattle.

Restriction enzyme analysis. Determination of the number and size of DNA fragments obtained when a particular DNA molecule is cut with a particular restriction enzyme.

Reticuloendothelial system. This defense system, also called the mononuclear phagocytic system, consists of macrophages and a network of specialized cells of the spleen, thymus, and other lymphoid tissues.

Reticuloendotheliosis. Hyperplasia* of reticulo-endothelial tissue (now known as the system of mononuclear phagocytes). (see **Reticuloendothelial system**).
Ribotyping. A procedure for typing (identifying varieties) bacteria using ribosomal RNA to probe chromosomal DNA in Southern blots. Ribosomal RNA genes are scattered throughout the chromosomes of most bacteria.

Salpingitis. Inflammation of the fallopian tubes.
Seborrhea. Excessive secretion of sebum (from the sebaceous glands).
Secondary infection. An infection superimposed on an existing (primary) infection caused by another microorganism.
Sepsis. This denotes the presence of pathogenic microorganisms or their toxins in the blood or tissues.
Septic. (see **Sepsis**).
Septicemia. The presence of multiplying microorganisms in the blood.
Seroconversion. The development of demonstrable antibody in response to a disease or vaccine.
Serosanguineous. Fluid consisting of both blood and serum.
Serotype. A variety of microorganism identified by its distinct antigenic character.
Serotyping. It involves methods for determining the serotype.*
Serovar. A serologic or antigenic variety, synonymous with serotype, and used for some genera, e.g., *Salmonella* and *Leptospira* .
Shock. In general, a state of circulatory failure associated with reduced total blood volume and low blood pressure. It has various causes, including bacterial endotoxin.
Sialoadenitis. Inflammation of the salivary gland.
Somatic. In the expression "somatic type," somatic refers to cell wall antigen or lipopolysaccaride.
Spondylitis. Inflammation of the vertebrae.
Sporadic infection or disease. Scattered occurrence; usually individual cases, e.g., actinomycosis, actinobacillosis.
Stomatitis. An inflammatory process involving the mouth.
Subspecies. These are recognizable varieties within a species. They have a consistent difference or differences from the parent species and are identified by an additional Latin name.
Superinfection. (see **Secondary infection**).
Suppuration. The formation of pus.*
Syndrome. A group of clinical signs that characterize a particular disease.

T cells. These thymus-derived lymphocytes include a number of subtypes with various functions. T cells are involved in cell-mediated* as well as humoral immunity.*
Thoracocentesis. Aspiration of fluid from the thorax.
Thrombocytopenia. A lower than normal number of thrombocytes (platelets).
Thrombophlebitis. Inflammation of a vein owing to thrombus formation.
Thrombus. A blood clot formed within a blood vessel and remaining by attachment to its place of origin.
Thylakoid membranes. Membranous sacs that are widened portions of the lamellae of chloroplasts.
Titer. The highest dilution at which an antibody can be detected in serologic tests.
Toxemia. Toxin in the blood leading to a toxic state.
Toxoid. An exotoxin that has been modified by treatment (usually formalin) to destroy its toxicity but not its antigenicity.
Transtracheal aspiration. The passage of a needle and plastic catheter into the trachea to obtain lower respiratory tract secretions free of extraneous microorganisms. Sterile fluid may be introduced to facilitate sampling.
Typhlitis. Inflammation of the cecum.
Typhlocolitis. Inflammation of the cecum and colon.

Uremia. The accumulation in the blood during severe kidney disease of urinary constituents that are normally eliminated in the urine. A severe toxic condition results.
Urethritis. Inflammation of the urethra, the tube that carries urine from the kidney to the bladder.
Urolithiasis. Presence of calculi in the urinary tract.
Uveitis. Inflammation of the iris, ciliary body, and choroid.

Vasculitis. Inflammation of a blood or lymph vessel.
Vector. An arthropod or other agent that carries microorganisms from one infected animal to another.
Vertical transmission. The transmission of microorganisms from a female to its offspring.
Vesicle. A small blister or bulla containing fluid.
Villi. These are minute, elongated, vascular projections from the intestinal mucosa, the outside boundary of which consist of epithelial cells. They are involved in the absorption of nutrients.

INDEX

Page numbers in *italics* indicate figures; page numbers followed by a t indicate tables.